DIAGNOSTIC TESTS

A Prescriber's Guide to
Test Selection
and Interpretation

DIAGNOSTIC TESTS

A Prescriber's Guide to Test Selection and Interpretation

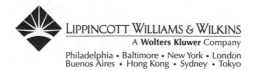

LIPPINCOTT WILLIAMS & WILKINS
A **Wolters Kluwer** Company

Philadelphia • Baltimore • New York • London
Buenos Aires • Hong Kong • Sydney • Tokyo

STAFF

Publisher
Judith A. Schilling McCann, RN, MSN

Editorial Director
H. Nancy Holmes

Clinical Director
Joan M. Robinson, RN, MSN

Senior Art Director
Arlene Putterman

Editors
William Welsh (associate editor),
Stacey Ann Folin, David P. Lenker

Clinical Editors
Bonnie L. McGonigle, RN, MSN, CRRN, CRNP;
Joanne Bartelmo, RN, MSN, CCRN;
Patricia Berlin Malay, BS, MSN, FNP, MA

Copy Editors
Kimberly Bilotta (supervisor),
Scotti Cohn, Tom DeZego, Heather Ditch,
Shana Harrington, Elizabeth Mooney,
Dona Hightower Perkins, Marcia Ryan,
Dorothy P. Terry, Pamela Wingrod

Designers
Susan Hopkins Rodzewich (book designer),
Debra Moloshok (project manager)

Digital Composition Services
Diane Paluba (manager), Joyce Rossi Biletz
(senior desktop assistant), Donna S. Morris

Manufacturing
Patricia K. Dorshaw (senior manager),
Beth Janae Orr (book production coordinator)

Editorial Assistants
Danielle J. Barsky, Beverly Lane, Linda Ruhf

Indexer
Barbara E. Hodgson

**Library of Congress
Cataloging-in-Publication Data**

Diagnostic tests : a prescriber's guide to test selection and interpretation.
    p. ; cm.
Includes bibliographical references and index.
    1. Diagnosis—Handbooks, manuals, etc. 2. Function tests—Handbooks, manuals, etc.
    [DNLM: 1. Diagnostic Tests, Routine. WB 200 D5365 2003] I. Lippincott Williams & Wilkins.
  RC71.D525 2003
  616.07'5—dc21
  ISBN 1-58255-234-7 (pbk. : alk. paper)
                    2003006251

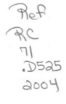
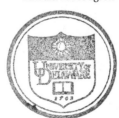

Contents

Contributors and consultants

Roseanne Baughman, RN, MSN, CRNP
Nurse Practitioner
Central Bucks Internal Medicine
Doylestown, Pa.

Deborah Becker, RN, MSN, CRNP, BC
Associate Director, Adult Acute Care Nurse
  Practitioner Program
University of Pennsylvania School of
  Nursing
Philadelphia

Garry Brydges, RN, MSN, ACNP-C, SRNA
Medical Consultant
Houston

Marilyn M. Cooksey, RN, MSN, PhD
Associate Professor of Nursing
William Carey College
Gulfport, Miss.

Jennifer Elizabeth DiMedio, RN, MSN, CRNP
Family Nurse Practitioner
University of Pennsylvania: West Chester
  Family Practice

Diane Dixon, PA-C, MA, MMSc, PhD(c)
Assistant Professor
University of South Alabama
Mobile, Ala.

Shelba Durston, RN, MSN, CCRN
Adjunct Faculty
San Joaquin Delta College
Stockton, Calif.
Staff Nurse
San Joaquin General Hospital
French Camp, Calif.

René A. Jackson, RN, BSN
Special Procedures Nurse
Charlotte Regional Medical Center
Punta Gorda, Fla.

Kay Luft, RN, MN, CCRN
Assistant Professor
Saint Luke's College
Kansas City, Mo.

Samir Ouzomgi, PhD
Associate Professor of Mathematics
Pennsylvania State University
Abington

Lisa A. Salamon, MSN, CNS, RNC
Clinical Nurse Specialist
Cleveland Clinic Foundation

Bruce Austin Scott, MSN, APRN, BC
Nursing Instructor
San Joaquin Delta College
Stockton, Calif.
Staff Nurse
University of California, Davis, Medical
  Center
Sacramento, Calif.

Daniel Vetrosky, PA-C, MEd, PhD(c)
Assistant Professor and Academic
  Coordinator
University of South Alabama
Mobile

Paul Zakrzewski, D.O.
Physician
Doylestown (Pa.) Hospital

Foreword

When a patient comes to you seeking professional help for an illness, he's depending on your medical expertise to make him well. For many patients, an important part of the assessment process is diagnostic testing, a field that presents prescribers with a rather daunting triple challenge:
1. an ever-widening range of diseases to treat
2. an ever-increasing number of diagnostic tests due to technological improvements and a more thorough understanding of many physiologic processes
3. cost-effectiveness mandated by rising health care costs.

Diagnostic Tests: A Prescriber's Guide to Test Selection and Interpretation is the book you need to meet these challenges.

Diagnostic tests and procedures now number in the hundreds, and each one possesses benefits that others like it do not. It's up to you to manage their many uses, not only for the initial diagnosis, but also for further testing to evaluate progress or problems. Do you order the test that's more reliable, the test that's cheaper, or the test that's less invasive? It's imperative that you choose correctly. Choosing the appropriate tests and interpreting their results knowledgeably often proves the difference between success and failure.

Fortunately, *Diagnostic Tests: A Prescriber's Guide to Test Selection and Interpretation* can help simplify the selection process for you. This all-new reference makes ordering diagnostic tests and interpreting their results a lot less complicated by covering the subject from every angle.

This book is comprised of five major sections. Part one, which is divided into two chapters, provides a broad overview of diagnostic testing. Chapter 1, Fundamentals of diagnostic tests, explains the theoretical underpinnings of diagnostic testing. Abstract concepts, such as *sensitivity, specificity, prevalence, thresholds,* and *odds ratios,* take on real importance when you understand how they influence a test's reliability. Chapter 2, Laboratory guidelines to diagnostic tests, walks you through the entire testing process, from patient preparation and education to posttest care.

Part two provides an in-depth look at more than 300 diagnostic tests that reflect the current trends in clinical pathology and laboratory medicine. Each entry starts with a general description of the test, including its purpose and relative cost, then moves on to patient preparation, normal findings and reference values, abnormal findings (and their significance), and factors that can interfere with proper test administration and accuracy.

Part three helps you move forward with test selection and interpretation by mapping out the clinical decision-making process. Using your patient's primary sign or symptom as a starting point, you'll advance through various test findings until reaching an accurate differential diagnosis that you — and your patient — can place confidence in.

Part four covers ECG interpretation. You'll review how to read and interpret single-lead and 12-lead ECGs. Common arrhythmias are covered in detail, as well as features that distinguish various other cardiac abnormalities, such as left and right bundle-branch block and pericarditis. Whether you're caring for a patient who's suffering from coronary artery disease, digoxin toxicity, or hypothermia, you'll be able to expertly assess the results of his ECGs and provide the best possible care.

Part five presents key diagnostic findings for more than 500 major disorders, arranged alphabetically. You'll find this section especially useful as a quick-reference tool when you need to instantly remind yourself of a disease's characteristic diagnostic results. It can also serve as an ideal cross-reference that links specific disorders to their typical test batteries. It's an invaluable resource, and I have no doubt that you'll return to it often.

Diagnostic Tests: A Prescriber's Guide to Test Selection and Interpretation emphasizes key points in a variety of ways. Sidebars filled with insightful information abound. Eye-catching icons call your attention to some of the most important information. *Alert!* highlights special precautions you need to consider when ordering a test, including contraindications and potential complications. *Age issue* discusses age-specific differences in patient preparation, monitoring, and test results. Appendices include charts on therapeutic drug monitoring guidelines, drugs that interfere with test results, laboratory value changes in elderly patients, and a quick-reference guide to laboratory test results.

Diagnostic Tests: A Prescriber's Guide to Test Selection and Interpretation is a comprehensive resource that no prescriber should be without. It will improve your skills and increase your confidence. It's the right book at the right time for identifying the right test, and I have no doubt that it will become an indispensable resource.

Anthony J. Dean, MD
Assistant Professor of Emergency Medicine
University of Pennsylvania Medical Center
Philadelphia

PART ONE

Overview of diagnostic tests

CHAPTER 1

Fundamentals of diagnostic tests

Diagnostic tests are indispensable medical tools and, as a practitioner, you frequently make clinical decisions on the basis of their results. However, despite the health care community's reliance upon them, diagnostic tests are far from perfect. Test results can be ambiguous, and improper interpretations may further cloud a patient's clinical picture. This is why every practitioner needs an understanding of basic test characteristics.

This chapter provides an overview of how evidence-based medicine, the current model for patient care, is incorporated into diagnostic testing. It covers the characteristics of diagnostic testing, its uses and clinical applications as well as the theoretical underpinnings for its use in practice. Armed with this information, you can use diagnostic tests more efficiently and place greater confidence in the results.

Uses of diagnostic tests

Diagnostic tests are used for a variety of purposes, including screening, confirming or ruling out diagnoses, and disease man-

agement, and all of their uses serve an important medical role. (See *Purposes of diagnostic testing.*)

Screening

Screening is the process of testing a large population whose members are considered to be at significant risk for a particular disease. A screening test is administered to every member of the designated at-risk population, even to those who appear to be symptom-free.

Though valuable, the use of screening tests is contentious. Because of their costs and the need to respond to a positive result even when it's likely to be a false-positive, their use demands care. Ideal screening tests should be able to detect the disease (even in its early stages), relatively non-painful, and relatively inexpensive: goals that are usually difficult to meet and unrealistic.

The broad scope of screening tests has even made the use of popular tests controversial. Screening mammography for breast cancer in women is a common preventative procedure among practitioners and their patients, but some insurance companies are reluctant to include it under their

Purposes of diagnostic testing

Selecting the appropriate diagnostic test depends on the purpose of the test itself and its overall benefit to the patient, among other factors. Listed below are purposes and appropriate examples.

PURPOSE	EXAMPLE
To be utilized for secondary health prevention	Order screening mammograms for women over age 40 with a strong family history of breast cancer.
To be utilized for specific situational testing	Order DNA testing to establish evidence in specific criminal cases or to establish identity.
To establish a diagnosis	Order a urine culture to identify a specific antigen to diagnose a urinary tract infection.
To evaluate a current treatment	Order routine prothrombin times to monitor the effectiveness of anticoagulant therapy.
To establish differential diagnoses	Order a complete blood cell count, erythrocyte sedimentation rate, antinuclear antibody test, urinalysis, and an X-ray of selected joints to establish signs and symptoms of rheumatoid arthritis.
To evaluate disease severity	Order a glucose fasting test to evaluate diabetes mellitus.
To monitor disease progression and response to treatment	Order a computed tomography scan to evaluate cancer severity and monitor the effectiveness of prescribed treatments.

list of covered services, and its value — based on the theory that earlier detection allows less invasive therapy and results in better patient outcomes — is still a matter of debate. Because of this, you should advise your patients to check with their insurance companies before undergoing any screening tests.

Confirming or ruling out diagnoses

Another use of diagnostic testing is to either confirm or rule out a suspected diagnosis. For example, when a skin lesion is multicolored or has irregular borders, performing a first-line procedure such as biop-

sy may rule out cancer. Alternative tests to confirm a diagnosis may be more invasive and more expensive, and their use might be restricted to only those patients who have a high probability of having the disease.

Managing disease

Testing also serves a variety of purposes once the diagnosis has been established. Tests are commonly repeated over time at specific intervals in order to compare test results with earlier reports. They're used to set prognosis and staging, to monitor disease progression, to assist in therapy selection, and to monitor the efficacy of medications.

Staging and prognosis
Tests can indicate the spread of disease as well as functional loss in organ systems. Test results can help you determine which medications to use, which surgical interventions to consider, and the patient's overall prognosis.

Monitoring disease progression
Tests can help determine whether the disease is progressing, in remission, recurring, or cured. A common example is a follow-up urine culture to determine if a urinary tract infection has been cured.

Selecting therapy
Diagnostic tests can help you decide on an appropriate course of therapy. Cultures to identify bacterial infections, for example, usually include testing for sensitivity of the pathogens to various antibiotics so that a particular antibiotic can be prescribed.

Monitoring drug therapy
Tests may be done to measure blood concentrations of medications. This is necessary for some medications in order to prevent toxicity from inordinately high concentrations of a medication and to prevent inadequate dosing. For example, aminoglycoside antibiotics can cause renal damage and ototoxicity at high concentrations. Yet, if concentrations fall below a certain level, aminoglycosides lose their therapeutic value.

Test characteristics

With so many diagnostic tests to choose from, it's helpful for practitioners to understand why one test might prove more valuable or reliable than a comparable test. Knowledge of test characteristics, including an understanding of sensitivity and specificity values and how they're reached, can go a long way in helping you select the right test for the right patient.

Sensitivity and specificity
No test is flawless, and the results of any given test in a specific situation can be inaccurate. To reduce ambiguity, many common laboratory tests have themselves been tested to determine quantitatively how often they're wrong. These measures determine a test's sensitivity and specificity.

Sensitivity measures how likely a test is to give a true positive result, or how likely it is that a diseased patient will have a positive result. The greater a test's sensitivity, the more likely the test will detect people who have the disease. Sensitivity is calculated by dividing the number of people who had the disease and tested positive by the total number of tested people known to have the disease.

Specificity measures how likely it is that a nondiseased patient will have a negative test result. It's calculated by dividing the number of people without the disease who tested negative by the total number of tested people who didn't have the disease. The higher the specificity, the lower the likelihood that the test result is a false-positive. (See *Measuring sensitivity and specificity*.)

Thus, if a test has a specificity of 80%, then it also has a 20% chance of returning a false-positive result. A test with a sensitivity of 74% also has a 26% chance of returning a false-negative result. Therefore, any result, either positive or negative, doesn't provide definitive information about whether the patient actually has the disease. Further testing is likely warranted,

Appropriate patient care includes picking the right test for the right patient. Knowledge of a test's sensitivity and specificity values can go a long way in helping you make the correct selection.

Sensitivity
A test's ability to accurately identify patients who have a particular disease is known as its *sensitivity*. To calculate this value, the number of patients with the disease testing positive is divided by the total number of tested patients with the disease. This value is then multiplied by 100 to obtain the percentage of sensitivity. For example:

$$\frac{80 \text{ patients with disease testing positive}}{100 \text{ tested patients with disease}} \times 100 = 80\% \text{ sensitivity}$$

Specificity
A test's ability to accurately identify patients who don't have a particular disease is known as its *specificity*. To calculate this value, the number of patients without the disease testing negative is divided by the total number of tested patients without the disease. This value is then multiplied by 100 to obtain the percentage of specificity. For example:

$$\frac{200 \text{ patients without disease testing negative}}{205 \text{ tested patients without disease}} \times 100 = 97.6\% \text{ specificity}$$

especially if the patient has symptoms that are strongly associated with the disorder.

The gold standard
Researchers arrive at values for sensitivity and specificity by comparing the test in question with its gold standard. A *gold standard* is a test that, if performed properly, is always positive when the disease is present and always negative when it isn't. It's the most definitive diagnostic method and establishes the "true" disease status. Pulmonary arteriography, for example, is the gold standard test for pulmonary embolism. All other diagnostic tests used to determine pulmonary embolism, such as the ventilation-perfusion ($\dot{V}/\dot{Q}$) scan, are then compared with pulmonary arteriography in order to calculate their sensitivity and specificity values.

Of course, this leads to the question of why the $\dot{V}/\dot{Q}$ scan is used at all if it can be inaccurate. Why not just use the always-reliable gold standard? While arteriography is the more dependable of the two tests, it's time-consuming and highly invasive, and it poses a greater risk to the patient than does the $\dot{V}/\dot{Q}$ scan. Other gold standard tests suffer from similar issues. Despite their reliability, they, too, are used as second-line tests.

Factors affecting sensitivity and specificity

A variety of factors can affect sensitivity and specificity. Patient populations (for testing both sensitivity and specificity) can differ, and reference standards can vary between laboratories and companies producing testing kits. Furthermore, the presence of coexisting disorders or complications of the primary disease can significantly affect the sensitivity and specificity values of a test. (See *Factors that can influence test results.*)

Measuring sensitivity and specificity also requires large, testable populations and adequate resources for performing the research involved, which is why not all diagnostic tests have established sensitivity and specificity rates. Generally, the most sensitive tests are best used to rule out a suspected disease because the number of false-negative results is minimized. In addition, the most specific tests are best used to confirm or exclude a suspected disease because the number of false-positive results is minimized.

PREVALENCE

Another factor that affects the situation in the clinical setting is prevalence. This is defined as the proportion of people in a given population who have a particular disease at a specified time. Prevalence is typically used in two ways: *Point* prevalence refers to a disease's prevalence at a point in time, and *period* prevalence refers to the number of people who have had the disease at any time during a certain period such as a single calendar year.

The way prevalence affects the use of sensitivity and specificity is this: A low prevalence in a given population means that fewer patients given the test will have true positive results. However, a low prevalence doesn't necessarily equate to a low number of false-positives. Although the sensitivity of a certain test may be very high, making the percentage of false-positives low, the actual number of false-positives in a large population (such as a screening population) would still be fairly high.

As an example, when screening for human immunodeficiency virus infection, the enzyme-linked immunosorbent assay (ELISA), which measures the presence of antibody in the serum to the virus, is generally the initial test performed. It's a highly sensitive test with a high specificity as well. Yet, if the test is performed in a population with a low prevalence of HIV, there are still a fair number of false-positive results, which is why positive specimens are commonly retested with another test that's even more specific than the ELISA — the Western blot test.

VALIDITY

The validity, or *accuracy*, of a diagnostic test is a measure of how well it corresponds to the true value of what's being measured. Validity depends upon properly calibrated laboratory equipment, the use of the correct reference ranges, and laboratory accordance with various quality control procedures. Bedside monitoring equipment must also be calibrated regularly for the same reason.

RELIABILITY

Reliability, or *precision*, is a measure of the likelihood that repeated testing of the same sample would give similar results. The reliability of a test depends on several factors: human judgment, equipment used, and sample size all can affect a test's final result. Laboratory personnel may interpret the same results differently, manual counts may not be as precise as machine counts, and sample size may vary. It's incumbent upon laboratories to employ quality control measures that will ensure that such differences, while usually insignificant, don't cause problems.

PREDICTIVE VALUES

The concept of predictive values is closely related to sensitivity and specificity. A positive predictive value is the probability of the disease being present if the test result is positive. Conversely, the negative predictive value of a test is the probability of the disease being absent if the test result is negative. From a clinical perspective, this determines how fully you can rely on the positive result of a particular test to confirm a suspected diagnosis. If testing is inconclusive or negative, other testing may be warranted in order to come to a more definitive diagnosis. (See *Determining predictive values,* page 8.)

REFERENCE RANGES

Normal reference ranges are based on data collected from apparently healthy persons and provide a standard for identifying results that indicate the presence of disease. Researchers calculate a range that represents the values for 95% of healthy people when they were tested, leaving a 5% chance that a value outside the reference range is normal for that particular person, especially if it's only slightly outside the normal range. You should be alerted to possible false-positives when the abnormal value is only slightly outside of the reference range.

Another factor to consider is individual norms. A result within the stated normal range may not be normal for a given patient. For example, the arterial blood gas results of a patient who usually has chronic elevated partial pressure of carbon dioxide level is trending lower to more normal levels. This would be considered abnormal for this patient. A practitioner just looking at values without knowing the patient's history may interpret the results as close to normal.

Determining predictive values

The ability of a screening test to correctly identify a particular disease is its predictive value, which is found through the use of true-positive and true-negative test results.

- A true-positive test result means that a person testing positive for a disease has it; a positive predicted value is the percentage of positive tests that are true positives.
- A true-negative test result means that the person testing negative for the disease doesn't have it; a negative predictive value is the percentage of negative tests that are true negatives.

The following tables demonstrate the methodology behind predictive values.

The methodology

TEST RESULT	WITH DISEASE	WITHOUT DISEASE	TOTAL
Positive test	A (true positive)	C (false positive)	A+C
Negative test	B (false negative)	D (true negative)	B+D
Total	A+B	C+D	A+B+C+D

The results

MEASURE	VALUE
Sensitivity	A/(A+B)
Specificity	D/(C+D)
Positive predictive	A/(A+C)
Negative predictive	D/(B+D)
Prevalence	(A+B)/(A+B+C+D)

The numbers

TEST RESULT	WITH DISEASE	WITHOUT DISEASE	TOTAL
Positive test	5	50	55
Negative test	200	20	220
Total	205	70	275

The results

MEASURE	VALUE
Sensitivity	2.44%
Specificity	28.57%
Positive predictive	9.09%
Negative predictive	9.09%
Prevalence	74.55%

Reference ranges vary depending on a variety of factors, including gender, age, weight, time of day, activity status, and posture. Furthermore, reference ranges vary from one laboratory to another, so you should be familiar with the laboratory and the ranges it uses.

Test deviations. A number of other factors can cause deviations from normal, even when reference ranges are considered. External influences on test deviation include medications and other ingested substances. Diuretics, for example, can affect sodium and potassium concentrations; cigarette smoking can elevate hepatic enzyme levels.

Test deviations may also be due to internal influences such as those stemming from a patient's physiologic status. For example, patients with gross lipemia may have falsely low sodium levels if the test methodology uses a step in which serum is diluted before the sodium is measured. You should be wary of unexpected abnormal test results and consider external and internal influences before pursuing the workup of the disease state suggested by the abnormal result.

Use of statistical data

Sensitivity and specificity measures are useful tools for interpreting test results, but they also indicate the limits of medical knowledge. Practitioners commonly base decisions on estimation after sifting through a variety of clinical factors. To help with this, researchers use statistical data from years of direct clinical experience to develop some basis for standardizing clinical decision making. This section explains some of the most widely used methods.

Pretest and posttest probability

Pretest probability refers to the probability that a patient has a specific disease before a test is done. The value for a pretest probability is based on the available clinical information about the patient — the history and physical examination — and on epidemiological information regarding populations at risk and prevalence.

Research has shown that small differences in pretest probability estimates aren't significant in determining posttest probability (predictive value); it's common practice for practitioners to estimate the pretest probability as high, medium, or low.

Posttest probability is a measure of the probability of the disease's presence after a test result is known. It's based on the estimated pretest probability and the known sensitivity and specificity of the test. The main value of the posttest probability measure is to help you decide when a particular test won't provide enough additional information to warrant using it.

Calculating pretest and posttest probabilities helps show that in some situations a particular diagnostic test may not be necessary. (See *Interpreting laboratory results*, page 10.)

Thresholds

Using pretest and posttest probabilities in clinical decision making is helpful when using certain thresholds, or cutoff points, for deciding when to treat a disease. When the probability of a certain disease rises above an assigned threshold level (using data from clinical research), the diagnosis is assumed and treatment is begun. The assigned threshold level is known as the test/treat threshold, and it's based on a comparison between the pretest probability of the disease being present and the suspicion of disease. If the pretest probability

Interpreting laboratory results

Calculation of posttest probability is completed using Bayes' formulas, which show the relationship between predictive value and the sensitivity and specificity values for that test for that particular disease and the prevalence of the disease for a particular population. The results are useful in determining whether ordering a particular test would be helpful.

Bayes' formula applied to predictive values:

$$\text{Positive predictive value} = \frac{\text{sensitivity} \times \text{prevalence}}{(\text{sensitivity} \times \text{prevalence}) + ([1 - \text{specificity}] \times [1 - \text{prevalence}])}$$

$$\text{Negative predictive value} = \frac{\text{specificity} \times (1 - \text{prevalence})}{(\text{specificity} \times [1 - \text{prevalence}]) + ([1 - \text{sensitivity}] \times \text{prevalence})}$$

Example:
Is a urinalysis necessary for a patient presenting with the classic signs of a urinary tract infection (UTI)? What is the probability of a UTI if the urinalysis is positive for pyuria? What would be done if the urinalysis is negative for pyuria?
Prevalence of UTI = 0.80
Sensitivity for pyuria = 0.80
Specificity for pyuria = 0.95

$$\text{Positive predictive value} = \frac{0.80 \times 0.80}{(0.80 \times 0.80) + ([1 - 0.95] \times [1 - 0.80])} = 0.98$$

$$\text{Negative predictive value} = \frac{0.95 \times (1 - 0.80)}{(0.95 \times [1 - 0.80]) + ([1 - 0.80] \times [0.80])} = 0.54$$

An abnormal test result (positive for pyuria) has a 0.98 probability of UTI but a negative test result still has a 0.46 (1 − 0.54) probability of UTI. Preforming a urinalysis in this case may not be helpful because a practitioner would still probably treat the patient despite a negative result.

is above the test/treat threshold, there may be no need for the test. If the probability is extremely low, doing the diagnostic test wouldn't be justified because a positive result would likely turn out to be false.

For example, a practitioner might prescribe antibiotics for pharyngitis if there's a 25% or greater chance that the cause is streptococcal infection. If a particular patient's pretest probability is high (60%), ordering a throat culture wouldn't be indicated because a negative test result wouldn't lower the posttest probability below 25%. Instead, antibiotics would be prescribed to treat streptococcal pharyngitis.

Odds ratios

Another way to use probabilities is the odds ratio approach. Odds are based on the probability that a particular outcome will occur versus the probability that it won't and is sometimes called the exposure-odds ratio. A probability of 75% (or 0.75) can also be stated as an odds ratio of 0.75:0.25 — or, using basic algebraic principles, 3:1. To convert an odds expression into a probability, first add both numbers in the expression. For a ratio of 4:1, add 4 and 1 for a sum of 5. Then finish the conversion by dividing the number on the left-hand side of the original ratio by the number you received by adding the ratio's numbers together:

$$4+1=5$$

$$4/5=0.8$$

Thus, a 4:1 odds ratio becomes a probability of 0.8, or 80%.

Decision analysis

The process of decision analysis can make applying the principles of probability easier and help you take multiple factors into account. Decision analysis also allows you to incorporate clinical outcomes that may occur. The process involves listing the options in a medical decision, assigning probabilities to the alternative actions, assigning values to the different outcomes, and then calculating which decision gives the greatest value. To complete a decision analysis, you need to draw a decision-analysis algorithm (decision tree) and complete the following steps:

- Assign probabilities to the various branches of the decision tree.
- Assign values to the outcomes at each of the levels.
- Determine the expected utility (by multiplying probability times utility).
- Select the decision with the highest expected utility.

The value of a decision tree is that it maps out the alternatives and possible outcomes for the clinical situation, but it's only as useful as the data on which it's based.

Utility values can be considered cost-benefit measures, and the utility of doing a test depends on how it affects quality of life for the patient and you. Utilities can be measured using any scale (such as 0 to 100), using life expectancy (live or die or average survival), or using quality adjusted life expectancy.

Other utilities that can be considered are morbidity, pain and suffering, functional status, and cost. Using the earlier example of performing a throat culture for pharyngitis, the decision to prescribe antibiotics without doing a throat culture is based on the following outcome factors: one-time use of antibiotics isn't dangerous or overly expensive for the patient, and nontreatment could result in life-threatening complications. The clinical decision would be different, however, if it were the patient's third case of pharyngitis in six months. The tree would change to reflect the dangers of antibiotic overuse and the lower pretest probability that the pharyngitis was caused by beta-hemolytic streptococcal infection.

Analysis

Safe, informed care is the result of a collaborative effort between you, the patient, and the patient's family. Health insurance restrictions and limited resources (personal and societal) have made cost considerations more relevant. These factors may include time lost from work, decreased productivity, transportation expenses, financial hardship of a prolonged illness, and other extraneous costs.

Another factor to consider is the necessity of testing and screening patients for diseases that occur at low prevalence rates, such as ovarian cancer, and the cost of following up with the patient if false-positive results turn out to be negative for the disease process. Such testing can exceed the costs of treating individuals who have the disease.

More economical screenings, such as diabetes screenings permitted with grant funding, may prove more prudent if individuals identified as positive for having the disease make changes in their lifestyle and diminish their chances of developing the disorder. The cost of pursuing and treating complications may far outweigh the cost of a simple blood test provided in a screening.

There are three kinds of economic analyses: cost identification, cost-benefit, and cost-effectiveness. *Cost identification analyses* examine the costs of one or more strategies of care (hospitalization, subacute care settings, home care, insurance or capitation, effect on society) with the goal of minimizing the cost of care from a given strategy. *Cost-benefit analyses* examine costs and health benefits on an economic scale, determining which strategy will provide the most with the least expense, thereby determining which strategy is most worthwhile. *Cost-effectiveness analysis* examines costs and health outcomes separately. When health outcomes are equal, the choice is based on cost. When costs are equal, the choice is based on health outcomes. However, when the favorable health outcomes of one strategy are complement-

ed by lower costs, that strategy is the best choice.

The amount of available resources also influences decision making. If resources are unlimited, the choice is simple; if resources are limited, calculation of marginal cost-effectiveness is necessary. This calculation is done by dividing the cost of a strategy by the health outcomes it achieves.

Diagnostic tests aren't perfect, and the various calculations described in this chapter represent attempts to quantify the factors involved in clinical decision making. While it isn't always possible or prudent to perform these calculations (to do this for every decision would bring the practice of health care to a grinding halt), it's useful to understand how the various values are arrived at and how they're used in creating protocols for testing and treatment.

CHAPTER 2

Laboratory guidelines to diagnostic tests

Laboratory guidelines set forth the basic principles that underlie many aspects of diagnostic testing, including patient preparation, specimen preparation, handling of specimens, and posttest care. An understanding of the basic facts can help assure accurate results. A practitioner may order the right test for the right patient, but won't obtain accurate results unless the test is carried out properly.

Patient preparation and education

Besides being knowledgeable about patient care, having the ability to gather vital patient information, and being able to make careful judgments, the ability to support the patient and his family is vital. An informed patient who feels like a valued member of the health care team will be better able to follow directions, tolerate the testing, and make decisions based on the results.

Prior to teaching, assess the patient's ability to hear or read instructions. Make sure the patient is using his usual adaptive devices, such as glasses or a hearing aid. Deliver precise instructions in a straightfor-

ward manner according to your patient's cognitive status. If English isn't his native language or he has trouble remembering the steps, provide verbal instructions along with written material that's age-appropriate, relevant, and in the patient's native language. For a patient who is illiterate or has difficulty comprehending the written materials, illustrations are beneficial.

If you're dealing with a patient from a culture you're unfamiliar with, it's often useful to engage the help of another staff member or a willing family member who can translate and help the practitioner anticipate special needs. First, however, to preserve patient confidentiality, make sure the patient agrees to the person selected to interpret; for instance, some patients may not want to discuss problems openly in front of a family member. If something about the test goes against the patient's beliefs, perhaps the testing can be adjusted to meet his needs (such as scheduling it for a different day if it interferes with beliefs or principles) or to substitute another test that's acceptable for both you and the patient.

If your patient wishes to know the reasons for certain instructions, which can sometimes be troubling, provide explana-

Choosing age-appropriate language for children

When explaining a laboratory test to a child, use words that he'll understand. Having a parent or other family member present is also helpful, but the careful selection of appropriate language is vital to effective communication.

TEST	CHILD'S INTERPRETATION	ALTERNATIVE
CAT scan (Computed tomography scan)	Scan a cat?	Tell the patient that this test will look at a part of his body. Also tell him what he needs to do and assure him that he won't be alone. ("You will need to lie down on a table, and the nurse will be right next to you.") Describe what he may hear or see in terms that he'll understand. ("The machine is going to make noises that sound like a picture being taken.")
I.V. injection (intravenous injection)	Ivy injection?	Be honest. Describe the test in simple terms and say that the needle may hurt a little.
Stool collection (stool culture)	Collecting chairs?	Use words familiar to the patient, such as "BM," "number two," "doody," or "poop."
Urine (urine specimen)	You're in?	Use words familiar to the patient, such as "pee," "number one," or "wee."
X-ray (radiography)	X-ray vision?	Describe to the patient what the machine looks like and the sounds that it will make. Also explain to the patient that the machine will take awesome pictures of the inside of his body.

tions that are accurate and address patient needs. Some patients wish to know the reasons for each step of the procedure; others don't. Adjust the depth and detail of the explanation to the patient's ability and desire to understand. Speak to children on their comprehension level, using simple concrete terms. Avoid words that conjure negative impressions of the testing procedure; substitute appropriate alternatives. (See *Choosing age-appropriate language for children.*)

Be aware of the special needs of a patient who has physical or emotional limitations, such as severe stress, alarming diagnoses, chronic conditions, neurologic conditions, altered level of consciousness, and physical or cognitive impairment. Offer the patient special attention and communication because such stressors can influence outcome, compliance, and positive response to procedures.

When a patient responds inappropriately, take time to let the patient express himself before intervening. Try to identify the specific source of his anxiety, although he may not be able to verbalize it easily. Encouraging dialogue about the patient's fears and apprehensions can help him ventilate feelings, and a thorough explanation of the procedure, including what the patient will and won't experience, can help to alleviate his fear of the unknown. Using imagery or relaxation techniques can be helpful, and most helpful of all is the presence of a caring professional.

In addition to describing pretest preparation, the actual testing procedure, and posttest care, explain to the patient how long it usually takes to get the test results and who will be explaining the results to him. Also, don't assume that a patient will remember everything he's told, even if his comprehension of the instructions appears strong. Because most of the information is new to him, he may need to hear explanations repeated at some point.

Safe, effective, informed care employs basic concepts. (See *Basics of informed care*.) A collaborative approach to patient preparation is essential to promote communication and ensure compliance. It's also important to assess risk factors and modify the approach to testing and patient care accordingly. (See *Assessing risks*, page 16.)

You should have an understanding of the test involved and its normal values. Test results will vary with the procedures used, interfering factors, and patient preparation, and you need to be ready to spot and account for deviations.

In addition to the information elicited by a history and physical examination, you also need to identify prior reactions to tests, especially tests involving injected dyes or contrast material. Unusual reactions to sedatives, such as somnolence, confusion, or agitation, should also be investigated. If

Basics of informed care

There are central concepts that every practitioner providing diagnostic services needs to be aware of in order to ensure appropriate care. These concepts include:
- proper patient preparation
- adherence to standards and guidelines
- consideration of culture, gender, and age differences
- effective and clear communication with the patient, other staff, and ancillary departments
- team approach to test management
- proper outcome evaluation
- treatment, monitoring, and counseling procedures appropriate to test outcomes
- documentation and maintenance of proper testing records.

significant, your findings may alter what test you order. Contraindicating factors, such as a patient's allergy to latex, iodine, certain medications, or contrast media, can also affect a test's administration.

Patient care will also vary after completion of the test. It's important to convey testing concepts and information while providing reassurance and support to the patient and his family.

Documentation should include what was explained to the patient, the patient's response, and educational materials supplied. A well-documented record can provide the practitioner with invaluable information. For instance, if a patient later experiences difficulty, a review of the records may indicate what was and wasn't effective in pretest care. This may be useful both in planning follow-up care for that patient and in planning approaches to pretest care

No matter how many pretest precautions are put into place, complications can occur. Some of the most common factors that can increase a patient's risk for complications include:

- age 70 or older
- history of weakness, fatigue, unsteady gait, balance problems, falls, or daily use of walker, cane, wheelchair, or other assistive devices
- severe vision problems or hearing impairment
- history of serious chronic illness
- allergy to latex, contrast iodine, radioactive agents, or medications
- presence of infection or increased risk for infection (such as human immunodeficiency virus infection, organ transplantation, chemotherapy, radiation therapy)
- neuromuscular condition, seizure disorders, paresthesias
- gastric motility dysfunction
- uncontrolled pain
- impaired judgment or illogical thinking
- aggressive or antisocial behavior
- use of diuretics, sedatives, analgesics, or other prescription or over-the-counter drugs
- alcohol or illegal drug use or addiction.

for other patients. Careful documentation will also improve audit and accreditation outcomes, reimbursement rates, and legal issue outcomes.

Specimen collection

A delicate procedure, specimen collection can result in costly mistakes when the wrong equipment and supplies are used. Incorrect technique also can contribute to erroneous test outcomes. Communication errors, however, are the biggest culprits when it comes to faulty specimen collection, so it's important for practitioners, staff members, and patients to communicate clearly. Following established procedures and guidelines can help avoid errors. (See *Checklist for minimizing errors.*)

Safety considerations

The first safety consideration, of course, is to identify the appropriate patient before performing the procedure. If you don't know the patient personally, check the patient's wristband and ask the patient to verify his name. If the patient is unable to respond, or if the identification is illegible, ask attending staff to verify the patient's identity.

The next consideration involves standard precautions for your own safety. Standard precautions, also known as universal precautions, are the current standard of care for specimen collection and handling. They're based on the recognition that any patient could have undiagnosed hepatitis B, human immunodeficiency virus, or other infectious diseases. All specimen collection, therefore, should be done as if all patient contact involves exposure to unidentified pathogens. The standard-setting agency for such precautions is the Occupational Safety and Health Administration (OSHA), but individual facilities may have additional policies and procedures that supplement OSHA standards. (See *Sources of standards*, page 18.)

When preparing standards, OSHA considers recommendations made by the Centers for Disease Control and Prevention (CDC). They call for the specimen to be obtained, processed, transported, and stored properly for a given test. Protocols

Checklist for minimizing errors

Many factors can impact test results and lead to inappropriate treatment and costly retesting. To avoid errors, use the following checklist to ensure that you're providing the proper care.

Patient factors

- Patient's age and gender appropriate for the test
- Patient followed pretest instructions, including dietary restrictions
- Patient questioned about drug or alcohol use
- Patient understands the testing process
- Patient's stress level won't affect test results
- Patient's drug therapy won't affect test results
- Patient's illness won't affect test results
- Patient's pregnancy status isn't a precaution and won't affect test results

Procedural factors

- Correct patient receiving the correct test
- Patients and significant others instructed on their responsibilities and made aware of necessary restrictions
- Appropriate consent forms obtained
- Patient preparation correct and complete
- Medications administered or withheld (as applicable)

- Patient in appropriate position or at appropriate activity at time of specimen collection
- Appropriate contrast media used
- Length of the procedure identified and necessary accommodations made for patient and staff
- Sample collection complete (especially timed specimens and specimens involving a number or samples)
- Specimen collected at the correct time of day (if applicable)
- Specimen volume correct
- Specimen handled correctly
- Specimen labeled correctly
- Blood samples not hemolyzed or traumatized
- Specimen not old or deteriorating
- Correct preservative or correct lack of preservative
- Specimen promptly delivered or stored
- Conscious sedation, oxygen, and anesthesia ready (if appropriate)
- Critical, panic, or STAT specimens treated accordingly
- Documentation correct and complete

for collection, handling, and transporting of specific specimens are established by the particular agency to ensure valid results and maintain patient safety.

The standards establish the type of specimen needed for a test and the method for obtaining it. In some instances, special equipment and supplies may be necessary, such as testing kits or sterile containers. Collection may also require direct supervision, as with specimens obtained for drug screening.

Timing of the collection is important in some tests, such as those for timed peak and trough levels for therapeutic drug monitoring, fasting specimens, or 2-hour postprandial blood glucose testing. An ill-timed specimen will invalidate results in these tests. In addition, legal and forensic specimens may be collected as evidence in legal proceedings, criminal investigations, and after the death of the patient. They may include tests, such as DNA specimens and drug and alcohol levels. These tests involve specific legal implications, and witnessed collections may be involved.

Standard precautions taken during specimen collection involve safety considerations, infection control, and appropriate equipment. Below are examples of the required equipment for just a few diagnostic tests:

■ *Stool and urine specimens* — These collections require clean, dry containers and kits. Timed urine collections may need special containers, specific additives, and refrigeration during or after collection. Midstream kits are available for clean-catch urine specimens.

■ *Oral and sputum specimens* — These specimens require specific techniques as well as special kits and preservatives to ensure proper collection and storage, depending on what type of specimen is obtained.

■ *Blood specimens* — Equipment, such as needles, collection tubes, syringes, tourniquets, needle disposal containers, lancets, antimicrobial skin preparation equipment, and adhesive bandages are often needed. Tubes are color-coded; some have additives to prevent deterioration, prevent coagulation, or block certain enzyme in the specimen. (See *Adapting collection technique to the patient.*)

Standard precautions
Most tests require standard precautions such as personal protective equipment. Wear disposable gloves when collecting and handling specimens, touching blood or other body fluids (for example suctioning), or touching mucous membranes or nonintact skin. The potential for air or water droplet dispersion mandates use of goggles and gowns in addition to gloves.

Prepare for procedures, especially those involving sharp instruments, by arranging all the necessary disposable equipment within arm's reach before the procedure begins. Don't recap used needles and other sharp instruments; dispose of them immediately in specially designated, punctureproof containers to avoid injury. When obtaining blood cultures, changing needles isn't necessary and may be hazardous.

After obtaining the specimen, dispose of gloves in the proper biohazard waste container and wash your hands. If a spill occurs, clean it up with designated solutions, usually a 10% bleach solution, or according to facility policy.

Dispose of biohazardous waste appropriately. Pour liquids slowly and carefully to prevent splashing. Place specimens in receptacles specifically designed for them, with the caps tightly sealed and marked with biohazard tags. If a splash occurs, follow safety procedures according to the type of biohazardous waste.

Specimen identification

Equally important is using the right collection tube (or tubes) for the specimen. Prepared test tubes are marked by the color of the stopper at the top and may contain anticoagulants or preservatives. (See *Guide to color-top collection tubes,* page 20.) If you're collecting multiple samples, fill sterile tubes (for bacteriologic tests) first, followed by color-top tubes. The generally recommended order for color-top tubes is red-topped (tubes without additives), then blue-topped, then green-topped, then lavender-topped.

After obtaining the specimen, label it with the patient's name and identification number according to facility policy. Generally, this involves labeling the actual container instead of just the lid because the lid is removed and can be misplaced in the laboratory with other specimens.

Gently invert any tubes containing anticoagulants or preservatives to allow the contents to mix. Place arterial blood gas and other sensitive specimen samples on ice according to facility policy. Remember that exposure to sunlight, air, or other substances — as well as warming and cooling — can alter specimen integrity.

Specimen transport

Transport specimens to the laboratory by means of an appropriate medium and in a timely fashion or store specimens properly as indicated. Failure to do so can result in specimen deterioration. Certain specimens,

---

AGE ISSUE ✱ ✱ ✱ ✱

Adapting collection technique to the patient

Medical equipment may be becoming increasingly specialized, but most equipment usage remains dependent upon a patient's age, condition, and ability and willingness to cooperate. For example, pediatric equipment may be just right for drawing blood from a small, elderly patient with fragile veins. Pediatric tubes may be equally appropriate for a critically ill patient who has already lost a significant amount of blood such as a multitrauma victim. And in an incontinent adult who is unable to accommodate test requirements, using a catheter can produce a sterile urine specimen.

---

such as oral and sputum samples and specimens labeled STAT must be delivered to the laboratory and processed immediately.

If the specimen needs to be mailed or transported to another facility or a specialty laboratory located in another city or distant area, it needs to be collected, packaged, labeled, and transported according to specific facility instructions; some specimens require delivery within an exact time frame. Containers for such transport are securely closed, made watertight for collection to minimize contamination during transport, and placed into a second durable, watertight container. Then this container is placed into a sturdy strong outer shipping container for transport and the container clearly labeled as biomedical material. If the package becomes damaged or leaks, federal regulation mandates that it be isolated and the CDC Office of Health and Safety in Atlanta be notified.

Guide to color-top collection tubes

The correct tube must be selected according to the sample needed for the test. Below is a list of common tubes used for blood sample collection with the type of additives in the vial and its purpose.

TUBE COLOR	DRAW VOLUME	ADDITIVE	PURPOSE
Black	2.7 or 4.5 ml	Sodium citrate	Coagulation studies on plasma
Blue	2.7 or 4.5 ml	Sodium citrate and citric acid	Coagulation studies on plasma
Gray	3 to 10 ml	Glycolytic inhibitor, such as sodium fluoride, powdered oxalate, or glycolytic-microbial inhibitor	Glucose determinations on serum or plasma
Green	2 to 15 ml	Heparin (sodium, lithium, or ammonium)	Plasma studies
Lavender	2 to 10 ml	Ethylenediaminetetraacetic acid	Whole-blood studies
Red	2 to 20 ml	None	Serum studies
Yellow	12 ml	Acid citrate dextrose	Whole-blood studies

Throughout the testing procedure, remember to maintain patient confidentiality. Relay information only on a need-to-know basis, with secure and protected access to information permitted only to select individuals.

Laboratory methods

The laboratory handles the specimen according to policy, standards, and procedures for the test being performed. Testing methods commonly include smears, stains, cultures, tissue biopsy, and serology.

Smears

Specimens for smears are obtained by applying a cotton-tipped swab to the tissue surface. The laboratory technician prepares a smear by rolling a small quantity of the specimen across a glass slide in a very thin layer that individual cells can be easily identified and examined. The specimen is usually "fixed" by passing the specimen area of the slide through the flame of a Bunsen burner. Smears are used to observe cell morphology and structure. A common example is the white blood cell differential count.

Stains

Stains are applied to fixed specimens in order to highlight certain cells or parts of cells, making them easy to identify. Probably the most used stain is the Gram stain, a procedure for identifying and differentiating types of bacteria — gram-positive or gram-negative, depending on whether they take up the stains applied and turn the color of the stain. The distinction is based on differences in cell wall structure; it's important not only for general identification, but also because the two groups have similar characteristics, including susceptibility to certain antibiotics (most of which act by disrupting cell wall structures). An example is chorionic villi sampling, which detects fetal chromosomal and biochemical disorders when performed during the first trimester of pregnancy.

Cultures

Culturing involves placing a sample of the specimen in an environment where the microorganisms infecting the tissue can grow and be identified. The specimen may be put into a liquid solution (usually in a test tube), or onto a Petri dish, a flat circular dish partially filled with the nutritive medium agar. The medium is always prepared in accordance with the specific needs of the cells to be identified. Generally, cultures require 48 to 72 hours to come to fruition; however, some cultures, such as fungi, require greater periods of time.

Tissue biopsy

Diagnosing bone infection (osteomyelitis), certain types of viral or fungal infections (often in the skin), and certain types of cancer requires a larger tissue sample. These cases rely on tissue biopsy. Excisional biopsy removes the entire lesion or affected area; incisional biopsy removes only part of the lesion. Types of incisional biopsy include:

■ punch biopsy, done by using a special cutting tool that removes a small (2 to 6 mm) diameter, full thickness skin sample

■ shave biopsy, used to remove a superficial portion of the skin that's raised above the surrounding skin level. It's commonly used to ascertain the presence or absence of malignant cells; however, it doesn't allow accurate determination of the full depth of the lesion.

■ elliptical biopsy, used when a slightly larger sample is desired. With a scalpel, two semi-elliptical incisions are made around the lesion.

■ pinch biopsy, performed by holding the lesion with a hemostat and snipping off the suspended piece of tissue. This is similar to a shave biopsy; however, it generally isn't used for potentially cancerous lesions because it doesn't ensure a full-thickness sample, which is needed for staging the cancer and determining proper treatment.

Serology

Some diseases are identified by the presence in serum of antibodies to the offending organism or molecule. Serologic testing involves inducing antigen-antibody reactions in the specimen. It's used to identify certain types of infections (especially viral), autoimmune disorders, and neoplasms.

Posttest concerns

After the test, inform the patient of the results in a timely and supportive fashion. Depending on the test involved and the procedure used, monitor the patient for complications and provide follow-up care as appropriate.

Test results

The time it takes to complete a diagnostic test varies, depending partly on the specific test ordered and the way the laboratory processes it. Interdepartmental and interdisciplinary collaboration can ensure that results become available to practitioner, patient, and staff as soon as possible.

Some tests, such as cultures, require time for the material under consideration to grow; this is usually 48 to 72 hours but can take as long as 4 weeks. A bone biopsy requires 24 to 48 hours for decalcification before histological sections can be prepared and examined microscopically. Other tests, such as hemoglobin values, can be available within minutes. Inform the patient as to how long it will take to receive test results and who will relay that information to him.

Normal test result ranges can vary from laboratory to laboratory according to the population tested, the manner of specimen collection and preservation, and the laboratory method employed. Laboratories specify their own normal ranges. Many factors can influence test outcomes, including the patient's age, gender, race, environment, posture, diurnal and other cyclic variations, fasting or postprandial state, hydration, nutritional status, drugs, exercise, mental status, and compliance with test protocols. Interpretation of the results requires taking all of these factors into consideration.

Posttest complications

Complications can occur from a number of variables, including the patient's particular condition, the pretest preparation, and the collection of the specimen itself. For example, rapid recovery from invasive tests requires that a patient have normal coagulation function and tissue healing ability. Because this usually isn't the case, many patients require careful monitoring and specific interventions to assure their recovery and to prevent complications.

Potential posttest complications include the following.

■ *Vascular:* Arterial puncture (needed for arterial blood gas sampling and cardiac catheterization) is especially hazardous due to the high pressures within the arterial system that make clotting more difficult. Pressure should be applied to the puncture site for a specified length of time and the patient assessed frequently for hematoma, particularly after femoral punctures with large-bore needles.

■ *Allergic reactions:* Patients may experience an allergic reaction to dyes or radioactive material. Observation for signs of allergic reaction (agitation, skin redness or itching, wheezing) is imperative. The first exposure to the allergen may be relatively mild as the body develops an immune readiness to the allergen. The second or third exposure may quickly result in an anaphylactic reaction, which is why it's vitally important to observe patients for signs of allergy after each test. If the patient has received proper pretest care, previous reactions will already be documented.

■ *Reactions to sedatives:* Patients are commonly given sedation to reduce anxiety associated with the testing. Sometimes the sedative is taken orally, but usually it's given I.V. because of the rapid onset and ability of practitioners to control serum levels. Patients recover consciousness at different rates depending on renal and hepatic function, age, weight, and sex — an important point to remember when deciding if a patient is ready to be discharged (for outpatient procedures) or when to perform other activities that require his full physical and cognitive abilities, including the ability to make informed decisions about his care. (See *Making informed decisions.*)

Posttest assessments include observing behaviors and monitoring activity as well as listening for any complaints and investigating concerns in an appropriate manner. Some patients may require closer, lengthier monitoring and observation; this is true for those who have had an invasive procedure because they're at risk for bleeding, circulatory problems, and infection. In addition, patients receiving sedation (including I.V. conscious sedation), drugs, contrast media (such as iodine or barium), or radioactive medications need to be evaluated and treated according to established protocols.

Follow-up care

Follow-up care involves careful assessment of the patient's condition, including monitoring vital signs and observing the site of entry (for invasive tests). The appropriate length of time for patient observation is determined by data from others who have undergone such testing and adjusted for specific patient situations. For example, a patient who has had conscious sedation or contrast media needs to be monitored for reactions for a specific period of time (minutes to hours, depending on the test involved and the patient's reaction). Puncture sites should be observed for several days for redness, swelling or induration, and increasing rather than decreasing soreness — any of which could indicate infection. For such lengthy monitoring, patient and family need to clearly understand discharge instructions.

Documentation

Documentation of all care given, including pretest and posttest care and patient education, is vital. If problems arise, this documentation provides a sound basis for understanding what happened and determining how future problems can be prevented. It also provides important information for quality control evaluations, reimbursement by insurance companies (who typically require records to be submitted before rendering payment) and, in some cases, defending a practitioner's decisions and clinical care.

Laboratory and diagnostic procedures

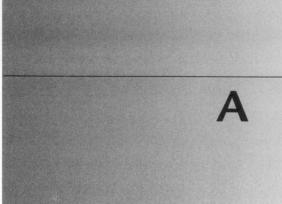

A

ABO blood typing

ABO blood typing classifies blood according to the presence of major antigens A and B on red blood cell (RBC) surfaces and according to serum antibodies anti-A and anti-B. ABO blood typing using forward and reverse methods is required before transfusion to prevent a lethal reaction.

In forward typing, the patient's RBCs are mixed with anti-A serum, and then with anti-B serum; the presence or absence of agglutination determines the blood group. In reverse typing, the results of the forward method are verified by mixing the patient's serum with known group A and group B cells. Blood group determination is confirmed when the results of forward and reverse typing match perfectly. (See *ABO blood types*.)

Purpose
■ To establish blood group according to the ABO system
■ To check compatibility of donor and recipient blood before transfusion

Cost
Inexpensive

Patient preparation
■ Tell the patient that this test determines his blood group.
■ If the patient is scheduled for a transfusion, explain that after his blood group is known, it can be matched with the right donor blood.
■ Tell the patient that the test requires a blood sample. Explain who will perform the venipuncture and when.
■ Explain to the patient that he may experience discomfort from the needle puncture and the tourniquet.
■ Check the patient's history for recent administration of blood, dextran, or I.V. contrast media.

Findings
In forward typing, if agglutination occurs when the patient's RBCs are mixed with anti-A serum, the A antigen is present and the blood is typed A. If agglutination occurs when the patient's RBCs are mixed with anti-B serum, the B antigen is present and the blood is typed B. If agglutination occurs in both mixes, A and B antigens are present and the blood is typed AB. If it doesn't occur in either mix, no antigens are present and the blood is typed O.

ABO blood types

ABO recipient-donor compatibility

RECIPIENT'S BLOOD TYPE	COMPATIBLE DONOR TYPE
A	A, O
B	B, O
AB	A, B, AB, O
O	O

ABO blood types in U.S. population

BLOOD TYPE	PERCENT	BLOOD TYPE	PERCENT
O$^+$	38%	B$^+$	9%
O$^-$	7%	B$^-$	2%
A$^+$	34%	AB$^+$	3%
A$^-$	6%	AB$^-$	1%

Note: Distribution may differ for specific ethnic and racial groups

In reverse typing, if agglutination occurs when B cells are mixed with the patient's serum, anti-B is present and the blood is typed A. If agglutination occurs when A cells are mixed, anti-A is present and the blood is typed B. If agglutination occurs when A and B cells are mixed, anti-A and anti-B are present and the blood is typed O. If agglutination doesn't occur when A and B cells are mixed, neither anti-A nor anti-B is present and the blood is typed AB.

Interfering factors

■ Recent administration of dextran or I.V. contrast media, causing cellular aggregation resembling antibody-mediated agglutination
■ Hemolysis due to rough handling of the sample

■ Blood transfusion or pregnancy in the past 3 months (possibility of lingering antibodies)

Acetylcholine receptor antibodies

The acetylcholine receptor antibodies test is the most useful immunologic test for confirming acquired (autoimmune) myasthenia gravis, a disorder of neuromuscular transmission. In myasthenia gravis, antibodies block and destroy acetylcholine receptor sites, causing muscle weakness that can be either generalized or localized to the ocular muscles.

Two test methods — a binding assay and a blocking assay — are now available to determine the relative concentration of acetylcholine antibodies in serum. The blocking assay is specific for the autoimmune form of myasthenia gravis and useful for research. Determination of acetylcholine antibodies by either method also helps monitor immunosuppressive therapy for myasthenia, although antibody levels don't usually parallel the severity of disease.

Purpose
■ To confirm diagnosis of myasthenia gravis
■ To monitor the effectiveness of immunosuppressive therapy for myasthenia gravis

Cost
Moderately expensive

Patient preparation
■ Explain to the patient that this test helps confirm myasthenia gravis and also assesses the effectiveness of treatment as appropriate.
■ Tell the patient that the test requires a blood sample. Explain who will perform the venipuncture and when.
■ Explain to the patient that he may experience discomfort from the needle puncture and the tourniquet.
■ Check the patient's history for immunosuppressive drugs that may affect test results, and note such use on the laboratory request.

Normal findings
Normal serum is negative for acetylcholine receptor-binding antibodies and acetylcholine receptor-blocking antibodies.

Abnormal findings
Positive acetylcholine receptor antibodies in symptomatic adults confirm the diagnosis of myasthenia gravis. Patients who have only ocular symptoms have lower antibody titers than those who have generalized symptoms.

Interfering factors
■ Thymectomy, thoracic duct drainage, immunosuppressive therapy, and plasmapheresis (possible decrease)
■ Amyotrophic lateral sclerosis (possible false-positive)

Acid perfusion

The lower esophageal sphincter normally prevents gastric reflux. However, if this sphincter is incompetent, the recurrent backflow of acidic juices (and of bile salts, if the pyloric sphincter is also incompetent) into the esophagus inflames the esophageal mucosa. This inflammation, esophagitis, manifests in burning epigastric or retrosternal pain that may radiate to the back or arms.

The acid perfusion test, also called the *Bernstein test,* helps to distinguish pain caused by esophagitis from pain caused by angina pectoris or other disorders. It requires perfusion of saline and acidic solutions into the esophagus through a nasogastric tube.

Purpose
■ To distinguish chest pains caused by esophagitis from those caused by cardiac disorders

Cost
Expensive

Patient preparation
■ Tell the patient that this test helps determine the cause of heartburn.

- Explain the following restrictions to the patient: no antacids for 24 hours before the test, no food for 12 hours before the test, and no fluids or smoking for 8 hours before the test.
- Describe the test to the patient, including who will perform it, where it will take place, and its expected duration.
- Tell the patient that the test involves passing a tube through his nose into the esophagus. Explain that he may experience some discomfort, a desire to cough, or a gagging sensation during tube passage.
- Tell the patient that liquid is slowly perfused through the tube into the esophagus.
- Tell the patient to immediately report any pain or burning during perfusion to the technician administering the test.
- Tell the patient that his pulse and blood pressure will be taken just prior to the test.
- Tell the patient to report heartburn to the technician administering the test.
- Obtain informed consent if necessary.

Normal findings

Absence of pain or burning during perfusion of either solution indicates a healthy esophageal mucosa.

Abnormal findings

In patients with esophagitis, the acidic solution causes pain or burning, and the normal saline solution should produce no adverse effects. Occasionally, both solutions cause pain in patients with esophagitis, but they may cause no pain in patients with asymptomatic esophagitis.

Interfering factors

- Failure to adhere to pretest restrictions
- Acid pump inhibitors, adrenergic blockers, anticholinergics, reserpine, corticosteroids, and histamine-2 blockers.

Activated clotting time

Activated clotting time (ACT), or automated coagulation time, measures whole blood clotting time. Activated clotting time is commonly performed during procedures that require extracorporeal circulation, such as cardiopulmonary bypass, ultrafiltration, hemodialysis, and extracorporeal membrane oxygenation (ECMO) as well as other invasive procedures, such as cardiac catheterization and percutaneous transluminal coronary angioplasty.

Purpose
- To monitor the effect of heparin
- To monitor the effect of protamine in heparin neutralization
- To detect severe deficiencies in clotting factors (except factor VII)

Cost
Moderately expensive

Patient preparation
- Explain to the patient that this test is used to monitor the effect of heparin on the blood's ability to coagulate.
- Tell the patient that the test requires two blood samples, and that the first sample will be disregarded so that any heparin in the tubing doesn't interfere with the results. Explain who will perform the venipuncture and when.
- Explain to the patient that he may experience discomfort from the needle puncture and the tourniquet.

Reference values
In a non-anticoagulated patient, normal activated clotting time is 107 seconds plus or minus 13 seconds (SI, 107 ± 13 s). During cardiopulmonary bypass, heparin is titrated to maintain an activated clotting

time between 400 and 600 seconds (SI, 400 to 600 s). During ECMO, heparin is titrated to maintain the activated clotting time between 220 and 260 seconds (SI, 220 to 260 s).

Interfering factors
■ Failure to send the sample to the laboratory immediately or to place it on ice
■ Failure to draw at least 5 ml waste to avoid sample contamination when drawing the sample from a venous access device that's used for heparin infusion

Adrenocorticotropic hormone

The adrenocorticotropic hormone test measures the plasma levels of corticotropin (also known as *adrenocorticotropic hormone* or *ACTH*) by radioimmunoassay. Corticotropin stimulates the adrenal cortex to secrete cortisol and, to a lesser degree, androgens and aldosterone. It also has some melanocyte-stimulating activity, increases the uptake of amino acids by muscle cells, promotes lipolysis by fat cells, stimulates pancreatic beta cells to secrete insulin, and may contribute to the release of growth hormone. Corticotropin levels vary diurnally, peaking between 6 a.m. and 8 a.m. and ebbing between 6 p.m. and 11 p.m.

The corticotropin test may be ordered for patients with signs of adrenal hypofunction (insufficiency) or hyperfunction (Cushing's syndrome). Corticotropin suppression or stimulation testing is usually necessary to confirm diagnosis. The instability and unavailability of corticotropin greatly limit this test's diagnostic significance and reliability.

Purpose
■ To facilitate differential diagnosis of primary and secondary adrenal hypofunction
■ To aid differential diagnosis of Cushing's syndrome

Cost
Moderately expensive

Patient preparation
■ Explain to the patient that this test helps determine if his hormonal secretion is normal.
■ Tell the patient that he must fast and limit his physical activity for 10 to 12 hours before the test.
■ Tell the patient that the test requires a blood sample. Explain who will perform the venipuncture and when.
■ Explain to the patient that he may experience discomfort from the needle puncture and the tourniquet.
■ Check the patient's history for medications that may affect the accuracy of test results, and withhold these medications for 48 hours or longer before the test. If they must be continued, note this on the laboratory request.
■ Instruct the patient to eat a diet low in carbohydrates for 2 days before the test. This requirement may vary, depending on the laboratory.
■ Tell the patient that the test will be done between 6 a.m. and 8 a.m. (peak secretion) to detect adrenal hypofunction, or between 6 p.m. and 11 p.m. (low secretion) to detect suspected Cushing's syndrome.

Normal findings
Mayo Medical Laboratories sets corticotropin baseline values at less than 120 pg/ml (SI, < 26.4 pmol/L) at 6 a.m. to 8 a.m.), but these values may vary, depending on the laboratory.

Abnormal findings

A higher-than-normal corticotropin level may indicate primary adrenal hypofunction (Addison's disease), in which the pituitary gland attempts to compensate for the unresponsiveness of the target organ by releasing excessive corticotropin.

A low-normal corticotropin level suggests secondary adrenal hypofunction resulting from pituitary or hypothalamic dysfunction. The primary determinant may be panhypopituitarism, absence of corticotropin-releasing hormone in the hypothalamus, or chronic blunting of corticotropin levels by long-term corticosteroid therapy.

In suspected Cushing's syndrome, an elevated corticotropin level suggests Cushing's disease, in which pituitary dysfunction (due to adenoma) causes continuous hypersecretion of corticotropin and, consequently, continuously elevated cortisol levels without diurnal variations. Moderately elevated corticotropin levels suggest pituitary-dependent adrenal hyperplasia and nonadrenal tumors such as oat cell carcinoma of the lungs.

A low-normal corticotropin level implies adrenal hyperfunction due to adrenocortical tumor or hyperplasia.

Interfering factors

- Failure to observe pretest restrictions
- Corticosteroids, including cortisone and its analogues (decrease)
- Drugs that increase endogenous cortisol secretion, such as amphetamines, calcium gluconate, estrogens, ethanol, and spironolactone (decrease)
- Lithium (decreases cortisol levels and may interfere with corticotropin secretion)
- Menstrual cycle and pregnancy
- Radioactive scan performed within 1 week before the test

- Acute stress (including hospitalization and surgery) and depression (increase)

Alanine aminotransferase

The alanine aminotransferase (ALT) test is used to measure serum levels of ALT, one of two enzymes that catalyze a reversible amino group transfer reaction in the Krebs cycle. ALT is necessary for tissue energy production. ALT is found primarily in the liver, with lesser amounts in the kidneys, heart, and skeletal muscles, and is a sensitive indicator of acute hepatocellular disease.

Purpose

- To detect and evaluate treatment of acute hepatic disease, especially hepatitis and cirrhosis without jaundice
- To distinguish between myocardial and hepatic tissue damage (used with aspartate aminotransferase)
- To assess hepatotoxicity of some drugs

Cost

Inexpensive

Patient preparation

- Explain to the patient that this test is used to assess liver function.
- Tell the patient that the test requires a blood sample. Explain who will perform the venipuncture and when.
- Explain to the patient that he may experience discomfort from the needle puncture and the tourniquet.
- Restrict medications the patient is taking that may affect test results. If they must be continued, note this on the laboratory request.

Normal findings

Serum ALT levels range from 8 to 50 U/L (SI, 0.14 to 0.85 μkat/L).

Abnormal findings

Very high serum ALT levels (up to 50 times normal) suggest viral or severe drug-induced hepatitis or other hepatic disease with extensive necrosis. Moderate to high levels may indicate infectious mononucleosis, chronic hepatitis, intrahepatic cholestasis or cholecystitis, early or improving acute viral hepatitis, or severe hepatic congestion due to heart failure.

Slight to moderate elevations of serum ALT may appear in any condition that produces acute hepatocellular injury, such as active cirrhosis and drug-induced hepatitis. Marginal elevations occasionally occur in acute myocardial infarction, reflecting secondary hepatic congestion or the release of small amounts of ALT from myocardial tissue.

Interfering factors

■ Hemolysis due to rough handling of the sample
■ Barbiturates, chlorpromazine, griseofulvin, isoniazid, methyldopa, nitrofurantoin, para-aminosalicylic acid, phenothiazines, phenytoin, salicylates, tetracycline, and other drugs that cause hepatic injury by competitively interfering with cellular metabolism (false-high)
■ Narcotic analgesics, such as codeine, meperidine, and morphine (possible false-high due to increased intrabiliary pressure)
■ Ingestion of lead or exposure to carbon tetrachloride (sharp increase due to direct injury to hepatic cells)

Aldosterone, serum

The blood aldosterone test measures serum aldosterone levels by quantitative analysis and radioimmunoassay. Aldosterone regulates ion transport across cell membranes to promote reabsorption of sodium and chloride in exchange for potassium and hydrogen ions. Consequently, it helps to maintain blood pressure and volume and to regulate fluid and electrolyte balance. This test identifies aldosteronism and, when supported by plasma renin levels, distinguishes between the primary and secondary forms of this disorder. (See *Sites of adrenal hormone production*.)

Purpose

■ To aid diagnosis of primary and secondary aldosteronism, adrenal hyperplasia, hypoaldosteronism, and salt-losing syndrome

Cost

Expensive

Patient preparation

■ Explain to the patient that this test helps determine if symptoms are due to improper hormonal secretion.
■ Tell the patient that the test requires a blood sample. Explain who will perform the venipuncture and when.
■ Explain to the patient that he may experience discomfort from the needle puncture and the tourniquet.
■ Instruct the patient to maintain a low-carbohydrate, normal-sodium diet (135 mEq or 3 g/day) for at least 2 weeks or, preferably, for 30 days before the test.
■ Withhold all drugs that alter fluid, sodium, and potassium balance — especially diuretics, antihypertensives, steroids, hormonal contraceptives, and estrogens — for

Sites of adrenal hormone production

The adrenal glands are paired structures located retroperitoneally on top of each kidney. Each gland consists of the three-layer cortex and the medulla. The outer layer of the cortex, the zona glomerulosa, produces aldosterone; the first inner layer, the zona fasciculata, produces cortisol; the next inner layer, the zona reticularis, secretes sex hormones (primarily androgens); and the medulla stores catecholamines (epinephrine and norepinephrine).

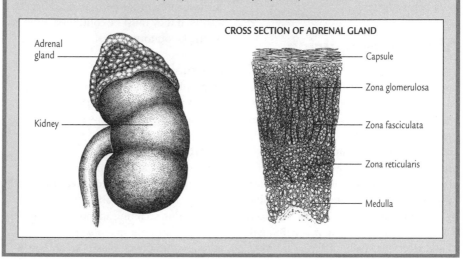

CROSS SECTION OF ADRENAL GLAND

Adrenal gland
Kidney

Capsule
Zona glomerulosa
Zona fasciculata
Zona reticularis
Medulla

at least 2 weeks or, preferably, for 30 days before the test.

■ Withhold all renin inhibitors, such as propranolol, for 1 week before the test. If they must be continued, note this on the laboratory request.

■ Tell the patient to avoid licorice for at least 2 weeks before the test because it produces an aldosterone-like effect.

Normal findings

Laboratory values vary with time of day and posture — upright postures have higher values. In upright individuals, normal is 7 to 30 ng/dl (SI, 190 to 832 pmol/L). In supine individuals, values are 3 to 16 ng/dl (SI, 80 to 440 pmol/L).

Abnormal findings

Excessive aldosterone secretion may indicate a primary or secondary disease. Primary aldosteronism (Conn's syndrome) may result from adrenocortical adenoma or carcinoma or from bilateral adrenal hyperplasia. Secondary aldosteronism can result from renovascular hypertension, heart failure, cirrhosis of the liver, nephrotic syndrome, idiopathic cyclic edema, and the third trimester of pregnancy.

Low serum aldosterone levels may indicate primary hypoaldosteronism, salt-losing syndrome, eclampsia, or Addison's disease.

Interfering factors

■ Failure to observe pretest restrictions of diet, medications, or physical activity

- Some antihypertensives such as methyldopa that promote sodium and water retention (possible decrease)
- Diuretics (possible increase)
- Some corticosteroids, such as fludrocortisone, that mimic mineralocorticoid activity (possible decrease)
- Radioactive scan performed within 1 week before the test

Aldosterone, urine

The urine aldosterone test measures urine levels of aldosterone, the principal mineralocorticoid secreted by the adrenal cortex. Aldosterone promotes retention of sodium and excretion of potassium by the renal tubules, thereby helping to regulate blood pressure and fluid and electrolyte balance. In turn, aldosterone secretion is controlled by the renin-angiotensin system. This feedback mechanism is vital to maintaining fluid and electrolyte balance. Urine aldosterone levels, measured through radioimmunoassay, are usually evaluated after measurement of serum electrolyte and renin levels.

Purpose
- To aid diagnosis of primary and secondary aldosteronism

Cost
Moderately expensive

Patient preparation
- Explain to the patient that this test evaluates hormonal balance.
- Instruct the patient to maintain a normal sodium diet (3 g/day) before the test and to avoid sodium-rich foods, such as bacon, barbecue sauce, corned beef, bouillon cubes or powder, pickles, snack foods (potato chips), and olives.
- Advise the patient to avoid strenuous physical exercise and stressful situations during the collection period.
- Tell the patient that the test requires collection of urine during a 24-hour period, and teach him the proper collection technique (placed on ice or refrigerated during collection period).
- Restrict medications that may affect test results. If they must be continued, note this on the laboratory request.

Normal findings
Normally, urine aldosterone levels range from 3 to 19 µg/24 hours (SI, 8 to 51 nmol/d).

Abnormal findings
Elevated urine aldosterone levels suggest primary or secondary aldosteronism. The primary form usually arises from an aldosterone-secreting adenoma of the adrenal cortex but may also result from adrenocortical hyperplasia. Secondary aldosteronism, the more common form, results from external stimulation of the adrenal cortex such as that produced when the renin-angiotensin system is activated by hypertensive and edematous disorders.

Disorders that may result in secondary aldosteronism are malignant hypertension, heart failure, cirrhosis of the liver, nephrotic syndrome, and idiopathic cyclic edema.

Low urine aldosterone levels may result from Addison's disease, salt-losing syndrome, and toxemia of pregnancy. These levels normally rise during pregnancy but rapidly decline following parturition.

Interfering factors
- Failure to maintain normal dietary sodium intake as well as excess intake of licorice or glucose
- Failure to avoid strenuous physical exercise and emotional stress before the test

(possible increase due to stimulation of adrenocortical secretions)
■ Radioactive scan performed within 1 week before the test
■ Failure to collect all urine during the collection period or to properly store the specimen
■ Failure to send the specimen to the laboratory immediately after collection
■ Antihypertensive drugs (possible decrease due to sodium and water retention)
■ Diuretics and most steroids (possible increase due to sodium excretion)
■ Some corticosteroids, such as fludrocortisone, which mimic mineralocorticoid activity (possible decrease)

Alkaline phosphatase

The alkaline phosphatase (ALP) test is used to measure serum levels of ALP, an enzyme that influences bone calcification as well as lipid and metabolite transport. ALP measurements reflect the combined activity of several ALP isoenzymes found in the liver, bones, kidneys, intestinal lining, and placenta. Bone and liver ALP are always present in adult serum, with liver ALP most prominent except during the third trimester of pregnancy (when the placenta originates about half of all ALP). The intestinal variant of ALP can be a normal component (in less than 10% of normal patterns; almost exclusively in the sera of blood groups B and O), or it can be an abnormal finding associated with hepatic disease.

Purpose
■ To detect and identify skeletal diseases primarily characterized by marked osteoblastic activity

■ To detect focal hepatic lesions causing biliary obstruction, such as tumor or abscess
■ To assess response to vitamin D in the treatment of rickets
■ To supplement information from other liver function studies and GI enzyme tests

Cost
Inexpensive

Patient preparation
■ Explain to the patient that this test is used to assess liver and bone function.
■ Instruct the patient to fast for at least 8 hours before the test because fat intake stimulates intestinal ALP secretion.
■ Tell the patient that the test requires a blood sample. Explain who will perform the venipuncture and when.
■ Explain to the patient that he may experience discomfort from the needle puncture and the tourniquet.

Normal findings
Total serum ALP levels normally range from 30 to 85 IU/ml (SI, 42 to 128 U/L).

Abnormal findings
Although significant ALP elevations are possible with diseases that affect many organs, they usually indicate skeletal disease or extrahepatic or intrahepatic biliary obstruction causing cholestasis. Many acute hepatic diseases cause serum ALP elevations before they affect serum bilirubin levels.

Moderate increases in serum ALP levels may reflect acute biliary obstruction from hepatocellular inflammation in active cirrhosis, mononucleosis, and viral hepatitis. Moderate increases are also seen in osteomalacia and deficiency-induced rickets.

Sharp elevations in serum ALP levels may indicate complete biliary obstruction by malignant or infectious infiltrations or fibrosis, most common in Paget's disease and, occasionally, in biliary obstruction, extensive bone metastasis, and hyperparathyroidism. Metastatic bone tumors resulting from pancreatic cancer raise serum ALP levels without a concomitant rise in serum alanine aminotransferase levels.

Isoenzyme fractionation and additional enzyme tests (gamma glutamyl transferase, lactate dehydrogenase, 5'-nucleotidase, and leucine aminopeptidase) are sometimes performed when the cause of serum ALP elevations is in doubt. Rarely, low levels of serum ALP are associated with hypophosphatasia and protein or magnesium deficiency.

Interfering factors
■ Recent ingestion of vitamin D (possible increase due to effect on osteoblastic activity)
■ Recent infusion of albumin prepared from placental venous blood (marked increase)
■ Drugs that influence liver function or cause cholestasis, such as barbiturates, chlorpropamide, hormonal contraceptives, isoniazid, methyldopa, phenothiazines, phenytoin, and rifampin (possible mild increase)
■ Halothane sensitivity (possible drastic increase)
■ Clofibrate (decrease)
■ Healing long-bone fractures (possible increase)
■ Third trimester of pregnancy (possible increase)
■ Age and sex (increase in infants, children, adolescents, and individuals over age 45)

Alpha$_1$-antitrypsin

A protein produced by the liver, alpha$_1$-antitrypsin (also known as *AAT*) is believed to inhibit the release of protease into body fluids by dying cells and is a major component of alpha$_1$-globulin. AAT is measured using radioimmunoassay or isoelectric focusing. Congenital absence or deficiency of AAT has been linked to high susceptibility to emphysema.

Purpose
■ To screen for high-risk emphysema patients
■ A nonspecific method of detecting inflammation, severe infection, and necrosis
■ To test for congenital AAT deficiency

Cost
Inexpensive

Patient preparation
■ Explain to the patient that this test is used to diagnose respiratory or liver disease as well as inflammation, infection, or necrosis.
■ Tell the patient to avoid smoking, hormonal contraceptives, and steroids for at least 24 hours before the test and to fast for at least 8 hours before the test.
■ Tell the patient that the test requires a blood sample. Explain who will perform the venipuncture and when.
■ Explain to the patient that he may experience discomfort from the needle puncture and the tourniquet.

Normal findings
Serum AAT levels vary by age, but the normal range is 110 to 200 mg/dl (SI, 1.10 to 2.0 g/L).

Abnormal findings

Decreased serum AAT levels may occur in early-onset emphysema and cirrhosis, nephrotic syndrome, malnutrition, congenital alpha$_1$-globulin deficiency and, transiently, in the neonate. If clinically indicated, patients with serum AAT levels lower than 125 mg/dl (SI, 1.25 g/L) should be phenotyped to confirm homozygous and heterozygous deficiencies. (Heterozygous patients don't seem to be at increased risk for early emphysema.)

Increased serum AAT levels can occur in chronic inflammatory disorders, necrosis, pregnancy, acute pulmonary infections, hyaline membrane disease in infants, hepatitis, systemic lupus erythematosus, and rheumatoid arthritis.

Interfering factors

- Corticosteroids and hormonal contraceptives (possible false-high)
- Smoking or failure to fast for 8 hours before the test (possible false-high)

Alpha-fetoprotein

Alpha-fetoprotein (AFP) is a glycoprotein produced by fetal tissue and tumors that differentiate from midline embryonic structures. During fetal development, AFP levels in serum and amniotic fluid rise. AFP crosses the placenta and appears in maternal serum.

Elevated serum AFP levels in patients who aren't pregnant may occur in cancers such as hepatocellular carcinoma or certain nonmalignant conditions such as ataxia-telangiectasia. In these conditions, AFP assays are more useful for monitoring response to therapy than for diagnosis. Serum AFP levels are best determined by enzyme immunoassay on amniotic fluid or serum.

Purpose

- To monitor the effectiveness of therapy in malignant conditions, such as hepatomas and germ cell tumors, and certain nonmalignant conditions such as ataxia-telangiectasia
- To screen for the need for amniocentesis or high-resolution ultrasonography in a pregnant woman

Cost

Inexpensive

Patient preparation

- As appropriate, explain to the patient that this test helps in monitoring fetal development, screens for a need for further testing, helps detect possible congenital defects in the fetus, and monitors her response to therapy by measuring a specific blood protein.
- Tell the patient that the test requires a blood sample. Explain who will perform the venipuncture and when.
- Explain to the patient that she may experience discomfort from the needle puncture and the tourniquet.

Normal findings

When testing by immunoassay, serum AFP values are less than 15 ng/ml (SI, < 15 mg/L) in men and nonpregnant women. Values in maternal serum are less than 2.5 multiples of the median for fetal gestational age.

Abnormal findings

Elevated maternal serum AFP levels may suggest neural tube defects or other tube anomalies. Maternal AFP levels rise sharply in the maternal blood of about 90% of women carrying a fetus with anencephaly and in 50% of those carrying a fetus with spina bifida. Definitive diagnosis requires ultrasonography and amniocentesis. High serum AFP levels may indicate intrauterine death. Sometimes, high levels indicate other anomalies, such as duodenal atresia, omphalocele, tetralogy of Fallot, and Turner's syndrome.

Elevated serum AFP levels occur in 70% of nonpregnant patients with hepatocellular carcinoma. Elevated levels are also related to germ cell tumor of gonadal, retroperitoneal, or mediastinal origin. Serum AFP levels rise in ataxia-telangiectasia and sometimes in cancer of the pancreas, stomach, or biliary system and in nonseminiferous testicular tumors. Transient modest elevations can occur in nonneoplastic hepatocellular disease, such as alcoholic cirrhosis and acute or chronic hepatitis. Elevation of serum AFP levels after remission suggests tumor recurrence.

Other congenital anomalies, such as Down syndrome and other chromosomal disorders, may be associated with low maternal serum AFP levels. In hepatocellular carcinoma, a gradual decrease in serum AFP levels indicates a favorable response to therapy. In germ cell tumors, serum AFP levels and serum human chorionic gonadotropin levels should be measured concurrently.

Interfering factors
■ Multiple pregnancies (possible false-positive)

Amebiasis, sputum

Parasitic infestation is rare in North America but may result from exposure to *Ascaris lumbricoides, Echinococcus granulosus, Entamoeba histolytica, Necator americanus, Paragonimus westermani,* or *Strongyloides stercoralis.* A sputum specimen is obtained by expectoration or tracheal suctioning to evaluate for parasites.

Purpose
■ To identify pulmonary parasites

Cost
Inexpensive

Patient preparation
■ Explain to the patient that this test helps identify parasitic pulmonary infection
■ Tell the patient that the test requires a sputum specimen (preferably in the morning) or, if necessary, tracheal suctioning.
■ Teach the patient how to expectorate by taking three deep breaths and forcing a deep cough.
■ Inform the patient that he'll experience discomfort from the catheter during tracheal suctioning as appropriate.
■ Restrict medications that may affect test results. If they must be continued, note this on the laboratory request.

Normal findings
Normally, no parasites or ova are present.

Abnormal findings
The parasite identified indicates the type of pulmonary infection and the presence and stage of intestinal infection.
■ *A. lumbricoides* larvae and adults: pneumonitis
■ *E. granulosus* cysts of larval stage: hydatid disease
■ *E. histolytica* trophozoites: pulmonary amebiasis
■ *N. americanus* larvae: hookworm disease
■ *P. westermani* ova: paragonimiasis
■ *S. stercoralis* larvae: strongyloidiasis

Interfering factors
■ Improper collection technique
■ Failure to send the specimen to the laboratory immediately after collection
■ Recent therapy with antihelmintics or amebicides

Amebiasis, stool

Examination of a stool specimen can detect several types of intestinal parasites. Some of these parasites live in nonpathogenic symbiosis; others cause intestinal disease. In North America, the most common parasites include the roundworms *Ascaris lumbricoides* and *Necator americanus* (also called *hookworms*); the tapeworms *Diphyllobothrium latum, Taenia saginata,* and *Taenia solium* (rare); the amoeba *Entamoeba histolytica;* and the flagellate *Giardia lamblia.* Cyclospora can also be detected in stool examination for ova and parasites.

Purpose
■ To confirm or rule out intestinal parasitic infection and disease

Cost
Inexpensive

Patient preparation
■ Explain to the patient that this test detects intestinal parasitic infection.
■ Instruct the patient to avoid treatments with castor or mineral oil, bismuth, magnesium or antidiarrheal compounds, barium enemas, and antibiotics for 7 to 10 days before the test.
■ Tell the patient that the test requires three stool specimens — one every other day or every third day. Up to six specimens may be required to confirm the presence of *E. histolytica.*
■ Check the patient's history for recent diet and travel information if he has diarrhea. Also check the patient's history for antiparasitic drugs, such as carbarsone, diiodohydroxyquin, metronidazole, paromomycin, and tetracycline, within 2 weeks of the test.

Normal findings
Normally, no parasites or ova appear in the stool.

Abnormal findings
The presence of *E. histolytica* confirms amebiasis; *G. lamblia,* giardiasis. However, the extent of infection depends on the degree of tissue invasion. If amebiasis is suspected but stool examinations are negative, specimen collection after a saline cathartic using buffered sodium biphosphate or during a sigmoidoscopy may be necessary. If giardiasis or the presence of *Strongyloides stercoralis* is suspected but stool examinations are negative, examination of duodenal contents may be necessary.

The number of worms is usually correlated with the patient's clinical symptoms to distinguish between helminth infestation and helminth diseases. Eosinophilia may also indicate parasitic infection.

Helminths may migrate from the intestinal tract, producing pathologic changes in other parts of the body, resulting in peritonitis or pneumonitis. Hookworms can cause hypochromic microcytic anemia secondary to bloodsucking and hemorrhage, especially in patients with iron-deficient diets. The tapeworm *D. latum* may cause megaloblastic anemia by removing vitamin B_{12}.

Interfering factors
■ Castor or mineral oil, bismuth, magnesium or antidiarrheal compounds, and barium enema
■ Improper collection technique, collection of too few specimens, or contamination of the specimen with urine (possible false-negative)
■ Radiographic contrast media given to the patient within 5 to 10 days prior to specimen collection

Ammonia, plasma

The plasma ammonia test measures plasma levels of ammonia, a nonprotein nitrogen compound that helps maintain acid-base balance. Most ammonia is absorbed from the intestinal tract, where it's produced by bacterial action on protein; a smaller amount of ammonia is produced in the kidneys from hydrolysis of glutamine. Normally, the body uses the nitrogen fraction of ammonia to rebuild amino acids and then converts the ammonia to urea in the liver for excretion by the kidneys. In diseases such as cirrhosis of the liver, ammonia can bypass the liver and accumulate in the blood. Therefore, measurement of plasma ammonia levels may help indicate the severity of hepatocellular damage.

Purpose

■ To help monitor the progression of severe hepatic disease and the effectiveness of therapy

■ To recognize impending or established hepatic coma (See *Recognizing hepatic coma.*)

Cost

Inexpensive

Patient preparation

■ Explain to the patient (or a responsible family member if the patient is comatose) that this test evaluates liver function and that he must fast overnight before the test.

■ Tell the patient that the test requires a blood sample. Explain who will perform the venipuncture and when.

- Explain to the patient that he may experience discomfort from the needle puncture and the tourniquet.
- Check the patient's medication history for drugs that may influence plasma ammonia levels.

Normal findings
Normally, plasma ammonia levels are less than 50 µg/dl (SI, < 36 µmol/L).

Abnormal findings
Elevated plasma ammonia levels are common in patients with severe hepatic disease, such as cirrhosis and acute hepatic necrosis, and may lead to hepatic coma. Elevated levels are also possible in patients with Reye's syndrome, severe congestive heart failure, GI hemorrhage, and erythroblastosis fetalis.

Interfering factors
- Acetazolamide, ammonium salts, furosemide, heparin, thiazides, and valproic acid (possible increase)
- Parenteral nutrition (possible increase)
- Portacaval shunt (possible increase)
- Kanamycin, lactulose, neomycin, and tetracycline (possible decrease)
- Smoking, poor venipuncture technique, and exposure to ammonia cleaners (possible increase)

Amniocentesis

Amniocentesis, or *amniotic fluid analysis*, is the transabdominal needle aspiration of 10 to 20 ml of amniotic fluid for laboratory analysis. This test can be performed only when the amniotic fluid level reaches 150 ml, usually after the 16th week of pregnancy. Amniocentesis is indicated if the mother is over age 35; has a family history of genetic, chromosomal, or neural tube defects; or has had a previous miscarriage. Potential complications include spontaneous abortion, trauma to the fetus or placenta, bleeding, premature labor, infection, and Rh sensitization from fetal bleeding into the maternal circulation. Abnormal test results or failure of the tissue cultures to grow may necessitate repetition of the test.

Another method of detecting fetal chromosomal and biochemical disorders in early pregnancy is chorionic villi sampling. (See *Chorionic villi sampling*, pages 42 and 43.)

Purpose
- To detect fetal abnormalities, particularly chromosomal and neural tube defects
- To detect hemolytic disease of the neonate
- To diagnose metabolic disorders, amino acid disorders, and mucopolysaccharidosis
- To determine fetal age and maturity, especially pulmonary maturity
- To assess fetal health by detecting the presence of meconium or blood or measuring amniotic levels of estriol and fetal thyroid hormone
- To identify fetal gender when one or both parents are carriers of a sex-linked disorder

Cost
Expensive

Patient preparation
- Explain to the patient that this test detects fetal abnormalities.
- Tell the patient that the test requires a specimen of amniotic fluid and who will perform the test.
- Explain to the patient that a stinging sensation may be felt as local anesthetic is injected.

Chorionic villi sampling

Chorionic villi sampling (CVS) is a prenatal test for quick detection of fetal chromosomal and biochemical disorders that's performed during the first trimester of pregnancy. Preliminary results may be available within hours, complete results within a few days. In contrast, amniocentesis can't be performed before the 16th week of pregnancy, and the results aren't available for at least 2 weeks. Thus, CVS can detect fetal abnormalities as much as 10 weeks sooner than amniocentesis.

The chorionic villi are fingerlike projections that surround the embryonic membrane and eventually give rise to the placenta. Cells obtained from an appropriate specimen are of fetal, rather than maternal, origin and thus can be analyzed for fetal abnormalities.

Collection time
Specimens are best obtained between the 8th and 10th weeks of pregnancy. Before 7 weeks, the villi cover the embryo and make selective sampling difficult. After 10 weeks, maternal cells begin to grow over the villi, and the amniotic sac begins to fill the uterine cavity, making the procedure difficult and potentially dangerous.

Collection method
To collect a chorionic villi specimen, place the patient in the lithotomy position. The physician checks the placement of the patient's uterus bimanually, and then inserts a Graves' speculum and swabs the cervix with an antiseptic solution. If necessary, he may use a tenaculum to straighten an acutely flexed uterus, permitting cannula insertion. Guided by ultrasound and possibly, endoscopy, he directs the catheter through the cannula to the villi. Suction is applied to the catheter to remove about 30 mg of tissue from the villi. The specimen is withdrawn, placed in a Petri dish, and examined with a dissecting microscope. Part of the specimen is then cultured for further testing.

Interpretation
CVS can be used to detect about 200 diseases prenatally. For example, direct analysis of rapidly dividing fetal cells can detect chromosome disorders, deoxyribonucleic acid analysis

■ Advise the patient that normal test results can't guarantee a normal fetus because some fetal disorders are undetectable.
■ Obtain informed consent if appropriate.
■ Inform the patient that she'll need to void just before the test to minimize the risk of puncturing the bladder and aspirating urine instead of amniotic fluid.

Normal findings
Normal amniotic fluid is clear but may contain white flecks of vernix caseosa when the fetus is near term. For a detailed analysis of the appearance and components of amniotic fluid. (See *Amniotic fluid analysis,* page 44.)

Abnormal findings
Blood, which is found in about 10% of amniocenteses, results from a faulty tap and doesn't indicate an abnormality. "Port wine" fluid, on the other hand, may be a sign of abruptio placentae, and blood of fetal origin may indicate damage to the fetal, placental, or umbilical cord vessels by the amniocentesis needle. (See *Apt test,* page 45.)

can detect hemoglobinopathies, and lysosomal enzyme assays can screen for lysosomal storage disorders such as Tay-Sachs disease.

The test appears to provide reliable results except when the specimen contains too few cells or the cells fail to grow in culture. Patient risks for this procedure appear to be similar to those for amniocentesis: a small chance of spontaneous abortion, cramps, infection, and bleeding. However, recent research reports an incidence of limb malformation in neonates when CVS has been performed.

Unlike amniocentesis, CVS can't detect complications in cases of Rh sensitization, uncover neural tube defects, or determine pulmonary maturity. However, it may prove to be the best way to detect other serious fetal abnormalities early in pregnancy.

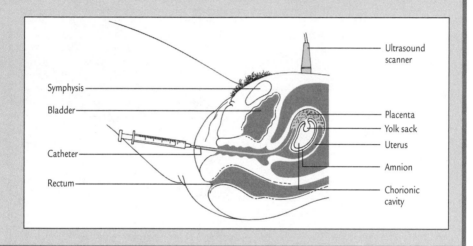

Large amounts of bilirubin, a breakdown product of red blood cells, may indicate hemolytic disease of the neonate. Normally, the bilirubin level increases from the 14th to the 24th week of pregnancy, then declines as the fetus matures, essentially reaching zero at term. Testing for bilirubin usually isn't performed until the 26th week because that's the earliest time successful therapy for Rh sensitization can begin.

Meconium, a semisolid viscous material found in the fetal GI tract, consists of mucopolysaccharides, desquamated cells, vernix, hair, and cholesterol. Meconium passes into the amniotic fluid when hypoxia causes fetal distress and relaxation of the anal sphincter. Meconium is a normal finding in breech presentation. Serial amniocentesis may show a clearing of meconium over a 2- to 3-week period. If meconium is present during labor, the neonate's nose and throat require thorough cleaning to prevent meconium aspiration.

Creatinine, a product of fetal urine, increases in the amniotic fluid as the fetal kidneys mature. Generally, the creatinine value exceeds 2 mg/dl in a mature fetus.

Amniotic fluid analysis

TEST	NORMAL FINDINGS	FETAL IMPLICATION OF ABNORMAL FINDINGS
Color	Clear, with white flecks of vernix caseosa in a mature fetus	Blood of maternal origin is usually harmless. "Port wine" fluid may indicate abruptio placentae. Fetal blood may indicate damage to the fetal, placental, or umbilical cord vessels.
Bilirubin	■ *Early:* < 0.075 mg/dl (SI, < 1.3 Umol/L) ■ *Term:* < 0.025 mg/dl (SI, < 0.41 Umol/L)	High levels indicate hemolytic disease of the neonate in isoimmunized pregnancy.
Meconium	Absent (except in breech presentation)	Presence indicates fetal hypotension or distress.
Creatinine	> 2mg/dl (SI, > 177 µmol/L)	Decreased levels may indicate immature fetus (less than 37 weeks).
Lecithin-sphingomyelin ratio	> 2:1	Less than 2:1 indicates pulmonary immaturity and subsequent increased risk of respiratory distress syndrome.
Phosphatidylglycerol	Present	Absence indicates pulmonary immaturity.
Glucose	< 45 mg/dl (SI, < 2.3 mmol/L)	Excessive increases at term or near term indicate hypertrophy of fetal pancreas and subsequent neonatal hypoglycemia.
Alpha-fetoprotein	Variable, depending on gestational age and laboratory technique	Inappropriate increases indicate neural tube defects, such as spina bifida or anencephaly, impending fetal death, congenital nephrosis, or contamination by fetal blood.
Chromosome	Normal karyotype	Abnormal karyotype may indicate fetal sex and chromosome disorders.
Acetylcholinesterase	Absent	Presence may indicate neural tube defects, exomphalos, or other serious malformations.

Alpha-fetoprotein (AFP) is a fetal alpha globulin produced first in the yolk sac and later in the parenchymal cells of the liver and GI tract. Fetal serum AFP levels are about 150 times higher than amniotic fluid levels; maternal serum AFP levels are far lower than amniotic fluid levels. High amniotic fluid levels indicate neural tube defects, but the fetal serum AFP level may remain normal if the defect is small and closed. Elevated fetal serum AFP levels may also occur in multiple pregnancy; in disorders, such as omphalocele, atresia, exomphalos, and Turner's syndrome; and in impending fetal death.

The amount of uric acid in the amniotic fluid increases as the fetus matures, but these levels fluctuate widely and can't accurately predict maturity. Laboratory studies indicate that severe erythroblastosis fetalis, familial hyperuricemia, and Lesch-Nyhan syndrome tend to increase the level of uric acid.

Estrone, estradiol, estriol, and estriol conjugates appear in amniotic fluid in varying amounts. Levels of estriol, the most prevalent estrogen, increase substantially at term. Severe erythroblastosis fetalis decreases the estriol level.

The type II cells lining the fetal lung alveoli produce lecithin slowly in early pregnancy and then markedly increase production around the 35th week.

The sphingomyelin level parallels that of lecithin until the 35th week, when it gradually decreases. Measuring the ratio of lecithin to sphingomyelin (L:S) confirms fetal pulmonary maturity (L:S ratio > 2) or suggests a risk of respiratory distress (L:S ratio < 2). However, fetal respiratory distress may develop in the fetus of a patient with diabetes, even though the L:S ratio is greater than 2, a level that usually indicates pulmonary maturity.

Fetal phosphatidylglycerol levels are present with pulmonary maturity; phosphatidylinositol levels decrease.

Measuring glucose levels in the fluid can aid in assessing glucose control in the patient with diabetes, but this isn't routinely performed. A level greater than 45 mg/dl (SI, > 2.6 mmol/L) indicates poor maternal and fetal control. Insulin levels normally increase slightly from the 27th to the 40th week but increase sharply (up to 27 times normal) in a poorly controlled patient with diabetes.

Apt test

Blood in the amniotic fluid can be of maternal or fetal origin. The Apt test, which is based on the premise that fetal hemoglobin is alkali-resistant and adult hemoglobin changes to alkaline hematin after the addition of alkali, can differentiate between the two. This test may be performed on all bloody amniotic fluid specimens.

The test's procedure consists of diluting 1 ml of amniotic fluid with water until it turns pink. The technician centrifuges for 10 minutes, and decants the supernatant. He then adds five parts supernatant to one part 0.25 N (1%) sodium hydroxide, and observes for 1 to 2 minutes. Fetal blood appears red; maternal blood, yellow-brown. A repeat of the test using known maternal blood confirms test results.

Laboratory analysis can identify at least 25 different enzymes (usually in low concentrations) in amniotic fluid. The enzymes have few known clinical implications, although elevated acetylcholinesterase levels may occur with neural tube defects, exomphalos, and other serious malformations.

When the mother carries an X-linked disorder, determination of fetal sex is important. If chromosome karyotyping identifies a male fetus, there's a 50% chance he'll be affected; a female fetus won't be affected but has a 50% chance of being a carrier.

Interfering factors
■ Failure to place the specimen in an appropriate amber or foil-covered tube (possible decrease in bilirubin).
■ Blood or meconium in the fluid (effect on L:S ratio)

■ Maternal blood in the fluid (possible decrease in creatinine)
■ Any amount of fetal blood in the fluid specimen (possible doubling of maternal AFP concentrations)
■ Several disorders that aren't associated with pregnancy, including infectious mononucleosis, cirrhosis, hepatic cancer, teratoma, endodermal sinus tumor, gastric carcinoma, pancreatic carcinoma, and subacute hereditary tyrosinemia (possible increase in maternal AFP levels)

Amylase, serum

An enzyme that's synthesized primarily in the pancreas and salivary glands, amylase (alpha-amylase) helps to digest starch and glycogen in the mouth, stomach, and intestine. In cases of suspected acute pancreatic disease, measurement of serum or urine amylase is the most important laboratory test.

Purpose
■ To diagnose acute pancreatitis
■ To distinguish between acute pancreatitis and other causes of abdominal pain that require immediate surgery
■ To evaluate possible pancreatic injury caused by abdominal trauma or surgery

Cost
Inexpensive

Patient preparation
■ Explain to the patient that this test is used to assess pancreatic function.
■ Inform the patient that he needn't fast before the test but must abstain from alcohol.
■ Tell the patient that the test requires a blood sample. Explain who will perform the venipuncture and when.

■ Explain to the patient that he may experience discomfort from the needle puncture and the tourniquet.
■ Restrict medications that may affect test results. If they must be continued, note this on the laboratory request.

Normal findings
Normal serum amylase levels range from 25 to 85 U/L (SI, 0.39 to 1.45 µkat/L) for adults age 18 and older.

Abnormal findings
After the onset of acute pancreatitis, amylase levels begin to rise within 2 hours, peak within 12 to 48 hours, and return to normal within 3 to 4 days. Determination of urine amylase levels should follow normal serum amylase results to rule out pancreatitis. Moderate serum amylase elevations may accompany obstruction of the common bile duct, pancreatic duct, or ampulla of Vater; pancreatic injury from a perforated peptic ulcer; pancreatic cancer; and acute salivary gland disease. Impaired kidney function may increase serum amylase levels.

Amylase levels may be slightly elevated in a patient who is asymptomatic or responding unusually to therapy.

Decreased amylase levels can occur in patients with chronic pancreatitis, pancreatic cancer, cirrhosis, hepatitis, and toxemia of pregnancy.

Interfering factors
■ Ingestion of ethyl alcohol (possible false-high)
■ Aminosalicylic acid, asparaginase, azathioprine, corticosteroids, cyproheptadine, narcotic analgesics, hormonal contraceptives, rifampin, sulfasalazine, and thiazide or loop diuretics (possible false-high)
■ Recent peripancreatic surgery, perforated ulcer or intestine, abscess, spasm of the

sphincter of Oddi or, rarely, macroamylasemia (possible false-high)

Anaerobic culture

Some anaerobes die when exposed to oxygen. To facilitate anaerobic collection and culturing, tubes filled with carbon dioxide (CO_2) or nitrogen are used for oxygen-free transport. After specimen collection, the swab is quickly replaced in the inner tube and the plunger is depressed. This separates the inner tube from the stopper, forcing it into the larger tube and exposing the specimen to the CO_2-rich environment.

Purpose
■ To obtain specimen collection to test for anaerobes

Cost
Inexpensive

Patient preparation
■ Explain to the patient that the purpose of the test is to determine if he has an infection.

Normal findings
Normal flora may be present in the specimen from the site obtained or has no evidence of growth.

Abnormal findings
Presence of anaerobes in the specimen (such as gas gangrene) indicates an abnormal finding.

Interfering factors
■ Contamination of the specimen with organisms due to inadequate collection.

Androstenedione

The androstenedione test helps identify disorders related to altered hormone levels, such as female virilization syndromes and polycystic ovary (Stein-Leventhal) syndrome. Androstenedione is a precursor of aldosterone, cortisol, estrogen, and testosterone. Tumors of the ovaries or adrenal glands can secrete excessive amounts of androstenedione, which then converts to testosterone, resulting in virilizing symptoms, such as hirsutism and sterility.

Increased androstenedione production may induce premature sexual development in children. It may produce renewed ovarian stimulation, endometriosis, bleeding, and polycystic ovaries in postmenopausal women. In obese women, increased levels of estrogen can lead to menstrual irregularities. In men, overproduction of androstenedione may cause feminizing signs such as gynecomastia.

Purpose
■ To help determine the cause of gonadal dysfunction, menstrual or menopausal irregularities, virilizing symptoms, and premature sexual development

Cost
Moderately expensive

Patient preparation
■ Explain to the patient that this test determines the cause of her symptoms.
■ Tell the patient that the test requires a blood sample. Explain who will perform the venipuncture and when.
■ Explain to the patient that she may experience discomfort from the needle puncture and the tourniquet.
■ If appropriate, explain to the patient that the test should be done 1 week before

or after her menstrual period and that it may be repeated.

■ Restrict steroid and pituitary-based hormones. If they must be continued, note this on the laboratory request.

Normal findings

Normal androstenedione values by radioimmunoassay are:

■ *females:* 85 to 275 ng/dl (SI, 3.0 to 9.6 nmol/L)

■ *males:* 75 to 205 ng/dl (SI, 2.6 to 7.2 nmol/L).

Abnormal findings

Elevated androstenedione levels are associated with polycystic ovary syndrome; Cushing's syndrome; ovarian, testicular, and adrenocortical tumors; ectopic corticotropin–producing tumors; late-onset congenital adrenal hyperplasia; and ovarian stromal hyperplasia. Elevated androstenedione levels result in increased estrone levels, causing premature sexual development in children; menstrual irregularities in premenopausal women; bleeding, endometriosis, and polycystic ovaries in postmenopausal women; and feminizing signs, such as gynecomastia, in men. Decreased androstenedione levels occur in hypogonadism.

Interfering factors

■ Steroids and pituitary hormones (possible increase)

Angiotensin-converting enzyme

The angiotensin-converting enzyme (ACE) test is used to measure serum levels of angiotensin-converting enzyme, which is found in lung capillaries and, in lesser con- centrations, blood vessels and kidney tissue. Its primary function is to help regulate arterial pressure by converting angiotensin I to angiotensin II. Measurement of ACE is of little use in diagnosing hypertension.

Purpose

■ To aid diagnosis of sarcoidosis, especially pulmonary sarcoidosis

■ To monitor response to therapy in sarcoidosis

■ To help confirm Gaucher's disease or Hansen's disease

Cost

Inexpensive

Patient preparation

■ Explain to the patient that this test is used to diagnose sarcoidosis, Gaucher's disease, or Hansen's disease or, if appropriate, to check response to treatment for sarcoidosis.

■ Tell the patient that the test requires a blood sample. Explain who will perform the venipuncture and when.

■ Explain to the patient that he may experience discomfort from the needle puncture and the tourniquet.

■ Inform the patient that he must fast for 12 hours before the test.

■ Note the patient's age on the laboratory request. If the patient is under age 20, the test may have to be postponed because patients under age 20 have variable ACE levels.

Normal findings

In the colorimetric assay, normal values for serum ACE in patients age 20 and older range from 8 to 52 U/L (SI, 0.14 to 0.88 µkat/L).

Abnormal findings

Elevated serum ACE levels may indicate sarcoidosis, Gaucher's disease, or Hansen's disease, but results must be correlated with the patient's clinical condition. In some patients, elevated serum ACE levels may result from hyperthyroidism, diabetic retinopathy, or hepatic disease.

Serum ACE levels decline as the patient responds to steroid or prednisone therapy for sarcoidosis.

Interfering factors

■ Failure to fast before the test (may cause significant lipemia of the sample)
■ Use of a collection tube with ethylenediaminetetraacetic acid (possible decrease)
■ Failure to freeze the specimen and place it on dry ice (possible false-low due to ACE degradation)

Anion gap

Total concentrations of cations and anions are usually equal, making serum electrically neutral. Measuring the gap between measured cation and anion levels provides information about the level of anions (including sulfate, phosphate, organic acids such as ketone bodies and lactic acid, and proteins) that aren't routinely measured in laboratory tests. In metabolic acidosis, measuring the anion gap helps to identify the type of acidosis and possible causes. Further tests are usually needed to determine the specific cause of metabolic acidosis. (See *Anion gap and metabolic acidosis*.)

Purpose

■ To distinguish types of metabolic acidosis
■ To monitor renal function and total parenteral nutrition

Anion gap and metabolic acidosis

Metabolic acidosis with a normal anion gap (8 to 14 mEq/L [SI, 8 to 14 mmol/L]) occurs in conditions characterized by loss of bicarbonate, such as:
■ hypokalemic acidosis associated with renal tubular acidosis, diarrhea, or ureteral diversions
■ hyperkalemic acidosis caused by acidifying agents (for example, ammonium chloride or hydrochloric acid), hydronephrosis, or sickle cell nephropathy.

Metabolic acidosis with an increased anion gap (greater than 14 mEq/L) occurs in conditions characterized by accumulation of organic acids, sulfates, or phosphates, such as:
■ renal failure
■ ketoacidosis associated with starvation, diabetes mellitus, or alcohol abuse
■ lactic acidosis
■ ingestion of toxins, such as salicylates, methanol, ethylene glycol (antifreeze), and paraldehyde.

Cost

Inexpensive

Patient preparation

■ Explain to the patient that this test is used to determine the cause of acidosis.
■ Tell the patient that the test requires a blood sample. Explain who will perform the venipuncture and when.
■ Explain to the patient that he may experience discomfort from the needle puncture and the tourniquet.
■ Restrict medications that may affect test results. If they must be continued, note this on the laboratory request.

Normal findings

Normally, the anion gap ranges from 8 to 14 mEq/L (SI, 8 to 14 mmol/L).

Abnormal findings

A normal anion gap doesn't rule out metabolic acidosis. It may occur in hyperchloremic acidoses, renal tubular acidosis, and severe bicarbonate-wasting conditions, such as biliary or pancreatic fistulas and poorly functioning ileal loops.

When acidosis results from loss of bicarbonate in the urine or other body fluids — the anion gap remains unchanged — it's called *normal anion gap acidosis.*

An increased anion gap indicates an increase in one or more of the unmeasured anions (sulfate, phosphates, organic acids such as ketone bodies and lactic acid, and proteins). This may occur with acidoses that are characterized by excessive organic or inorganic acids, such as lactic acidosis or ketoacidosis.

When acidosis results from an accumulation of metabolic acids — as occurs in lactic acidosis, for example — the anion gap increases (> 14 mEq/L) with the increase in unmeasured anions. Metabolic acidosis caused by such an accumulation is known as *high anion gap acidosis.*

A decreased anion gap is rare but may occur with hypermagnesemia and paraprotein enemia states, such as multiple myeloma and Waldenström's macroglobulinemia.

Interfering factors

■ Chlorpropamide, diuretics, lithium, and vasopressin (possible decrease due to decreased serum sodium levels)
■ Antihypertensives and corticosteroids (possible increase due to increased serum sodium levels)
■ Acetazolamide, ammonium chloride, dimercaprol, ethylene glycol, methicillin, methyl alcohol, paraldehyde, and salicylates (possible increase due to decreased serum bicarbonate levels)
■ Corticotropin, cortisone, mercurial or chlorthiazide diuretics, and excessive ingestion of alkalis or licorice (possible decrease due to increased serum bicarbonate levels)
■ Ammonium chloride, boric acid, cholestyramine, oxyphenbutazone, phenylbutazone, and excessive I.V. infusion of sodium chloride (possible decrease due to increased serum chloride levels)
■ Bicarbonates, ethacrynic acid, furosemide, thiazide diuretics, and prolonged I.V. infusion of dextrose 5% in water (possible increase due to decreased serum chloride levels)
■ Iodine absorption from wounds packed with povidone-iodine or excessive use of magnesium-containing antacids, especially by patients with renal failure (possible false-low)

Antibody screening

Also called the *indirect Coombs' test,* the antibody screening test detects unexpected circulating antibodies in the patient's serum. After incubating the serum with group O red blood cells (RBCs), which are unaffected by anti-A or anti-B antibodies, an antiglobulin (Coombs') serum is added. Agglutination occurs if the patient's serum contains an antibody to one or more antigens on the red cells.

The antibody screening test detects 95% to 99% of the circulating antibodies. After this screening procedure detects them, the antibody identification test can determine the specific identity of the antibodies present.

Purpose

■ To detect unexpected circulating anti-bodies to RBC antigens in the recipient's or donor's serum before transfusion
■ To determine the presence of anti-D antibody in maternal blood
■ To evaluate the need for $Rh_o(D)$ immune globulin
■ To aid diagnosis of acquired hemolytic anemia

Cost

Inexpensive

Patient preparation

■ As appropriate, explain to the prospective blood recipient that the antibody screening test helps evaluate the possibility of a transfusion reaction or to determine if fetal antibodies are in her blood and if treatment is needed.
■ If the test is being performed because the patient is anemic, explain to him that it helps identify the specific type of anemia.
■ Tell the patient that the test requires a blood sample. Explain who will perform the venipuncture and when.
■ Explain to the patient that he may experience discomfort from the needle puncture and the tourniquet.
■ Check the patient's history for recent administration of blood, dextran, or I.V. contrast media, which can produce a false positive.

Normal findings

Normally, agglutination doesn't occur, indicating that the patient's serum contains no circulating antibodies other than anti-A or anti-B.

Abnormal findings

A positive result indicates the presence of unexpected circulating antibodies to RBC antigens. Such a reaction demonstrates donor and recipient incompatibility.

A positive result in a pregnant patient with Rh-negative blood may indicate the presence of antibodies to the Rh factor from an earlier transfusion with incompatible blood or from a previous pregnancy with an Rh-positive fetus.

A positive result indicates that the fetus may develop hemolytic disease of the neonate. As a result, repeated testing throughout the pregnancy is necessary to evaluate progressive development of circulating antibody levels.

Interfering factors

■ Previous administration of dextran or I.V. contrast media (causing aggregation resembling agglutination)
■ Blood transfusion or pregnancy within the past 3 months (possible presence of antibodies)

Antidiuretic hormone

Antidiuretic hormone (ADH), also called *vasopressin*, promotes water reabsorption in response to increased osmolality (water deficiency with high concentration of sodium and other solutes). In response to decreased osmolality (water excess), reduced secretion of ADH allows increased excretion of water to maintain fluid balance. Along with aldosterone, ADH helps regulate sodium, potassium, and fluid balance. It also stimulates vascular smooth-muscle contraction, causing an increase in arterial blood pressure.

This relatively rare test is a quantitative analysis of serum ADH levels. It may be ordered as part of dehydration or hypertonic saline infusion testing, which determines the body's response to states of hyperosmolality.

Purpose

■ To aid in the differential diagnosis of pituitary diabetes insipidus, nephrogenic diabetes insipidus (congenital or familial), and syndrome of inappropriate antidiuretic hormone (SIADH)

Cost

Inexpensive

Patient preparation

■ Explain to the patient that this test, used to measure hormonal secretion levels, may aid in identifying the cause of his symptoms.

■ Instruct the patient to fast and limit physical activity for 10 to 12 hours before the test.

■ Tell the patient that the test requires a blood sample. Explain who will perform the venipuncture and when.

■ Explain to the patient that he may experience discomfort from the needle puncture and the tourniquet.

■ Restrict medications that may cause SIADH before the test. If they must be continued, note this on the laboratory request.

■ Instruct the patient to lie down and relax for 30 minutes before the test.

Reference values

ADH values range from 1 to 5 pg/ml (SI, 1 to 5 mg/L). It may also be evaluated in light of serum osmolality; if serum osmolality is < 285 mOsm/kg, ADH is normally < 2 pg/ml (SI, 2 mg/L); if > 290 mOsm/kg, ADH may range from 2 to 12 pg/ml (SI, 2 to 12 mg/L).

Abnormal findings

Absent or below-normal ADH levels indicate Hand-Schüller-Christian disease, head trauma, metastatic disease, neurosurgical procedures, pituitary diabetes insipidus, resulting from a neurohypophyseal or hypo-thalamic tumor, sarcoidosis, syphilis, tuberculosis, or viral infection.

Normal serum ADH levels in the presence of signs of diabetes insipidus (such as polydipsia, polyuria, and hypotonic urine) may indicate the nephrogenic form of the disease, marked by renal tubular resistance to ADH; however, levels may rise if the pituitary gland tries to compensate.

Elevated serum ADH levels may also indicate SIADH, possibly as a result of acute porphyria, Addison's disease, bronchogenic carcinoma, circulatory shock, cirrhosis of the liver, hypothyroidism, infectious hepatitis, or severe hemorrhage.

Interfering factors

■ Failure to observe pretest restrictions of diet, medications, or physical activity

■ Anesthetics, carbamazepine, chlorothiazide, chlorpropamide, cyclophosphamide, estrogen, hypnotics, lithium, morphine, oxytocin, tranquilizers, and vincristine (increase)

■ Stress, pain, and positive-pressure ventilation (increase)

■ Alcohol and negative-pressure ventilation (decrease)

■ Radioactive scan performed within 1 week before the test

Anti-insulin antibodies

Some patients with diabetes form antibodies to the insulin they take. These antibodies bind with some of the insulin, making less insulin available for glucose metabolism and necessitating increased insulin dosages. This is known as insulin resistance.

Performed on the blood of a patient with diabetes who's receiving insulin, the anti-insulin antibody test detects insulin antibodies. Insulin antibodies are immunoglobulins, called anti-insulin Ab. The most common type of anti-insulin Ab is immunoglobulin (Ig) G, but anti-insulin Ab is also found in the other four classes of immunoglobulins — IgA, IgD, IgE, and IgM. IgM may cause insulin resistance, and IgE has been associated with allergic reactions.

Purpose
- To determine insulin allergy
- To confirm insulin resistance
- To determine if hypoglycemia is caused by insulin overuse

Cost
Inexpensive

Patient preparation
- Inform the patient that this test is used to determine the most appropriate treatment for his diabetes and to determine if he has insulin resistance or an allergy to insulin.
- Tell the patient that the test requires a blood sample. Explain to the patient who will perform the venipuncture and when.
- Explain to the patient that he may feel some discomfort from the needle puncture and the tourniquet.
- Inform the patient that he doesn't have to fast before the test.
- Ask the patient if he has had a radioactive test recently, and if so note this on the laboratory request.

Normal findings
There should be less than 3% binding of the patient's serum with labeled beef, human, and pork insulin.

Abnormal findings
Elevated levels may occur in insulin antibody or resistance and in factitious hyperglycemia.

Interfering factors
- Radioactive test performed within 1 week before the test

Antinuclear antibodies

In such conditions as systemic lupus erythematosus (SLE), scleroderma, and certain infections, the body's immune system may perceive portions of its own cell nuclei as foreign and may produce antinuclear antibodies (ANAs). Specific ANAs include antibodies to deoxyribonucleic acid (DNA), nucleoprotein, histones, nuclear ribonucleoprotein, and other nuclear constituents.

Because they don't penetrate living cells, ANAs are harmless but sometimes form antigen-antibody complexes that cause tissue damage (as in SLE). Because of multiorgan involvement, test results aren't diagnostic and can only partially confirm clinical evidence. (See *Incidence of antinuclear antibodies in various disorders*, page 54.)

Purpose
- To screen for SLE (failure to detect ANAs essentially rules out active SLE)
- To monitor the effectiveness of immunosuppressive therapy for SLE

Cost
Inexpensive

Patient preparation
- Explain to the patient that this test evaluates the immune system and that further testing is usually required for diagnosis.
- If appropriate, inform the patient that the test will be repeated to monitor his response to therapy.
- Tell the patient that the test requires a blood sample. Explain who will perform the venipuncture and when.

Incidence of antinuclear antibodies in various disorders

The chart below indicates the percentage of patients with certain disorders whose serum contains antinuclear antibodies (ANAs). About 40% of elderly people and 5% of the general population also have positive ANA findings.

DISORDER	POSITIVE ANA
Systemic lupus erythematosus (SLE)	95% to 100%
Lupoid hepatitis	95% to 100%
Felty's syndrome	95% to 100%
Progressive systemic sclerosis (scleroderma)	75% to 80%
Drug-associated SLE-like syndrome (hydralazine, procainamide, isoniazid)	Approximately 50%
Sjögren's syndrome	40% to 75%
Rheumatoid arthritis	25% to 60%
Healthy family member of SLE patient	Approximately 25%
Chronic discoid lupus erythematosus	15% to 50%
Juvenile arthritis	15% to 30%
Polyarteritis nodosa	15% to 25%
Miscellaneous diseases	10% to 50%
Dermatomyositis, polymyositis	10% to 30%
Rheumatic fever	Approximately 5%

■ Explain to the patient that he may experience discomfort from the needle puncture and the tourniquet.

■ Check the patient's history for drugs that may affect test results, such as hydralazine, isoniazid, and procainamide and notify the laboratory.

Normal findings

Test results are reported as positive (with pattern and serum titer noted) or negative.

Abnormal findings

Although this test is a sensitive indicator of ANAs, it isn't specific for SLE. Low titers may occur in patients with viral diseases, chronic hepatic disease, collagen vascular disease, and autoimmune diseases and in some healthy adults; the incidence increases with age. The higher the titer, the more specific the test is for SLE (titer often exceeds 1:256).

The pattern of nuclear fluorescence helps identify the type of immune disease present. A peripheral pattern is almost exclusively associated with SLE because it indicates the presence of anti-DNA antibodies; sometimes anti-DNA antibodies are measured by radioimmunoassay if ANA titers are high or a peripheral pattern is observed. A homogeneous, or diffuse, pattern is also associated with SLE as well as with related connective tissue disorders; a nucleolar pattern, with scleroderma; and a speckled, irregular pattern, with infectious mononucleosis and mixed connective tissue disorders (for example, SLE and scleroderma).

A single serum sample, especially one collected from a patient with collagen vascular disease, may contain antibodies to several parts of the cell's nucleus. In addition, as serum dilution increases, the fluorescent pattern may change because different antibodies are reactive at different titers.

Interfering factors

■ Most commonly hydralazine, isoniazid, and procainamide, but also chlorpromazine, clofibrate, ethosuximide, gold salts, griseofulvin, hormonal contraceptives, mephenytoin, methyldopa, methysergide, para-aminosalicylic acid, penicillin, phenylbutazone, phenytoin, primidone, propylthiouracil, quinidine, reserpine, streptomycin, sulfonamides, tetracyclines, and trimethadione (possible production of a syndrome resembling SLE)

Antistreptolysin-O

The antistreptolysin-O test measures the relative serum concentrations of the antibody to streptolysin O (known as *ASO*). A serum sample is diluted with a commercial preparation of streptolysin O and incubated. After the addition of human red blood cells, the tube is reincubated and examined visually. Failure of hemolysis to develop indicates recent streptococcal infection.

Purpose

■ To confirm recent or ongoing streptococcal infection
■ To help diagnose rheumatic fever and poststreptococcal glomerulonephritis in the presence of clinical symptoms
■ To distinguish between rheumatic fever and rheumatoid arthritis when joint pains are present

Cost
Inexpensive

Patient preparation
■ Explain to the patient that this test detects an immunologic response to certain bacteria (streptococci). If the test is to be repeated at regular intervals to identify active and inactive states of rheumatic fever or to confirm acute glomerulonephritis, tell the patient that measuring changes in antibody levels helps determine the effectiveness of therapy.
■ Tell the patient that the test requires a blood sample. Explain who will perform the venipuncture and when.
■ Explain to the patient that he may experience discomfort from the needle puncture and the tourniquet.
■ Check the patient's history for drugs that may suppress the streptococcal antibody responses. If such drugs must be continued, note this on the laboratory request.

Normal findings
Even healthy people have some detectable ASO titers from previous minor streptococcal infections. Normal ASO titers are as follows:
■ *School-age children:* 170 Todd units/ml
■ *Preschoolers and adults:* 85 Todd units/ml

Abnormal findings
High ASO titers usually occur only after prolonged or recurrent infections. Generally, a titer higher than 166 Todd units is considered a definite elevation. A low ASO titer is good evidence for the absence of active rheumatic fever. A higher ASO titer indicates the presence of a streptococcal infection. Serial titers, determined at 10- to 14-day intervals, provide more reliable information than a single titer. An increase in titer 2 to 5 weeks after the acute infection,

which peaks 4 to 6 weeks after the initial increase, confirms poststreptococcal disease.

Interfering factors
■ Streptococcal skin infections, seldom producing abnormal ASO titers even with poststreptococcal disease (probable false-negative)
■ Antibiotic or corticosteroid therapy (possible suppression of the streptococcal antibody response)

Antithrombin III

The antithrombin III test measures levels of antithrombin III (AT III). This protein inhibits the activity of factors II, IX, X, XI, and XII by inactivating thrombin and inhibiting coagulation. Normally, a balance exists between AT III and thrombin; an AT III deficiency increases coagulation.

AT III may be evaluated by a functional clotting assay or by synthetic substrates. Exogenous heparin is added to a fresh, citrated blood sample to accelerate AT III activity. Then excess thrombin (factor X) is added to the plasma. The amount of factor X not activated by AT III is quantitated by clotting time or spectrophotometrically and is compared with a normal control.

Purpose
■ To detect the cause of impaired coagulation, especially hypercoagulation

Cost
Moderately expensive

Patient preparation
■ Tell the patient that this test will help determine the cause of blood coagulation problems.

■ Tell the patient that the test requires a blood sample. Explain who will perform the venipuncture and when.
■ Explain to the patient that he may experience discomfort from the venipuncture and the tourniquet.

Normal findings
Reference values may vary for each laboratory but should lie between 80% and 120% of normal activity.

Abnormal findings
Decreased AT III levels can indicate disseminated intravascular coagulation or thromboembolic, hypercoagulation, or hepatic disorders. Slightly decreased levels can result from use of hormonal contraceptives. Elevated levels can result from kidney transplantation and use of oral anticoagulants or anabolic steroids.

Interfering factors
■ Surgery (decrease)
■ Heparin therapy for 3 days or longer (decrease)
■ Hormonal contraceptives
■ Performed during last trimester of pregnancy or early postpartum period

Arterial blood gas analysis

Arterial blood gas (ABG) analysis is used to measure the partial pressure of arterial oxygen (Pao_2) and partial pressure of arterial carbon dioxide ($Paco_2$) and the pH of an arterial sample. Oxygen content (O_2CT), arterial oxygen saturation (Sao_2), and bicarbonate (HCO_3^-) values are also measured. A blood sample for ABG analysis may be drawn by percutaneous arterial puncture or from an arterial line.

Purpose
- To evaluate efficiency of pulmonary gas exchange
- To assess integrity of the ventilatory control system
- To determine the acid-base level of the blood
- To monitor respiratory therapy

Cost
Moderately expensive

Patient preparation
- Explain to the patient that this test is used to evaluate how well the lungs are delivering oxygen to blood and eliminating carbon dioxide.
- Tell the patient that the test requires a blood sample. Explain who will perform the arterial puncture and when.
- Tell the patient that he must breathe normally during the test. Explain that he may experience a brief cramping or throbbing pain at the puncture site.
- Inform the patient that the laboratory technician has to wait at least 20 minutes before he can draw arterial blood when starting, changing, or discontinuing oxygen therapy; after initiating or changing settings of mechanical ventilation; or after extubation.

Normal findings
Normal ABG values fall within the following ranges:
- Pao_2: 80 to 100 mm Hg (SI, 10.6 to 13.3 kPa)
- $Paco_2$: 35 to 45 mm Hg (SI, 4.7 to 5.3 kPa)
- pH: 7.35 to 7.45 (SI, 7.35 to 7.45)
- O_2CT: 15% to 23% (SI, 0.15 to 0.23)
- Sao_2: 94% to 100% (SI, 0.94 to 1.00)
- HCO_3^-: 22 to 25 mEq/L (SI, 22 to 25 mmol/L)

Abnormal findings
Low Pao_2, O_2CT, and Sao_2 levels and a high $Paco_2$ level may result from conditions that impair respiratory function, such as respiratory muscle weakness or paralysis, respiratory center inhibition (from head injury, brain tumor, or drug abuse), and airway obstruction (possibly from mucus plugs or a tumor). Similarly low readings may result from bronchiole obstruction caused by asthma or emphysema, from an abnormal ventilation-perfusion ratio due to partially blocked alveoli or pulmonary capillaries, or from alveoli that are damaged or filled with fluid because of disease, hemorrhage, or near drowning.

When inspired air contains insufficient oxygen, Pao_2, O_2CT, and Sao_2 decrease, but $Paco_2$ may be normal. Such findings are common in pneumothorax, impaired diffusion between alveoli and blood (due to interstitial fibrosis, for example), or an arteriovenous shunt that permits blood to bypass the lungs.

Low O_2CT level — with normal Pao_2, Sao_2 and, possibly, $Paco_2$ values — may result from severe anemia, decreased blood volume, and reduced hemoglobin oxygen-carrying capacity.

In addition to clarifying blood oxygen disorders, ABG values can give considerable information about acid-base disorders. (See *Acid-base disorders*, page 58.)

Interfering factors
- Venous blood in the sample (possible decrease in Pao_2 and increase in $Paco_2$)
- Bicarbonate, ethacrynic acid, hydrocortisone, metolazone, prednisone, and thiazides (possible increase in $Paco_2$)
- Acetazolamide, methicillin, nitrofurantoin, and tetracycline (possible decrease in $Paco_2$)
- Fever (possible false-high Pao_2 and $Paco_2$)

Acid-base disorders

DISORDERS AND ABG FINDINGS	POSSIBLE CAUSES	SIGNS AND SYMPTOMS
Respiratory acidosis (excess CO_2 retention) pH < 7.35 (SI, < 7.35) HCO_3^- > 26 mEq/L (SI, > 25 mmol/L) (if compensating) $Paco_2$ > 45 mm Hg (SI, > 5.3 kPa)	■ Central nervous system depression from drugs, injury, or disease ■ Asphyxia ■ Hypoventilation due to pulmonary, cardiac, musculoskeletal, or neuromuscular disease	■ Diaphoresis, headache, tachycardia, confusion, restlessness, apprehension
Respiratory alkalosis (excess CO_2 excretion) pH > 7.45 (SI, > 7.45) HCO_3^- < 22 mEq/L (SI, < 22 mmol/L) (if compensating) $Paco_2$ < 35 mm Hg (SI, < 4.7 kPa)	■ Hyperventilation due to anxiety, pain, or improper ventilator settings ■ Respiratory stimulation caused by drugs, disease, hypoxia, fever, or high room temperature ■ Gram-negative bacteria	■ Rapid, deep breathing; paresthesia; light-headedness; twitching; anxiety; fear
Metabolic acidosis (HCO_3^- loss, acid retention) pH < 7.35 (SI, < 7.35) HCO_3^- < 22 mEq/L (SI, < 22 mmol/L) $Paco_2$ > 35 mm Hg (SI, > 4.7 kPa) (if compensating)	■ HCO_3^- depletion due to renal disease, diarrhea, or small bowel fistulas ■ Excessive production of organic acids due to hepatic disease, endocrine disorders, hypoxia, shock, and drug intoxication	■ Rapid, deep breathing; fruity breath; fatigue; headache; lethargy; drowsiness; nausea; vomiting; coma (severe)
Metabolic alkalosis (HCO_3^- retention, acid loss) pH > 7.45 (SI, > 7.45) HCO_3^- > 26 mEq/L (SI, > 26 mmol/L) $Paco_2$ > 45 mmHg (SI, > 5.3 kPa)	■ Inadequate excretion of acids due to renal disease ■ Loss of hydrochloric acid from prolonged vomiting or gastric suctioning ■ Loss of potassium due to increased renal excretion or steroid overdose ■ Excessive alkali ingestion	■ Slow, shallow breathing; hypertonic muscles; restlessness; twitching; confusion; irritability; apathy; tetany; seizures; coma (if severe)

Aspartate aminotransferase

Aspartate aminotransferase (AST) is one of two enzymes that catalyze the conversion of the nitrogenous portion of an amino acid to an amino acid residue. It's essential to energy production in the Krebs cycle. AST is found in the cytoplasm and mitochondria of many cells, primarily in the liver, heart, skeletal muscles, kidneys, pancreas, and red blood cells. It's released into serum in proportion to cellular damage.

Purpose
■ To aid detection and differential diagnosis of acute hepatic disease
■ To monitor patient progress and prognosis in cardiac and hepatic diseases
■ To aid diagnosis of myocardial infarction in correlation with creatine kinase and lactate dehydrogenase levels

Cost
Moderately expensive

Patient preparation
■ Explain to the patient that this test is used to assess heart and liver function.
■ Inform the patient that the test usually requires a venipuncture for 3 successive days.
■ Inform the patient that he may experience pain from the needle punctures and the tourniquet.
■ Restrict medications that may affect test results. If they must be continued, note this on the laboratory request.

Normal findings
AST levels range from 8 to 46 U/L (SI, 0.14 to 0.78 µkat/L) in males and from 7 to 34 U/L (SI, 0.12 to 0.58 µkat/L) in females. Normal values for infants are typically higher.

Abnormal findings
AST levels fluctuate in response to the extent of cellular necrosis, being transiently and minimally increased early in the disease process and extremely increased during the most acute phase. Depending on when the initial specimen is drawn, AST levels may increase, indicating increasing disease severity and tissue damage, or decrease, indicating disease resolution and tissue repair.

Maximum AST elevations (> 20 times normal) may indicate acute viral hepatitis, severe skeletal muscle trauma, extensive surgery, drug-induced hepatic injury, or severe passive liver congestion.

High AST levels (10 to 20 times normal) may indicate severe myocardial infarction, severe infectious mononucleosis, or alcoholic cirrhosis. High AST levels also occur during the prodromal or resolving stages of conditions that cause maximum AST elevations.

Moderate to high AST levels (5 to 10 times normal) may indicate dermatomyositis, Duchenne's muscular dystrophy, or chronic hepatitis. Moderate to high AST levels also occur during prodromal and resolving stages of diseases that cause high AST elevations.

Low to moderate AST levels (2 to 5 times normal) occur at some time during the preceding conditions or diseases or may indicate hemolytic anemia, metastatic hepatic tumors, acute pancreatitis, pulmonary emboli, delirium tremens, or fatty liver. AST levels rise slightly after the first few days of biliary duct obstruction.

Interfering factors
■ Failure to draw the specimen as scheduled (may miss peak)
■ Antitubercular agents, chlorpropamide, dicumarol, erythromycin, methyldopa, opioids, pyridoxine, and sulfonamides; large doses of acetaminophen, salicylates, or vitamin A; and many other drugs known to affect the liver (increase)
■ Strenuous exercise and muscle trauma due to I.M. injections (increase)

Atrial natriuretic factor, plasma

The plasma atrial natriuretic factor (ANF) test, a radioimmunoassay measures the plasma level of ANF, a vasoactive and natriuretic hormone that's secreted from the heart when expansion of blood volume stretches atrial tissue. An extremely potent natriuretic agent and vasodilator, ANF (also known as *atrial natriuretic hormone, atrionatriuretic peptide,* and *atriopeptin*) rapidly produces diuresis and increases the glomerular filtration rate.

The role of ANF in regulating extracellular fluid volume, blood pressure, and sodium metabolism appears critical. It promotes sodium excretion, inhibits the renin-angiotensin system's effect on aldosterone secretion, and decreases atrial pressure by decreasing venous return, thereby reducing blood pressure and volume.

Purpose
■ To confirm heart failure
■ To identify asymptomatic cardiac volume overload

Cost
Moderately expensive

Patient preparation
■ As appropriate, explain the purpose of the test to the patient.
■ Inform the patient that he must fast before the test.
■ Tell the patient that the test requires a blood sample. Explain who will perform the venipuncture and when.
■ Explain to the patient that he may experience discomfort from the needle puncture and the tourniquet.
■ Check the patient's history for use of medications that can influence test results. Restrict beta-adrenergic blockers, calcium antagonists, diuretics, vasodilators, and cardiac glycosides for 24 hours before sample collection; note this on the laboratory request.

Normal findings
ANF levels normally range from 20 to 77 pg/ml (SI, 4 to 27 pmol/L).

Abnormal results
Markedly elevated ANF levels are found in patients with frank heart failure and significantly elevated cardiac filling pressure.

Interfering factors
■ Cardiovascular drugs, including beta-adrenergic blockers, calcium antagonists, cardiac glycosides, diuretics, and vasodilators

B

Bacterial meningitis antigen

The bacterial meningitis antigen test can detect specific antigens of *Streptococcus pneumoniae, Neisseria meningitidis,* and *Haemophilus influenzae type B,* the principal etiologic agents in meningitis. It can be performed on samples of serum, cerebrospinal fluid (CSF), urine, pleural fluid, and joint fluid, but CSF and urine are preferred.

Purpose
■ To identify the etiologic agent in meningitis
■ To aid diagnosis of bacterial meningitis, especially when the Gram stain and culture are negative

Cost
Moderately expensive

Patient preparation
■ Explain to the patient the purpose of the test, as appropriate.
■ Inform the patient that this test requires a specimen of urine or CSF. Explain how the sample will be obtained, including who will perform the procedure and when.

■ Explain to the patient that he may experience discomfort from the needle puncture.
■ Advise the patient that a headache is the most common complication of lumbar puncture, but that his cooperation during the test minimizes such an effect.
■ Obtain informed consent if necessary.

Normal findings
Normally, results are negative for bacterial antigens.

Abnormal findings
Positive results identify the specific bacterial antigen: *S. pneumoniae, N. meningitidis, H. influenzae* type B, or group B streptococci.

Interfering factors
■ Previous antimicrobial therapy
■ Failure to maintain sterility during specimen collection

Barium enema

Also called *lower GI examination,* barium enema is the radiographic examination of the large intestine after rectal instillation of barium sulfate (single-contrast technique) or barium sulfate and air (double-contrast technique). It's indicated in patients with histories of altered bowel habits, lower abdominal pain, or the passage of blood, mucus, or pus in the stool. It may also be indicated after colostomy or ileostomy; in these patients, barium (or barium and air) is instilled through the stoma. Complications include perforation of the colon, water intoxication, barium granulomas and, rarely, intraperitoneal and extraperitoneal extravasation of barium and barium embolism.

The single-contrast technique provides a profile view of the large intestine; the double-contrast technique provides profile and frontal views. The latter technique best detects small intraluminal tumors (especially polyps), the early mucosal changes of inflammatory disease, and the subtle intestinal bleeding caused by ulcerated polyps or the shallow ulcerations of inflammatory disease.

Although barium enema clearly outlines most of the large intestine, proctosigmoidoscopy provides the best view of the rectosigmoid region. Barium enema should precede the barium swallow and upper GI and small-bowel series because barium ingested in the latter procedure may take several days to pass through the GI tract and thus may interfere with subsequent X-ray studies.

ALERT! ▼ ▼ ▼ ▼ ▼ ▼ ▼ ▼ ▼
Barium enema is contraindicated in patients with tachycardia, fulminant ulcerative colitis associated with systemic toxicity and megacolon, toxic megacolon, or suspected perforation. This test should be performed cautiously in patients with obstruction, acute inflammatory conditions (such as ulcerative colitis and diverticulitis), acute vascular insufficiency of the bowel, acute fulminant bloody diarrhea, and suspected pneumatosis cystoides intesti-

nalis. Barium enema is also contraindicated in a patient who is pregnant because of the radiation's possible teratogenic effects.

Purpose
■ To aid diagnosis of colorectal cancer and inflammatory disease
■ To detect polyps, diverticula, and structural changes in the large intestine

Cost
Expensive

Patient preparation
■ Explain to the patient that this test permits examination of the large intestine through X-ray films taken after a barium enema.
■ Describe the test to the patient, including who will perform it and where it will take place.
■ Explain to the patient that he may experience some cramping or an urge to defecate during the procedure.
■ Instruct the patient to carefully follow the prescribed bowel preparation, which may include diet, laxatives, or an enema.
■ Stress that accurate test results depend on the patient's cooperation with prescribed dietary restrictions and bowel preparation. A common bowel preparation technique includes restricted intake of dairy products and maintenance of a liquid diet for 24 hours before the test. A bowel preparation is supplied by the radiography department (a GoLYTELY preparation isn't recommended because it leaves the bowel too wet and the barium won't coat the walls of the bowel), and prescribed enemas are administered until return is clear.
■ Tell the patient not to eat breakfast before the procedure; if the test is scheduled for late afternoon (or delayed), tell him that he may have clear liquids.

- Tell the patient that he'll receive a mild cathartic or an enema after the procedure and that his stool will be light colored for 24 to 72 hours.

Normal findings

In the single-contrast enema, the intestine is uniformly filled with barium, and colonic haustral markings are clearly apparent. The intestinal walls collapse as the barium is expelled, and the mucosa has a regular, feathery appearance on the postevacuation film. In the double-contrast enema, the intestine is uniformly distended with air and has a thin layer of barium providing excellent detail of the mucosal pattern. As the patient is assisted to various positions, the barium collects on the dependent walls of the intestine by the force of gravity.

Abnormal findings

Although most colonic cancers occur in the rectosigmoid region and are best detected by proctosigmoidoscopy, X-ray films may reveal adenocarcinoma and, rarely, sarcomas occurring higher in the intestine. Carcinoma usually appears as a localized filling defect, with a sharp transition between the normal and the necrotic mucosa. If it's circumferential, it will have an "apple core" appearance. These characteristics help distinguish carcinoma from the more diffuse lesions of inflammatory disease, but endoscopic biopsy may be necessary to confirm the diagnosis.

X-ray studies demonstrate and define the extent of inflammatory disease. Ulcerative colitis usually originates in the anal region and ascends through the intestine; granulomatous colitis usually originates in the cecum and terminal ileum and descends through the intestine. However, biopsy may be necessary to confirm diagnosis.

Barium X-ray films may also reveal saccular adenomatous polyps, broad-based villous polyps, structural changes in the intestine (such as intussusception, telescoping of the bowel, sigmoid volvulus [360-degree turn or greater], and sigmoid torsion [up to 180-degree turn]), gastroenteritis, irritable colon, vascular injury due to arterial occlusion, and selected cases of acute appendicitis.

Interfering factors

- Inadequate bowel preparation (possible poor imaging)
- Barium retained from previous studies (possible poor imaging)
- The patient's inability to retain barium enema

Barium swallow

Barium swallow (*esophagography*) is the cineradiographic, radiographic, or fluoroscopic examination of the pharynx and the fluoroscopic examination of the esophagus after ingestion of thick and thin mixtures of barium sulfate. This test, most commonly performed as part of the upper GI series, is indicated in patients with histories of dysphagia and regurgitation. Further testing is usually required for definitive diagnosis. (See *Gastroesophageal reflux scanning,* page 64.)

Cholangiography and the barium enema test, if necessary, should precede the barium swallow because ingested barium may obscure anatomic detail on the X-rays.
ALERT! ▼ ▼ ▼ ▼ ▼ ▼ ▼ ▼
Barium swallow is usually contraindicated in patients with intestinal obstruction as well as in patients who are pregnant because of possible teratogenic effects.

Gastroesophageal reflux scanning

When results of a barium swallow are inconclusive, gastroesophageal reflux scanning may be done to evaluate esophageal function and detect reflux. This test delivers less radiation than a barium swallow and is a much more sensitive indicator of reflux. It also allows reflux to be measured without insertion of an esophageal tube — an important consideration in testing infants, small children, and other patients for whom intubation is contraindicated.

Procedure

The patient is instructed to fast after midnight before the test to clear stomach contents that impede passage of the imaging agent. As the test begins, the patient is placed in a supine or upright position and is asked to swallow a solution containing a radiopharmaceutical such as technetium 99m sulfur colloid (^{99m}Tc). A gamma counter placed over the patient's chest records passage of the ^{99m}Tc through the esophagus into the stomach to determine transit time and to evaluate esophageal function.

If gastroesophageal reflux is suspected, the patient is repositioned as his stomach distends, and continuous recordings visualize reflux and estimate its quantity. Depending on hospital policy, manual pressure may be applied to the patient's upper abdomen, and recordings may be taken at specific intervals.

Findings and contraindications

Normally, ^{99m}Tc descends through the esophagus in about 6 seconds; radioactivity is then detected only in the stomach and small bowel. However, diffuse spasm of the esophagus, achalasia, or other esophageal motility disorders may prolong transit time. In gastroesophageal reflux, radioactivity may be detected in the esophagus.

As with other radionuclide studies, this scan is usually contraindicated during pregnancy and lactation. It can be modified for use in infants and children.

Purpose

■ To diagnose hiatal hernia, diverticula, and varices
■ To detect strictures, ulcers, tumors, polyps, and motility disorders

Cost

Expensive

Patient preparation

■ Explain to the patient that this test evaluates the function of the pharynx and esophagus.
■ Instruct the patient to fast after midnight the night before the test. Inform the patient that he may also be given a restricted diet for 2 to 3 days before the test.

AGE ISSUE ✳ ✳ ✳ ✳ ✳
If the patient is an infant, make sure his parents understand to delay feeding to ensure complete digestion of barium.

■ Describe the test to the patient, including who will perform it and where it will take place.
■ Tell the patient that he will need to drink a preparation to outline his GI system and that X-rays will be taken.
■ Withhold antacids, histamine-2 blockers, and proton pump inhibitors if gastric reflux is suspected.

When intestinal disease is strongly suspected, the GI motility study may follow the upper GI and small bowel series. This study, which evaluates intestinal motility and the integrity of the mucosal lining, records the passage of barium through the lower digestive tract.

About 6 hours after barium ingestion, the head of the barium column is usually in the hepatic flexure, and the tail is in the terminal ileum. The barium completely opacifies the large intestine by 24 hours after ingestion. Because the amount of barium passing through the large intestine isn't sufficient to fully extend the lumen, spot films taken 24, 48, or 72 hours after barium ingestion prove inferior to the barium enema. However, when spot films suggest intestinal abnormalities, the barium enema and colonoscopy can provide more specific results, confirming diagnostic information.

■ Instruct the patient to drink plenty of fluids after the test, unless contraindicated, to help eliminate the barium. Tell him that he may receive a cathartic.

■ Inform the patient that stools will be chalky and light colored for 24 to 72 hours.

Normal findings

After the barium sulfate is swallowed, the bolus pours over the base of the tongue into the pharynx. A peristaltic wave propels the bolus through the entire length of the esophagus in about 2 seconds. When the peristaltic wave reaches the base of the esophagus, the cardiac sphincter opens, allowing the bolus to enter the stomach. After passage of the bolus, the cardiac sphincter closes. Normally, the bolus evenly fills and distends the lumen of the pharynx and esophagus, and the mucosa appears smooth and regular.

Abnormal findings

Barium swallow may reveal hiatus hernia, diverticula, and varices. Aspiration into the lungs will also be revealed. Although strictures, tumors, polyps, ulcers, and motility disorders (pharyngeal muscular disorders, esophageal spasms, and achalasia) may be detected, definitive diagnosis commonly requires endoscopic biopsy or, for motility disorders, manometric studies. (See *GI motility study*.)

Interfering factors

■ Aspiration of barium into lungs due to poor swallowing reflex

Bilirubin, serum

The serum bilirubin test is used to measure serum levels of bilirubin, the predominant pigment in bile. Bilirubin is the major product of hemoglobin catabolism. Serum bilirubin measurements are especially significant in neonates because elevated unconjugated bilirubin can accumulate in the brain, causing irreparable damage.

Purpose

■ To evaluate liver functions

■ To aid differential diagnosis of jaundice and monitor its progress

■ To aid diagnosis of biliary obstruction and hemolytic anemia

■ To determine whether a neonate requires an exchange transfusion or phototherapy because of dangerously high unconjugated bilirubin levels

Cost
Inexpensive

Patient preparation
■ Explain to the patient that this test is used to evaluate liver function and the condition of red blood cells.
■ Tell the patient that the test requires a blood sample. Explain who will perform the venipuncture and when.
■ Explain to the patient that he may experience discomfort from the needle puncture and the tourniquet.
■ Instruct the patient that he need not restrict fluids but should fast for at least 4 hours before the test.

AGE ISSUE ✳ ✳ ✳ ✳ ✳
Fasting isn't necessary if the patient is a neonate. Tell the parents or a responsible family member that a small amount of blood will be drawn from the patient's heel. Explain who will perform the venipuncture and when.

Reference values
In adults, normal indirect serum bilirubin levels are 1.1 mg/dl (SI, 19 µmol/L), and direct serum bilirubin levels are < 0.5 mg/dl (SI, < 6.8 µmol/L). In neonates, total serum bilirubin levels are 2 to 12 mg/dl (SI, 34 to 205 µmol/L).

Abnormal findings
Elevated indirect serum bilirubin levels usually indicate hepatic damage. High levels of indirect bilirubin are also likely in severe hemolytic anemia. If hemolysis continues, both direct and indirect bilirubin levels may rise. Other causes of elevated indirect bilirubin levels include congenital enzyme deficiencies such as Gilbert's disease.

Elevated direct serum bilirubin levels usually indicate biliary obstruction. If obstruction continues, both direct and indirect bilirubin levels may rise. In severe chronic hepatic damage, direct bilirubin concentrations may return to normal or near-normal levels, but indirect bilirubin levels remain elevated.

ALERT! ▼ ▼ ▼ ▼ ▼ ▼ ▼ ▼
In neonates, total bilirubin levels of 15 mg/dl (SI, 257 µmol/L) or more indicate the need for an exchange transfusion.

Interfering factors
■ Exposure of the sample to direct sunlight or ultraviolet light (possible decrease)
■ Hemolysis due to rough handling of the sample

Bilirubin, urine

The urine bilirubin screening test, based on a color reaction with a specific reagent, detects water-soluble direct (conjugated) bilirubin in the urine. Detectable amounts of bilirubin in the urine may indicate liver disease caused by infections, biliary disease, or hepatotoxicity. When combined with urobilinogen measurements, the bilirubin test helps identify disorders that can cause jaundice. The analysis can be performed at the bedside, using a bilirubin reagent strip, or in the laboratory.

Purpose
■ To help identify the cause of jaundice
■ To compare urine and serum bilirubin levels and other liver enzyme tests

Cost
Inexpensive

Patient preparation
■ Explain to the patient that this test helps determine the cause of jaundice.

Comparative values of bilirubin and urobilinogen

CAUSES OF JAUNDICE	Indirect bilirubin	Direct bilirubin	Bilirubin	Uro-bilinogen	Uro-bilinogen
	SERUM		URINE		STOOL
Unconjugated hyperbilirubinemia					
Hemolytic disorders: hemolytic anemia, erythroblastosis fetalis	↑	N	O	N↑	↑
Gilbert's disease: constitutional hepatic dysfunction	↑↑	N	O	N↓	N↓
Crigler-Najjar syndrome: congenital hyperbilirubinemia	↑↑↑	N	O	N↓	N↓
Conjugated hyperbilirubinemia					
Extrahepatic obstruction: calculi, tumor, scar tissue in common bile duct or hepatic excretory duct	N	↑	+	↓O	↓O
Hepatocellular disorders: viral, toxic, or alcoholic hepatitis; cirrhosis; parenchymal injury	↑	↑	+	↓N↑	N↑
Hepatocanalicular disorders or intrahepatic obstruction: drug-induced cholestasis; some familial defects, such as Dubin-Johnson and Rotor's syndromes; viral hepatitis; and primary biliary cirrhosis	↑	↑	+	↓N↑	N↑

Key:

↑	Increased	O	Absent
N↑	May be increased	+	Present
↑↑	Moderately increased	N↓	Normal or reduced
↑↑↑	Markedly increased	↓O	Decreased or absent
N	Normal	↓N↑	Variable

■ Inform the patient that he need not restrict food or fluids before the test.

■ Tell the patient that the test requires a random urine specimen.

■ Restrict medications that may affect test results. If they must be continued, note this on the laboratory request.

Normal findings

Normally, bilirubin isn't found in urine in a routine screening test.

Abnormal findings

High concentrations of direct bilirubin in urine may be evident from the specimen's appearance (dark, with a yellow foam). To diagnose jaundice, however, the presence or absence of direct bilirubin in urine must be correlated with serum test results and with urine and fecal urobilinogen levels. (See *Comparative values of bilirubin and urobilinogen*.)

Interfering factors

■ Phenazopyridine, phenothiazine derivatives (chlorpromazine and acetophenazine maleate) (false-positive)
■ Large amounts of ascorbic acid and nitrite (false-negative if using dipstick testing, such as chemstrip or N-multistix)
■ Exposure of specimen to room temperature or light (decrease due to bilirubin degradation)

Blood culture

A blood culture is performed to isolate and aid identification of the pathogens in bacteremia (bacterial invasion of the bloodstream) and septicemia (systemic spread of such infection). It requires inoculating a culture medium with a blood sample and incubating it.

Purpose

■ To confirm bacteremia
■ To identify the causative organism in bacteremia and septicemia

Cost

Moderately expensive

Patient preparation

■ Explain to the patient that this procedure is used to help identify the organism causing his symptoms.
■ Tell the patient that the test requires multiple blood samples. Explain who will perform the venipunctures and when.
■ Explain to the patient that he may experience discomfort from the needle punctures and the tourniquet.
■ Indicate the tentative diagnosis on the laboratory request, and note any current or recent antimicrobial therapy.

ALERT! ▼ ▼ ▼ ▼ ▼ ▼ ▼ ▼ ▼
Whenever possible, blood cultures should be collected prior to administration of antimicrobial agents.

Normal findings

Normally, blood cultures are negative for pathogens.

Abnormal findings

Positive blood cultures don't necessarily confirm pathologic septicemia. Mild, transient bacteremia may occur during the course of many infectious diseases or may complicate other disorders. Persistent, continuous, or recurrent bacteremia reliably confirms the presence of serious infection. To detect most causative agents, blood cultures are ideally drawn on 2 consecutive days.

Isolation of most organisms takes about 72 hours; negative cultures are held for 1 or more weeks before being reported negative. Common blood pathogens include *Streptococcus pneumoniae* and other *Streptococcus* species, *H. influenzae, S. aureus, Pseudomonas aeruginosa, Bacteroides, Brucella,* Enterobacteriaceae, coliform bacilli, and *C. albicans*. Although 2% to 3% of cultured blood samples are contaminated by skin bacteria, such as *S. epidermidis,* diphtheroids, and *Propionibacterium,* these organisms may be clinically significant when isolated from multiple cultures or from immunocompromised patients. Debilitated or immunocompromised patients may have isolates of *C. albicans*. In patients with human immunodeficiency virus infection, *M. tuberculosis* and *M. avium* complex may be isolated as well as other mycobacterium species on a less frequent basis.

Interfering factors

■ Previous or current antimicrobial therapy (possible false-negative)

- Removal of culture bottle caps at the bedside (possible prevention of anaerobic growth)
- Use of incorrect bottle and media (possible prevention of aerobic growth)

Blood urea nitrogen

The blood urea nitrogen (BUN) test is used to measure the nitrogen fraction of urea, the chief end product of protein metabolism. Formed in the liver from ammonia and excreted by the kidneys, urea constitutes 40% to 50% of the blood's nonprotein nitrogen. The BUN level reflects protein intake and renal excretory capacity but is a less reliable indicator of uremia than the serum creatinine level.

Purpose
- To evaluate kidney function and aid diagnosis of renal disease
- To aid assessment of hydration

Cost
Inexpensive

Patient preparation
- Tell the patient that this test is used to evaluate kidney function.
- Inform the patient that he need not restrict food and fluids but should avoid a diet high in meat.
- Tell the patient that the test requires a blood sample. Explain who will perform the venipuncture and when.
- Explain to the patient that he may experience discomfort from the needle puncture and the tourniquet.
- Restrict medications that may affect test results. If they must be continued, note this on the laboratory request.

Reference values
BUN values normally range from 8 to 20 mg/dl (SI, 2.9 to 7.5 mmol/L), with slightly higher values in elderly patients.

Abnormal findings
Elevated BUN levels occur in renal disease, reduced renal blood flow (due to dehydration, for example), urinary tract obstruction, and increased protein catabolism (such as burn injuries).

Low BUN levels occur in severe hepatic damage, malnutrition, and overhydration.

Interfering factors
- Hemolysis due to rough handling of the sample
- Chloramphenicol (possible decrease)
- Aminoglycosides, amphotericin B, methicillin (increase due to nephrotoxicity)

Bone densitometry

Bone densitometry assesses bone mass quantitatively. This noninvasive technique, also known as *dual energy X-ray absorptiometry*, uses a radiography tube to measure bone mineral density and exposes the patient to only minimal radiation. Computers analyze the detected images to determine bone mineral status. The computer calculates the size and thickness of the bone as well as its volumetric density to determine its potential resistance to mechanical stress.

This test can scan the lumbar spine and the proximal femur, two sites at high risk for fractures. It's precise enough to scan three lumbar vertebrae and the introchanteric area of the hip. Scanning the distal forearm is also useful because research has shown a high correlation between bone mineral density of this area of the forearm and the bone mineral density of the spine and femur.

The value and reliability of bone densitometry as a predictor of fractures are under investigation. Controversy exists regarding the scanning site and whether bone loss occurs as a general phenomenon or occurs first in the spine. Also, large-scale studies are being conducted to establish an "at-risk" level of bone density to help predict fractures.

ALERT! ▼ ▼ ▼ ▼ ▼ ▼ ▼ ▼ ▼
Bone densitometry is contraindicated during pregnancy.

Purpose
■ To determine bone mineral density
■ To identify people at risk for osteoporosis
■ To evaluate a patient's clinical response to therapy aimed at reducing the rate of bone loss.

Cost
Moderately expensive

Patient preparation
■ Reassure the patient that the test is painless and that exposure to radiation is minimal.
■ Tell the patient who will perform the test and where it will be done.
■ Tell the patient a detector measures the bone's absorption of the radiation and registers a digital readout. The scan is usually completed in less than 10 minutes.

Normal findings
The results of the scan are analyzed by a computer program according to the patient's age, sex, and height.

Abnormal findings
Values other than normal for the patient's age, sex, race, and height are considered abnormal and may reveal estrogen deficiency in postmenopausal women, hyperparathyroidism, radiographic osteopenia, and vertebral abnormalities.

Interfering factors
■ Osteoarthritis, fractures, the size of the region to be scanned, and fat tissue distribution
■ Metallic prosthetic devices or surgical implants

Bone marrow aspiration and biopsy

Bone marrow, the soft tissue contained in the medullary canals of long bone and in the interstices of cancellous bone, may be removed by aspiration or needle biopsy under local anesthesia. In aspiration biopsy, a fluid specimen in which pustulae of marrow are suspended is removed from the bone marrow. In needle biopsy, a core of marrow — cells, not fluid — is removed. These methods are often used concurrently to obtain the best possible marrow specimens. Because bone marrow is the major site of hematopoiesis, histologic and hematologic examination of its contents provide reliable diagnostic information about blood disorders.

ALERT! ▼ ▼ ▼ ▼ ▼ ▼ ▼ ▼ ▼
Bone marrow aspiration and biopsy are contraindicated in patients with severe bleeding disorders.

Purpose
■ To diagnose thrombocytopenia, leukemias, granulomas, and aplastic, hypoplastic, and pernicious anemias
■ To diagnose primary and metastatic tumors
■ To determine the cause of infection

■ To aid staging of disease such as Hodgkin's disease
■ To evaluate the effectiveness of chemotherapy and help monitor myelo-suppression

Cost
Expensive

Patient preparation
■ Describe the procedure to the patient, and answer any questions. Explain that the test permits microscopic examination of a bone marrow specimen. (See *Common sites of bone marrow aspiration and biopsy,* page 72.)
■ Explain to the patient who will perform the biopsy and where it will be done.
■ Explain to the patient that more than one specimen may be required and that a blood sample will be collected before the biopsy. Explain who will perform the venipuncture and when.
■ Explain to the patient that he may experience discomfort from the needle puncture and the tourniquet.
■ Obtain informed consent if necessary.
■ Check the patient's history for hypersensitivity to the local anesthetic. Inform the patient that a local anesthetic will be given but he may still feel some pressure on insertion or a pulling pain on removal of the marrow. Tell him a mild sedative may be administered 1 hour before the test.

AGE ISSUE ✻ ✻ ✻ ✻ ✻
Preparation of children requires additional steps. Before the biopsy, explain the equipment on the tray to the child. Encourage the parents to get involved by helping hold the child still and reassuring him. Tell the child that he'll feel some pain when the bone marrow is aspirated and that it's okay to cry or yell if he wants to, but the pain will go away quickly.

Normal findings
Yellow marrow contains fat cells and connective tissue; red marrow contains hematopoietic cells, fat cells, and connective tissue. In addition, special stains that detect hematologic disorders produce these normal findings: the iron stain, which measures hemosiderin (storage iron), has a +2 level; the Sudan black B (SBB) stain, which shows granulocytes, is negative; and the periodic acid–Schiff (PAS) stain, which detects glycogen reactions, is negative.

Abnormal findings
Histologic examination of a bone marrow specimen can help detect myelofibrosis, granulomas, lymphomas, or cancer. Hematologic analysis, including the differential count and the myeloid-erythroid ratio, can implicate a wide range of disorders. (See *Bone marrow: Normal values and implications of abnormal findings,* pages 73 and 74.)

In an iron stain, decreased hemosiderin levels may indicate a true iron deficiency. Increased levels may accompany other types of anemias or blood disorders. A positive SBB stain can differentiate acute myelogenous leukemia from acute lymphoblastic leukemia (negative SBB), or it may indicate granulation in myeloblasts. A positive PAS stain may indicate acute or chronic lymphocytic leukemia, amyloidosis, thalassemia, lymphoma, infectious mononucleosis, iron-deficiency anemia, or sideroblastic anemia.

Interfering factors
■ Failure to obtain a representative specimen
■ Failure to use a fixative (for histologic analysis)
■ Failure to send the specimen to the laboratory immediately

(Text continues on page 74.)

Common sites of bone marrow aspiration and biopsy

The *posterior superior iliac spine* (1) is usually the site preferred for bone marrow aspiration and biopsy because no vital organs or vessels are located nearby. With the patient lateral with one leg flexed, the practitioner inserts the needle several centimeters lateral to the iliosacral junction, entering the bone plane crest with the needle directed downward and toward the anterior inferior spine or entering a few centimeters below the crest at a right angle to the surface of the bone.

The *sternum* (2) involves the greatest risks but is commonly used for marrow aspiration because it's near the surface, the cortical bone is thin, and the marrow cavity contains numerous cells and relatively little fat or supporting bone. For this procedure, the patient is supine on a firm bed or examining table with a small pillow beneath the shoulders to elevate the chest and lower the head. The practitioner secures the needle guard 3 to 4 mm from the tip of the needle to avoid accidental puncture of the heart or a major vessel. Then he inserts the needle at the midline of the sternum at the second intercostal space.

The *spinous process* (3) is the preferred site if multiple punctures are necessary, marrow is absent at other sites, or the patient objects to sternal puncture. For this procedure, the patient sits on the edge of the bed, leaning over the bedside stand; if he's uncooperative, he may be placed in the prone position with restraints. The practitioner selects the spinous process of the third or fourth lumbar vertebra and inserts the needle at the crest or slightly to one side, advancing the needle in the direction of the bone plane.

The *tibia* (4) is the site of choice for infants under 1 year of age. The infant is placed in a prone position on a bed or examining table with a sandbag beneath the leg. The foot is taped to the surface of the table, or an assistant holds the leg stationary by placing a hand under it. The practitioner inserts the needle about ⅜" (1 cm) below the tibial tuberosity and slightly toward the medial side, being careful to angle the needle point toward the foot to avoid epiphyseal injury.

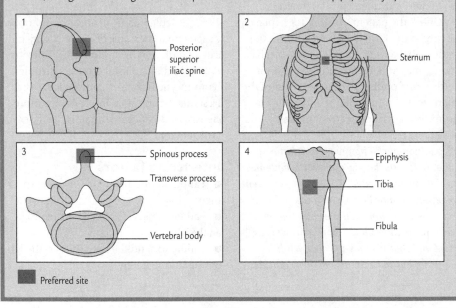

1 — Posterior superior iliac spine

2 — Sternum

3 — Spinous process / Transverse process / Vertebral body

4 — Epiphysis / Tibia / Fibula

■ Preferred site

Bone marrow: Normal values and implications of abnormal findings

CELL TYPES	NORMAL MEAN VALUES			CLINICAL IMPLICATIONS
	Adults	Children	Infants	
Normoblasts, total	25.6%	23.1%	8.0%	*Elevated values:* polycythemia vera
Pronormoblasts	0.2% to 1.3%	0.5%	0.1%	*Depressed values:* vitamin B_{12} or folic acid deficiency; hypoplastic
Basophilic	0.5% to 2.4%	1.7%	0.34%	or aplastic anemia
Polychromatic	17.9% to 29.2%	18.2%	6.9%	
Orthochromatic	0.4% to 4.6%	2.7%	0.54%	
Neutrophils, total	56.5%	57.1%	32.4%	*Elevated values:* acute myeloblastic or chronic myeloid leukemia
Myeloblasts	0.2% to 1.5%	1.2%	0.62%	
Promyelocytes	2.1% to 4.1%	1.4%	0.76%	*Depressed values:* lymphoblastic, lymphatic, or monocytic leukemia; aplastic anemia
Myelocytes	8.2% to 15.7%	18.3%	2.5%	
Metamyelocytes	9.6% to 24.6%	23.3%	11.3%	
Bands	9.5% to 15.3%	0	14.1%	
Segmented	6.0% to 12.0%	12.9%	3.6%	
Eosinophils	3.1%	3.6%	2.6%	*Elevated values:* bone marrow carcinoma, lymphadenoma, myeloid leukemia, eosinophilic leukemia, pernicious anemia (in relapse)
Plasma cells	1.3%	0.4%	0.02%	*Elevated values:* myeloma, collagen disease, infection, antigen sensitivity, cancer
Basophils	0.01%	0.06%	0.07%	*Elevated values:* no relation between basophil count and symptoms *Depressed values:* no relationship between basophil count and symptoms

(continued)

CELL TYPES	NORMAL MEAN VALUES			CLINICAL IMPLICATIONS
	Adults	Children	Infants	
Lymphocytes	16.2%	16.0%	49.0%	*Elevated values:* B- and T-cell chronic lymphocytic leukemia, other lymphatic leukemia, lymphoma, mononucleosis, aplastic anemia, macroglobulinemia
Megakaryocytes	0.1%	0.1%	0.05%	*Elevated values:* old age, chronic myeloid leukemia, polycythemia vera, megakaryocytic myelosis, infections, autoimmune thrombocytopenic purpura, thrombocytopenia *Depressed values:* pernicious anemia
Myeloiderythroid ratio	2:1 to 4:1	2.9:1	4.4:1	*Elevated values:* myeloid leukemia, infection, leukemoid reactions, depressed hematopoiesis *Depressed values:* agranulocytosis, hematopoiesis after hemorrhage or hemolysis, iron deficiency anemia, polycythemia vera

Bronchoscopy

Bronchoscopy allows direct visualization of the larynx, trachea, and bronchi through a flexible fiber-optic bronchoscope or a rigid metal bronchoscope. Although a flexible fiber-optic bronchoscope allows a wider view and is used more often, the rigid metal bronchoscope is required to remove foreign objects, excise endobronchial lesions, and control massive hemoptysis. A brush, biopsy forceps, or catheter may be passed through the bronchoscope to obtain specimens for cytologic examination. Bronchoscopy may require fluoroscopic guidance for distal evaluation of lesions for a transbronchial biopsy in alveolar areas.

Purpose

■ To visually examine a tumor, an obstruction, secretions, bleeding, or a foreign body in the tracheobronchial tree

■ To help diagnose bronchogenic carcinoma, tuberculosis, interstitial pulmonary disease, and fungal or parasitic pulmonary infection by obtaining a specimen for bacteriologic and cytologic examination

■ To remove foreign bodies, malignant or benign tumors, mucus plugs, and excessive secretions from the tracheobronchial tree

Cost

Expensive

Patient preparation

- Explain to the patient that this test is used to examine the lower airways.
- Describe the procedure to the patient, and instruct him to fast for 6 to 12 hours before the test.
- Tell the patient who will perform the test, where it will be done, and that a chest X-ray and blood studies will be performed before the bronchoscopy and afterward if appropriate.
- Advise the patient that he may receive a sedative I.V. to help him relax. If the procedure isn't being performed under general anesthesia, inform the patient that a local anesthetic will be sprayed into his nose and mouth to suppress the gag reflex and that it may have an unpleasant taste.
- Reassure the patient that his airway won't be blocked during the procedure and that oxygen will be administered through the bronchoscope.
- Obtain informed consent if necessary.
- Check the patient's history for hypersensitivity to the anesthetic.
- Tell the patient who has had a biopsy to refrain from clearing his throat and coughing after the procedure, which may dislodge the clot at the biopsy site and cause hemorrhaging.
- Tell the patient that food and fluids will be restricted for 1 to 2 hours after the procedure. Also, reassure him that hoarseness, loss of voice, and sore throat are temporary.

Normal findings

The trachea normally consists of smooth muscle containing C-shaped rings of cartilage at regular intervals, and it's lined with ciliated mucosa. The bronchi appear structurally similar to the trachea; the right bronchus is slightly larger and more vertical than the left. Smaller segmental bronchi branch off the main bronchi.

Abnormal findings

Bronchial wall abnormalities include inflammation, swelling, protruding cartilage, ulceration, enlargement of the mucous gland orifices or submucosal lymph nodes, and tumors. Endotracheal abnormalities include stenosis, compression, ectasia (dilation of tubular vessel), irregular bronchial branching, and abnormal bifurcation due to diverticulum. Abnormal substances in the trachea or bronchi include blood, secretions, calculi, and foreign bodies. Results of tissue and cell studies may indicate interstitial pulmonary disease, bronchogenic carcinoma, tuberculosis, or other pulmonary infections. Correlation of radiographic, bronchoscopic, and cytologic findings with clinical signs and symptoms is essential.

Interfering factors

- Failure to observe pretest restrictions
- Failure to place specimens in the appropriate containers or to send them to the laboratory immediately

C

Calcitonin, plasma

The plasma calcitonin test, a radioimmunoassay measures plasma levels of calcitonin (also known as thyrocalcitonin), a polypeptide hormone secreted by interstitial or parafollicular cells called specialized C cells of the thyroid gland in response to rising plasma calcium levels. While the exact role of calcitonin in normal human physiology hasn't been fully determined, calcitonin is known to inhibit bone resorption by osteoclasts and osteocytes and to increase calcium excretion by the kidneys. Therefore, calcitonin acts as an antagonist to parathyroid hormone and lowers serum calcium levels.

The usual clinical indication for this test is suspected medullary carcinoma of the thyroid, which causes hypersecretion of calcitonin without associated hypocalcemia. Equivocal results require provocative testing with I.V. pentagastrin or calcium to rule out this disease. (See *Calcitonin stimulation tests.*)

Purpose
■ To aid diagnosis of thyroid medullary carcinoma or ectopic calcitonin-producing tumors (rare)

Cost
Inexpensive

Patient preparation
■ Explain to the patient that this test helps evaluate thyroid function.
■ Instruct the patient to observe an overnight fast because eating may interfere with calcium homeostasis and, subsequently, calcitonin levels.
■ Tell the patient that the test requires a blood sample. Explain who will perform the venipuncture and when.
■ Explain to the patient that he may experience discomfort from the needle puncture and the tourniquet.

Reference values
Normal basal plasma calcitonin levels are:
■ *Males:* 40 pg/ml (SI, 40 ng/L)
■ *Females:* 20 pg/ml (SI, 20 ng/L).
  Values after provocative testing with 4-hour calcium infusion are:
■ *Males:* 190 pg/ml (SI, 190 ng/L)
■ *Females:* 130 pg/ml (SI, 130 ng/L)
  Values after provocative testing with pentagastrin infusion are:
■ *Males:* 110 pg/ml (SI, 110 ng/L)
■ *Females:* 30 pg/ml (SI, 30 ng/L).

Abnormal findings

Elevated plasma calcitonin levels in the absence of hypocalcemia usually indicate medullary carcinoma of the thyroid. Transmitted as an autosomal dominant trait, this disease may occur as part of multiple endocrine neoplasia. Occasionally, increased calcitonin levels may be associated with ectopic calcitonin production resulting from oat cell carcinoma of the lung or from breast carcinoma.

Interfering factors

■ Failure to observe an overnight fast before the test

Calcium and phosphates

The calcium and phosphates test measures the urine levels of calcium and phosphates, elements essential for the formation and resorption of bone. Urine calcium and phosphate levels generally parallel serum levels.

Normally absorbed in the upper intestine and excreted in stool and urine, calcium and phosphates help maintain tissue and fluid pH, electrolyte balance in cells and extracellular fluids, and permeability of cell membranes. Calcium promotes enzymatic processes, aids blood coagulation, and lowers neuromuscular irritability; phosphates aid carbohydrate metabolism.

Purpose

■ To evaluate calcium and phosphate metabolism and excretion
■ To monitor treatment of calcium or phosphate deficiency

Cost
Inexpensive

Patient preparation

■ Explain to the patient that this test measures the amount of calcium and phosphates in the urine.
■ Encourage the patient to be as active as possible before the test.
■ Tell the patient the test requires urine collection over a 24-hour period, and review proper technique.
■ Instruct the patient to consume a diet that contains about 130 mg of calcium/24 hours for 3 days before the test or provide a copy of the diet for the patient to follow at home.
■ Restrict medications that may affect test results. If they must be continued, note this on the laboratory request.

Disorders that affect urine calcium and urine phosphorus levels

DISORDER	URINE CALCIUM LEVEL	URINE PHOSPHATE LEVEL
Hyperparathyroidism	Elevated	Elevated
Vitamin D intoxication	Elevated	Suppressed
Metastatic carcinoma	Elevated	Normal
Sarcoidosis	Elevated	Suppressed
Renal tubular acidosis	Elevated	Elevated
Multiple myeloma	Elevated or normal	Elevated or normal
Paget's disease	Normal	Normal
Milk-alkali syndrome	Suppressed or normal	Suppressed or normal
Hypoparathyroidism	Suppressed	Suppressed
Acute nephrosis	Suppressed	Suppressed or normal
Chronic nephrosis	Suppressed	Suppressed
Acute nephritis	Suppressed	Suppressed
Renal insufficiency	Suppressed	Suppressed
Osteomalacia	Suppressed	Suppressed
Steatorrhea	Suppressed	Suppressed

Reference values

Normal values depend on dietary intake. For a normal diet, urine calcium levels for a 24-hour period range from 100 to 300 mg/ 24 hours (SI, 2.50 to 7.50 mmol/d). Normal excretion of phosphate is less than 1,000 mg/24 hours.

Abnormal findings

A variety of disorders may affect calcium and phosphorus levels. (See *Disorders that affect urine calcium and urine phosphorus levels.*)

Interfering factors

■ Failure to collect all urine during the test period
■ Parathyroid hormones (increases excretion of phosphates and decreases urinary excretion of calcium)
■ Thiazide diuretics (decreases excretion of calcium)
■ Prolonged inactivity and ingestion of corticosteroids, sodium phosphate, calcitonin (increases excretion of calcium)
■ Vitamin D (increases phosphate absorption and excretion)

Calcium, serum

The serum calcium test is the most frequently performed test for evaluation of serum calcium levels. Approximately 1% of the total calcium in the body circulates in the blood. Of this, about 50% is bound to plasma proteins and 40% is ionized, or free. Evaluation of serum calcium levels measures the total amount of calcium circulating in the blood. Evaluation of ionized calcium levels measures the fraction of serum calcium that's in the ionized form, which is the most physiologically active form of serum calcium. The other 99% of the calcium in the body is stored in the bones and teeth. Serum calcium is needed for the proper function of many metabolic processes, muscle contraction, cardiac function, transmission of nerve impulses, blood clotting, and stability of plasma membrane permeability.

Parathyroid hormone (PTH), vitamin D, and calcitonin are the three substances that regulate calcium balance. PTH is secreted in response to low calcium levels and promotes movement from bone to plasma. PTH also activates vitamin D in the liver and kidney. The activated vitamin D circulates in the blood and promotes the absorption of dietary calcium from the small intestine. Calcitonin, produced by the thyroid gland, is secreted in response to high serum calcium levels and promotes movement of calcium from the blood to the bones.

Purpose
- To evaluate endocrine function, calcium metabolism, and acid-base balance
- To guide therapy in patients with renal failure, renal transplant, endocrine disorders, malignancies, cardiac disease, and skeletal disorders

Cost
Inexpensive

Patient preparation
- Explain to the patient that this test determines his blood calcium level.
- Tell the patient that the test requires a blood sample. Explain who will perform the venipuncture and when.
- Explain to the patient that he may experience discomfort from the needle puncture and the tourniquet.

Reference values
- *Total calcium:* 8.2 to 10.2 mg/dl (SI, 2.05 to 2.54 mmol/L) in adults; 8.6 to 11.2 mg/dl (SI, 2.15 to 2.79 mmol/L) in children
- *Ionized calcium:* 4.65 to 5.28 mg/dl (SI, 1.1 to 1.25 mmol/L).

Abnormal findings
Abnormally high serum calcium levels, or hypercalcemia, may occur in patients with hyperparathyroidism and parathyroid tumors (because of oversecretion of PTH), Paget's disease of the bone, multiple myeloma, metastatic carcinoma, multiple fractures, or prolonged immobilization. Elevated serum calcium levels may also result from inadequate excretion of calcium, as in adrenal insufficiency and renal disease; from excessive calcium ingestion; or from overuse of antacids such as calcium carbonate.

Low calcium levels, or hypocalcemia, may result from hypoparathyroidism, total parathyroidectomy, or malabsorption. Decreased serum levels of calcium may follow calcium loss in patients with Cushing's syndrome, renal failure, acute pancreatitis, or peritonitis.

Interfering factors
- Excessive ingestion of vitamin D or its derivatives (dihydrotachysterol, calcitriol) or the use of androgens, calciferol-activated

calcium salts, progestins-estrogens, or thiazide diuretics (possible increase)
- Chronic laxative use, excessive transfusions of citrated blood, and administration of acetazolamide, corticosteroids, or mithramycin
- Prolonged application of a tourniquet (may cause venous stasis and falsely increase calcium results)

Candida antibodies

Commonly present in the body, *Candida albicans* is a saprophytic yeast that can become pathogenic when the environment favors proliferation or the host's defenses have been significantly weakened. Candidiasis is usually limited to the skin and mucous membranes but may cause life-threatening systemic infection. Susceptibility to candidiasis is associated with antibacterial, antimetabolic, and corticosteroid therapy as well as with immunologic defects, pregnancy, obesity, diabetes, and debilitating diseases.

AGE ISSUE * * * * *
Oral candidiasis is common and benign in children; in adults, it may be an early indication of acquired immunodeficiency syndrome.

Diagnosis of candidiasis is usually made by culture or histologic study. When such diagnosis can't be made, identifying *Candida* antibodies may be helpful in diagnosing systemic candidiasis. Be cautioned that serologic testing to detect antibodies in candidiasis isn't reliable, and investigators continue to disagree about its usefulness.

Purpose
- To aid diagnosis of candidiasis when culture or histologic study can't confirm the diagnosis

Cost
Inexpensive

Patient preparation
- Explain to the patient the purpose of the test.
- Tell the patient that the test requires a blood sample. Explain who will perform the venipuncture and when.
- Explain to the patient that he may experience discomfort from the needle puncture and the tourniquet.
- Note recent antimicrobial therapy on the laboratory request form.

Normal findings
A normal test result is negative for *Candida* antibodies.

Abnormal findings
A positive test for *C. albicans* antibodies is common in patients with disseminated candidiasis. However, this test yields a significant percentage of false-positive results.

Interfering factors
- Hemolysis due to rough handling of the sample

Carbon dioxide content, total

Carbon dioxide (CO_2) is present in the body as an end product of metabolic processes as well as being present in small amounts in the air. When the pressure of CO_2 in the red cells exceeds 40 mm Hg, CO_2 flows out of the cells and dissolves in plasma. At this point, it combines with water to form carbonic acid, which in turn dissociates into hydrogen and bicarbonate ions.

This total CO_2 measures the total concentration of all such forms of CO_2 in serum, plasma, or whole blood samples.

Because about 90% of CO_2 in serum is in the form of bicarbonate, this test is a close approximation of bicarbonate levels. Total CO_2 content reflects the efficiency of the carbonic acid-bicarbonate buffer system, which maintains acid-base balance and normal pH. However, this test isn't highly accurate in measuring acid-base balance because exposure to air affects the CO_2 level in the specimen. For maximum clinical significance, test results must be considered with both pH and arterial blood gas values.

Purpose
■ To help evaluate acid-base balance

Cost
Inexpensive

Patient preparation
■ Explain to the patient that this test measures the amount of CO_2 in the blood.
■ Tell the patient that the test requires a blood sample. Explain who will perform the venipuncture and when.
■ Explain to the patient that he may experience discomfort from the needle puncture and the tourniquet.
■ Check the patient's history for use of medications that may influence CO_2 blood levels.

Reference values
Normally, total CO_2 levels range from 22 to 26 mEq/L (SI, 22 to 26 mmol/L). Levels may vary, depending on sex and age.

Abnormal findings
High CO_2 levels may occur in metabolic alkalosis (due to excessive ingestion or retention of base bicarbonate), respiratory acidosis (from hypoventilation, for example, as in emphysema or pneumonia), primary aldosteronism, and Cushing's syndrome. CO_2 levels may also be elevated after excessive loss of acids, as in severe vomiting and continuous gastric drainage.

Decreased CO_2 levels are common in metabolic acidosis (such as diabetic acidosis or renal tube acidosis caused by renal failure). Decreased total CO_2 levels in metabolic acidosis also result from loss of bicarbonate (as in severe diarrhea or intestinal drainage). Levels may also fall below normal in respiratory alkalosis (for example, from hyperventilation after trauma).

Interfering factors
■ Excessive use of corticotropin, cortisone, or thiazide diuretics or with excessive ingestion of alkalis or licorice (possible increase)
■ Use of salicylates, paraldehyde, methicillin, dimercaprol, ammonium chloride, or acetazolamide and after ingestion of ethylene glycol or methyl alcohol (possible decrease)
■ Underfilling of the collection tube (allows CO_2 to escape, resulting in inaccurate levels)

Carcinoembryonic antigen

Carcinoembryonic antigen (CEA) is a protein normally found in embryonic entodermal epithelium and fetal GI tissue. Production of CEA stops before birth, but it may begin again later if a neoplasm develops. Because CEA levels are also raised by biliary obstruction, alcoholic hepatitis, chronic heavy smoking, and other conditions, this test can't be used as a general indicator of cancer. The measurement of enzyme CEA levels by immunoassay is useful for staging and monitoring treatment of certain cancers, while other tests are used to diagnose certain types of cancer.

Purpose

■ To monitor the effectiveness of cancer therapy
■ To assist in preoperative staging of colorectal cancers, assess adequacy of surgical resection, and test for recurrence of colorectal cancers

Cost

Inexpensive

Patient preparation

■ Explain to the patient that this test detects and measures a special protein that isn't normally present in adults.
■ Inform the patient that the test will be repeated to monitor the effectiveness of therapy, if appropriate.
■ Tell the patient that the test requires a blood sample. Explain who will perform the venipuncture and when.
■ Explain to the patient that he may experience discomfort from the needle puncture and the tourniquet.

Reference values

Normal serum CEA values are less than 5 ng/ml (SI, < 5 mg/L).

Abnormal findings

Persistent elevation of CEA levels suggests residual or recurrent tumor. If levels exceed normal before surgical resection, chemotherapy, or radiation therapy, their return to normal within 6 weeks suggests successful treatment.

High CEA levels are characteristic in various malignant conditions, particularly entodermally derived neoplasms of the GI organs and lungs, and in certain nonmalignant conditions, such as benign hepatic disease, hepatic cirrhosis, alcoholic pancreatitis, and inflammatory bowel disease.

Elevated CEA concentrations may occur in nonendodermal carcinomas, such as breast and ovarian cancers.

Interfering factors

■ Chronic cigarette smoking (possible increase)

Cardiac blood pool imaging

Cardiac blood pool imaging evaluates regional and global ventricular performance after I.V. injection of human serum albumin or red blood cells tagged with the isotope technetium 99m pertechnetate. In first-pass imaging, a scintillation camera records the radioactivity emitted by the isotope in its initial pass through the left ventricle. Higher counts of radioactivity occur during diastole because the ventricle contains more blood; lower counts occur during systole as the blood is ejected. The portion of isotope that's ejected during each heartbeat can then be calculated to determine the ejection fraction; the presence and size of intracardiac shunts can also be determined. In addition, left ventricular regional wall motion may also be evaluated.

Gated cardiac blood pool imaging, performed after first-pass imaging or as a separate test, has several forms; however, most forms use signals from an electrocardiogram (ECG) to trigger the scintillation camera. In two-frame gated imaging, the camera records left ventricular end-systole and end-diastole for 500 to 1,000 cardiac cycles; superimposition of these gated images allows assessment of left ventricular contraction to find areas of dyskinesia or akinesia.

In multiple-gated acquisition (MUGA) scanning, the camera records 14 to 64 points of a single cardiac cycle, yielding sequential images that can be studied like motion picture films to evaluate regional wall motion and determine the ejection fraction and other indices of cardiac function. In the stress MUGA test, the same test is performed at rest and after exercise to detect changes in ejection fraction and cardiac output. In the nitro MUGA test, the scintillation camera records points in the cardiac cycle after the sublingual administration of nitroglycerin to assess the drug's effect on ventricular function.

Blood pool imaging is more accurate and involves less risk to the patient than left ventriculography in assessing cardiac function.

ALERT! ▼ ▼ ▼ ▼ ▼ ▼ ▼ ▼ ▼
Cardiac blood pool imaging is contraindicated during pregnancy.

Purpose
■ To evaluate left ventricular function
■ To detect aneurysms of the left ventricle and other myocardial wall-motion abnormalities (areas of akinesia or dyskinesia)
■ To detect intracardiac shunting

Cost
Expensive

Patient preparation
■ Explain to the patient that this test permits assessment of the heart's left ventricle.
■ Tell the patient who will perform the test and where it will take place.
■ Inform the patent that he'll be given an I.V. injection of a radioactive tracer and that a detector positioned above his chest will record the circulation of this tracer through the heart. Reassure him that the tracer poses no radiation hazard and rarely produces adverse effects.
■ Explain to the patient that he may experience discomfort from the needle puncture but that the imaging procedure itself is painless.
■ Tell the patient that he needs to remain silent and motionless during imaging unless otherwise instructed.
■ Obtain informed consent if necessary.

Reference values
The left ventricle contracts symmetrically, and the isotope appears evenly distributed in the scans. The normal ejection fraction is 55% to 65%.

Abnormal findings
Patients with coronary artery disease usually have asymptomatic blood distribution to the myocardium, which produces segmental abnormalities of ventricular wall motion; such abnormalities may also result from preexisting conditions such as myocarditis. In contrast, patients with cardiomyopathy exhibit globally reduced ejection fractions.

In patients with left-to-right shunts, the recirculating radioisotope prolongs the downslope of the curve of scintigraphic data; early arrival of activity in the left ventricle or aorta signifies a right-to-left shunt.

Interfering factors
None significant

Cardiac catheterization

Cardiac catheterization involves passing a catheter into the right or left side of the heart. Catheterization can determine blood pressure and blood flow in the chambers of the heart, permit collection of blood samples, and record films of the heart's ventricles (contrast ventriculography) or arteries (coronary arteriography or angiography).

In catheterization of the left side of the heart, a catheter is inserted into an artery in the antecubital fossa or into the femoral artery through a puncture or cutdown procedure. Guided by fluoroscopy, the catheter is advanced retrograde through the aorta into the coronary artery orifices and left ventricle. Then, a contrast medium is injected into the ventricle, permitting radiographic visualization of the ventricle and coronary arteries and filming (cineangiography) of heart activity.

Catheterization of the left side of the heart assesses the patency of the coronary arteries, mitral and aortic valve function, and left ventricular function. It aids diagnosis of left ventricular enlargement, aortic stenosis and insufficiency, aortic root enlargement, mitral insufficiency, aneurysm, and intracardiac shunt.

In catheterization of the right side of the heart, the catheter is inserted into an antecubital vein or the femoral vein and is advanced through the inferior vena cava or right atrium into the right side of the heart and the pulmonary artery. Catheterization of the right side of the heart assesses tricuspid and pulmonic valve function and pulmonary artery pressures.

ALERT! ▼ ▼ ▼ ▼ ▼ ▼ ▼ ▼ ▼
Coagulopathy, impaired renal function, and debilitation usually contraindicate catheterization of both sides of the heart. Unless a temporary pacemaker is inserted to counteract induced ventricular asystole, left bundle-branch block contraindicates catheterization of the right side of the heart.

Purpose
■ To evaluate valvular insufficiency or stenosis, septal defects, congenital anomalies, myocardial function and blood supply, and cardiac wall motion

Cost
Very expensive

Patient preparation
■ Explain to the patient that this test evaluates the function of the heart and its vessels.
■ Instruct the patient to restrict food and fluids for at least 6 hours before the test but

to continue his prescribed drug regimen unless directed otherwise.
■ Describe the test to the patient, including who will perform it and where it will take place.
■ Obtained informed consent if necessary.
■ Inform the patient that he may receive a mild sedative but will remain conscious during the procedure. Tell him that he'll lie on a padded table as the camera rotates so his heart can be examined from different angles.
■ Inform the patient that he'll have an I.V. needle inserted in his arm to administer medication. Assure him that the electrocardiography (ECG) electrodes attached to his chest during the procedure will cause no discomfort.
■ Tell the patient that the catheter will be inserted into an artery or a vein in his arm or leg; if the skin above the vessel is hairy, it'll be shaved and cleaned with an antiseptic.
■ Explain to the patient that he'll experience a transient stinging sensation when a local anesthetic is injected to numb the incision site for catheter insertion and that he may experience pressure as the catheter moves along the blood vessel. Assure him that these sensations are normal.
■ Inform the patient that injection of a contrast medium through the catheter may produce a hot, flushing sensation or nausea that quickly passes; instruct him to follow directions to cough or breathe deeply.
■ Explain to the patient that he'll be given medication if he experiences chest pain during the procedure and may also receive nitroglycerin periodically to dilate coronary vessels and aid visualization. Reassure him that complications, such as MI or thromboembolism, are rare. (See *Complications of cardiac catheterization.*)
■ Inform the patient that bed rest will be enforced for 8 hours. If the femoral route is

Complications of cardiac catheterization

Because cardiac catheterization is an invasive test that's usually performed on high-risk patients, it poses a greater risk than most other diagnostic tests. Although complications are rare, they're potentially life-threatening and require careful observation during the procedure.

Keep in mind that some complications are common to *both* left-sided and right-sided heart catheterization; others result only from catheterization of one side. In either case, complications require that you carefully document the complication and its treatment.

COMPLICATIONS AND POSSIBLE CAUSES	SIGNS AND SYMPTOMS
Left- or right-sided catheterization	
Myocardial infarction	
■ Emotional stress induced by procedure ■ Blood clot dislodged by catheter tip travels to a coronary artery (left-sided heart catheterization only) ■ Air embolism	■ Chest pain, possibly radiating to left arm, back, or jaw ■ Cardiac arrhythmias ■ Diaphoresis, restlessness, or anxiety ■ Thready pulse ■ Fever ■ Peripheral cyanosis, causing cool skin
Arrhythmias	
■ Cardiac tissue irritated by catheter	■ Irregular heartbeat ■ Irregular apical pulse ■ Palpitations
Cardiac tamponade	
■ Perforation of heart wall by catheter	■ Sudden shock ■ Arrhythmias ■ Increased heart rate ■ Decreased blood pressure ■ Chest pain ■ Diaphoresis and cyanosis ■ Distant heart sounds
Infection (systemic)	
■ Poor aseptic technique ■ Catheter contaminated during manufacture, storage, or use	■ Fever ■ Increased pulse rate ■ Chills and tremors ■ Unstable blood pressure
Hypovolemia	
■ Diuresis from contrast medium used in angiography	■ Increased urine output ■ Hypotension

(continued)

COMPLICATIONS AND POSSIBLE CAUSES	SIGNS AND SYMPTOMS
Left- or right-sided catheterization *(continued)*	
Hematoma or blood loss at insertion site ■ Bleeding at insertion site from vein or artery damage	■ Bloody dressing ■ Limb swelling ■ Decreased blood pressure ■ Increased heart rate
Reaction to contrast medium ■ Allergy to iodine	■ Fever ■ Agitation ■ Hives ■ Itching ■ Decreased urine output, indicating kidney failure
Pulmonary edema ■ Excessive fluid administration	■ *Early stage:* tachycardia, tachypnea, dependent crackles, diastolic (S_3) gallop ■ *Acute stage:* dyspnea; rapid, noisy respirations; cough with frothy, blood-tinged sputum; cyanosis with cold, clammy skin; tachycardia; hypertension
Infection at insertion site ■ Poor aseptic technique	■ Swelling, warmth, redness, and soreness at site ■ Purulent discharge at site
Left-sided catheterization	
Arterial embolus or thrombus in limb ■ Injury to artery during catheter insertion, causing blood clot ■ Plaque dislodged from artery wall by catheter	■ Slow or faint pulse distal to insertion site ■ Loss of warmth, sensation, and color in arm or leg distal to insertion site
Stroke ■ Blood clot or plaque dislodged by catheter tip travels to brain	■ Hemiplegia ■ Aphasia ■ Lethargy, confusion, decreased level of consciousness
Right-sided catheterization	
Thrombophlebitis ■ Vein damaged during catheter insertion	■ Hard, sore, cordlike, warm vein; may look like a red line above catheter insertion site ■ Swelling at site

COMPLICATIONS AND POSSIBLE CAUSES	SIGNS AND SYMPTOMS
Right-sided catheterization *(continued)*	
Pulmonary embolism	
■ Blood clot or plaque dislodged by catheter tip travels to lungs	■ Shortness of breath ■ Tachypnea ■ Increased heart rate ■ Chest pain
Vagal response	
■ Vagus nerve endings irritated in sinoatrial node, atrial muscle tissue, or atrioventricular junction ■ Complete heart block	■ Hypotension ■ Decreased heart rate ■ Nausea

to be used, tell the patient that his leg will be extended for 6 to 8 hours; if the antecubital fossa is to be used, let him know that his arm will be extended for at least 3 hours.

■ Document the patient's history for hypersensitivity to shellfish, iodine, or the contrast media used in other diagnostic tests.

■ Discontinue any anticoagulant therapy to reduce the risk of complications from venous bleeding.

ALERT! ▼ ▼ ▼ ▼ ▼ ▼ ▼ ▼ ▼

If the patient has valvular heart disease, prophylactic antimicrobial therapy may be indicated to guard against subacute bacterial endocarditis.

Normal findings

Cardiac catheterization should reveal no abnormalities of heart chamber size or configuration, wall motion or thickness, direction of blood flow, or valve motion; the coronary arteries should have a smooth and regular outline and vessels should be patent.

Cardiac catheterization provides information on pressures in the heart's chambers and vessels. Higher pressures than normal are clinically significant; lower pressures, except in shock, usually aren't significant. (See *Normal pressure curves*, page 88, and *Upper limits of normal pressures in cardiac chambers and great vessels in recumbent adults*, page 89.)

Abnormal findings

Common abnormalities confirmable by cardiac catheterization include coronary artery disease (CAD), myocardial incompetence, valvular heart disease, and septal defects.

In CAD, catheterization shows constriction of the lumen of the coronary arteries. Constriction greater than 70% is especially significant, particularly in proximal lesions. Narrowing of the left main coronary artery and occlusion or narrowing high in the left anterior descending artery are often indications for revascularization surgery. (This lesion responds best to coronary artery bypass grafting.)

Impaired wall motion can indicate myocardial incompetence from CAD, aneurysm, cardiomyopathy, or congenital anomalies. Comparing the size of the left

Normal pressure curves

Chambers of the right side of the heart

Two pressure complexes are represented for each chamber. Complexes at the far right in this diagram represent simultaneous recordings of pressures from the right atrium, right ventricle, and pulmonary artery.

Chambers of the left side of the heart

Overall pressure configurations are similar to those of the right side of the heart, but pressures in the left side of the heart are significantly higher because systemic flow resistance is much greater than pulmonary resistance.

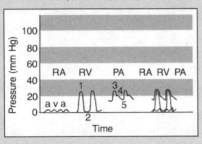

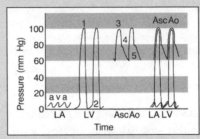

Key:

PA = Pulmonary artery
RV = Right ventricle
RA = Right atrium
a wave = Contraction
v wave = Passive filling
LV = Left ventricle

LA = Left atrium
AscAo = Ascending aorta
1 = RV peak systolic pressure
2 = RV end-diastolic pressure
3 = PA peak systolic pressure
4 = PA dicrotic notch
5 = PA diastolic pressure

ventricle in systole and diastole helps assess the efficiency of cardiac muscle contraction, segmental wall motion, chamber size, and ejection fraction. An ejection fraction under 35% generally increases the risk of complications and decreases the probability of successful surgery.

Valvular heart disease is indicated by a gradient, or difference in pressures, above and below a heart valve. For example, systolic pressure measurements on both sides of a stenotic aortic valve show a gradient across the valve. The higher the gradient, the greater the degree of stenosis. If left ventricular systolic pressure measures 200 mm Hg and aortic systolic pressure measures 120 mm Hg, the gradient across

the valve is 80 mm Hg. Because these pressures should normally be equal during systole, when the aortic valve is open, a gradient of this magnitude indicates the need for corrective surgery. Incompetent valves can be visualized during ventriculography by watching retrograde flow of the contrast medium across the valve during systole.

Septal defects (both atrial and ventricular) can be confirmed by measuring blood oxygen content in both sides of the heart. Elevated blood oxygen levels on the right side indicate a left-to-right atrial or ventricular shunt; decreased oxygen levels on the left side indicate a right-to-left shunt.

Cardiac output can be measured by analyzing blood oxygen levels in the cardiac

Upper limits of normal pressures in cardiac chambers and great vessels in recumbent adults

CHAMBER OR VESSEL	PRESSURE (mm Hg)
Right atrium	6 (mean)
Right ventricle	30/6*
Pulmonary artery	30/12* (mean, 18)
Left atrium	12 (mean)
Left ventricle	140/12*
Ascending aorta	140/90* (mean, 105)
Pulmonary artery wedge	Almost identical (±1 to 2 mm Hg) to left atrial mean pressure

* Peak systolic and end-diastolic

chambers. This may be accomplished by drawing blood from cardiac chambers or by injecting contrast medium into the venous circulation and measuring its concentration as it moves past a thermodilution catheter.

Interfering factors
■ Improperly functioning equipment and poor technique
■ Patient anxiety (increase in heart rate and cardiac chamber pressures)

Cardiac magnetic resonance imaging

A great asset in the diagnosis of cardiac disorders, magnetic resonance imaging (MRI) has the ability to see through bone and delineate fluid-filled soft tissue in great detail as well as produce images of organs and vessels in motion.

MRI relies on the magnetic properties of the atom. Hydrogen, the most abundant and magnetically sensitive of the body's atoms, is most commonly selected for MRI studies. The scanner uses a powerful magnetic field and radiofrequency (RF) energy to produce images based on the hydrogen (primarily water) content of body tissues. Exposed to an external magnetic field, positively charged electrons align uniformly in the field. RF energy is directed at the atoms, knocking them out of this magnetic alignment and causing them to precess, or spin. When the RF pulse is discontinued, the atoms realign themselves with the magnetic field, emitting RF energy as a tissue-specific signal based on the relative density of nuclei and the realignment time. These signals are monitored by the MRI computer, which processes them and displays information as a high-resolution video image.

MRI is contraindicated in patients with pacemakers, intracranial aneurysm clips, or other ferrous metal implants. Ventilators, I.V. infusion pumps, and other metallic or computer-based equipment also can't be used in the MRI area. Make sure the patient doesn't have any surgically implanted joints, pins, clips, valves, or pumps containing metal because such objects could be attracted to the strong MRI magnet. Ask if the patient has ever worked with metals or has any metal in his eyes. Some facilities may have a checklist that covers all pertinent questions. If he does have such devices, he won't be able to undergo the test.

Purpose

■ To identify anatomic sequelae related to myocardial infarction, such as formation of ventricular aneurysm, ventricular wall thinning, and mural thrombus
■ To detect and evaluate cardiomyopathy or pericardial disease
■ To identify paracardiac or intracardiac masses
■ To detect congenital heart disease, such as atrial or ventricular septal defects and the degree of malposition of the great vessel
■ To identify vascular disease, such as thoracic aneurysm and thoracic dissection
■ To assess the structure of the pulmonary vasculature

Cost

Very expensive

Patient preparation

■ Explain to the patient that this test assesses the function and structure of the heart.
■ Tell the patient who will perform the test, where it will be done, and that it takes up to 90 minutes.

■ Explain to the patient that although MRI is painless, he may experience discomfort because he must remain still inside a small space throughout the test. Ask if claustrophobia is an issue; if so, the patient might not be able to tolerate the procedure or might need sedation.
■ Inform the patient that he'll be positioned on a narrow bed that slides into a large cylinder that houses the MRI magnets. Tell him that the scanner will make clicking, whirring, and thumping noises as it moves but he'll be able to communicate with the technician at all times.
■ Obtain informed consent if appropriate.

Normal findings

MRI should reveal no anatomic or structural dysfunctions in cardiovascular tissue.

Abnormal findings

MRI can detect cardiomyopathy and pericardial disease as well as atrial or ventricular septal defects and other congenital defects. The test is also useful for identifying paracardiac or intracardiac masses and evaluating the extent of pericardial or vascular disease.

Interfering factors

■ Excessive patient movement (can blur images)

Cerebral angiography

Cerebral angiography involves injecting a contrast medium to allow radiographic examination of the cerebral vasculature. Possible injection sites include the femoral, carotid, and brachial arteries. Because it allows visualization of four vessels (the carotid and the vertebral arteries), the femoral artery is used most often.

Usually, this test is performed on patients with suspected abnormality of the cerebral vasculature; abnormalities may be suggested by intracranial computed tomography, lumbar puncture, magnetic resonance imaging, or magnetic resonance angiography.

ALERT! ▼ ▼ ▼ ▼ ▼ ▼ ▼ ▼ ▼

Check the patient's history for hypersensitivity to iodine, iodine-containing substances (such as shellfish), or other contrast media. Cerebral angiography is contraindicated in these patients, and in patients with hepatic, renal, or thyroid disease.

Purpose

■ To detect cerebrovascular abnormalities, such as aneurysm or arteriovenous malformation, thrombosis, narrowing, or occlusion
■ To study vascular displacement caused by tumor, hematoma, edema, herniation, vasospasm, increased intracranial pressure (ICP), or hydrocephalus
■ To locate clips applied to blood vessels during surgery and to evaluate the postoperative status of affected vessels

Cost

Very expensive

Patient preparation

■ Explain to the patient that this test shows blood circulation in the brain.
■ Describe the test to the patient, including who will perform it and where it will take place.
■ Tell the patient to fast for 8 to 10 hours before the test.
■ Order pretest blood work to determine bleeding tendency or kidney function. Anticoagulants may need to be discontinued for 3 days before the test.

■ Tell the patient that a sedative and an anticholinergic drug may be administered 30 to 45 minutes before the test if needed.
■ Tell the patient that he'll be positioned on an X-ray table with his head immobilized and that a local anesthetic will be administered

AGE ISSUE ✳ ✳ ✳ ✳ ✳

Some patients — especially children — receive a general anesthetic and will need to be monitored closely.

■ Explain to the patient that he'll feel a transient burning sensation as the medium is injected; a warm, flushed feeling; transient headache; a salty or metallic taste in his mouth; or nausea and vomiting after the dye is injected.
■ Obtain informed consent if necessary.
■ Inform the patient that he'll be on bed rest with his neurologic status monitored for 6 hours and the affected extremity immobilized and monitored carefully. The patient is usually discharged the same day.

Normal findings

During the arterial phase of perfusion, the contrast medium fills and opacities superficial and deep arteries and arterioles; it opacities superficial and deep veins during the venous phase. The finding of apparently normal (symmetrical) cerebral vasculature must be correlated with the patient's history and clinical status.

Abnormal findings

Changes in the caliber of vessel lumina suggest vascular disease, possibly due to spasms, plaques, fistulas, arteriovenous malformation, or arteriosclerosis. Diminished blood flow to vessels may be related to increased ICP.

Vessel displacement may reflect the presence and size of a tumor, areas of edema, or obstruction of the cerebrospinal fluid pathway. Cerebral angiography may also show circulation within a tumor, often giving precise information on the tumor's position and nature. Meningeal blood supply originating in the external carotid artery may indicate an extracerebral tumor but usually designates a meningioma. Such a tumor may arise outside the brain substance, but it may still be within the cerebral hemisphere.

Disorientation and weakness or numbness in the extremities may indicate thrombosis or hematoma; arterial spasms may produce symptoms of transient ischemic attacks.

Interfering factors
■ Head movement during the test (possible poor imaging)
■ Failure to remove metallic objects from the X-ray field (possible poor imaging)

Cerebrospinal fluid analysis

For qualitative analysis, cerebrospinal fluid (CSF) is most commonly obtained by lumbar puncture (usually between the third and fourth lumbar vertebrae) and, rarely, by cisternal or ventricular puncture. A CSF specimen may also be obtained during other neurologic tests such as myelography. Infection at the puncture site contraindicates removal of CSF; in a patient with increased intracranial pressure, CSF should be removed with extreme caution because the rapid reduction in pressure that follows withdrawal of fluid can cause cerebellar tonsillar herniation and medullary compression.

Normally, the CSF pressure is recorded and the appearance of the specimen is checked. Three tubes are collected routinely and are sent to the laboratory for analysis of protein, sugar, and cells as well as for

serologic testing, such as the Venereal Disease Research Laboratory test for neurosyphilis. A separate specimen is also sent to the laboratory for culture and sensitivity testing. Electrolyte analysis and Gram stain may be ordered as supplementary tests. CSF electrolyte levels are of special interest in patients with abnormal serum electrolyte levels or CSF infection and in those receiving hyperosmolar agents.

Purpose
■ To measure CSF pressure as an aid in detecting obstruction of CSF circulation
■ To aid diagnosis of viral or bacterial meningitis, subarachnoid or intracranial hemorrhage, tumors, brain abscesses, neurosyphilis, or chronic central nervous system infections
■ To check for Alzheimer's disease

Cost
Very expensive

Patient preparation
■ Describe the procedure to the patient, and explain that this test analyzes the fluid around the spinal cord. Tell him who will perform the procedure and where it will take place.
■ Advise the patient that a headache is the most common adverse effect of a lumbar puncture, but reassure him that his cooperation during the test helps minimize this effect.
■ Tell the patient that he may need to be supine or with his head elevated 30 degrees for 8 hours after lumbar puncture.
■ Obtain informed consent if necessary.

Findings
For a summary of normal and abnormal findings in CSF analysis, see *Analysis of cerebrospinal fluid.*

Analysis of cerebrospinal fluid

TEST	NORMAL	ABNORMAL	IMPLICATIONS
Pressure	50 to 180 mm H$_2$O	Increase	Increased intracranial pressure
		Decrease	Spinal subarachnoid obstruction above puncture site
Appearance	Clear, colorless	Cloudy	Infection
		Xanthochromic or bloody	Subarachnoid, intracerebral, or intraventricular hemorrhage; spinal cord obstruction; traumatic tap (usually noted only in initial specimen)
		Brown, orange, or yellow	Elevated protein levels, RBC breakdown (blood present for at least 3 days)
Protein	15 to 50 mg/dl (SI, 0.15 to 0.5 g/L)	Marked increase	Tumors, trauma, hemorrhage, diabetes mellitus, polyneuritis, blood in cerebral spinal fluid (CSF)
		Marked decrease	Rapid CSF production
Gamma globulin	3% to 12% of total protein	Increase	Demyelinating disease, neurosyphilis, Guillain-Barré Syndrome
Glucose	50 to 80 mg/dl (SI, 2.8 to 4.4 mmol/L)	Increase	Systemic hyperglycemia
		Decrease	Systemic hypoglycemia, bacterial or fungal infection, meningitis, mumps, postsubarachnoid hemorrhage
Cell count	0 to 5 white blood cells	Increase	Active disease: meningitis, acute infection, onset of chronic illness, tumor, abscess, infarction, demyelinating disease
	No red blood cells (RBCs)	RBCs	Hemorrhage or traumatic lumbar puncture
VDRL, test for syphilis, and other serologic tests	Nonreactive	Positive	Neurosyphilis
Chloride	118 to 130 mEq/L (SI, 118 to 130 mmol/L)	Decrease	Infected meninges
Gram stain	No organisms	Gram-positive or gram-negative organisms	Bacterial meningitis

Interfering factors

■ Patient position and activity (possible increase or decrease)
■ Crying, coughing, or straining (possible increase)
■ Delay between collection time and laboratory testing (possible invalidation of test results, especially cell counts)

Cervical punch biopsy

Cervical punch biopsy is the excision by sharp forceps of a tissue specimen from the cervix for histologic examination. Generally, multiple biopsies are done to obtain specimens from all areas with abnormal tissue or from the squamocolumnar junction and other sites around the cervical circumference.

Biopsy sites are selected by direct visualization of the cervix with a colposcope, which is the most accurate method, or by Schiller's test, which stains normal squamous epithelium a dark mahogany but fails to color abnormal tissue. (For information on other biopsies done to detect gynecologic disorders, see *Endometrial and ovarian biopsies.*)

Purpose

■ To evaluate suspicious cervical lesions
■ To diagnose cervical cancer

Cost

Expensive

Patient preparation

■ Describe the procedure to the patient, and explain that it provides a cervical tissue specimen for microscopic study.
■ Tell the patient who will perform the biopsy and where it will be done. Explain that she may experience discomfort during and after the procedure and that someone must accompany her home.
■ Obtain informed consent if necessary.
■ Instruct the patient to avoid strenuous exercise for 8 to 24 hours after the biopsy. Also, if a tampon was inserted after the biopsy, tell her to leave it in place for 8 to 24 hours. Inform her that some bleeding may occur, but to report heavy bleeding (heavier than menstrual). Warn the patient against using tampons, which can irritate the cervix and provoke bleeding. She should also avoid douching and refrain from sexual intercourse for up to 2 weeks, as appropriate.
■ Inform the patient that a foul-smelling, gray-green vaginal discharge is normal for several days after the biopsy and may persist for 3 weeks.

Normal findings

Cervical tissue should be composed of columnar and squamous epithelial cells, loose connective tissue, and smooth-muscle fibers, with no dysplasia or abnormal cell growth.

Abnormal findings

Histologic examination of a cervical tissue specimen identifies abnormal cells and differentiates the tissue as intraepithelial neoplasia or invasive cancer. If the cause of an abnormal Papanicolaou test isn't demonstrated by cervical biopsy or if the specimen shows advanced dysplasia or carcinoma in situ, a cone biopsy is performed in the operating room under general anesthesia. A cone biopsy garners a larger tissue

Endometrial and ovarian biopsies

METHOD	PURPOSE	SPECIAL CONSIDERATIONS
Endometrial biopsy ■ Dilatation and curettage (D&C) ■ Endometrial washing (by jet irrigation, aspiration, or brushing)	■ To evaluate uterine bleeding ■ To diagnose suspected endometrial cancer ■ To diagnose a missed abortion	■ Time of menstrual cycle affects accuracy of biopsy results. ■ Type of specimen obtained depends on patient's age and disorder. ■ Endometrial washing requires no anesthesia and can be done in a physician's office. ■ D&C by endometrial washing may follow a negative biopsy. ■ Specimens obtained by D&C may be processed as frozen sections.
Ovarian biopsy ■ Transrectal or transvaginal fine-needle biopsy ■ Aspiration biopsy during laparoscopy	■ To detect an ovarian tumor ■ To determine the spread of cancer	■ Fine-needle biopsy may follow palpation, laparoscopy, or computed tomography that detects an abnormal ovary. ■ Aspiration during laparoscopy is particularly useful for young women who are infertile or who have lesions that appear benign.

specimen and allows a more accurate evaluation of dysplasia.

Interfering factors

■ Failure to obtain representative specimens or to place them in the preservative immediately

Chest radiography

In chest radiography, X-rays or electromagnetic waves penetrate the chest and cause an image to form on specially sensitized film. Normal pulmonary tissue is radiolucent, whereas abnormalities — such as infiltrates, foreign bodies, fluids, and tumors — appear as densities on the film. A chest X-ray is most useful when compared with prior films to detect changes. (See *Se-*

lected clinical implications of chest X-ray films, pages 96 and 97.)

ALERT! ▼ ▼ ▼ ▼ ▼ ▼ ▼ ▼ ▼

Chest radiography is usually contraindicated during the first trimester of pregnancy; however, when radiography is absolutely necessary, a lead apron placed over the patient's abdomen can shield the fetus.

Purpose

■ To detect pulmonary disorders (pneumonia, atelectasis, pneumothorax, pulmonary bullae, pleurisy, and tumors) or mediastinal abnormalities (tumors and cardiac disease such as heart failure)
■ To determine correct placement of pulmonary catheters, endotracheal tubes, and other chest tubes
■ To determine the location and size of lesions or foreign bodies (coins, broken central lines) that were swallowed or aspirated

Selected clinical implications of chest X-ray films

Chest X-rays can reveal needed information to help identify abnormalities, which can hasten treatment to prevent patient deterioration. Abnormalities and their complications are reviewed below with their corresponding anatomic locations.

NORMAL ANATOMIC LOCATION AND APPEARANCE	POSSIBLE ABNORMALITY	IMPLICATIONS
Trachea Visible midline in the anterior mediastinal cavity; translucent tubelike appearance	■ Deviation from midline ■ Narrowing with hourglass appearance and deviation to one side	■ Tension pneumothorax, atelectasis, pleural effusion, consolidation, mediastinal nodes or, in children, enlarged thymus ■ Substernal thyroid *or* stenosis secondary to trauma
Heart Visible in the anterior left mediastinal cavity; solid appearance due to blood contents; edges may be clear in contrast with surrounding air density of the lung	■ Shift ■ Hypertrophy of right heart ■ Cardiac borders obscured by stringy densities ("haggy heart")	■ Atelectasis, pneumothorax ■ Cor pulmonale, heart failure ■ Cystic fibrosis
Aortic knob Visible as water density; formed by the arch of the aorta	■ Solid densities, possibly indicating calcifications ■ Tortuous shape	■ Atherosclerosis ■ Atherosclerosis
Mediastinum (mediastinal shadow) Visible as the space between the lungs; shadowy appearance that widens at the hilum of the lungs	■ Deviation to nondiseased side; deviation to diseased side by traction ■ Gross widening	■ Pleural effusion or tumor, fibrosis or collapsed lung ■ Neoplasms of esophagus, bronchi, lungs, thyroid, thymus, peripheral nerves, lymphoid tissue; aortic aneurysm; mediastinitis; cor pulmonale
Ribs Visible as thoracic cavity encasement	■ Break or misalignment ■ Widening of intercostal spaces	■ Fractured sternum or ribs ■ Emphysema
Spine Visible midline in the posterior chest; straight bony structure	■ Spinal curvature ■ Break or misalignment	■ Scoliosis, kyphosis ■ Fractures

Selected clinical implications of chest X-ray films *(continued)*

NORMAL ANATOMIC LOCATION AND APPEARANCE	POSSIBLE ABNORMALITY	IMPLICATIONS
Clavicles Visible in upper thorax; intact and equidistant in properly centered X-ray films	■ Break or misalignment	■ Fractures
Hila (lung roots) Visible above the heart, where pulmonary vessels, bronchi, and lymph nodes join the lungs; appear as small, white, bilateral densities	■ Shift to one side ■ Accentuated shadows	■ Atelectasis ■ Pneumothorax, emphysema, pulmonary abscess, tumor, enlarged lymph nodes
Mainstem bronchus Visible; part of the hila with translucent tubelike appearance	■ Spherical or oval density	■ Bronchogenic cyst
Bronchi Usually not visible	■ Visible	■ Bronchial pneumonia
Lung fields Usually not visible throughout, except for the blood vessels	■ Visible ■ Irregular	■ Atelectasis ■ Resolving pneumonia, infiltrates, silicosis, fibrosis, metastatic neoplasm
Hemidiaphragm Rounded, visible; right side ⅜″ to ¾″ (1 to 2 cm)	■ Elevation of diaphragm (difference in elevation can be measured on inspiration and expiration to detect movement) ■ Flattening of diaphragm ■ Unilateral elevation of either side ■ Unilateral elevation of left side only	■ Active tuberculosis, pneumonia, pleurisy, acute bronchitis, active disease of the abdominal viscera, bilateral phrenic nerve involvement, atelectasis ■ Asthma, emphysema ■ Possible unilateral phrenic nerve paresis ■ Perforated ulcer (rare), gas distention of stomach or splenic flexure of colon, free air in abdomen

■ To help assess pulmonary status
■ To evaluate response to interventions

Cost
Moderately expensive

Patient preparation
■ Explain to the patient that this test assesses respiratory status.
■ Describe the test to the patient, including who will perform it and when it will take place.

■ Explain to the patient that he'll be asked to take a deep breath and to hold it momentarily while the film is being taken to provide a clearer view of pulmonary structures.

Findings

For an overview of normal and abnormal chest radiography findings, see the accompanying chart. For an accurate diagnosis, radiography findings must be correlated with the results of additional radiologic and pulmonary tests as well as physical assessment findings. For example, pulmonary hyperinflation with low diaphragm and generalized increased radiolucency may suggest emphysema but may also occur in a healthy person.

Interfering factors

■ Portable chest X-rays (possibly lower quality image than stationary X-rays)
■ Portable chest X-rays taken in the anteroposterior position (may show larger cardiac shadowing than other X-rays due to shorter distance between beam and anterior structures)
■ Patient supine (hides fluid levels that are visible in decubitus views)
■ Age and sex of the patient
■ Patient's inability to take a full inspiration
■ Underexposure or overexposure of films
■ Incorrect view of the area (for example, lateral film views reveal infiltrates [pneumonia, atelectasis] that may not be seen in anteroposterior views or posteroanterior views because of heart obstruction)

Chest tomography

Also called *laminagraphy, planigraphy, stratigraphy,* or *body section roentgenography,* chest tomography provides clearly focused radiographic images of selected body sections otherwise obscured by shadows of overlying or underlying structures. In this procedure, the X-ray tube and film move around the patient in opposite directions (a motion called the linear tube sweep), producing exposures in which a selected body plane appears sharply defined and the areas above and below it are blurred. Some facilities have spiral computed tomography (CT) available to further evaluate chest lesions when other tests are inconclusive. In more modern facilities, CT has superseded plain film tomography.

ALERT! ▼ ▼ ▼ ▼ ▼ ▼ ▼ ▼ ▼
Tomography is contraindicated during pregnancy.

Purpose

■ To demonstrate pulmonary densities (for cavitation, calcification, and presence of fat), tumors (especially those obstructing the bronchial lumen), or lesions (especially those located deep within the mediastinum such as at lymph nodes at the hilum)
■ To evaluate severity of disease such as emphysema

Cost

Expensive

Patient preparation

■ Explain to the patient that this test helps evaluate lesions inside the chest.
■ Describe the test to the patient, including who will perform it and where it will take place.
■ Warn the patient that the equipment is noisy because of rapidly moving metal-on-metal parts and that the X-ray tube swings overhead.

Normal findings

A normal chest tomogram shows structures equivalent to those seen on a normal chest radiograph film.

Abnormal findings

Central calcification in a nodule suggests a benign lesion; an irregularly bordered tumor suggests malignancy; a sharply defined tumor suggests granuloma or nonmalignancy. Evaluation of the hilum can help differentiate blood vessels from nodes, detect tumor extension into the hilar lung area, and identify bronchial dilation, stenosis, and endobronchial lesions. Tomography can also identify extension of a mediastinal lesion to the ribs or spine.

Interfering factors

■ Failure to remove all metallic objects within the X-ray field (possible poor imaging)
■ Uncooperative patient

Chlamydia

The most common sexually transmitted disease in the United States, chlamydia is caused by the organism *Chlamydia trachomatis*. Identification of this parasite requires cultivation in the laboratory. After incubation, *Chlamydia*-infected cells can be detected by fluorescein isothiocyanate–conjugated monoclonal antibodies or by iodine stain. Detection in cell cultures of *C. psittaci* and *C. pneumoniae* requires specific technical manipulations and reagents; deoxyribonucleic acid detection may also be performed in women who may be susceptible to the infections, whether they have symptoms or not.

Culture is the detection method of choice, but rapid noncultural (antigen detection) procedures are also available.

Purpose

■ To confirm infections caused by *C. trachomatis*

Cost

Moderately expensive

Patient preparation

■ Explain the purpose of the test to the patient.
■ Describe the procedure for collecting a specimen for culture.
■ If the specimen will be collected from the patient's genital tract, instruct the patient not to urinate for 3 to 4 hours before the specimen is taken.
■ Tell a female patient not to douche for 24 hours before the test.
■ Tell a male patient that he may experience some burning and pressure as the culture is taken but that the discomfort will subside after a few minutes.
ALERT! ▼ ▼ ▼ ▼ ▼ ▼ ▼ ▼ ▼
In patients suspected of being sexually abused, be sure specimens are processed by culture rather than by antigen detection methods.
■ Advise the patient to avoid all sexual contact until after test results are available.

Normal findings

Normally, no *C. trachomatis* appears in the culture.

Abnormal findings

A positive culture confirms *C. trachomatis* infection.

Interfering factors

■ Using an antimicrobial drug within a few days before specimen collection (possible inability to recover *C. trachomatis*)
■ In males, voiding within 1 hour of specimen collection; in females, douching within 24 hours of specimen collection (fewer organisms available for culture)

- Failure to use proper collection technique
- Contamination of the specimen due to fecal material in a rectal culture

Chloride

The chloride test is used to measure serum levels of chloride, the major extracellular fluid anion. Chloride helps maintain osmotic pressure of blood and, therefore, helps regulate blood volume and arterial pressure. Chloride levels also affect acid-base balance. Chloride is absorbed from the intestines and excreted primarily by the kidneys.

Purpose
- To detect acid-base imbalance (acidosis or alkalosis) and to aid evaluation of fluid status and extracellular cation-anion balance

Cost
Inexpensive

Patient preparation
- Explain to the patient that the test is used to evaluate the chloride content of blood.
- Tell the patient that the test requires a blood sample. Explain who will perform the venipuncture and when.
- Explain to the patient that he may experience discomfort from the needle puncture and the tourniquet.
- Restrict medications that may affect test results. If they must be continued, note this on the laboratory request.

Reference values
Normally, serum chloride levels range from 100 to 108 mEq/L (SI, 100 to 108 mmol/L) in adults.

Abnormal findings
Chloride levels are inversely related to bicarbonate levels, reflecting acid-base balance. Excessive loss of gastric juices or other secretions containing chloride may cause hypochloremic metabolic alkalosis; excessive chloride retention or ingestion may lead to hyperchloremic metabolic acidosis.

Elevated serum chloride levels may result from severe dehydration, complete renal shutdown, head injury (producing neurogenic hyperventilation), and primary aldosteronism.

Low chloride levels are usually associated with low sodium and potassium levels. Possible underlying causes include prolonged vomiting, gastric suctioning, intestinal fistula, chronic renal failure, and Addison's disease. Heart failure or edema resulting in excess extracellular fluid can cause dilutional hypochloremia.

Interfering factors
- Hemolysis due to rough handling of the sample
- Use of ammonium chloride, cholestyramine, boric acid, oxyphenbutazone, or phenylbutazone and excessive I.V. infusion of sodium chloride (possible increase)
- Use of thiazide diuretics, ethacrynic acid, furosemide, or bicarbonates and prolonged I.V. infusion of dextrose 5% in water (decrease)

Cholecystography, oral

Oral cholecystography is the radiographic examination of the gallbladder after administration of a contrast medium. This test is commonly replaced by nuclear medicine technetium 99m-labeled scan, ultrasound, and computerized tomography. It's indicated in patients with signs of biliary tract disease (such as right upper quadrant epigastric pain, fat intolerance, and jaundice) and is most commonly used to confirm gallbladder disease.

After the contrast medium is ingested, it's absorbed by the small intestine, filtered by the liver, excreted in the bile, and then concentrated and stored in the gallbladder. Full gallbladder opacification usually occurs 12 to 14 hours after ingestion, at which time a series of X-rays are done to record gallbladder appearance. Additional information is obtained by giving the patient a fat stimulus, causing the gallbladder to contract and empty the contrast-laden bile into the common bile duct and small intestine. X-rays are then taken to record this emptying and to evaluate patency of the common bile duct.

Oral cholecystography should precede barium studies because retained barium may cloud subsequent X-rays.

ALERT! ▼ ▼ ▼ ▼ ▼ ▼ ▼ ▼ ▼
Oral cholecystography is contraindicated in patients with severe renal or hepatic damage and in those with a hypersensitivity to iodine, seafood, or contrast media. The test is also contraindicated in patients who are pregnant because of the radiation's possible teratogenic effects.

Purpose
- To detect gallstones
- To aid diagnosis of inflammatory disease and tumors of the gallbladder

Cost
Very expensive

Patient preparation
- Explain to the patient that this procedure permits examination of the gallbladder through X-rays taken after ingestion of a contrast medium.

- Describe the test to the patient, including who will perform it and where it will take place.
- Instruct the patient to eat a normal meal at noon the day before the test and a fat-free meal in the evening. The former stimulates release of bile from the gallbladder, preparing it to receive the contrast-laden bile; the latter inhibits gallbladder contraction, promoting accumulation of bile.
- Instruct the patient to restrict food and fluids after the evening meal, except water.
- Tell the patient that he'll receive an oral contrast agent after the evening meal, as necessary; water, cigarettes, and gum need to be withheld afterward.
- Tell the patient that he'll be placed on an X-ray table and that X-rays will be taken of his gallbladder.
- Document the patient's history for hypersensitivity to iodine, seafood, or contrast media used for other diagnostic tests.
- Inform the patient about the adverse effects of dye ingestion: diarrhea (common) and, rarely, nausea, vomiting, abdominal cramps, and dysuria. Tell him to report such signs and symptoms immediately if they develop.
- Tell the patient that he may receive an enema the morning of the test to clear the GI tract of interfering shadows that may obscure the gallbladder.

Normal findings
The gallbladder is normally opacified and appears pear shaped, with smooth, thin walls. Although its size is variable, its basic structure — neck, infundibulum, body, and fundus — is clearly outlined on film.

Abnormal findings
When the gallbladder is opacified, filling defects (typically appearing within the lumen as negative shadows that show mobil-

ity) indicate the presence of gallstones. Fixed defects, on the other hand, may indicate the presence of cholesterol polyps or a benign tumor such as an adenomyoma.

When the gallbladder fails to opacify or when only faint opacification occurs, inflammatory disease such as cholecystitis — with or without gallstone formation — may be present. Gallstones may obstruct the cystic duct and prevent the contrast medium from entering the gallbladder; inflammation may impair the concentrating ability of the gallbladder mucosa and prevent or diminish opacification.

If the gallbladder fails to contract after stimulation by a fatty meal, cholecystitis or common bile duct obstruction may be the cause. If the X-rays are inconclusive, oral cholecystography will need to be repeated the following day.

Interfering factors

■ Failure to follow dietary restrictions
■ Failure to ingest the full dose of contrast medium or partial loss of contrast medium through vomiting or diarrhea (possible invalid test results)
■ Inadequate absorption of the contrast medium in the small intestine or barium retained from previous studies (possible invalid test results)
■ Decreased excretion of the contrast medium into the bile due to impaired hepatic function and moderate jaundice (possible poor imaging)

Cholesterol

The quantitative analysis of serum cholesterol measures the circulating levels of free cholesterol and cholesterol esters; it reflects the level of the two forms in which this biochemical compound appears in the body.

Cholesterol, a structural component in cell membranes and plasma lipoproteins, is absorbed from the diet and synthesized in the liver and other body tissues. The body uses cholesterol for numerous functions, including steroid and hormone synthesis (sex hormones as well as adrenal steroids), cell membrane biogenesis, and formation of bile acids. The human body can produce all the cholesterol it requires, although researchers estimate that 20% to 40% is obtained through diet. A diet high in saturated fat raises cholesterol levels by stimulating absorption of lipids, including cholesterol, from the intestine; a diet low in saturated fat lowers cholesterol levels. High serum cholesterol levels may be associated with an increased risk of atherosclerosis-related diseases, especially coronary artery disease (CAD).

ALERT! ▼ ▼ ▼ ▼ ▼ ▼ ▼ ▼ ▼
Cholesterol levels shouldn't be measured immediately after a myocardial infarction (MI) because of falsely low readings. In these patients, cholesterol levels should be evaluated 3 months after the MI.

Purpose

■ To assess the risk of atherosclerosis and CAD
■ To evaluate fat metabolism
■ To aid in monitoring the effects of other disease processes, such as nephrotic syndrome, diabetes mellitus, pancreatitis, hepatic disease, and hypothyroidism and hyperthyroidism
■ To assess the efficacy of lipid-lowering drug therapy

Cost

Inexpensive

Patient preparation

■ Explain to the patient that this test determines the body's fat metabolism to detect disorders of blood lipids that may indicate risk of atherosclerotic diseases, especially CAD.

■ Tell the patient that fasting isn't necessary for isolated cholesterol checks or screening, but that it is required if part of a lipid profile. If fasting is required, instruct the patient to abstain from food and drink for 12 hours before the test.
■ Tell the patient that the test requires a blood sample. Explain who will perform the venipuncture and when.
■ Explain to the patient that he may experience discomfort from the needle puncture and the tourniquet.
■ Restrict medications that may affect test results. If they must be continued, note this on the laboratory request.

Reference values

Total cholesterol levels vary with age and sex. Total cholesterol values for adults and children are as follows:
■ *Adults:* desirable: < 200 mg/dl (SI, < 5.2 mmol/L); borderline high: 200 to 239 mg/dl (5.2 to 6.2 mmol/L); high: ≥ 239 mg/dl (SI, ≥ 6.2 mmol/L).
■ *Children and adolescents ages 12 to 18:* desirable: < 170 mg/dl (SI, < 4.39 mmol/ L); borderline high: 170 to 199 mg/dl (SI, 4.40 to 5.16 mmol/L); high: ≥ 200 mg/dl (SI, ≥ 5.17 mmol/L).

Abnormal findings

The cholesterol level needs to be evaluated in the context of the entire risk factor analysis for each individual patient. If the level is abnormal, a second cholesterol test should be completed in 1 week to verify the results. Marked fluctuations can occur from day to day. A decision to begin treatment will be based on the number of risk factors and a patient's prior cardiovascular history.

An elevated serum cholesterol level (hypercholesterolemia) may indicate an increased risk for CAD as well as incipient hepatitis, lipid disorders, bile duct blockage, nephrotic syndrome, obstructive jaundice, pancreatitis, and hypothyroidism. Hypercholesterolemia associated with increased intake of fats and cholesterol-rich foods requires dietary changes and, possibly, medication to retard absorption of cholesterol.

A low serum cholesterol level (hypocholesterolemia) is commonly associated with malnutrition, cellular necrosis of the liver, or hyperthyroidism. Abnormal cholesterol levels commonly require further testing to pinpoint the causative disorder, depending on the type of abnormality and the presence of overt signs. Abnormal levels associated with cardiovascular diseases, for example, may require lipoprotein phenotyping.

ALERT! ▼ ▼ ▼ ▼ ▼ ▼ ▼ ▼ ▼
If a genetic lipid disorder is discovered, family members should be screened for cholesterol abnormalities.

Interfering factors

■ Failure to follow dietary restrictions
■ Cholestyramine, clofibrate, colestipol, dextrothyroxine, haloperidol, neomycin, niacin, and chlortetracycline (possible decrease)
■ Epinephrine, chlorpromazine, trifluoperazine, hormonal contraceptives, and trimethadione (possible increase)
■ Androgens (variable effect)
■ Various antibiotics (possible false-low)
■ Various vitamins (possible false-high)
■ Pregnancy (possible increase)
■ Time of year (may cause higher values in winter and fall and lower values in spring and summer)
■ Emotional stress
■ Menstrual cycle

Chromosome analysis

Chromosome analysis studies the relationship between the microscopic appearance of chromosomes and an individual's phenotype — the expression of the genes in physical, biochemical, or physiologic traits.

Ideally, chromosomes are studied during metaphase, the middle phase of mitosis, when new cell poles appear. During metaphase, colchicine (a cell poison) is added to arrest cell division. Cells are harvested, stained, and then examined under a microscope. These cells are then photographed to record the karyotype — the systematic arrangement of chromosomes in groupings according to size and shape.

Only rapidly dividing cells, such as bone marrow or neoplastic cells, permit direct, immediate study. In other cells, mitosis is stimulated by the addition of phytohemagglutinin. Indications for the test determine the specimen required (blood, bone marrow, amniotic fluid, skin, or placental tissue) and the specific analytic procedure.

Purpose
■ To identify chromosomal abnormalities, such as hypoploidy or hyperploidy, as the underlying cause of malformation, maldevelopment, or disease

Cost
Very expensive

Patient preparation
■ Explain to the patient or a responsible family member, if appropriate, the purpose of this test.
■ Tell the patient who will perform the test and what kind of specimen will be required. (See *Percutaneous umbilical blood sampling.*)

■ Inform the patient when results will be available, according to the specimen required.

Normal findings
The normal cell contains 46 chromosomes: 22 pairs of nonsex chromosomes (autosomes) and 1 pair of sex chromosomes (Y for the male-determining chromosome, X for the female-determining chromosome). On a karyotype, chromosomes are arranged according to size and the location of their primary constrictions, or centromeres. The centromere may be medial (metacentric), slightly to one end of the chromosome (submetacentric), or entirely to one end (acrocentric). The largest chromosomes are displayed first; the others are arranged in order of decreasing size, with the two sex chromosomes traditionally placed last. By convention, the centromere is always placed at the top in a karyotype. Thus, if the two pairs of chromosomal arms are of unequal length, the arm above the centromere will be shorter. The letter "p" designates the short arm; the letter "q," the long arm.

Special stains identify individual chromosomes and locate and enumerate particular portions of chromosomes. Trypsin, alkali, heat denaturation, and Giemsa stain are used for visible light microscopy; quinacrine stain, for ultraviolet microscopy. These techniques produce nonuniform staining of each chromosome in a repetitive, banded pattern. The mechanism of chromosome banding is unknown, but seems related to primary deoxyribonucleic acid sequence and protein composition of the chromosome.

Abnormal findings
Implications of chromosome analysis results depend on the specimen and indica-

Percutaneous umbilical blood sampling

Useful in chromosomal analysis, percutaneous umbilical blood sampling (PUBS) provides a fetal blood sample for karyotype, direct Coombs' test, or complete blood cell count. PUBS, sometimes called cordocentesis, can also be used to determine fetal blood type, check blood gas levels and acid-base status, and identify and treat isoimmunization.

To obtain a percutaneous umbilical blood sample, a needle is inserted transabdominally (using ultrasound guidance) into a fetal umbilical vessel. A blood sample is then tested to ensure that fetal and not maternal blood has been drawn. Possible complications include blood leakage at the puncture site, fetal bradycardia, or infection.

tions for the test. (See *Chromosome analysis findings,* page 106 and 107.)

Chromosomal abnormalities may be numerical or structural. Any numerical deviation from the norm of 46 chromosomes is called aneuploidy. Less than 46 chromosomes is called hypoploidy; more than 46, hyperploidy. Special designations exist for whole multiples of the haploid number 23: diploidy for the normal somatic number of 46, triploidy for 69, tetraploidy for 92, and so forth.

When the deviation occurs within a single pair of chromosomes, the suffix "-somy" is used, as in trisomy for the presence of three chromosomes instead of the usual pair or monosomy for the presence of only one chromosome.

Aneuploidy most commonly follows failure of the chromosomal pair to separate (nondisjunction) during anaphase, the mitotic stage that follows metaphase. It may also result from anaphase lag, in which one of the normally separated chromosomes fails to move to a pole and is left out of the daughter cells.

If nondisjunction or anaphase lag occurs during meiosis, the cells of the zygote will all be the same. Errors in mitotic division after zygote formation will produce more than one cell line (mosaicism).

Structural chromosomal abnormalities result from chromosome breakage. Intrachromosomal rearrangement occurs within a single chromosome in the following forms:
- *Deletion:* loss of an end (terminal) or middle (interstitial) portion of a chromosome
- *Inversion:* end-to-end reversal of a chromosome segment, which may be pericentric inversion (including the centromere) or paracentric inversion (occurring in only one arm of the chromosome)
- *Ring chromosome formation:* breakage of both ends of a chromosome and reunion of the ends
- *Isochromosome formation:* abnormal splitting of the centromere in a transverse rather than a longitudinal plane.

Interchromosomal rearrangements (of more than one chromosome, usually two) also occur. The most common rearrangement is translocation, or exchange, of genetic material between two chromosomes. Translocations may be balanced, in which the cell neither loses nor gains genetic material; unbalanced, in which a piece of genetic material is gained or lost from each cell; reciprocal (in children), in which two chromosomes exchange material; or Robertsonian, in which two chromosomes

Chromosome analysis findings

SPECIMEN AND INDICATION	RESULT	IMPLICATIONS
Blood ▪ To evaluate abnormal appearance of development suggesting chromosomal irregularity	▪ Abnormal chromosome number (aneuploidy) or arrangement	▪ Identifies specific chromosomal abnormality
▪ To evaluate couples with history of miscarriages or to identify balanced translocation carriers having unbalanced offspring	▪ Normal chromosomes ▪ Parental balanced translocation carrier	▪ Miscarriage unrelated to parental chromosomal abnormality ▪ Increased risk of repeated abortion or unbalanced offspring indicates need for amniocentesis in future pregnancies
▪ To detect chromosomal rearrangements in rare genetic diseases predisposing patient to malignant neoplasms	▪ Chromosomal rearrangements, gaps, and breaks	▪ Occurs in Bloom's syndrome, Fanconi's syndrome, telangiectasia; patient predisposed to malignant neoplasms
Blood or bone marrow ▪ To identify Philadelphia chromosome and confirm chronic myelogenous leukemia	▪ Translocation of chromosome 22q (long arm) to another chromosome (often chromosome 9) ▪ Aneuploidy (usually due to abnormalities in chromosomes 8 and 12) ▪ Trisomy 21	▪ Aids diagnosis of chronic myelogenous leukemia ▪ Occurs in acute myelogenous leukemia ▪ Occasionally occurs in chronic lymphocytic leukemia cells
Skin ▪ To evaluate abnormal appearance or development, suggesting chromosomal irregularity	▪ All chromosomal abnormalities are possible	▪ Same as chromosomal abnormality in blood; rarely, mosaic individual has normal blood but abnormal skin chromosomes
Amniotic fluid ▪ To evaluate developing fetus with possible chromosomal abnormality	▪ All chromosomal abnormalities are possible	▪ Same as chromosomal abnormality in blood or fetus
Placental tissue ▪ To evaluate products of conception after a miscarriage to determine if abnormality is fetal or placental in origin	▪ All chromosomal abnormalities are possible	▪ More than 50% of aborted tissue is chromosomally abnormal

SPECIMEN AND INDICATION	RESULT	IMPLICATIONS
Tumor tissue ■ For research purposes only	■ Many chromosomal abnormalities are possible	■ Although malignant tumors aren't associated with specific chromosomal aberrations, most are aneuploid (usually hyperploid)

join to form one combined chromosome, with little or no loss of material.

Interfering factors
■ Chemotherapy (possible abnormal results due to chromosome breaks)
■ Contamination of tissue with bacteria, fungus, or a virus (possible inhibition of culture growth)
■ Inclusion of maternal cells in a specimen obtained by amniocentesis, with subsequent culturing (possible false results)

Cold agglutinins

Cold agglutinins are antibodies, usually of the immunoglobulin (Ig) M type, that cause red blood cells (RBCs) to aggregate at low temperatures. They may occur in small amounts in healthy people. Transient elevations of these antibodies develop during certain infectious diseases, notably primary atypical pneumonia. This test reliably detects such pneumonia within 1 to 2 weeks after onset.

Patients with high cold agglutinin titers, such as those with primary atypical pneumonia, may develop acute transient hemolytic anemia after repeated exposure to

cold; patients with persistently high titers may develop chronic hemolytic anemia.

Purpose
■ To help confirm primary atypical pneumonia
■ To provide additional diagnostic evidence for cold agglutinin disease associated with many viral infections and lymphoreticular cancer
■ To detect cold agglutinins in patients with suspected cold agglutinin disease

Cost
Inexpensive

Patient preparation
■ Explain to the patient that this test detects antibodies in the blood that attack RBCs after exposure to low temperatures.
■ Inform the patient that the test will be repeated to monitor his response to therapy if appropriate.
■ Tell the patient that the test requires a blood sample. Explain who will perform the venipuncture and when.
■ Explain to the patient that he may feel discomfort from the needle puncture and the tourniquet.
■ Document the patient's use of antimicrobial drugs because the use of such drugs

may interfere with the development of cold agglutinins.

Normal findings

Cold agglutinin screening results are reported as negative or positive. A positive result, indicating the presence of cold agglutinin, is titered. A normal titer is less than 1:64.

Abnormal findings

High titers may occur as primary phenomena or secondary to infections or lymphoreticular cancer. They may be present in infectious mononucleosis, cytomegalovirus infection, hemolytic anemia, multiple myeloma, scleroderma, malaria, cirrhosis of the liver, congenital syphilis, peripheral vascular disease, pulmonary embolism, trypanosomiasis, tonsillitis, staphylococcemia, scarlatina, influenza and, occasionally, pregnancy. Chronically elevated titers are most commonly associated with pneumonia and lymphoreticular cancer; an acute transient elevation typically accompanies many viral infections.

Extremely high titers (1:2,000 or higher) can occur with idiopathic cold agglutinin disease that precedes lymphoma development. Patients with titers this high are susceptible to intravascular agglutination, which causes significant clinical problems.

Interfering factors

■ Hemolysis due to rough handling of the sample (possible false-low)
■ Refrigeration of the sample before serum is separated from RBCs (possible false-low)
■ Antimicrobial drugs

Colonoscopy

Colonoscopy uses a flexible fiber-optic video endoscope to permit visual examination of the lining of the large intestine. It's indicated for patients with a history of constipation or diarrhea, persistent rectal bleeding, and lower abdominal pain when the results of proctosigmoidoscopy and a barium enema test are negative or inconclusive.

ALERT! ▼ ▼ ▼ ▼ ▼ ▼ ▼ ▼ ▼
Although it's usually a safe procedure, colonoscopy can cause perforation of the large intestine, excessive bleeding, and retroperitoneal emphysema. This procedure is contraindicated in pregnant women near term, in patients who have had recent acute myocardial infarction or abdominal surgery, and in patients who have ischemic bowel disease, acute diverticulitis, peritonitis, fulminant granulomatous colitis, perforated viscus, or fulminant ulcerative colitis. For these patients or for screening purposes, a virtual colonoscopy may be an option to help visualize polyps early before they become concerns.

Purpose

■ To detect or evaluate inflammatory and ulcerative bowel disease
■ To locate the origin of lower GI bleeding
■ To aid diagnosis of colonic strictures and benign or malignant lesions
■ To evaluate the colon postoperatively for recurrence of polyps and malignant lesions

Cost

Very expensive

Patient preparation

■ Tell the patient that this test permits examination of the lining of the large intestine.

- Instruct the patient to maintain a clear liquid diet for 24 to 48 hours before the test and to take nothing by mouth after midnight the night before the procedure.
- Describe the procedure to the patient. Tell the patient who will perform it and where it will be done.
- Explain to the patient that the large intestine must be thoroughly cleaned to be clearly visible and he'll be administered a laxative or a gallon of GoLYTELY solution in the evening. Tell him he may also receive a suppository or tap-water enema.
- Inform the patient that an I.V. line will be started before the procedure and he'll receive a sedative. Explain that he should arrange for someone to drive him home.
- Document the patient's medical history of allergies, medications, and information pertinent to the current complaint.
- Obtain informed consent if necessary.

Normal findings

Normally, the mucosa of the large intestine beyond the sigmoid colon appears light pink-orange and is marked by semilunar folds and deep tubular pits. Blood vessels are visible beneath the intestinal mucosa, which glistens from mucus secretions.

Abnormal findings

Visual examination of the large intestine, coupled with histologic and cytologic test results, may indicate proctitis, granulomatous or ulcerative colitis, Crohn's disease, and malignant or benign lesions. Diverticular disease or the site of lower GI bleeding can be detected through colonoscopy alone.

Interfering factors

- Fixation of the sigmoid colon due to inflammatory bowel disease, surgery, or radiation therapy (may hinder passage of the colonoscope)

- Blood from acute colonic hemorrhage (hinders visualization)
- Insufficient bowel preparation or barium retained in the intestine from previous diagnostic studies (makes accurate visual examination impossible)

Colposcopy

In colposcopy, the cervix and vagina are visually examined by an instrument containing a magnifying lens and a light (colposcope). This test is primarily used to evaluate abnormal cytology or grossly suspicious lesions and to examine the cervix and vagina after a positive Papanicolaou (Pap) test.

During the examination, a biopsy may be performed and photographs taken of suspicious lesions with the colposcope and its attachments. Risks of biopsy include bleeding (especially during pregnancy) and infection.

Purpose

- To help confirm cervical intraepithelial neoplasia or invasive carcinoma after a positive Pap test
- To evaluate vaginal or cervical lesions
- To monitor conservatively treated cervical intraepithelial neoplasia
- To monitor patients whose mothers received diethylstilbestrol during pregnancy

Cost

Expensive

Patient preparation

- Explain to the patient that this test magnifies the image of the vagina and cervix, providing more information than a routine vaginal examination.
- Tell the patient who will perform the examination, where it will be done, and that it's safe and painless.

■ Tell the patient that a biopsy may be performed during colposcopy and that this may cause minimal but easily controlled bleeding and mild cramping.
■ Obtain informed consent if necessary.

Normal findings

Surface contour of the cervical vessels should be smooth and pink; columnar epithelium appears grapelike. Different tissue types are sharply demarcated.

Abnormal findings

Abnormal colposcopy findings include white epithelium (leukoplakia) or punctate and mosaic patterns, which may indicate underlying cervical intraepithelial neoplasia; keratinization in the transformation zone, which may indicate cervical intraepithelial neoplasia or invasive carcinoma; and atypical vessels, which may indicate invasive carcinoma.

Other abnormalities visible on colposcopic examination include inflammatory changes (usually from infection), atrophic changes (usually from aging or, less commonly, the use of hormonal contraceptives), erosion (probably from increased pathogenicity of vaginal flora due to changes in vaginal pH), and papilloma and condyloma (possibly from viruses).

Histologic study of the biopsy specimen confirms colposcopic findings. If the results of the examination and biopsy are inconsistent with the results of the Pap test and biopsy of the squamocolumnar junction, conization of the cervix for biopsy may be indicated.

Interfering factors

■ Failure to clean the cervix of menstrual blood or foreign materials, such as creams and medications (possible obstruction to visualization)

Complement assays

Complement is a collective term for a system of at least 15 serum proteins designed to destroy foreign cells and help remove foreign materials. Complement deficiency can increase susceptibility to infection and predispose patients to other diseases. Complement assays are indicated in patients with known or suspected immunomediated disease or repeatedly abnormal response to infection. Various laboratory methods are used to evaluate and measure total complement and its components; hemolytic assay, laser nephelometry, and radial immunodiffusion are the most common.

Although complement assays provide valuable information about the patient's immune system, the results must be considered in light of serum immunoglobulin and autoantibody tests for a definitive diagnosis of immunomediated disease or abnormal response to infection.

Purpose

■ To help detect immunomediated disease and genetic complement deficiency
■ To monitor effectiveness of therapy

Cost

Moderately expensive

Patient preparation

■ Explain to the patient that this test measures a group of proteins that fight infection.
■ Advise the patient that he need not restrict food or fluids.
■ Tell the patient that the test requires a blood sample. Explain who will perform the venipuncture and when.
■ Tell the patient that he may experience discomfort from the needle puncture and the tourniquet.

- If the patient is scheduled for C1q assay, check and document his history of recent heparin therapy.

Reference values
Normal values for complement range as follows:
- *total complement:* 25 to 110 U/ml (SI, 0.25 to 1.1 g/L)
- *C3:* 70 to 150 mg/dl (SI, 0.7 to 1.5 g/L)
- *C4:* 15 to 45 mg/dl (SI, 0.15 to 0.45 g/L).

Abnormal findings
Complement abnormalities may be genetic or acquired; acquired abnormalities are most common. Depressed total complement levels (which are clinically more significant than elevations) may result from excessive formation of antigen-antibody complexes, insufficient synthesis of complement, inhibitor formation, or increased complement catabolism and are characteristic in such conditions as systemic lupus erythematosus (SLE), acute poststreptococcal glomerulonephritis, and acute serum sickness. Low levels may also occur in some patients with advanced cirrhosis of the liver, multiple myeloma, hypogammaglobulinemia, or rapidly rejecting allografts.

Elevated total complement may occur in obstructive jaundice, thyroiditis, acute rheumatic fever, rheumatoid arthritis, acute myocardial infarction, ulcerative colitis, and diabetes.

C1 esterase inhibitor deficiency is characteristic in hereditary angioedema, the most common genetic abnormality associated with complement; C3 deficiency is characteristic in recurrent pyogenic infection and disease activation in SLE; C4 deficiency is characteristic in SLE and rheumatoid arthritis. C4 is increased in autoimmune hemolytic anemia.

Interfering factors
- Hemolysis due to rough handling of the sample
- Failure to send the sample to the laboratory immediately
- Recent heparin therapy

Computed tomography

A computed tomography (CT) scan combines radiologic and computer technology to produce tissue analysis. A series of tomograms is translated by a computer and displayed on a monitor, representing cross-sectional images of various layers of tissue. This technique can reconstruct cross-sectional, horizontal, sagittal, and coronal plane images. (See *Spiral CT,* page 112.)

Hundreds of thousands of readings of radiation levels absorbed by the tissues may be combined to depict anatomic slices of varying thickness. Use of an I.V. or oral contrast medium during the procedure can accentuate differences in tissue density.

ALERT! ▼ ▼ ▼ ▼ ▼ ▼ ▼ ▼ ▼
This test is usually contraindicated during pregnancy and in patients with severe renal or hepatic disease or are hypersensitive to iodine.

Purpose
- To produce tissue analysis and images not readily seen on standard radiographs

Cost
Very expensive

Patient preparation
- Explain to the patient the purpose of the test.
- Tell the patient who will perform the test and where it will take place.
- Inform the patient that he'll be placed on an adjustable table, which is positioned

Spiral CT

The spiral (helical) computed tomography (CT) scan is produced while the X-ray tube rotates continuously around the patient, forming a spiral path through the patient. This path represents a contiguous volumetric data set, covering a specific volume of the patient's anatomy with no spatial or temporal gaps. The patient continuously moves through the slip-ring gantry, and no two data points are taken in exactly the same plane.

Benefits include increased speed (spiral CT is typically 8 to 10 times faster than conventional CT), improved image quality and diagnostic accuracy, and reduced radiation exposure. The improved speed — the scan can usually be obtained during a single breath hold — is especially beneficial for the elderly, pediatric, and critically ill populations, in which scanning commonly proves difficult.

There are disadvantages. Spiral CT delivers a limited amount of milliamperes, which can result in a grainier image than conventional CT (more common in larger patients). In addition, artifacts ("pseudothrombi") can be created in the infrahepatic inferior vena cava by the admixture of unopacified blood and contrast medium flowing in from the renal veins. These disadvantages are being resolved with improved equipment and technique.

inside a scanning gantry, and that he'll be asked to remain still during the procedure.
■ Depending on the specific CT scan, the patient may be given an oral or I.V. contrast medium. If an I.V. contrast medium is used, tell him that he may feel transient discomfort from the needle puncture and a feeling of warmth or flushing. Tell him that these feelings usually subside in 2 minutes.

ALERT! ▼ ▼ ▼ ▼ ▼ ▼ ▼ ▼ ▼
Tell the patient to immediately report a feeling of nausea, vomiting, dizziness, headache, or hives.

Findings
Values will differ depending upon the area being scanned and the disorder of the patient.

Interfering factors
■ Use of oral or I.V. contrast media in previous diagnostic tests may obscure the images.
■ Inability of the patient to remain still during the test may provide inaccurate results.

Coombs' test, direct

The direct Coombs' test detects immunoglobulins (antibodies) on the surface of red blood cells (RBCs). These immunoglobulins coat RBCs when they become sensitized to an antigen, such as the Rh factor.

In this test, antiglobulin (Coombs') serum added to saline-washed RBCs results in agglutination if immunoglobulins or complement is present. This test is "direct" because it requires only one step—the addition of Coombs' serum to washed cells.

Purpose
■ To diagnose hemolytic disease of the neonate (HDN)
■ To investigate hemolytic transfusion reactions
■ To aid differential diagnosis of hemolytic anemias, which may be congenital or may result from an autoimmune reaction or use of certain drugs

Cost

Moderately expensive

Patient preparation

- If the patient is a neonate, explain to the parents that this test helps diagnose HDN.
- If the patient is suspected of having hemolytic anemia, explain that the test determines whether the condition results from an abnormality in the body's immune system, the use of certain drugs, or some unknown cause.
- Inform the adult patient that he need not fast before the test.
- Tell the patient (or a neonate's parents) that the test requires a blood sample. Explain who will perform the venipuncture and when.
- Tell the patient that he may experience discomfort from the needle puncture and the tourniquet.
- Restrict medications that may affect test results, including cephalosporins, chlorpromazine, diphenylhydantoin, ethosuximide, hydralazine, isoniazid, levodopa, mefenamic acid, melphalan, methyldopa, penicillin, procainamide, quinidine, rifampin, streptomycin, sulfonamides, and tetracyclines. If they must be continued, note this on the laboratory request.
- Tell the patient to resume his usual medication schedule after the test is completed.

Normal findings

A negative test, in which neither antibodies nor complement appear on the RBCs, is normal.

Abnormal findings

A positive test on umbilical cord blood indicates that maternal antibodies have crossed the placenta and coated fetal RBCs, causing HDN. Transfusion of compatible blood lacking the antigens to these maternal antibodies may be necessary to prevent anemia.

In other patients, a positive test result may indicate hemolytic anemia and help differentiate between autoimmune and secondary hemolytic anemia, which can be drug-induced or associated with an underlying disease. A positive test can also indicate sepsis.

A weakly positive test may suggest a transfusion reaction in which the patient's antibodies react with transfused RBCs containing the corresponding antigen.

Interfering factors

- Hemolysis due to rough handling of the sample
- Cephalosporins, chlorpromazine, diphenylhydantoin, dipyrone, ethosuximide, hydralazine, isoniazid, levodopa, mefenamic acid, melphalan, methyldopa, penicillin, procainamide, quinidine, rifampin, streptomycin, sulfonamides, and tetracyclines (positive test results, possibly due to immune hemolysis)

Corneal staining

Corneal staining with fluorescein dye allows a detailed view of the anterior part of the eye that can't ordinarily be seen during slit-lamp examination. A special attachment is used during the slit-lamp examination to enhance visualization.

Purpose

- To detect the depth and pattern of injuries to the corneal surface of the eye
- To diagnose corneal injuries

Cost

Moderately expensive

Patient preparation

■ Describe the procedure to the patient. Explain that this test evaluates the eye surface and is painless.
■ Tell the patient who will perform the test and where it will take place.
■ Ask the patient for a detailed history of the eye injury and symptoms associated with the injury.
■ Ask the patient to remove his glasses or contact lenses before the test.
■ Inform the patient that he may have blurring of vision, but it will gradually disappear within 2 hours. Tell the patient that he should arrange for someone to drive him home.

Normal findings

The normal cornea is convex in shape and has a smooth, shiny appearance. No scratches or indentations are noted.

Abnormal findings

Abnormal findings include corneal scratches, abrasions, ulcerations, and keratitis.

Interfering factors

■ The patient's inability to remain still during the examination
■ Allergy to the fluorescein dye

Corticotropin

The corticotropin test measures the plasma levels of corticotropin (also known as *adrenocorticotropic hormone* or *ACTH*) by radioimmunoassay. Corticotropin stimulates the adrenal cortex to secrete cortisol and, to a lesser degree, androgens and aldosterone. It also has some melanocyte-stimulating activity, increases the uptake of amino acids by muscle cells, promotes lipolysis by fat cells, stimulates pancreatic beta cells to secrete insulin, and may contribute to the release of growth hormone. Corticotropin

levels vary diurnally, peaking between 6 a.m. and 8 a.m. and ebbing between 6 p.m. and 11 p.m.

The corticotropin test may be ordered for patients with signs of adrenal hypofunction (insufficiency) or hyperfunction (Cushing's syndrome). Corticotropin suppression or stimulation testing is usually necessary to confirm diagnosis. The instability and unavailability of corticotropin greatly limit this test's diagnostic significance and reliability.

Cost

Expensive

Purpose

■ To facilitate differential diagnosis of primary and secondary adrenal hypofunction
■ To aid differential diagnosis of Cushing's syndrome

Patient preparation

■ Explain to the patient that this test helps determine if his hormonal secretion is normal.
■ Tell the patient to fast and limit his physical activity for 10 to 12 hours before the test.
■ Tell the patient that the test requires a blood sample. Explain who will perform the venipuncture and when.
■ Inform the patient that he may experience some discomfort from the needle puncture and the tourniquet.
■ Restrict medications that may affect test results. If they must be continued, note this on the laboratory request.
■ Instruct the patient to eat a diet low in carbohydrates for 2 days before the test. This requirement may vary, depending on the laboratory.

Reference values

Mayo Medical Laboratories sets baseline values for corticotropin at less than

120 pg/ml (SI, < 26.4 pmol/L) at 6 a.m. to 8 a.m., but these values may vary, depending on the laboratory.

Abnormal findings

A higher-than-normal corticotropin level may indicate primary adrenal hypofunction (Addison's disease), in which the pituitary gland attempts to compensate for the unresponsiveness of the target organ by releasing excessive corticotropin. The underlying cause of adrenocortical hypofunction may be idiopathic atrophy of the adrenal cortex or partial destruction of the gland by granuloma, neoplasm, amyloidosis, or inflammatory necrosis.

A low-normal corticotropin level suggests secondary adrenal hypofunction resulting from pituitary or hypothalamic dysfunction. The primary determinant may be panhypopituitarism, absence of corticotropin-releasing hormone in the hypothalamus, or chronic blunting of corticotropin levels by long-term corticosteroid therapy.

In suspected Cushing's syndrome, an elevated corticotropin level suggests Cushing's disease, in which pituitary dysfunction (due to adenoma) causes continuous hypersecretion of corticotropin and, consequently, continuously elevated cortisol levels without diurnal variations. Moderately elevated corticotropin levels suggest pituitary-dependent adrenal hyperplasia and nonadrenal tumors such as oat cell carcinoma of the lungs.

A low-normal corticotropin level implies adrenal hyperfunction due to adrenocortical tumor or hyperplasia.

Interfering factors

- Failure to observe pretest restrictions
- Corticosteroids, including cortisone and its analogues (decrease)
- Drugs that increase endogenous cortisol secretion, such as amphetamines, calcium gluconate, estrogens, ethanol, and spironolactone (decrease)
- Lithium carbonate (decreases cortisol levels and may interfere with corticotropin secretion)
- Menstrual cycle and pregnancy
- Radioactive scan performed within 1 week before the test
- Acute stress (including hospitalization and surgery) and depression (increase)

Corticotropin, rapid

The rapid corticotropin test (also known as the *rapid ACTH test* or *cosyntropin test*) is gradually replacing the 8-hour corticotropin stimulation test as the most effective diagnostic tool for evaluating adrenal hypofunction. Using cosyntropin, the rapid corticotropin test provides faster results and causes fewer allergic reactions than the 8-hour test, which uses natural corticotropin from animal sources.

This test requires prior determination of baseline cortisol levels to evaluate the effect of cosyntropin administration on cortisol secretion. An unequivocally high morning cortisol level rules out adrenal hypofunction and makes further testing unnecessary.

Purpose

- To aid in identification of primary and secondary adrenal hypofunction

Cost

Expensive

Patient preparation

- Explain to the patient that this test helps determine if his condition is due to a hormonal deficiency.
- Inform the patient that he may be required to fast for 10 to 12 hours before the

test and must relax and rest quietly for 30 minutes before the test.
■ Tell the patient that the test takes at least 1 hour to perform.
■ Restrict corticotropin and all steroid medications before the test. If they must be continued, note this on the laboratory request.
■ Inform the patient that he may experience discomfort from the needle puncture and the tourniquet.
■ Instruct the patient to resume his normal diet and medications after the test is completed.

Reference values
Normally, cortisol levels rise after 30 to 60 minutes to a peak of 18 mg/dl (SI, 500 mmol/L) or more than 60 minutes after the cosyntropin injection. Generally, doubling the baseline value indicates a normal response.

Abnormal findings
A normal result excludes adrenal hypofunction (insufficiency). In patients with primary adrenal hypofunction (Addison's disease), cortisol levels remain low. Thus, the rapid corticotropin test provides an effective method of screening for adrenal hypofunction. If test results show subnormal increases in cortisol levels, prolonged stimulation of the adrenal cortex may be required to differentiate between primary and secondary adrenal hypofunction.

Interfering factors
■ Failure to observe pretest restrictions
■ Hemolysis due to rough handling of the sample
■ Estrogens and amphetamines (increase in plasma cortisol)
■ Smoking and obesity (possible increase in plasma cortisol)

■ Lithium carbonate (decrease in plasma cortisol)
■ Radioactive scan performed within 1 week before the test

Cortisol, free, urine

Used as a screen for adrenocortical hyperfunction, the free urine cortisol test measures urine levels of the portion of cortisol not bound to the corticosteroid-binding globulin transcortin. It's one of the best diagnostic tools for detecting Cushing's syndrome.

Unlike a single measurement of plasma cortisol, radioimmunoassay determinations of free cortisol levels in a 24-hour urine specimen reflect overall secretion levels instead of diurnal variations. Concurrent measurements of plasma cortisol and corticotropin, with urine 17-hydroxycorticosteroids and the dexamethasone suppression test, may be used to confirm the diagnosis.

Purpose
■ To aid diagnosis of Cushing's syndrome
■ To evaluate adrenal cortical function

Cost
Moderately expensive

Patient preparation
■ Explain to the patient that this test helps evaluate adrenal gland function.
■ Inform the patient that he need not restrict food or fluids before the test but he should avoid stressful situations and excessive physical exercise during the collection period.
■ Tell the patient the test requires collection of urine over a 24-hour period.
■ Teach the patient the proper collection technique for a 24-hour urine specimen.

■ Restrict medications that may affect test results. If they must be continued, note this on the laboratory request.

Reference values
Normal free urine cortisol values are less than 50 µg/24 hours (SI, < 138 mmol/24 h).

Abnormal findings
Elevated free urine cortisol levels may indicate Cushing's syndrome resulting from adrenal hyperplasia, adrenal or pituitary tumor, or ectopic corticotropin production. Hepatic disease and obesity, which can raise plasma cortisol levels, generally don't appreciably raise urine levels of free cortisol. Low levels have little diagnostic significance and don't necessarily indicate adrenocortical hypofunction.

Interfering factors
■ Failure to collect all urine during the test period or to properly store the specimen
■ Pregnancy (possible increase)
■ Aldactone, amphetamines, danazol, morphine, hormonal contraceptives, phenothiazines, prolonged steroid therapy, and reserpine (possible increase)
■ Dexamethasone, ethacrynic acid, ketoconazole, and thiazides (decrease)

Cortisol, plasma

Cortisol, the principal glucocorticoid secreted by the zona fasciculata of the adrenal cortex, primarily in response to corticotropin stimulation, helps metabolize nutrients, mediate physiologic stress, and regulate the immune system. Cortisol secretion normally follows a diurnal pattern: Levels rise during the early morning hours and peak around 8 a.m., then decline to very low levels in the evening and during the early phase of sleep. Production of this hormone is influenced by physical or emotional stress, which activates corticotropin. Thus, intense heat or cold, infection, trauma, exercise, obesity, and debilitating disease influence cortisol secretion.

This radioimmunoassay, a quantitative analysis of plasma cortisol levels, is usually ordered for patients with signs of adrenal dysfunction, but dynamic tests, suppression tests for hyperfunction, and stimulation tests for hypofunction are generally required to confirm the diagnosis.

Purpose
■ To aid in the diagnosis of Cushing's disease, Cushing's syndrome, Addison's disease, and secondary adrenal insufficiency

Cost
Inexpensive

Patient preparation
■ Explain to the patient that this test helps determine if his symptoms are due to improper hormonal secretion.
■ Instruct the patient to maintain a normal-sodium diet for 3 days before the test and to fast and limit physical activity for 10 to 12 hours before the test.
■ Tell the patient that the test requires a blood sample. Explain who will perform the venipuncture and when.
■ Explain to the patient that he may experience discomfort from the needle puncture and the tourniquet.
■ Restrict all medications that may interfere with plasma cortisol levels, such as estrogens, androgens, and phenytoin, for 48 hours before the test. If the patient is receiving replacement therapy and is dependent on exogenous steroids for survival, note this on the laboratory request as well

as any other medications that must be continued.

■ Make sure the patient is relaxed and recumbent for at least 30 minutes before the test.

Reference values

Normally, plasma cortisol levels range from 9 to 35 µg/dl (SI, 250 to 690 nmol/L) in the morning and from 3 to 12 µg/dl (SI, 80 to 330 nmol) in the afternoon; the afternoon level is usually half the morning level.

Abnormal findings

Increased plasma cortisol levels may indicate adrenocortical hyperfunction in Cushing's disease (a rare disease due to basophilic adenoma of the pituitary gland) or in Cushing's syndrome (glucocorticoid excess from any cause). In most patients with Cushing's syndrome, the adrenal cortex tends to secrete independently of any natural rhythm. Thus, absence of diurnal variations in cortisol secretion is a significant finding in almost all patients with Cushing's syndrome; in these patients, little difference in values, if any, is found between morning samples and those taken in the afternoon. Diurnal variations may also be absent in otherwise healthy persons who are under considerable emotional or physical stress.

Decreased cortisol levels may indicate primary adrenal hypofunction (Addison's disease), usually due to idiopathic glandular atrophy (a presumed autoimmune process). Tuberculosis, fungal invasion, and hemorrhage can cause adrenocortical destruction. Low cortisol levels resulting from secondary adrenal insufficiency may occur in conditions of impaired corticotropin secretion, such as hypophysectomy, postpartum pituitary necrosis, craniopharyngioma, or chromophobe adenoma.

Interfering factors

■ Failure to observe restrictions of diet, medications, or physical activity
■ Pregnancy or use of hormonal contraceptives (possible false-high)
■ Obesity, stress, or severe hepatic or renal disease (possible false-high)
■ Androgens and phenytoin (possible decrease)
■ Radioactive scan performed with the week before the test's administration
■ Hemolysis caused by rough handling of the sample

C-peptide assay

Connecting peptide (C-peptide) is a biologically inactive peptide chain formed during the proteolytic conversion of proinsulin to insulin in the pancreatic beta cells. It has no insulin effect, either biologically or immunologically. This is important because circulating insulin is measured by immunologic assay. As insulin is released into the bloodstream, the C-peptide chain splits off from the hormone.

Purpose

■ To determine the cause of hypoglycemia by distinguishing between endogenous hyperinsulinism or insulinoma (elevated C-peptide levels) and surreptitious insulin injection (decreased C-peptide levels)
■ To indirectly measure insulin secretion in the presence of circulating insulin antibodies, which interfere with insulin assays but not with C-peptide assays
■ To detect residual tissue (some C-peptide present) after total pancreatectomy for carcinoma
■ To indicate the remission phase (some C-peptide present) of diabetes mellitus
■ To determine beta-cell function in patients with diabetes mellitus; absence of

C-peptide indicates no beta-cell function, and presence indicates residual beta-cell function

Cost
Moderately expensive

Patient preparation
- Explain to the patient that the purpose of the test is to determine the cause of low blood sugar as appropriate.
- Tell the patient that the test requires a blood sample. Explain who will perform the venipuncture and when.
- Explain to the patient that he may experience discomfort from the needle puncture and the tourniquet.
- Tell the patient he must fast, except for water, for 8 to 12 hours before the test.
- Restrict medications that may affect test results. If they must be continued, note this on the laboratory request.

Reference values
Serum C-peptide levels generally parallel those of insulin. Normal fasting values range from 0.78 to 1.89 ng/ml (SI, 0.26 to 0.63 mmol/L). An insulin:C-peptide ratio may be performed to differentiate insulinoma from factitious hypoglycemia. A ratio of 1.0 or less indicates increased, endogenous insulin secretion; a ratio of 1.0 or more indicates exogenous insulin.

Abnormal findings
Increased values occur in patients with endogenous hyperinsulinism (insulinemia), who have had pancreas or B-cell transplant, renal failure, and non–insulin-dependent diabetes mellitus (type 2).

Decreased values occur in those with factitious hypoglycemia (surreptitious insulin administration), radical pancreatectomy, and insulin-dependent diabetes mellitus (type 1).

Interfering factors
- Failure to adhere to dietary restrictions
- Oral hypoglycemic drug ingestion (increased value)

C-reactive protein

C-reactive protein (CRP) is an abnormal protein that appears in the blood during an inflammatory process. It's absent from the blood serum of healthy people. This protein is mainly synthesized in the liver and is found in many body fluids (pleural, peritoneal, pericardial, synovial). It appears in the blood 18 to 24 hours after onset of tissue damage with levels that increase up to 1,000-fold and then decline rapidly when the inflammatory process regresses. CRP has been found to increase before rises in antibody titers and erythrocyte sedimentation rate (ESR) levels occur, and also decreases sooner than ESR levels.

Purpose
- To evaluate inflammatory disease course and severity in conditions where there is tissue necrosis (myocardial infarction [MI], malignancy, rheumatoid arthritis)
- To monitor acute inflammatory phases of rheumatoid arthritis and rheumatic fever so early treatment can be initiated
- To help interpret ESR
- To monitor the wound healing process of internal incisions, burns, and organ transplantation

Cost
Inexpensive

Patient preparation
- Explain to the patient that this test is used to identify the presence of infection or to monitor treatment.

- Inform the patient that he needs to restrict all fluids except for water for 8 to 12 hours before the test.
- Tell the patient who will perform the venipuncture and when.
- Explain to the patient that he may experience slight discomfort from the needle puncture and the tourniquet.
- Restrict medications that may affect test results. If they must be continued, note this on the laboratory request.
- Instruct the patient that he may resume his usual diet and medications discontinued before the test as appropriate.

Reference values

C-reactive protein usually isn't present in the blood, but in adults, results may be reported as < 0.8 mg/dl (SI, < 8 mg/L).

Abnormal findings

Increased levels may occur in rheumatoid arthritis, rheumatic fever, MI, cancer (active, widespread), acute bacterial and viral infections, inflammatory bowel disease, Hodgkin's disease, and systemic lupus erythematosus.

Increased levels may also be detected postoperatively. (Levels begin to decline after the fourth postoperative day.)

Interfering factors

- Steroids and salicylates (false normal level)
- Hormonal contraceptives (false increase)
- Pregnancy (third trimester) and intrauterine contraceptive devices (increase)

Creatine kinase

Creatine kinase (CK) is an enzyme that catalyzes the creatine-creatinine metabolic pathway in muscle cells and brain tissue. Because of its intimate role in energy production, CK reflects normal tissue catabolism; increased serum levels indicate trauma to cells.

Fractionation and measurement of three distinct CK isoenzymes — CK-BB (CK_1), CK-MB (CK_2), and CK-MM (CK_3) — have replaced the use of total CK levels to accurately localize the site of increased tissue destruction. CK-BB is most often found in brain tissue. CK-MM and CK-MB are found primarily in skeletal and heart muscle. In addition, subunits of CK-MB and CK-MM, called isoforms or isoenzymes, can be assayed to increase the test's sensitivity.

Purpose

- To detect and diagnose acute myocardial infarction (MI) and reinfarction (CK-MB primarily used)
- To evaluate possible causes of chest pain and to monitor the severity of myocardial ischemia after cardiac surgery, cardiac catheterization, and cardioversion (CK-MB primarily used)
- To detect early dermatomyositis, and musculoskeletal disorders that aren't neurogenic in origin, such as Duchenne muscular dystrophy (total CK primarily used)

Cost

Inexpensive

Patient preparation

- Tell the patient that this test is used to assess myocardial and musculoskeletal function.
- Tell the patient that the test requires multiple blood samples to detect fluctuations in serum levels. Explain who will perform the venipunctures and when.
- Explain to the patient that he may experience discomfort from the needle punctures and the tourniquet.
- If the patient is being evaluated for musculoskeletal disorders, advise him to avoid exercising for 24 hours before the test.

- Restrict medications that may affect test results. If they must be continued, note this on the laboratory request.

Reference values

Total CK values determined by ultraviolet or kinetic measurement range from 55 to 170 U/L (SI, 0.94 to 2.89 μkat/L) for men and from 30 to 135 U/L (SI, 0.51 to 2.3 μkat/L) for women. CK levels may be significantly higher in muscular people.

AGE ISSUE ✳ ✳ ✳ ✳ ✳
Infants up to age 1 have levels two to four times higher than adult levels, possibly reflecting birth trauma and striated muscle development.

Normal ranges for isoenzyme levels are as follows: CK-BB, undetectable; CK-MB, less than 5% (SI, <0.05); CK-MM, 90% to 100% (SI, 0.9 to 1.00).

Abnormal findings

CK-MM makes up 99% of total CK normally present in serum. Detectable CK-BB isoenzyme may indicate, but doesn't confirm, a diagnosis of brain tissue injury, widespread malignant tumors, severe shock, or renal failure.

CK-MB levels greater than 5% of total CK indicate myocardial infarction (MI), especially if the lactate dehydrogenase 1 and 2 (LD_1/LD_2) isoenzyme ratio is greater than 1 (flipped LD). In acute MI and after cardiac surgery, CK-MB begins to increase within 2 to 4 hours, peaks within 12 to 24 hours, and usually returns to normal within 24 to 48 hours; persistent elevations and increasing levels indicate ongoing myocardial damage. Total CK follows roughly the same pattern but increases slightly later. CK-MB levels may not increase in heart failure or during angina pectoris not accompanied by myocardial cell necrosis. Serious skeletal muscle injury that occurs in certain muscular dystrophies, polymyositis, and severe myoglobinuria may produce a

mild CK-MB increase because a small amount of this isoenzyme is present in some skeletal muscles.

Increasing CK-MM values follow skeletal muscle damage from trauma, such as surgery and I.M. injections, and from diseases, such as dermatomyositis and muscular dystrophy (values may be 50 to 100 times normal). A moderate increase in CK-MM levels develops in patients with hypothyroidism; sharp increases occur with muscle activity caused by agitation, such as during an acute psychotic episode.

Total CK levels may be increased in patients with severe hypokalemia, carbon monoxide poisoning, malignant hyperthermia, and alcoholic cardiomyopathy. They may also be increased after seizures and, occasionally, in patients who have suffered pulmonary or cerebral infarctions. Troponin-I and cardiac troponin C are present in the contractile cells of cardiac myocardial tissue, and are released with injury to the myocardial tissue. Troponin levels increase within 1 hour of the infarction and may remain elevated for up to 14 days. (See *Serum protein and isoenzyme levels after MI*, page 122.)

Interfering factors

- Failure to send the sample to the laboratory immediately or to refrigerate the serum if testing will be delayed more than 2 hours (possible decrease in concentration)
- Failure to draw the samples at the scheduled time (may miss peak levels)
- Halothane and succinylcholine, alcohol, lithium, large doses of aminocaproic acid, I.M. injections, cardioversion, invasive diagnostic procedures, recent vigorous exercise or muscle massage, severe coughing, and trauma (increase in total CK)
- Surgery through skeletal muscle (increase in total CK)

Serum protein and isoenzyme levels after MI

Because they're released by damaged tissue, serum proteins and isoenzymes (catalytic proteins that vary in concentration in specific organs) can help identify the compromised organ and assess the extent of damage after myocardial infarction (MI). The serum protein and isoenzyme determinations listed below are most significant after MI.

Isoenzymes

- *Creatine kinase-MB (CK-MB):* in the heart muscle and a small amount in skeletal muscle
- *Lactate dehydrogenase 1 and 2 (LD$_1$, LD$_2$):* in the heart, brain, kidneys, liver, skeletal muscles, and red blood cells (RBCs)

Proteins

- Troponin-I and troponin-T (the cardiac contractile proteins) have greater sensitivity than CK-MB in detecting myocardial injury.

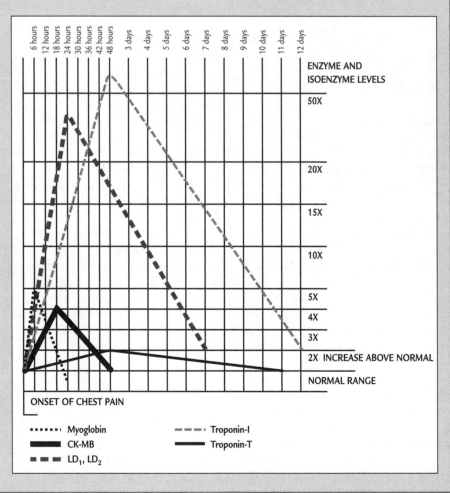

Creatinine clearance

An anhydride of creatine, creatinine is formed and excreted in constant amounts by an irreversible reaction and functions solely as the main end product of creatine. Creatinine production is proportional to total muscle mass and is relatively unaffected by urine volume or normal physical activity or diet.

An excellent diagnostic indicator of renal function, the creatinine clearance test determines how efficiently the kidneys are clearing creatinine from the blood. The rate of clearance is expressed in terms of the volume of blood (in milliliters) that can be cleared of creatinine in 1 minute. Creatinine levels become abnormal when more than 50% of the nephrons have been damaged.

Purpose
- To assess renal function (primarily glomerular filtration)
- To monitor progression of renal insufficiency

Cost
Moderately expensive

Patient preparation
- Explain to the patient that this test assesses kidney function.
- Inform the patient that he may need to avoid meat, poultry, fish, tea, or coffee for 6 hours before the test, and to avoid strenuous physical exercise during the collection period.
- Tell the patient the test requires a timed urine specimen and at least one blood sample. Explain who will perform the venipuncture and when, and that more than one venipuncture may be necessary.
- Explain to the patient that he may experience discomfort from the needle puncture and the tourniquet.
- Restrict medications that may affect test results. If they must be continued, note this on the laboratory request.
- Tell the patient that a timed urine specimen will be a collected at 2, 6, 12, or 24 hours in a bottle containing a preservative.

Reference values
Normal creatinine clearance varies with age; in males, it ranges from 94 to 140 mL/min/1.73m² (SI, 0.91 to 1.35 mL/s/m²); in females, 72 to 110 mL/min/1.73m² (SI, 0.69 to 1.06 mL/s/m²)

Abnormal findings
Low creatinine clearance may result from reduced renal blood flow (associated with shock or renal artery obstruction), acute tubular necrosis, acute or chronic glomerulonephritis, advanced bilateral chronic pyelonephritis, advanced bilateral renal lesions (which may occur in polycystic kidney disease, renal tuberculosis, and cancer), nephrosclerosis, heart failure, or severe dehydration.

High creatinine clearance can suggest poor hydration.

Interfering factors
- Failure to observe restrictions, to collect all urine during the test period, to properly store the specimen, or to send the sample to the laboratory immediately after the collection is completed
- Amphotericin B, thiazide diuretics, furosemide, and aminoglycosides (possible decrease)
- High-protein diet, strenuous exercise (increase)

Creatinine, serum

The serum creatinine test provides a more sensitive measure of renal damage than blood urea nitrogen levels. Creatinine is a nonprotein end product of creatine metabolism that appears in serum in amounts proportional to the body's muscle mass.

Purpose
- To assess glomerular filtration
- To screen for renal damage

Cost
Inexpensive

Patient preparation
- Explain to the patient that this test is used to evaluate kidney function.
- Tell the patient that the test requires a blood sample. Explain who will perform the venipuncture and when.
- Explain to the patient that he may experience discomfort from the needle puncture and the tourniquet.
- Restrict medications that may affect test results. If they must be continued, note this on the laboratory request.

Reference values
Creatinine concentrations normally range from 0.8 to 1.2 mg/dl (SI, 62 to 115 µmol/L) in males and 0.6 to 0.9 mg/dl (SI, 53 to 97 µmol/L) in females.

Abnormal findings
Elevated serum creatinine levels generally indicate renal disease that has seriously damaged 50% or more of the nephrons. Elevated levels may also be associated with gigantism and acromegaly.

Interfering factors
- Ascorbic acid, barbiturates, and diuretics (possible increase)
- Exceptionally large muscle mass, such as that found in athletes (possible increase despite normal renal function)
- Sulfabromopthalein or phenosulfaphthalein given within the 24 hours previous to the test's administration (may elevate creatinine levels if the test is based on the Jaffé reaction)
- Diet high in meat (possible increase)

Cryoglobulins

Cryoglobulins are abnormal serum proteins that precipitate at low laboratory temperatures (39.2° F [4° C]) and redissolve after being warmed. Their presence in the blood (cryoglobulinemia) is usually associated with immunologic disease, but can also occur without known immunopathology. If patients with cryoglobulinemia are subjected to cold, they may experience Raynaud-like symptoms (pain, cyanosis, and coldness of fingers and toes), which generally result from precipitation of cryoglobulins in cooler parts of the body. In some patients, for example, cryoglobulins may precipitate at temperatures as high as 86° F (30° C); such temperatures are possible in some peripheral blood vessels.

The cryoglobulin test involves refrigerating a serum sample at 33.8° F (1° C) for 24 hours and observing for formation of a heat-reversible precipitate. Such a precipitate requires further study by immunoelectrophoresis or double diffusion to identify cryoglobulin components.

Purpose
- To detect cryoglobulinemia in patients with Raynaud-like vascular symptoms

Cost
Moderately expensive

Diseases associated with cryoglobulinemia

This chart indicates typical serum levels and diseases associated with the three types of cryoglobulins.

TYPE OF CRYOGLOBULIN	SERUM LEVEL	ASSOCIATED DISEASES
Type I Monoclonal cryoglobulin	> 5 mg/ml	■ Myeloma ■ Waldenström's macroglobulinemia ■ Chronic lymphocytic leukemia
Type II Mixed cryoglobulin	> 1 mg/ml	■ Rheumatoid arthritis ■ Sjögren's syndrome ■ Mixed essential cryoglobulinemia
Type III Mixed polyclonal cryoglobulin	< 1 mg/ml (50% below 80 µg/ml)	■ Systemic lupus erythematosus ■ Rheumatoid arthritis ■ Sjögren's syndrome ■ Infectious mononucleosis ■ Cytomegalovirus infections ■ Acute viral hepatitis ■ Chronic active hepatitis ■ Primary biliary cirrhosis ■ Poststreptococcal glomerulonephritis ■ Infective endocarditis ■ Leprosy ■ Kala-azar ■ Tropical splenomegaly syndrome

Patient preparation

■ Explain to the patient that this test detects antibodies in blood that may cause sensitivity to low temperatures.
■ Instruct the patient to fast for 4 to 6 hours before the test.
■ Tell the patient that the test requires a blood sample. Explain who will perform the venipuncture and when.
■ Explain to the patient that he may experience discomfort from the needle puncture and the tourniquet.

ALERT! ▼ ▼ ▼ ▼ ▼ ▼ ▼ ▼ ▼
Tell the patient to avoid cold temperatures or contact with cold objects if the test is positive for cryoglobulins.

Normal findings

Normally, serum is negative for cryoglobulins. Positive results are reported as a percentage based on the amount of sample cryoprecipitation.

Abnormal findings

The presence of cryoglobulins in the blood confirms cryoglobulinemia. This finding doesn't always indicate the presence of clinical disease. (See *Diseases associated with cryoglobulinemia*.)

Interfering factors

■ Failure to adhere to dietary restrictions

■ Failure to keep the sample at 98.6° F (37° C) before centrifugation (possible loss of cryoglobulins)
■ Reading the sample before the 72-hour precipitation period ends (possible incorrect analysis of results because some cryoglobulins take several days to precipitate)

Cystometry

Cystometry assesses the bladder's neuromuscular function by measuring efficiency of the detrusor muscle reflex, intravesical pressure and capacity, and the bladder's reaction to thermal stimulation by instillation of physiologic saline solution or sterile water instilled into the bladder through a catheter. Because results from cystometry can be ambiguous, they're typically supported by results of other tests, such as cystourethrography, excretory urography, and voiding cystourethrography.

ALERT! ▼ ▼ ▼ ▼ ▼ ▼ ▼ ▼ ▼
Cystometry is contraindicated in patients with acute urinary tract infections because uninhibited contractions may cause erroneous readings and the test may lead to pyelonephritis and septic shock.

Purpose
■ To evaluate detrusor muscle function and tonicity
■ To help determine the cause of bladder dysfunction

Cost
Expensive

Patient preparation
■ Explain to the patient that this test evaluates bladder function.
■ Describe the procedure to the patient, including who will perform it, where it will take place, and its duration.

■ Tell the patient that he'll feel a strong urge to void during the test and may feel embarrassed or uncomfortable.
■ Obtain informed consent if necessary.
■ Restrict medications that may affect test results. If they must be continued, note this on the laboratory request.
■ Tell the patient to drink lots of fluids to relieve burning on urination, a common adverse effect of the procedure, unless contraindicated.
■ Tell the patient that short-term antibiotics are often given afterward to prevent infection.
■ Inform the patient that a sitz bath or warm tub bath may be administered if the patient experiences discomfort after the test.

Findings
For characteristic findings, see *Normal and abnormal cystometry findings.*

Interfering factors
■ Failure to follow instructions because of misunderstanding or embarrassment
■ Inability to urinate in the supine position
■ Concurrent use of drugs such as antihistamines (possible interference with bladder function)
■ Cystometry performed within 6 to 8 weeks after surgery for spinal cord injury (inconclusive results)

Cytomegalovirus antibody screen

After primary infection, cytomegalovirus (CMV) remains latent in white blood cells (WBCs). The presence of CMV antibodies indicates past infection with this virus. In an immunocompromised patient, CMV can be reactivated to cause active infection.

Normal and abnormal cystometry findings

Because cystometry assesses micturition and vesical function, it can aid diagnosis of neurogenic bladder dysfunction. The five main types of neurogenic bladder, as presented in the following chart, result from lesions of the central or peripheral nervous system.

Uninhibited neurogenic bladder results from a lesion to the upper motor neuron and causes frequent, often uncontrollable micturition in the presence of even a small amount of urine. A complete upper motor neuron lesion characterizes reflex neurogenic bladder and causes total loss of conscious sensation and vesical control.

FEATURE OR RESPONSE	NORMAL BLADDER FUNCTION	UNINHIBITED NEUROGENIC BLADDER (mildly spastic, incomplete upper motor neuron lesion)	REFLEX NEUROGENIC BLADDER (completely spastic, complete upper motor neuron lesion)
Micturition			
Start	+	+/0	0
Stop	+	0	0
Residual urine	0	0	+
Vesical sensation	+	+	0
First urge to void	150 to 200 ml	E (< 50 ml)	0
Bladder capacity	400 to 500 ml	↓	↓
Bladder contractions	0	+	+
Intravesical pressure	L	↑	↑
Bulbocavernosus reflex	+	+	↑
Saddle sensation	+	+	0
Bethanechol test (exaggerated response)	0	+	0
Ice water test	+	+	+
Anal reflex	+	+	+
Heat sensation and pain	+	+	0

(continued)

KEY
+ = Present/Positive
0 = Absent/Negative
↑ = Increased
↓ = Decreased
V = Variable
E = Early
D = Delayed
L = Low

In autonomous neurogenic bladder, a lower motor neuron lesion produces a flaccid bladder that fills without contracting. The patient can't perceive bladder fullness or initiate and maintain urination without applying external pressure.

Lower motor neuron lesions can cause sensory or motor paralysis of the bladder. In sensory paralysis, the patient experiences chronic urine retention because he can't perceive bladder fullness. In motor paralysis, the patient has full sensation but can't initiate or control urination.

FEATURE OR RESPONSE	AUTONOMOUS NEUROGENIC BLADDER (flaccid, incomplete lower motor neuron lesion)	SENSORY PARALYTIC BLADDER (lower motor neuron lesion)	MOTOR PARALYTIC BLADDER (lower motor neuron lesion)
Micturition			
Start	0	+	0
Stop	0	+	0
Residual urine	+	+	++
Vesical sensation	0	0	+
First urge to void	0	D	+
Bladder capacity	↑	↑ (< 1,000 ml)	V
Bladder contractions	0	0	0
Intravesical pressure	↓	↓	L
Bulbocavernosus reflex	0	+/↓/0	+
Saddle sensation	0	V	+
Bethanechol test (exaggerated response)	+	+	0
Ice water test	0	0	0
Anal reflex	0	V	V
Heat sensation and pain	0	0	+

KEY

+ = Present/Positive	↑ = Increased	V = Variable	D = Delayed
0 = Absent/Negative	↓ = Decreased	E = Early	L = Low

Administration of blood or tissue from a seropositive donor may cause active CMV infection in CMV-seronegative organ transplant recipients or neonates, especially those born prematurely.

Antibodies to CMV can be detected by several methods, including passive hemagglutination, latex agglutination, enzyme immunoassay, and indirect immunofluorescence. The complement fixation test is only 60% sensitive compared with other assays and shouldn't be used to screen for CMV antibodies. Screening tests for CMV antibodies are qualitative; they detect the presence of antibody at a single low dilution. In quantitative methods, several dilutions of the serum sample are tested to indicate acute infection with CMV.

Purpose
■ To detect CMV infection in donors and recipients of organs and blood and in immunocompromised patients
■ To screen for CMV infection in infants who require blood transfusions or tissue transplants

Cost
Moderately expensive

Patient preparation
■ Explain the purpose of the test to the patient or the parents of an infant.
■ Tell the patient that the test requires a blood sample and who will perform the venipuncture and when.
■ Tell him he may experience transient discomfort from the needle puncture and tourniquet.

Reference values
Patients who have never been infected with CMV have no detectable antibodies to the virus. Immunoglobulin (Ig) G and IgM are normally negative.

Abnormal findings
A serum sample collected early during the acute phase or late in the convalescent stage may not contain detectable IgG or IgM antibodies to CMV. Therefore, a negative result doesn't preclude recent infection. More than a single sample is needed to ensure accurate results.

A serum sample that tests positive for antibodies at this single dilution indicates that the patient has been infected with CMV and that his WBCs contain latent virus capable of being reactivated in an immunocompromised host. Immunosuppressed patients who lack antibodies to CMV should receive blood products or organ transplants from donors who are also seronegative. Patients with CMV antibodies don't require seronegative blood products.

Interfering factor
■ Hemolysis due to rough handling of the sample

D

Dexamethasone suppression

A standard screening test for Cushing's syndrome, the dexamethasone suppression test also helps diagnose major depression and monitor its treatment. Certain patients with major depression have high levels of circulating adrenal steroid hormones in their blood. Administration of dexamethasone, an oral corticosteroid, suppresses levels of circulating adrenal steroid hormones in normal people but fails to suppress them in patients with Cushing's syndrome and some forms of clinical depression.

Purpose
- To diagnose Cushing's syndrome
- To aid diagnosis of clinical depression

Cost
Very expensive

Patient preparation
- Explain to the patient the purpose of the test.
- Inform the patient that the test requires two blood samples drawn after administration of dexamethasone. Explain to him who will perform the venipunctures and when.
- Explain to the patient that he may experience discomfort from the needle punctures and the tourniquet.
- Restrict food and fluids for 10 to 12 hours before the test.

Reference values
A cortisol level of 5 g/dl (SI, 140 nmol/L) or greater indicates failure of dexamethasone suppression.

Abnormal findings
A normal test result doesn't rule out major depression, but an abnormal result strengthens a clinically based diagnosis. Failure of suppression occurs in patients with Cushing's syndrome, severe stress, and depression that's likely to respond to treatment with antidepressants.

Interfering factors
- Diabetes mellitus, pregnancy, and severe stress, such as trauma, severe weight loss, dehydration, and acute alcohol withdrawal (possible false-positive)
- Certain drugs, particularly barbiturates or phenytoin, within 3 weeks of the test (possible false-positive)

- Caffeine consumed after midnight the night before the test (possible false-positive)
- Failure to withhold corticosteroids, hormonal contraceptives, lithium, methadone, aspirin, diuretics, morphine, or MAO inhibitors for 24 to 48 hours before the test

Direct antiglobulin

The direct antiglobulin test detects immunoglobulins (antibodies) on the surface of red blood cells (RBCs). These immunoglobulins coat RBCs when they become sensitized to an antigen, such as the Rh factor.

In this test, antiglobulin (Coombs') serum added to saline-washed RBCs results in agglutination if immunoglobulins or complement is present. This test is "direct" because it requires only one step — the addition of Coombs' serum to washed cells.

Purpose
- To diagnose hemolytic disease of the neonate (HDN)
- To investigate hemolytic transfusion reactions
- To aid differential diagnosis of hemolytic anemias, which may be congenital or may result from an autoimmune reaction or use of certain drugs

Cost
Moderately expensive

Patient preparation
- If the patient is a neonate, explain to the parents that this test helps diagnose HDN.
- If the patient is suspected of having hemolytic anemia, explain to him that the test determines whether the condition results from an abnormality in the body's

immune system, the use of certain drugs, or some unknown cause.
- Inform the patient that he need not fast before the test.
- Tell the patient (or a neonate's parents) that the test requires a blood sample. Explain who will perform the venipuncture and when.
- Explain to the patient (or a neonate's parents) that he may experience discomfort from the needle puncture and the tourniquet if appropriate.
- Restrict medications that may affect test results, including quinidine, methyldopa, cephalosporins, sulfonamides, chlorpromazine, diphenylhydantoin, ethosuximide, hydralazine, levodopa, mefenamic acid, melphalan, penicillin, procainamide, rifampin, streptomycin, tetracyclines, and isoniazid. If they must be continued, note this on the laboratory request.

Normal findings
A negative test, in which neither antibodies nor complement appear on the RBCs, is normal.

Abnormal findings
A positive test on umbilical cord blood indicates that maternal antibodies have crossed the placenta and coated fetal RBCs, causing HDN. Transfusion of compatible blood lacking the antigens to these maternal antibodies may be necessary to prevent anemia.

In other patients, a positive test result may indicate hemolytic anemia and help differentiate between autoimmune and secondary hemolytic anemia, which can be drug-induced or associated with an underlying disease. A positive test can also indicate sepsis.

A weakly positive test may suggest a transfusion reaction in which the patient's antibodies react with transfused RBCs containing the corresponding antigen.

AGE ISSUE * * * * *

For a neonate, 5 ml of cord blood may be drawn into a tube with EDTA or additives after the cord is clamped and cut. Tell the parents of the neonate with HDN that further tests will be necessary to monitor anemia.

Interfering factors

■ Hemolysis due to rough handling of the sample

■ Quinidine, methyldopa, cephalosporins, sulfonamides, chlorpromazine, diphenylhydantoin, dipyrone, ethosuximide, hydralazine, levodopa, mefenamic acid, melphalan, penicillin, procainamide, rifampin, streptomycin, tetracyclines, and isoniazid (positive test results, possibly due to immune hemolysis)

Doppler ultrasonography

Doppler ultrasonography is a noninvasive test used to evaluate blood flow in the major veins and arteries of the arms and legs and in the extracranial cerebrovascular system using high frequency sound waves. An alternative to arteriography and venography, it's safer, less costly, and faster than invasive tests. The sound waves strike moving red blood cells and are reflected back to the transducer, allowing direct listening and graphic recording of blood flow. This test is always performed bilaterally.

Measurement of systolic pressure during this test is used to detect the presence, location, and extent of peripheral arterial occlusive disease. Changes in sound wave frequency during respiration are observed to detect venous occlusive disease. Compression maneuvers detect occlusion of the

veins and occlusion or stenosis of carotid arteries.

Pulse volume recorder testing may be performed with Doppler ultrasonography to record changes in blood volume or flow in an extremity or organ.

Purpose

■ To aid diagnosis of venous insufficiency and superficial and deep vein thromboses (popliteal, femoral, iliac)

■ To aid diagnosis of peripheral artery disease and arterial occlusion

■ To monitor patients who have had arterial reconstruction and bypass grafts

■ To detect abnormalities of carotid artery blood flow associated with conditions such as aortic stenosis

■ To evaluate possible arterial trauma

Cost

Expensive

Patient preparation

■ Explain to the patient that this test is used to evaluate blood flow in the arms and legs or neck and doesn't involve risk or discomfort.

■ Tell the patient that he'll be asked to move his arms to different positions and to perform breathing exercises as measurements are taken. A small ultrasonic probe resembling a microphone is placed at various sites along veins or arteries, and blood pressure is checked at several sites.

■ Consult with the vascular laboratory about special equipment or instructions.

Normal findings

Arterial waveforms of the arms and legs are triphasic, with a prominent systolic component and one or more diastolic sounds. The ankle-arm pressure index — the ratio between ankle systolic pressure and brachial systolic pressure — is normally equal to or greater than 1. (The ankle-arm pressure index is also known as arterial ischemia index, the ankle-brachial index, or the pedal-brachial index.) Proximal thigh pressure is normally 20 to 30 mm Hg higher than arm pressure, but pressure measurements at adjacent sites are similar. In the arms, pressure readings should remain unchanged despite postural changes.

Venous blood flow velocity is normally phasic with respiration and is of a lower pitch than arterial flow. Distal compression or release of proximal limb compression increases blood flow velocity. In the legs, abdominal compression eliminates respiratory variations, but release increases blood flow; Valsalva's maneuver also interrupts venous flow velocity.

In cerebrovascular testing, a strong velocity signal is present. In the common carotid artery, blood flow velocity increases during diastole due to low peripheral vascular resistance of the brain. The direction of periorbital arterial flow is normally anterograde out of the orbit.

Abnormal findings

Arterial stenosis or occlusion diminishes the blood flow velocity signal, with no diastolic sound and a less prominent systolic component distal to the lesion. At the lesion, the signal is high-pitched and, occasionally, turbulent. If complete occlusion is present and collateral circulation hasn't taken over, the velocity signal may be absent.

A pressure gradient exceeding 20 mm Hg at adjacent sites of measurement in the leg may indicate occlusive disease. Specifically, low proximal thigh pressure signifies common femoral or aortoiliac occlusive disease. An abnormal gradient between the proximal thigh and the above- or below-knee cuffs indicates superficial femoral or popliteal artery occlusive disease; an abnor-

mal gradient between the below-knee and ankle cuffs indicates tibiofibular disease. Abnormal gradients of arm and forearm pressure readings may indicate brachial artery occlusion.

An abnormal ankle-arm pressure index is directly proportional to the degree of circulatory impairment: mild ischemia, 1 to 0.75; claudication, 0.75 to 0.50; pain at rest, 0.50 to 0.25; and pregangrene, 0.25 to 0.

If venous blood flow velocity is unchanged by respirations, doesn't increase in response to compression or Valsalva's maneuver, or is absent, venous thrombosis is indicated. In chronic venous insufficiency and varicose veins, the flow velocity signal may be reversed. Confirmation of results may require venography.

Inability to identify Doppler signals during cerebrovascular examination implies total arterial occlusion. Reversed periorbital arterial flow indicates significant arterial occlusive disease of the extracranial internal carotid artery. In addition, the audible signal may take on the acoustic characteristics of a normal peripheral artery. Stenosis of the internal carotid artery causes turbulent signals. Collateral circulation can be assessed by compression maneuvers.

Oculoplethysmography, carotid phonoangiography, or carotid imaging can further evaluate cerebrovascular disease. Retrograde blood velocity in the vertebral artery can indicate subclavian steal syndrome. A weak velocity signal on comparison of contralateral vertebral arteries can indicate diffuse vertebral artery disease.

Interfering factors
- Uncooperative patient

D-xylose absorption

The D-xylose absorption test evaluates patients with symptoms of malabsorption, such as weight loss and generalized malnutrition, weakness, and diarrhea. D-xylose is a pentose sugar that's absorbed in the small intestine without the aid of pancreatic enzymes, passes through the liver without being metabolized, and is excreted in the urine. Because of its absorption in the small intestine without digestion, measurement of D-xylose in the urine and blood indicates the absorptive capacity of the small intestine.

Purpose
- To aid differential diagnosis of malabsorption
- To determine the cause of malabsorption syndrome

Cost
Moderately expensive

Patient preparation
- Tell the patient that this test helps evaluate digestive function by analyzing blood samples and urine specimens after ingestion of a sugar solution.
- Explain to the patient that he must fast overnight before the test and that he'll have to fast and remain in bed during the test.
- Tell the patient that he will be given D-xylose solution to drink and then several blood and urine samples will be taken. Explain who will perform the venipunctures and when.
- Explain to the patient that he may experience discomfort from the needle puncture and the tourniquet.
- Inform the patient that all his urine will be collected for 5 or 24 hours as ordered.
- Restrict medications that may affect test results, such as aspirin and indomethacin.

If they must be continued, note this on the laboratory request.

AGE ISSUE * * * * *
Because patients age 65 and older and those with borderline or elevated creatinine levels tend to have low 5-hour urine levels but normal 24-hour levels, establish the length of the collection period.

Reference values
- *Children:* blood concentration, more than 30 mg/dl in 1 hour; urine, 16% to 33% of ingested D-xylose excreted in 5 hours
- *Adults:* blood concentration, 25 to 40 mg/dl in 2 hours; urine, 3.5 g excreted in 5 hours (age 65 or older, > 5 g in 24 hours)

Abnormal findings
Depressed blood and urine D-xylose levels most commonly result from malabsorption disorders that affect the proximal small intestine, such as sprue and celiac disease. Depressed levels may also result from regional enteritis involving the jejunum, Whipple's disease, multiple jejunal diverticula, myxedema, diabetic neuropathic diarrhea, rheumatoid arthritis, alcoholism, severe heart failure, and ascites.

Interfering factors
- Failure to adhere to pretest restrictions
- Aspirin (decreased D-xylose excretion by the kidneys)
- Indomethacin (decreased intestinal D-xylose absorption)
- Failure to obtain a complete urine specimen or to collect blood samples at designated times
- Intestinal overgrowth of bacteria, renal insufficiency, or renal retention of urine (possible drop in urine levels)

E

Electro-encephalography

In electroencephalography (EEG), electrodes attached to areas of the patient's scalp record the brain's electrical activity and transmit this information to an electroencephalograph, which records the resulting brain waves on recording paper. The procedure may be performed in a special laboratory or by a portable unit at the bedside. Ambulatory recording EEGs are available for the patient to wear at home or the workplace to record the patient as he performs his normal daily activities. Continuous-video EEG recording is available on an inpatient basis for the identification of epileptic discharges during clinical events or for localization of a seizure focus during a surgical evaluation of epilepsy. Intracranial electrodes are surgically implanted to record EEG changes for localization of the seizure focus.

Purpose
■ To determine the presence and type of seizure disorder
■ To aid diagnosis of intracranial lesions, such as abscesses and tumors
■ To evaluate the brain's electrical activity in metabolic disease, cerebral ischemia, head injury, meningitis, encephalitis, mental retardation, psychological disorders, and drugs
■ To evaluate altered states of consciousness or brain death

Cost
Expensive

Patient preparation
■ Explain to the patient that this test records the brain's electrical activity.
■ Describe the procedure to the patient and his family members, and answer all questions.
■ Tell the patient that he must forgo caffeine 24 hours before the test but to otherwise eat regularly, because skipping the meal before the test can cause relative hypoglycemia and alter the brain wave pattern.
■ Explain to the patient that during the test electrodes will be attached to his scalp with a special paste. Assure him that the electrodes won't shock him.
■ Check the patient's medication history for drugs that may interfere with test results. Restrict anticonvulsants, tranquilizers,

barbiturates, and other sedatives for 24 to 48 hours before the test. Infants and young children occasionally require sedation to prevent crying and restlessness during the test, but sedation itself may alter test results.

■ A patient with a seizure disorder may require a "sleep EEG." In this case, tell the patient that he'll be awake the night before the test and receive a sedative to help him sleep during the test.

Normal findings

EEG records a portion of the brain's electrical activity as waves; some are irregular, whereas others demonstrate frequent patterns. Among the basic waveforms are the alpha, beta, theta, and delta rhythms.

Alpha waves occur at a frequency of 8 to 11 cycles/second in a regular rhythm. They're present only in the waking state when the patient's eyes are closed but he's mentally alert; usually, they disappear with visual activity or mental concentration. Beta waves (13 to 30 cycles/second) — generally associated with anxiety, depression, and use of sedatives — are seen most readily in the frontal and central regions of the brain. Theta waves (4 to 7 cycles/second) are most common in children and young adults and appear in the frontal and temporal regions. Delta waves (0.5 to 3.5 cycles/second) normally occur only in young children and during sleep.

Abnormal findings

Usually, about a 100′ to 200′ (30 to 61 m) strip of recordings is evaluated, with particular attention paid to basic waveforms, symmetry of cerebral activity, transient discharges, and responses to stimulation. A specific diagnosis depends on the patient's clinical status. (See *Comparing EEG tracings*.)

In patients with epilepsy, EEG patterns may identify the specific disorder. In absence seizures, the EEG shows spikes and waves at a frequency of 3 cycles/second. In generalized tonic-clonic seizures, it generally shows multiple, high-voltage, spiked waves in both hemispheres. In temporal lobe epilepsy, the EEG usually shows spiked waves in the affected temporal region. And in patients with focal seizures, it usually shows localized, spiked discharges.

In patients with intracranial lesions, such as tumors or abscesses, the EEG may show slow waves (usually delta waves but possibly unilateral beta waves). Vascular lesions, such as cerebral infarcts and intracranial hemorrhages, generally produce focal abnormalities in the injured area.

Generally, any condition that causes a diminishing level of consciousness alters the EEG pattern in proportion to the degree of consciousness lost. For example, in a patient with a metabolic disorder, an inflammatory process (such as meningitis or encephalitis), or increased intracranial pressure, the EEG shows generalized, diffuse, and slow brain waves.

The most pathologic finding of all is an absent EEG pattern — a "flat" tracing (except for artifacts) that may indicate brain death.

Interfering factors

■ Interference from extraneous electrical activity; head, body, eye, or tongue movement; or muscle contractions (possible production of excessive artifact)
■ Anticonvulsants, barbiturates, tranquilizers and other sedatives (possible masking of seizure activity)
■ Acute drug intoxication or severe hypothermia resulting in loss of consciousness (flat EEG)

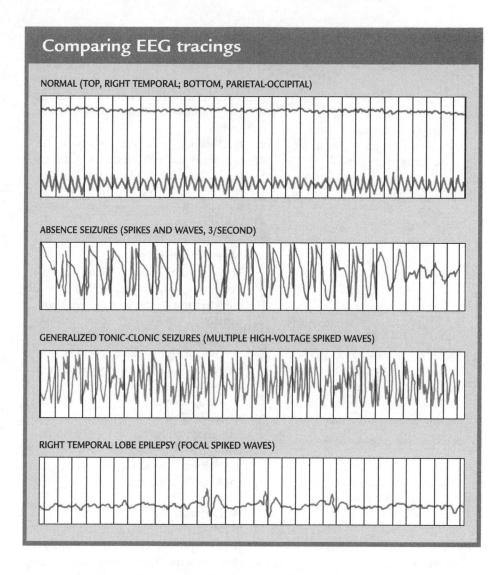

Comparing EEG tracings

NORMAL (TOP, RIGHT TEMPORAL; BOTTOM, PARIETAL-OCCIPITAL)

ABSENCE SEIZURES (SPIKES AND WAVES, 3/SECOND)

GENERALIZED TONIC-CLONIC SEIZURES (MULTIPLE HIGH-VOLTAGE SPIKED WAVES)

RIGHT TEMPORAL LOBE EPILEPSY (FOCAL SPIKED WAVES)

Electromyography

Electromyography records the electrical activity of selected skeletal muscle groups at rest and during voluntary contraction. It involves percutaneous insertion of a needle electrode into a muscle. An oscilloscope then measures the muscle's electrical discharge. Nerve conduction time is often measured simultaneously. (See *Nerve conduction studies*, page 138.)

ALERT! ▼ ▼ ▼ ▼ ▼ ▼ ▼ ▼ ▼
Electromyography is contraindicated in patients with bleeding disorders.

Purpose

■ To aid differentiation between primary muscle disorders, such as the muscular dystrophies, and secondary disorders

Nerve conduction studies

Nerve conduction studies aid diagnosis of peripheral nerve injuries and diseases affecting the peripheral nervous system such as peripheral neuropathies. To measure nerve conduction time, a nerve is stimulated electrically through the skin and underlying tissues. The patient experiences a mild electric shock with each stimulation. At a known distance from the point of stimulation, a recording electrode detects the response from the stimulated nerve.

The time between stimulation of the nerve and the detected response is measured on an oscilloscope. The speed of conduction along the nerve is then calculated by dividing the distance between the point of stimulation and the recording electrode by the time between stimulus and response. In peripheral nerve injuries and diseases such as peripheral neuropathies, nerve conduction time is abnormal.

■ To help assess diseases characterized by central neuronal degeneration such as amyotrophic lateral sclerosis
■ To aid diagnosis of neuromuscular disorders, such as myasthenia gravis and radiculomyopathies

Cost
Expensive

Patient preparation
■ Explain to the patient that this test measures the electrical activity of his muscles.
■ Tell the patient that there are usually no restrictions on food or fluids (in some cases, cigarettes, coffee, tea, and cola may be restricted for 2 to 3 hours before the test).

■ Describe the test, including who will perform it and where it will take place.
■ Advise the patient that a needle will be inserted into selected muscles and that he may experience mild discomfort. Reassure him that adverse effects and complications are rare.
■ Obtain informed consent if necessary.
■ Restrict medications that may affect test results, for example, cholinergics, anticholinergics, and skeletal muscle relaxants. If they must be continued, note this on the laboratory request.

Normal findings
At rest, a normal muscle exhibits minimal electrical activity. During voluntary contraction electrical activity increases markedly. A sustained contraction or one of increasing strength causes a rapid "train" of motor unit potentials that can be heard as a crescendo of sounds over the audio amplifier.

At the same time, the monitor displays a sequence of waveforms that vary in amplitude (height) and frequency. Waveforms that are close together indicate a high frequency, whereas waveforms that are far apart signify a low frequency.

Abnormal findings
In primary muscle diseases, such as muscular dystrophy, motor unit potentials are short (low amplitude), with frequent, irregular discharges. In disorders such as amyotrophic lateral sclerosis (as well as in peripheral nerve disorders), motor unit potentials are isolated and irregular but show increased amplitude and duration. In myasthenia gravis, motor unit potentials may initially be normal but progressively diminish in amplitude with continuing contractions. The interpreter distinguishes between waveforms that indicate a muscle disorder and those that indicate denerva-

tion. Findings must be correlated with the patient's history, clinical features, and the results of other neurodiagnostic tests.

Interfering factors
■ Patient's inability to comply with instructions
■ Drugs affecting myoneural junctions, such as cholinergics, anticholinergics, and skeletal muscle relaxants

Electrophysiology studies

Electrophysiology studies (also known as *His bundle electrography*) permit measurement of discrete conduction intervals by recording electrical conduction during the slow withdrawal of a bipolar or tripolar electrode catheter from the right ventricle through the His bundle to the sinoatrial node. The catheter is introduced into the femoral vein, passing through the right atrium and across the septal leaflet of the tricuspid valve.

ALERT! ▼ ▼ ▼ ▼ ▼ ▼ ▼ ▼
Electrophysiology studies are contraindicated in patients with severe coagulopathy, recent thrombophlebitis, or acute pulmonary embolism.

Purpose
■ To diagnose arrhythmias and conduction anomalies
■ To determine the need for an implanted pacemaker, an internal cardioverter-defibrillator, and cardioactive drugs and to evaluate their effects on the conduction system and ectopic rhythms
■ To locate the site of a bundle-branch block, especially in asymptomatic patients with conduction disturbances
■ To determine the presence and location of accessory conducting structures

Cost
Expensive

Patient preparation
■ Explain to the patient that this test will help evaluate his heart's conduction system.
■ Tell the patient not to eat or drink anything for at least 6 hours before the test.
■ Describe the test to the patient, including who will perform it and where it will take place.
■ Inform the patient that after his groin area is shaved, a catheter will be inserted into the femoral vein and an I.V. line may be started. Assure him that the electrocardiogram (ECG) electrodes attached to his chest during the test will cause no discomfort.
■ Explain to the patient that he'll experience a stinging sensation when a local anesthetic is injected to numb the incision site for catheter insertion. Tell him he may experience pressure on catheter insertion.
■ Inform the patient that he will be conscious during the test, and urge him to report any discomfort or pain to the person performing the test.
■ Obtain informed consent if necessary.
■ Tell the patient that he'll be monitored closely after the procedure and bed rest will be enforced for 4 to 6 hours.
■ Order a 12-lead resting ECG to assess for changes.

Reference values
Normal conduction intervals in adults are as follows: HV interval, 35 to 55 msec; AH interval, 45 to 150 msec; and PA interval, 20 to 40 msec.

Abnormal findings
■ A prolonged HV interval (the conduction time from the His bundle to the Purk-

inje fibers) can result from acute or chronic disease.

■ Atrioventricular nodal (AH interval) delays can stem from atrial pacing, chronic conduction system disease, carotid sinus pressure, recent myocardial infarction, and use of certain drugs.

■ Intra-atrial (PA interval) delays can result from acquired, surgically induced, or congenital atrial disease and atrial pacing.

Interfering factors

■ Malfunctioning recording equipment and improper catheter positioning

Epstein-Barr virus antibodies

Epstein-Barr virus (EBV), a member of the herpesvirus group, is the causative agent of heterophil-positive infectious mononucleosis, Burkitt's lymphoma, and nasopharyngeal carcinoma. Although the virus doesn't replicate in standard cell cultures, testing the patient's serum for heterophil antibodies (monospot test), which usually appear within the first 3 weeks of illness and then decline rapidly within a few weeks, can recognized most EBV infections.

In about 10% of adults and a larger percentage of children, the monospot test is negative, despite primary infection with EBV. Further, EBV has been associated with lymphoproliferative processes in immunosuppressed patients. These disorders occur with reactivated, rather than primary, EBV infections and therefore are also monospot-negative.

Alternatively, EBV-specific antibodies, which develop to several antigens of the virus during active infection, can be measured with a high level of sensitivity and specificity by indirect immunofluorescence.

Purpose

■ To provide a laboratory diagnosis of heterophil- (or monospot-) negative cases of infectious mononucleosis

■ To determine the antibody status to EBV of immunosuppressed patients with lymphoproliferative processes

Cost
Inexpensive

Patient preparation

■ Explain to the patient the purpose of the test.

■ Tell the patient that the test requires a blood sample. Explain who will perform the venipuncture and when.

■ Explain to the patient that he may experience discomfort from the needle puncture and the tourniquet.

Normal findings

Sera from patients who have never been infected with EBV have no detectable antibodies to the virus as measured by either the monospot test or the indirect immunofluorescence test. The monospot test is positive only during the acute phase of infection with EBV; the indirect immunofluorescence test detects and discriminates between acute and past infection with the virus.

Abnormal findings

EBV infection can be ruled out if no antibodies to EBV antigens are detected in the indirect immunofluorescence test. A positive monospot test or an indirect immunofluorescence test that's either immunoglobulin (Ig) M–positive or Epstein-Barr nuclear antigen (EBNA)–negative indicates acute EBV infection.

A monospot-negative result doesn't necessarily rule out acute or past infection with EBV. Conversely, IgG class antibody to viral capsid antigens and EBNAs (IgM-negative) indicates remote (more than 2 months) infection with EBV. Recognize that most cases of monospot-negative infectious mononucleosis are caused by cytomegalovirus infections.

Interfering factors
■ Hemolysis due to rough handling of the sample

Erythrocyte sedimentation rate

The erythrocyte sedimentation rate (ESR) measures the degree of erythrocyte settling in a blood sample during a specified time period. The ESR is a sensitive but nonspecific test that's frequently the earliest indicator of disease when other chemical or physical signs are normal. The ESR commonly increases significantly in widespread inflammatory disorders; elevators may be prolonged in localized inflammation and malignant disease.

Purpose
■ To monitor inflammatory or malignant disease
■ To aid detection and diagnosis of occult disease, such as tuberculosis, tissue necrosis, or connective tissue disease

Cost
Inexpensive

Patient preparation
■ Explain to the patient that this test is used to evaluate the condition of red blood cells.
■ Tell the patient that the test requires a blood sample. Explain who will obtain the venipuncture and when.

■ Explain to the patient that he may experience discomfort from the needle puncture and the tourniquet.
■ Inform the patient that food or fluids need not be restricted before the test.

Reference values
The ESR normally ranges from 0 to 10 mm/hour (SI, 0 to 10 mm/h) in males, 0 to 20 mm/hour (SI, 0 to 20 mm/h) in females, and 0 to 10 mm/hour (SI, 0 to 10 mm/h) in children. Rates gradually increase with age.

Abnormal findings
The ESR rises in pregnancy, anemia, acute or chronic inflammation, tuberculosis, paraproteinemias (especially multiple myeloma and Waldenström's macroglobulinemia), rheumatic fever, rheumatoid arthritis, and some malignant disease.

Polycythemia, sickle cell anemia, hyperviscosity, and low plasma fibrinogen or globulins levels tend to depress the ESR.

Interfering factors
■ Failure to use the proper anticoagulant and inadequate mixing of the sample and anticoagulant
■ Failure to send the sample to the laboratory immediately
■ Hemolysis due to rough handling or excessive mixing of the sample
■ Hemoconcentration due to prolonged tourniquet constriction
■ Testing delayed more than 3 hours after sample collection (may possibly decrease)

Erythropoietin

The erythropoietin test of renal hormone production measures erythropoietin (EPO) by immunoassay. It's used to evaluate anemia, polycythemia, and kidney tumors. It's also used to evaluate abuse of commercially prepared EPO by athletes who believe that the drug enhances performance.

Purpose
- To aid diagnosis of anemia, polycythemia, and kidney tumors
- To detect EPO abuse by athletes

Cost
Moderately expensive

Patient preparation
- Explain to the patient that this test determines if hormonal secretion is causing changes in his red blood cells (RBCs).
- Instruct the patient to fast for 8 to 10 hours before the test.
- Tell the patient that the test requires a blood sample. Explain who will perform the venipuncture and when.
- Explain to the patient that he may experience discomfort from the needle puncture and the tourniquet.

Reference values
The reference range for EPO is 5 to 36 mU/ml (SI, 5 to 36 IU/L).

Abnormal findings
Low levels of EPO appear in patients with anemia who have inadequate or absent hormone production. Congenital absence of EPO can occur. Severe renal disease may decrease EPO production.

Elevated EPO levels occur in anemias as a compensatory mechanism in the reestablishment of homeostasis. Inappropriate elevations (when the hematocrit is normal to high) are seen in polycythemia and EPO-secreting tumors.

Some athletes use EPO to enhance performance. The increased RBC volume conveys additional oxygen-carrying capacity to the blood. Adverse reactions include clotting abnormalities, headache, seizures, hypertension, nausea, vomiting, diarrhea, and rash.

Interfering factors
- Failure to collect a sample in the fasting state

Esophagogastroduodenoscopy

Esophagogastroduodenoscopy (EGD) permits visual examination of the lining of the esophagus, stomach, and upper duodenum using a flexible fiber-optic or video endoscope. It's indicated for patients with GI bleeding, hematemesis, melena, substernal or epigastric pain, gastroesophageal reflux disease, dysphagia, anemia, strictures, or peptic ulcer disease; those requiring foreign body retrieval; and postoperative patients with recurrent or new symptoms.

EGD eliminates the need for extensive exploratory surgery and can be used to detect small or surface lesions missed by radiography. Because the scope provides a channel for biopsy forceps or a cytology brush, it permits laboratory evaluation of abnormalities detected by radiography. Similarly, it allows removal of foreign bodies by suction (for small, soft objects) or by electrocautery snare or forceps (for large, hard objects).

ALERT! ▼ ▼ ▼ ▼ ▼ ▼ ▼ ▼
EGD is usually contraindicated in patients with Zenker's diverticulum; a large aortic aneurysm; recent ulcer perforation, known as suspected viscus perforation; and unstable cardiac or pulmonary conditions. EGD shouldn't be performed within 2 days after an upper GI series.

Purpose

■ To diagnose inflammatory disease, malignant and benign tumors, ulcers, Mallory-Weiss syndrome, and structural abnormalities
■ To evaluate the stomach and duodenum postoperatively
■ To obtain emergency diagnosis of duodenal ulcer or esophageal injury such as that caused by ingestion of chemicals

Cost

Expensive

Patient preparation

■ Explain to the patient that this procedure permits visual examination of the lining of the esophagus, stomach, and upper duodenum through the use of a scope.
■ Instruct the patient to fast for 6 to 12 hours before the test.
■ Inform the patient that a bitter-tasting local anesthetic will be sprayed into his mouth and throat and a mouth guard will be inserted; assure him that this won't obstruct his breathing.
■ Inform the patient that an I.V. line will be started and a sedative will be administered but he may still feel pressure and fullness. Drugs that retard peristalsis of the upper GI tract may be administered in some circumstances.
■ Obtain informed consent if necessary.
■ Tell the patient that after the test has been administered, food and fluids will be withheld until the gag reflex returns (usually in 1 hour), after which he'll be allowed fluids and a light meal.
■ Because of sedation, tell the outpatient to secure transportation home.

Normal findings

The smooth mucosa of the esophagus is normally yellow-pink and marked by a fine vascular network. A pulsation on the ante-rior wall of the esophagus between 8″ and 10″ (20.5 and 25.5 cm) from the incisor teeth represents the aortic arch. The orange-red mucosa of the stomach begins at the "Z" line, an irregular transition line slightly above the esophagogastric junction.

Unlike the esophagus, the stomach has rugal folds, and its blood vessels aren't visible beneath the gastric mucosa. The reddish mucosa of the duodenal bulb is marked by a few shallow longitudinal folds. The mucosa of the distal duodenum has prominent circular folds, is lined with villi, and appears velvety.

Abnormal findings

EGD, coupled with the results of histologic and cytologic tests, may indicate acute or chronic ulcers, benign or malignant tumors, and inflammatory disease, including esophagitis, gastritis, and duodenitis. This test may demonstrate diverticula, varices, Mallory-Weiss syndrome, esophageal rings, esophageal and pyloric stenoses, and esophageal hiatal hernia. Although EGD can evaluate gross abnormalities of esophageal motility, as occur in achalasia, manometric studies are more accurate.

Interfering factors

■ Patients taking anticoagulants (increased risk of bleeding)
■ Failure to adhere to pretest restrictions
■ Failure to send specimens to the laboratory immediately
■ Patient's inability to cooperate, preventing optimal visualization

Estrogens

Estrogens as well as progesterone are secreted by the ovaries. They're responsible for the development of secondary female sexu-

Predicting premature labor

A simple salivary test can help determine whether a pregnant woman is at risk for premature labor, a complication that's detrimental to the health of the premature infant. The test, known as the SalEst test, measures salivary levels of estriol, an estrogen that increases 1,000-fold during pregnancy. For women determined to be at risk, the SalEst test is 98% accurate in ruling out premature labor and delivery.

The test is performed on women between 22 and 36 weeks' gestation, using their saliva and the SalEst test kit. Estriol has been found to increase 2 to 3 weeks before the spontaneous onset of labor and delivery. A positive test indicates that the patient is at risk for premature labor. With this knowledge and evaluation by a physician, precautions can be instituted to decrease the risk of preterm labor and maintain fetal viability.

Purpose
- To determine sexual maturation and fertility
- To aid diagnosis of gonadal dysfunction, such as precocious or delayed puberty, menstrual disorders (especially amenorrhea), and infertility
- To determine fetal well-being
- To aid diagnosis of tumors known to secrete estrogen

Cost
Moderately expensive

Patient preparation
- Explain to the patient that this test helps determine if secretion of female hormones is normal and that the test may be repeated during the various phases of the menstrual cycle.
- Tell the patient that the test requires a blood sample. Explain who will perform the venipuncture and when.
- Explain to the patient that she may experience discomfort from the needle puncture and the tourniquet.
- Restrict all steroid and pituitary-based hormones. If they must be continued, note this on the laboratory request as well as her phase of menstrual cycle (if premenopausal).

Reference values
Normal serum estrogen levels for premenopausal women vary widely during the menstrual cycle, ranging from 26 to 149 pg/ml (SI, 90 to 550 pmol/L). The range for postmenopausal women is 0 to 34 pg/ml (SI, 0 to 125 pmol/L).

Serum estrogen levels in men range from 12 to 34 pg/ml (SI, 40 to 125 pmol/L). In children under age 6, the normal level of serum estrogen is 3 to 10 pg/ml (SI, 10 to 36 pmol/L). Estriol is secreted in large amounts by the placenta during pregnancy.

al characteristics and for normal menstruation. Levels are usually undetectable in children. These hormones are secreted by ovarian follicular cells during the first half of the menstrual cycle and by the corpus luteum during the luteal phase and during pregnancy. In menopause, estrogen secretion drops to a constant, low level.

This radioimmunoassay measures serum levels of estradiol, estrone, and estriol (the only estrogens that appear in serum in measurable amounts) and has diagnostic significance in evaluating female gonadal dysfunction. (See *Predicting premature labor*.)

Tests of hypothalamic-pituitary function may be required to confirm the diagnosis.

Levels range from 2 ng/ml (SI, 7 nmol/L) by 30 weeks' gestation to 30 ng/ml (SI, 105 nmol/L) by week 40.

Abnormal findings

Decreased estrogen levels may indicate primary hypogonadism, or ovarian failure, as in Turner's syndrome or ovarian agenesis; secondary hypogonadism such as in hypopituitarism; or menopause.

Abnormally high estrogen levels may occur with estrogen-producing tumors, in precocious puberty, and in severe hepatic disease, such as cirrhosis, that prevents clearance of plasma estrogens. High levels may also result from congenital adrenal hyperplasia (increased conversion of androgens to estrogen).

Interfering factors

- Pregnancy and pretest use of estrogens such as hormonal contraceptives (possible increase)
- Clomiphene, an estrogen antagonist (possible decrease)
- Steroids and pituitary-based hormones such as dexamethasone

Evoked potential

Evoked potential studies evaluate the integrity of visual, somatosensory, and auditory nerve pathways by measuring evoked potentials — the brain's electrical response to stimulation of the sensory organs or peripheral nerves. Evoked potentials are recorded as electronic impulses by surface electrodes attached to the scalp and skin over various peripheral sensory nerves. A computer extracts these low-amplitude impulses from background brain wave activity and averages the signals from repeated stimuli. (See *Visual and somatosensory evoked potentials*, pages 146 and 147.)

Two types of responses are measured:
- *Visual evoked potentials:* Produced by exposing the eye to a rapidly reversing checkerboard pattern, this type of response helps evaluate demyelinating diseases, traumatic injury, and puzzling visual complaints.
- *Somatosensory evoked potentials:* Produced by electrically stimulating a peripheral sensory nerve, this type of response helps diagnose peripheral nerve disease and locate brain and spinal cord lesions.

Purpose
- To aid diagnosis of nervous system lesions and abnormalities
- To assess neurologic function

Cost
Expensive

Patient preparation
- Tell the patient that this group of tests measures the electrical activity of his nervous system. Explain who will perform the test and where it will take place.
- Tell the patient that he'll sit in a reclining chair or lie on a bed. If visual evoked potentials will be measured, electrodes will be attached to his scalp; if somatosensory evoked potentials will be measured, electrodes will be placed on his scalp, neck, lower back, wrist, knee, and ankle.
- Assure the patient that the electrodes won't cause discomfort. Encourage him to relax; tension can affect neurologic function and interfere with test results.

Normal findings
Visual evoked potentials
On the waveform, the most significant wave is P100, a positive wave appearing about 100 msec after the pattern-shift stimulus is applied. The most clinically signifi-

(Text continues on page 148.)

Visual and somatosensory evoked potentials

Visual (pattern-shift) evoked potentials: In this test, visual neural impulses are recorded as they travel along the pathway from the eye to the occipital cortex. Wave P100 is the most significant component of the resultant waveform. Normal P100 latency is about 100 milliseconds after the application of a visual stimulus, as shown in the top diagram. Increased P100 latency, shown in the bottom diagram, is an abnormal finding, indicating a lesion along the visual pathway.

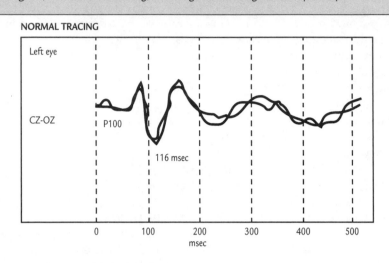

NORMAL TRACING

Left eye

CZ-OZ
P100

116 msec

0   100   200   300   400   500
msec

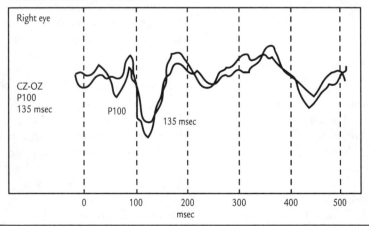

TRACING IN MULTIPLE SCLEROSIS

Right eye

CZ-OZ
P100
135 msec

P100
135 msec

0   100   200   300   400   500
msec

Key: CZ = vertex; OZ = midocciput

Visual and somatosensory evoked potentials *(continued)*

Somatosensory evoked potentials: These tests measure the conduction time of an electrical impulse traveling along a somatosensory pathway to the cortex. Interwave latency is the most significant component of the resultant waveform. On the set of upper- and lower-limb tracings shown below, the top tracings represent normal interwave latencies; the bottom tracings represent typical abnormal latencies found in a patient with multiple sclerosis. Because of the close correlation between waveforms and the anatomy of somatosensory pathways, such tracings allow precise location of lesions that produce conduction defects.

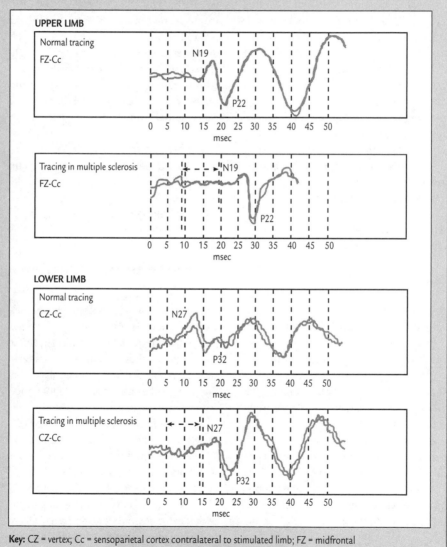

Key: CZ = vertex; Cc = sensoparietal cortex contralateral to stimulated limb; FZ = midfrontal

cant measurements are absolute P100 latency (the time between stimulus application and peaking of the P100 wave) and the difference between the P100 latencies of each eye. Because many physical and technical factors affect P100 latency, normal results vary greatly among laboratories and patients.

Somatosensory evoked potentials
Waveforms obtained vary, depending on locations of the stimulating and recording electrodes. The positive and negative peaks are labeled in sequence, based on normal time of appearance. For example, N19 is a negative peak normally recorded 19 msec after application of the stimulus. Each wave peak arises from a discrete location: N19 is generated mainly from the thalamus, P22 from the parietal sensory cortex, and so on. Interwave latencies (time between waves), rather than absolute latencies, are used as a basis for clinical interpretation. Latency differences between sides are significant.

Abnormal findings

Information from evoked potential studies is useful but insufficient to confirm a specific diagnosis. Test data must be interpreted in light of clinical information.

Visual evoked potentials
Generally, abnormal (extended) P100 latencies confined to one eye indicate a visual pathway lesion anterior to the optic chiasm. A lesion posterior to the optic chiasm usually doesn't produce abnormal P100 latencies. Because each eye projects to both occipital lobes, the unaffected pathway transmits sufficient impulses to produce a normal latency response. Bilateral abnormal P100 latencies have been found in patients with multiple sclerosis, optic neuritis, retinopathies, amblyopia (although abnormal latencies don't correlate well with impaired visual acuity), spinocerebellar degeneration, adrenoleukodystrophy, sar-

coidosis, Parkinson's disease, and Huntington's disease.

Somatosensory evoked potentials
Because somatosensory evoked potential components are assumed to be linked in series, an abnormal interwave latency indicates a conduction defect between the generators of the two peaks involved. This often allows precise location of a neurologic lesion. Abnormal upper-limb interwave latencies may indicate cervical spondylosis, intracerebral lesions, or sensorimotor neuropathies. Abnormalities in the lower limb demonstrate peripheral nerve and root lesions, such as those in Guillain-Barré syndrome, compressive myelopathies, multiple sclerosis, transverse myelitis, and traumatic spinal cord injury.

Interfering factors

■ Incorrect electrode placement or equipment failure
■ Patient tension, inability to relax, or failure to cooperate
■ Poor patient vision

Excretory urography

The cornerstone of a urologic workup, excretory urography (also called *intravenous pyelography*) requires I.V. administration of a contrast medium and allows visualization of the renal parenchyma, calyces, and pelvis as well as the ureters, bladder and, in some cases, the urethra.

In some facilities, a nonenhanced computed tomography scan of the urinary tract is commonly performed instead of this test if urinary tract calculi are suspected.

ALERT! ▼ ▼ ▼ ▼ ▼ ▼ ▼ ▼ ▼
This test may be contraindicated in patients with abnormal renal function (as evidenced by increased creatinine and blood urea nitro-

gen levels) and in children or elderly patients with actual or potential dehydration.

Purpose

■ To evaluate the structure and excretory function of the kidneys, ureters, and bladder

■ To support a differential diagnosis of renovascular hypertension

Cost

Expensive

Patient preparation

■ Explain to the patient that this test helps to evaluate the structure and function of the urinary tract.

■ Instruct the patient to fast for 8 hours before the test.

■ Tell the patient who will perform the test and where it will take place.

■ Explain to the patient that he may experience a transient burning sensation and metallic taste when the contrast medium is injected. Tell him to report any other sensations he experiences.

■ Warn the patient that the X-ray machine may make loud, clacking sounds during the test.

■ Obtain informed consent if necessary.

■ Document the patient's history for hypersensitivity to iodine, iodine-containing foods, or contrast media containing iodine.

■ Tell the patient that a laxative may be administered the night before the test to minimize poor resolution of X-ray films due to stool and gas in the GI tract.

ALERT! ▼ ▼ ▼ ▼ ▼ ▼ ▼ ▼ ▼
Premedication with corticosteroids may be indicated for patients with severe asthma or a history of sensitivity to the contrast medium.

Normal findings

The kidneys, ureters, and bladder show no gross evidence of soft- or hard-tissue lesions. Prompt visualization of the contrast medium in the kidneys demonstrates bilateral renal parenchyma and pelvicalyceal systems of normal conformity. The ureters and bladder should be outlined and the postvoiding radiograph should show no mucosal abnormalities and minimal residual urine.

Abnormal findings

Intravenous pyelography can demonstrate many abnormalities of the urinary system, including renal or ureteral calculi; abnormal size, shape, or structure of kidneys, ureters, or bladder; supernumerary or absent kidney; polycystic kidney disease associated with renal hypertrophy; redundant pelvis or ureter; space-occupying lesion; pyelonephrosis; renal tuberculosis; hydronephrosis; and renovascular hypertension.

Interfering factors

■ End-stage renal disease, stool or gas in the colon (possible poor imaging)

■ Insufficient injection of contrast medium, a recent barium enema, gastrointestinal or gallbladder series (possible poor imaging)

F

Febrile agglutination

Bacterial infections (such as tularemia, brucellosis, and the disorders caused by *Salmonella*) and rickettsial infections (such as Rocky Mountain spotted fever and typhus) sometimes cause fevers of undetermined origins (FUOs). In these infections and others in which microorganisms are difficult to isolate from blood or excreta, febrile agglutination tests can provide important diagnostic information.

The Weil-Felix test for rickettsial disease, Widal's test for *Salmonella,* and tests for brucellosis and tularemia are essentially the same. In these tests, a serum sample is mixed with a few drops of prepared antigens in normal saline solution on a slide and the reaction is observed.

Purpose
■ To support clinical findings in diagnosis of disorders caused by *Salmonella, Rickettsia, Francisella tularensis,* and *Brucella* organisms
■ To identify the cause of an FUO

Cost
Moderately expensive

Patient preparation
■ Explain to the patient that this test detects and quantifies microorganisms that may cause fever and other symptoms.
■ Tell the patient that the test requires a blood sample. Explain who will perform the venipuncture and when.
■ Explain to the patient that he may experience discomfort from the needle puncture and the tourniquet.
■ If appropriate, explain to the patient that this test requires a series of blood samples to detect a pattern of titers characteristic of the suspected disorder. Reassure him that a positive titer only suggests a disorder.
■ Note on the laboratory request when antimicrobial therapy began, if appropriate.

Reference values
Results are reported as negative or positive, and positive results are titered. Normal dilutions are:
■ *Salmonella* antibody: < 1:80
■ brucellosis antibody: < 1:80
■ tularemia antibody: < 1:40
■ rickettsial antibody: < 1:40.

Abnormal findings

Observed rise and fall of titers is crucial for detecting active infection. If this isn't possible, certain titer levels can suggest the disorder. For all febrile agglutinins, a fourfold increase in titers is strong evidence of infection.

The Weil-Felix test is positive for rickettsiae with antibodies to *Proteus,* 6 to 12 days after infection; titers peak in 1 month and usually drop to negative in 5 to 6 months. This test can't be used to diagnose rickettsialpox or Q fever because the antibodies of these diseases don't cross-react with *Proteus* antigens; the test shows positive titers in *Proteus* infections and, in such cases, is nonspecific for rickettsiae.

In *Salmonella* infection, H and O agglutinins usually appear in serum after 1 week, and titers rise for 3 to 6 weeks. O agglutinins usually fall to insignificant levels in 6 to 12 months. Agglutinin titers may remain elevated for years.

In brucellosis, titers usually rise after 2 to 3 weeks and reach their highest levels between 4 and 8 weeks. The absence of *Brucella* agglutinins doesn't rule out brucellosis. In tularemia, titers usually become positive during the second week of infection, exceed 1:320 by the 3rd week, peak within 4 to 7 weeks, and usually decline gradually 1 year after recovery.

Interfering factors

■ Vaccination or continuous exposure to bacterial or rickettsial infection, resulting in immunity (high titers)
■ Antibody cross-reaction with bacteria causing other infectious diseases, such as tularemia antibodies cross-reacting with *Brucella* antigens
■ Immunodeficiency (negative titers even during symptomatic infection due to inability to form antibodies)

■ Antibiotics (low titers early in the course of infection)
■ Elevated immunoglobulin levels due to hepatic disease or excessive drug use (high *Salmonella* titers)
■ Skin tests with *Brucella* antigen (possible high *Brucella* titers)
■ *Proteus* infections (possible positive Weil-Felix titers for rickettsial disease)

Fecal occult blood

Fecal occult blood is detected by microscopic analysis or by chemical tests for hemoglobin, such as the guaiac test. Normally, stool contains small amounts of blood (2 to 2.5 ml/day); therefore, tests for occult blood detect quantities larger than this. Clinical symptoms and preliminary blood studies suggest GI bleeding and indicate testing. Additional tests are required to pinpoint the origin of the bleeding. (See *Common sites and causes of GI blood loss,* page 152.)

Purpose
■ To detect GI bleeding
■ To aid early diagnosis of colorectal cancer

Cost
Inexpensive

Patient preparation
■ Explain to the patient that this test helps detect abnormal GI bleeding.
■ Instruct the patient to maintain a high-fiber diet and to refrain from eating red meats, turnips, and horseradish for 48 to 72 hours before the test and throughout the collection period.
■ Tell the patient that the test requires collection of three stool specimens. Occasionally, only a random specimen is collected.

Common sites and causes of GI blood loss

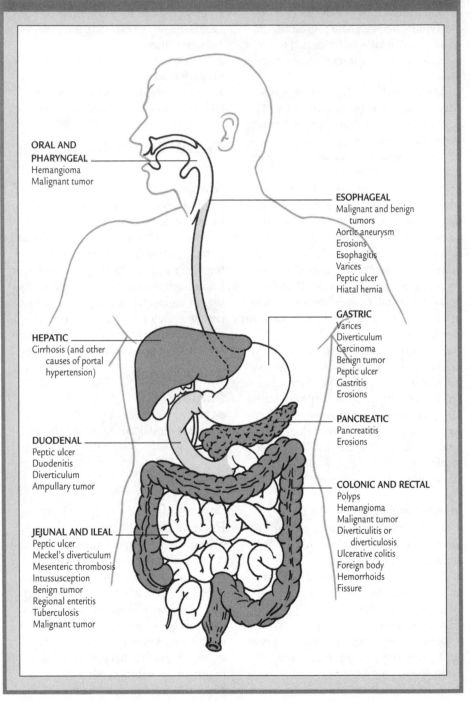

ORAL AND PHARYNGEAL
Hemangioma
Malignant tumor

ESOPHAGEAL
Malignant and benign
    tumors
Aortic aneurysm
Erosions
Esophagitis
Varices
Peptic ulcer
Hiatal hernia

GASTRIC
Varices
Diverticulum
Carcinoma
Benign tumor
Peptic ulcer
Gastritis
Erosions

HEPATIC
Cirrhosis (and other
    causes of portal
    hypertension)

PANCREATIC
Pancreatitis
Erosions

DUODENAL
Peptic ulcer
Duodenitis
Diverticulum
Ampullary tumor

COLONIC AND RECTAL
Polyps
Hemangioma
Malignant tumor
Diverticulitis or
    diverticulosis
Ulcerative colitis
Foreign body
Hemorrhoids
Fissure

JEJUNAL AND ILEAL
Peptic ulcer
Meckel's diverticulum
Mesenteric thrombosis
Intussusception
Benign tumor
Regional enteritis
Tuberculosis
Malignant tumor

■ Restrict medications that may affect test results. If they must be continued, note this on the laboratory request.

Normal findings

Less than 2.5 ml of blood should be present, resulting in a green reaction.

Abnormal findings

A positive test indicates GI bleeding, which may result from many disorders, such as varices, peptic ulcer, carcinoma, ulcerative colitis, dysentery, or hemorrhagic disease. This test is particularly important for early diagnosis of colorectal cancer. Further tests, such as barium swallow, analyses of gastric contents, and endoscopic procedures, are necessary to define the site and extent of the bleeding.

Interfering factors

■ Failure to observe pretest restrictions
■ Failure to test the specimen immediately
■ Bromides, colchicine, indomethacin, iron preparations, phenylbutazone, rauwolfia derivatives, and steroids (possible increase due to association with GI blood loss)
■ Ascorbic acid (false-normal, even with significant bleeding)
■ Ingestion of 2 to 5 ml of blood such as from bleeding gums
■ Active bleeding from hemorrhoids (possible false-positive)

Ferritin

Ferritin, a major iron-storage protein, normally appears in small quantities in serum. In healthy adults, serum ferritin levels are directly related to the amount of available iron stored in the body and can be measured accurately by radioimmunoassay.

Purpose

■ To screen for iron deficiency and iron overload
■ To measure iron storage
■ To distinguish between iron deficiency (a condition of low iron storage) and chronic inflammation (a condition of normal storage)

Cost

Inexpensive

Patient preparation

■ Explain to the patient that this test is used to assess the available iron stored in the body.
■ Tell the patient that the test requires a blood sample. Explain who will perform the venipuncture and when.
■ Explain to the patient that he may experience discomfort from the needle puncture and the tourniquet.
■ Review the patient's history of transfusion within the past 4 months.

Reference values

AGE ISSUE ✳ ✳ ✳ ✳ ✳
Normal serum ferritin values vary with age, as follows:
■ Neonates: *25 to 200 ng/ml (SI, 25 to 200 µg/L)*
■ 1 month: *200 to 600 ng/ml (SI, 200 to 600 µg/L)*
■ 2 to 5 months: *50 to 200 ng/ml (SI, 50 to 200 µg/L)*
■ 6 months to 15 years: *7 to 140 ng/ml (SI, 7 to 140 µg/L)*
■ Adult males: *20 to 300 ng/ml (SI, 20 to 300 µg/L)*
■ Adult females: *20 to 120 ng/ml (SI, 20 to 120 µg/L)*

Abnormal findings

High serum ferritin levels may indicate acute or chronic hepatic disease, iron overload, leukemia, acute or chronic infection or inflammation, Hodgkin's disease, or chronic hemolytic anemias. In these disorders, iron stores in the bone marrow may be normal or significantly increased. Serum ferritin levels are characteristically normal or slightly elevated in patients with chronic renal disease.

Low serum ferritin levels indicate chronic iron deficiency.

Interfering factors
■ Recent blood transfusion (possible false-high)

Fetal monitoring, external

In external fetal monitoring, a noninvasive test, an electronic transducer and a cardiotachometer amplify and record fetal heart rate (FHR) while a pressure-sensitive transducer (tocodynamometer) records uterine contractions. External fetal monitoring records the baseline FHR (average FHR over two contraction cycles or 10 minutes), periodic fluctuations in the baseline FHR, and beat-to-beat heart rate variability. External fetal monitoring is also used during other tests of fetal health, notably the nonstress test and the contraction stress test (CST).

Purpose
■ To measure FHR and the frequency of uterine contractions
■ To evaluate antepartum and intrapartum fetal health during stress and nonstress situations
■ To detect fetal distress
■ To determine the necessity for internal fetal monitoring

Cost
Expensive

Patient preparation
■ Explain to the patient that this test assesses fetal health.
■ Describe the procedure to the patient and answer all questions. Assure the patient that external fetal monitoring is painless and won't hurt the fetus or interfere with normal labor.
■ If monitoring is to be performed antepartum, instruct the patient to eat a meal just before the test to increase fetal activity, which decreases the test time.
■ If the patient is still smoking, advise her to abstain for 2 hours before testing because smoking decreases fetal activity.
■ Obtain informed consent if necessary.

Normal findings
Normal baseline FHR ranges from 120 to 160 beats/minute, with a variability of 5 to 25 beats/minute. For the antepartum nonstress test, the fetus is considered healthy and should remain so for another week if two fetal movements causing a heart rate acceleration of more than 15 beats/minute from baseline FHR occur in a 20-minute period. Nonstress testing is also done for postdate fetal well-being. A normal, healthy fetus usually has three rises in FHR within 10 to 15 minutes, but fetuses may sleep up to 45 minutes at a time. If there's no change in FHR in a 10-minute period, consider shaking the mother's abdomen gently, clapping loudly, or having the mother drink ice water or apple juice. If the FHR remains unchanged, a CST or biophysical profile test should be ordered. Observations of fetal movement, breathing, and muscle tone and the amniotic fluid index can help assessment.

For the CST, the fetus is assumed to be healthy and should remain so for another week if three contractions occur during a 10-minute period, with no late decelerations.

ALERT! ▼ ▼ ▼ ▼ ▼ ▼ ▼ ▼ ▼

During CST, fetal distress may occur with oxytocin infusion or nipple stimulation. (See Contraction stress test.*)*

Abnormal findings

Bradycardia (FHR < 120 beats/minute) may indicate fetal heart block, malposition, or hypoxia. Fetal bradycardia may also be drug-induced. Tachycardia (FHR > 160 beats/minute) may result from early fetal hypoxia; fetal infection or arrhythmia; prematurity; or maternal fever, tachycardia, hyperthyroidism, or use of vagolytic drugs.

Decreased variability (a fluctuation of < 5 beats/minute in the FHR) may be caused by fetal arrhythmia or heart block; fetal hypoxia, central nervous system malformation, or infections; or vagolytic drugs. FHR accelerations may result from early hypoxia. They may precede or follow variable decelerations and may indicate that the fetus is in a breech position. (See *Comparing decelerated fetal heart rates and uterine contractions,* page 156.)

For the antepartum nonstress test, a positive result (less than two accelerations of FHR that last longer than 15 seconds each, with a heart rate acceleration over 15 beats/minute) indicates an increased risk of perinatal morbidity and mortality and usually requires CST.

For CST, persistent late decelerations during two or more contractions may indicate increased risk of fetal morbidity or mortality. Hyperstimulation (long or frequent uterine contractions) or suspicious results require biophysical profile assessment. If findings are unsatisfactory, cesarean birth may be indicated.

Interfering factors

■ Maternal position, particularly if supine (possible artifactual fetal distress)

Contraction stress test

The contraction stress test measures the ability of the fetus to withstand the stress of contractions induced before actual labor begins. Late decelerations in the fetal heart rate in response to uterine contractions during this test may indicate that the placenta can't deliver enough oxygen to the fetus. Placental insufficiency may result from maternal vascular disease associated with diabetes mellitus, preeclampsia, or chronic hypertension. Intrauterine growth retardation, postmaturity syndrome, and Rh isoimmunization may also cause fetal compromise.

Because this test mimics labor, it's contraindicated in patients who have had a cesarean delivery or placenta previa in the past and in those likely to have premature labor (as in premature rupture of the membrane, multiple pregnancy, or incompetent cervix).

■ Drugs that affect the sympathetic and parasympathetic nervous systems (possible low FHR)
■ Excessive maternal or fetal activity (possible difficulty in recording uterine contractions or FHR)
■ Maternal obesity (possible difficulty due to density of abdominal wall)
■ Loose or dirty leads or transducer connections (possible production of artifacts)

Fetal monitoring, internal

Internal fetal monitoring is an invasive procedure that involves attaching an electrode to the fetal scalp to directly monitor

Comparing decelerated fetal heart rates and uterine contractions

Unlike variable decelerations, early and late decelerations in the fetal heart rate (FHR) correspond to uterine contractions.

Decelerations in FHR may be affected by uterine contractions. The three types of FHR decelerations — early, late, and variable — occur at different points in the contraction phase.

Early FHR decelerations occur at onset of uterine contraction and reach their lowest point at the peak of the contraction. In early deceleration, FHR returns to the average baseline by the end of the contraction. FHR produces a smooth wave pattern that mirrors the uterine contraction. A consistent relationship is seen between the fall in FHR and the uterine contractions. Early deceleration is usually benign and is most commonly caused by compression of the fetal head. This pattern often occurs with advanced dilation (more than 7 cm).

Late decelerations begin about 20 seconds after onset of a contraction and reach their lowest point well after the contraction has peaked. In late deceleration, FHR recovery occurs later than 15 seconds following the contraction. Although the FHR tracing in late deceleration resembles the smooth wave of early deceleration, its implications are far more serious. Late decelerations usually result from uteroplacental insufficiency and may lead to fetal death. When associated with increased variability or with tachycardia and no variability, late decelerations indicate fetal central nervous system depression and myocardial hypoxia.

Variable decelerations — sudden drops in the FHR — may occur at any time during a contraction. After the decline, baseline FHR recovery may be rapid or prolonged. Because the fall in FHR is unrelated to uterine contractions, wave patterns also vary. Variable decelerations occur in about 50% of all labors and are usually associated with transitory umbilical cord compression. However, a severe drop (to less than 70 beats/minute for more than 60 seconds) may indicate fetal acidosis, hypoxia, and low Apgar scores.

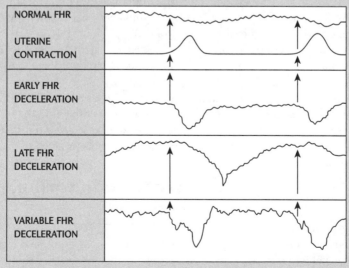

Normal intrauterine pressure readings during labor

STAGE OF LABOR	FREQUENCY (number of contractions per 10 minutes)	BASELINE PRESSURE (mm Hg)	PRESSURE DURING CONTRACTION (mm Hg)
Prelabor	1 to 2	None	25 to 40
First stage	3 to 5	8 to 12	30 to 40 (or more)
Second stage	5	10 to 20	50 to 80

fetal heart rate (FHR). A catheter introduced into the uterine cavity measures the frequency and pressure of uterine contractions. Internal fetal monitoring is performed only during labor, after the membranes have ruptured and the cervix has dilated 3 cm, with the fetal head lower than the –2 station and only if external monitoring provides inadequate data.

Internal fetal monitoring provides more accurate information about fetal health than external monitoring and is especially useful in determining if cesarean delivery is necessary. The procedure carries minimal risks to the mother (perforated uterus and intrauterine infection) and fetus (scalp abscess and hematoma).

ALERT! ▼ ▼ ▼ ▼ ▼ ▼ ▼ ▼ ▼
Internal fetal monitoring is contraindicated if there's uncertainty about the fetus's presenting part or a technical impediment to attaching the lead. If FHR patterns indicate fetal distress, fetal oxygenation often can be improved by loading maternal fluids to increase placental perfusion, turning the mother on her side (preferably left) to alleviate supine hypotension, and administering oxygen to the mother. If these measures return heart rate patterns to normal, labor may continue. If abnormal patterns persist, cesarean birth may be necessary.

Purpose
■ To monitor FHR, especially beat-to-beat variability (short-term variability)
■ To measure the frequency and pressure of uterine contractions to assess the progress of labor
■ To evaluate intrapartum fetal health
■ To supplement or replace external fetal monitoring

Cost
Expensive

Patient preparation
■ Explain to the patient that this test accurately assesses fetal health and uterine activity and that it doesn't necessarily mean that there's a problem.
■ Warn the patient that she may feel mild discomfort when the uterine catheter and scalp electrode are inserted.
■ Obtain informed consent if necessary.

Reference values
Normal FHR ranges from 120 to 160 beats/minute, with a variability of 5 to 25 beats/minute. (See *Normal intrauterine pressure readings during labor*.)

Abnormal findings

Bradycardia (FHR < 120 beats/minute) may indicate fetal heart block, malposition, or hypoxia. Fetal bradycardia may also result from maternal ingestion of certain drugs, such as propranolol and narcotic analgesics.

Tachycardia (FHR > 160 beats/minute) may result from early fetal hypoxia; fetal infection or arrhythmia; prematurity; or maternal fever, tachycardia, hyperthyroidism, or use of vagolytic drugs.

Decreased variability (fluctuation of < 5 beats/minute from baseline) may result from fetal arrhythmia or heart block; fetal hypoxia, central nervous system malformation, or infections; or from maternal use of narcotics or vagolytic drugs.

Early decelerations (slowing of FHR at the onset of a contraction with recovery to baseline no greater than 15 seconds after the contraction ends) are related to fetal head compression and usually ensure fetal health.

Late decelerations (slowing of FHR after a contraction begins, a lag time of more than 20 seconds, and a recovery time of more than 15 seconds) may be related to uteroplacental insufficiency, fetal hypoxia, or acidosis. Recurrent and persistently late decelerations with decreased variability usually indicate serious fetal distress, possibly resulting from conduction (spinal, caudal, or epidural) anesthesia or fetal hypoxia.

Variable decelerations (sudden precipitous drops in FHR unrelated to uterine contractions) are commonly related to cord compression. A severe drop in FHR (to less than 70 beats/minute for more than 60 seconds) with a decrease in variability indicates fetal distress and may result in a compromised neonate. Poor beat-to-beat variability without periodic patterns may indicate fetal distress, requir-

ing further evaluation, such as analysis of fetal blood gas levels.

Decreased intrauterine pressure during labor that's not progressing normally may require oxytocin stimulation. Elevated intrauterine pressure readings may indicate abruptio placentae or overstimulation from oxytocin, possibly resulting in fetal distress due to decreased placental perfusion.

Interfering factors

■ Drugs that affect parasympathetic and sympathetic nervous systems

Fibrinogen, plasma

The plasma fibrinogen test measures the plasma concentration of fibrinogen available for coagulation. Fibrinogen (factor I) originates in the liver and is converted to fibrin by thrombin during clotting. Because fibrin is necessary for clot formation, fibrinogen deficiency can produce mild-to-severe bleeding disorders.

ALERT! ▼ ▼ ▼ ▼ ▼ ▼ ▼ ▼ ▼
This test is contraindicated in patients with active bleeding and acute infection or illness, and in those who have received blood transfusions within 4 weeks.

Purpose

■ To aid the diagnosis of suspected clotting or bleeding disorders caused by fibrinogen abnormalities

Cost

Inexpensive

Patient preparation

■ Explain to the patient that this test is used to determine if his blood clots normally.

- Tell the patient that the test requires a blood sample. Explain who will perform the venipuncture and when.
- Explain to the patient that he may experience discomfort from the needle puncture and the tourniquet.
- Restrict medications that may affect test results. If they must be continued, note this on the laboratory request.

Reference values

Plasma fibrinogen levels normally range from 200 to 400 mg/dl (SI, 2 to 4 g/L).

Abnormal findings

Depressed plasma fibrinogen levels may indicate congenital afibrinogenemia; hypofibrinogenemia or dysfibrinogenemia; disseminated intravascular coagulation; fibrinolysis; severe hepatic disease; cancer of the prostate, pancreas, or lung; or bone marrow lesions. Obstetric complications or trauma may also cause low levels.

ALERT! ▼ ▼ ▼ ▼ ▼ ▼ ▼ ▼

Markedly decreased plasma fibrinogen levels impede the accurate interpretation of coagulation tests that have a fibrin clot as an end point.

Elevated levels may indicate cancer of the stomach, breast, or kidney, or inflammatory disorders, such as pneumonia or membranoproliferative glomerulonephritis.

Prolonged partial thromboplastin time, prothrombin time, and thrombin time may also indicate a fibrinogen deficiency.

Interfering factors

- Failure to fill the collection tube completely or to adequately mix the sample and anticoagulant, or failure to send the sample to the laboratory immediately
- Hemolysis due to rough handling of the sample or to excessive probing at the venipuncture site

- Heparin or hormonal contraceptives
- Third trimester of pregnancy (possible increase)
- Postoperative status (possible increase)

Fluorescein angiography

In fluorescein angiography, a special camera takes rapid-sequence photographs of the fundus following I.V. injection of sodium fluorescein (a contrast medium), thereby recording the appearance of blood vessels within the eye. This technique provides enhanced visibility of the microvascular structures of the retina and choroid, which permits evaluation of the entire retinal vascular bed, including retinal circulation.

Purpose

- To document retinal circulation when evaluating intraocular abnormalities, such as retinopathy, tumors, and circulatory or inflammatory disorders

Cost

Very expensive

Patient preparation

- Explain to the patient that this procedure takes about 30 minutes and evaluates the small blood vessels in the eyes. Explain that eyedrops will be instilled to dilate his pupils and that a dye will be injected into his arm. Tell him that his eyes will be photographed with a special camera before and after the injection. Stress that these are photographs, not X-rays.
- Obtain informed consent if necessary.
- Check the patient's history for glaucoma and hypersensitivity reactions or allergies, especially to contrast media and dilating eyedrops. If necessary, tell a patient with

glaucoma not to use miotic eyedrops on the day of the test.

■ Warn the patient that his skin may be discolored and urine may appear orange for 24 to 48 hours after the procedure and that near vision will be blurred for up to 12 hours; advise him to avoid direct sunlight and refrain from driving during this time.

Normal findings

After rapid injection into the antecubital vein, sodium fluorescein reaches the retina in 12 to 15 seconds (filling phase). As the choroidal vessels and choriocapillaries fill, the background of the retina fluoresces, taking on an evenly mottled appearance known as the choroidal flush. Then the dye fills the arteries (arterial phase). The arteriovenous phase lasts from the complete filling of the arteries and capillaries to the earliest evidence of dye in the veins. The time the arteries begin to empty to the time the veins fill and empty is known as the venous phase. Finally, the recirculation phase occurs 30 to 60 minutes after the injection, when the fluorescein — if at all present — is barely detectable in the retinal vessels. Normally, there's no leakage from the retinal vessels.

Abnormal findings

The varying and complex findings after fluorescein angiography require interpretation by a highly skilled ophthalmologist with extensive experience in the diagnosis of retinal disorders.

Abnormalities detected in the early filling phase may include microaneurysms, arteriovenous shunts, and neovascularization. The test may identify arterial occlusion by showing delayed or absent flow of the dye through the arteries, stenosis, and prolonged venous drainage. Venous occlusion may be associated with dilation of the vessels and fluorescein leakage. Chronic

obstruction may produce recanalization and collateral circulation.

In hypertensive retinopathy, abnormalities may include areas of increased vascular tortuosity, microaneurysms around zones of capillary nonperfusion, and generalized suffusion of the dye in the retina. Aneurysms and capillary hemangiomas may leak fluorescein and are commonly surrounded by hard yellow exudate. Tumors exhibit variable fluorescein patterns, depending on histologic type. Retinal edema or inflammation and fibrous tissue may show variable degrees of fluorescence. Papilledema produces vascular leakage in the disk area.

ALERT! ▼ ▼ ▼ ▼ ▼ ▼ ▼ ▼ ▼
Serious adverse effects (laryngeal edema, bronchospasm, and respiratory arrest) are possible. If a reaction occurs, make sure that it's noted in the patient's allergy history.

Interfering factors

■ Inadequate view of the fundus due to insufficient pupillary dilation (possible poor imaging)
■ Cataract, media opacity, or inability to keep eyes open and to maintain fixation (possible poor imaging)

Fluorescent treponemal antibody absorption

The fluorescent treponemal antibody absorption (FTA-ABS or simply FTA) test uses indirect immunofluorescence to detect antibodies to the spirochete *Treponema pallidum* in serum. This spirochete causes syphilis.

Although the FTA-ABS test is generally performed on a serum sample to detect primary or secondary syphilis, a cerebrospinal fluid (CSF) specimen is required to detect tertiary syphilis. Because antibody levels remain constant for long periods, the FTA-ABS test isn't recommended for monitoring response to therapy.

Purpose
■ To confirm primary and secondary syphilis
■ To screen for suspected false-positive results of Venereal Disease Research Laboratory test

Cost
Moderately expensive

Patient preparation
■ Explain to the patient that this test can confirm or rule out syphilis.
■ Tell the patient that the test requires a blood sample. Explain who will perform the venipuncture and when.
■ Explain to the patient that he may experience discomfort from the needle puncture and the tourniquet.

Normal findings
Normally, results of the FTA-ABS test are nonreactive.

Abnormal findings
The presence of treponemal antibodies in the serum — a reactive test result — doesn't indicate the stage or severity of infection. (The presence of these antibodies in CSF is strong evidence of tertiary neurosyphilis.) Elevated antibody levels appear in most patients with primary syphilis and in almost all patients with secondary syphilis. Higher antibody levels persist for several years, with or without treatment.

The absence of treponemal antibodies in the serum — a nonreactive test result — doesn't necessarily rule out syphilis. *T. pallidum* causes no detectable immunologic changes in the blood for 14 to 21 days after initial infection. Organisms may be detected earlier by examining suspicious lesions with a dark-field microscope. Low antibody levels and other nonspecific factors produce borderline findings. In such cases, repeated testing and a thorough review of the patient's history may be productive.

Although the FTA-ABS test is specific, some patients with nonsyphilitic conditions — such as systemic lupus erythematosus, genital herpes, and increased or abnormal globulins — and pregnant women may show minimally reactive levels. In addition, the FTA-ABS test doesn't always distinguish between *T. pallidum* and certain other treponemas, such as those that cause pinta, yaws, and bejel.

Interfering factors
■ Hemolysis due to rough handling of the sample

Folic acid

The folic acid test is a quantitative analysis of serum folic acid levels (also called *pteroylglutamic acid, folacin,* or *folate*) by radioisotope assay of competitive binding. It's commonly performed concomitantly with measurement of serum vitamin B_{12} levels. Like vitamin B_{12}, folic acid is a water-soluble vitamin that influences hematopoiesis, deoxyribonucleic acid synthesis, and overall body growth.

Normally, diet supplies folic acid in liver, kidney, yeast, fruits, leafy vegetables, fortified breads and cereals, eggs, and milk. Inadequate dietary intake may cause a deficiency, especially during pregnancy. Because of folic acid's vital role in hematopoiesis, the usual indication for this test is a suspected hematologic abnormality.

Purpose

■ To aid differential diagnosis of megaloblastic anemia, which may result from folic acid or vitamin B_{12} deficiency
■ To assess folate stores in pregnancy

Cost

Inexpensive

Patient preparation

■ Explain to the patient that this test determines the folic acid level in the blood.
■ Instruct the patient to fast overnight before the test.
■ Tell the patient that the test requires a blood sample. Explain who will perform the venipuncture and when.
■ Explain to the patient that he may experience discomfort from the needle puncture and the tourniquet.
■ Check the patient's history for drugs that may affect test results, such as phenytoin or pyrimethamine.

Reference values

Normally, serum folic acid values are 1.8 to 9 ng/ml (SI, 4 to 20 nmol/L).

Abnormal findings

Low serum levels may indicate hematologic abnormalities, such as anemia (especially megaloblastic anemia), leukopenia, and thrombocytopenia. The Schilling test is usually performed to rule out vitamin B_{12} deficiency, which also causes megaloblastic anemia. Decreased folic acid levels can also result from hypermetabolic states (such as hyperthyroidism), inadequate dietary intake, small-bowel malabsorption syndrome, hepatic or renal diseases, chronic alcoholism, or pregnancy.

Serum levels greater than normal may indicate excessive dietary intake of folic acid or folic acid supplements. Even when taken in large doses, this vitamin is nontoxic.

Interfering factors

■ Hemolysis due to rough handling of the sample
■ Alcohol; anticonvulsants, such as primidone; antimalarials; antineoplastics; hormonal contraceptives; phenytoin; pyrimethamine; (possible decrease)

Follicle-stimulating hormone

The follicle-stimulating hormone test of gonadal function, performed more often on women than on men, measures follicle-stimulating hormone (FSH) levels and is vital in infertility studies. Plasma FSH levels fluctuate widely in females; to obtain a true baseline level, daily testing may be necessary for 3 to 5 days.

Purpose

■ To aid in the diagnosis and treatment of infertility and disorders of menstruation such as amenorrhea
■ To aid in the diagnosis of precocious puberty in girls (before age 9) and in boys (before age 10)
■ To aid in the differential diagnosis of hypogonadism

Cost

Inexpensive

Patient preparation

■ Explain to the patient, or to the patient's parents if the patient is a minor, that this test helps determine if hormonal secretion is normal.
■ Tell the patient that the test requires a blood sample. Explain who will perform the venipuncture and when.

- Explain to the patient that she may experience discomfort from the needle puncture and the tourniquet.
- Restrict medications that may interfere with accurate determination of test results for 48 hours before the test. If they must be continued (for example, for infertility treatment), note this on the laboratory request; also note the phase of the menstrual cycle or if the patient is menopausal.

Reference values

Reference values vary greatly, depending on the patient's age, stage of sexual development, and — for a female — phase of her menstrual cycle. For menstruating females, approximate FSH values are as follows:
- *follicular phase:* 5 to 20 mIU/ml (SI, 5 to 20 IU/L)
- *ovulatory phase:* 15 to 30 mIU/ml (SI, 15 to 30 IU/L)
- *luteal phase:* 5 to 15 mIU/ml (SI, 5 to 15 IU/L).

Approximate FSH values for men range from 5 to 20 mIU/ml (SI, 5 to 20 IU/L); for menopausal women, 50 to 100 mIU/ml (SI, 50 to 100 IU/L).

Abnormal findings

Decreased FSH levels may cause male or female infertility: aspermatogenesis in men and anovulation in women. Low FSH levels may indicate secondary hypogonadotropic states, which can result from anorexia nervosa, panhypopituitarism, or hypothalamic lesions.

High FSH levels in women may indicate ovarian failure associated with Turner's syndrome or Stein-Leventhal syndrome. Elevated levels may occur in patients with precocious puberty (idiopathic or with central nervous system lesions) and in postmenopausal women. In men, abnormally high FSH levels may indicate destruction of the testes, testicular failure, seminoma, or

male climacteric. Congenital absence of the gonads and early-stage acromegaly may cause FSH levels to rise in both sexes.

Interfering factors

- Failure to observe pretest restrictions of medications
- Hemolysis due to rough handling of the sample
- Ovarian steroid hormones, such as estrogen and progesterone, related compounds, and phenothiazines such as chlorpromazine (possible decrease through negative feedback by inhibiting FSH flow from the hypothalamus and pituitary gland)
- Radioactive scan performed within 1 week before the test

Fungal serology

Most fungal organisms enter the body as spores inhaled into the lungs or infiltrated through wounds in the skin or mucosa. If the body's defenses can't destroy the organisms initially, the fungi multiply to form lesions; blood and lymph vessels may then spread the mycoses (diseases caused by a fungus) throughout the body. Most healthy people easily overcome initial mycotic infection, but elderly people and others with a deficient immune system are more susceptible to acute or chronic mycotic infection and to disorders secondary to such infection. Mycosis may be deep-seated or superficial: Deep-seated mycosis occurs primarily in the lungs; superficial mycosis, in the skin or mucosal linings.

Although cultures are usually performed to diagnose mycoses by identifying the causative organism, fungal serology tests occasionally provide the sole evidence for mycosis. Such serologic tests use immunodiffusion, complement fixation, precipitin, latex agglutination, or agglutination

Serum test methods for fungal infections

DISEASE AND NORMAL VALUES	CLINICAL SIGNIFICANCE OF ABNORMAL RESULTS
Blastomycosis Complement fixation: titers < 1:8	Titers ranging from 1:8 to 1:16 suggest infection; titers > 1:32 denote active disease. A rising titer in serial samples taken every 3 to 4 weeks indicates disease progression; a falling titer indicates regression. This test has limited diagnostic value because of a high percentage of false-negatives.
Immunodiffusion: negative	A more sensitive test for blastomycosis; detects 80% of infected people.
Coccidioidomycosis Complement fixation: titers < 1:2	Most sensitive test for this fungus. Titers ranging from 1:2 to 2:4 suggest active infection; titers > 1:16 usually denote active disease. Test may remain active in mild infections.
Immunodiffusion: negative	Most useful for screening, followed by complement fixation test for confirmation.
Precipitin titers < 1:16	Good screening test, titers > 1:16 usually indicate infection. About 80% of infected people show positive titers by 2 weeks; most revert to negative by 6 months. Early primary disease is shown by positive precipitin and negative complement fixation test. A positive complement fixation and negative precipitin test indicate chronic disease.
Histoplasmosis Complement fixation (histoplasmin): titers < 1:8	Titers ranging from 1:8 to 1:16 suggest infection; titers > 1:32 indicate active disease. Antibodies generally appear 10 to 21 days after initial infection. Test is positive in 10% to 15% of cases.
Complement fixation: titers < 1:18	Titers ranging from 1:8 to 1:16 suggest infection; titers > 1:32 indicate active disease. More sensitive than histoplasmin complement fixation test; gives positive results in 75% to 80% of cases. (Histoplasmin and yeast antigens are positive in 10% of cases.) A rising titer in serial samples taken every 2 to 3 weeks indicates progressive infection; a decreasing titer indicates regression.
Immunodiffusion (histoplasmin): negative	Appearance of both H and M bands indicates active infection. If the M band appears first and lasts longer than the H band, the infection may be regressing. The M band alone may indicate early infection, chronic disease, or a recent skin test.
Aspergillosis Complement fixation: titers < 1:8	Titers > 1:8 suggest infection; 70% to 90% of patients with known pulmonary aspergillosis or aspergillus allergy present antibodies. This test can't detect invasive aspergillosis because patients with this disease don't have antibodies; biopsy is required.
Immunodiffusion: negative	One or more precipitin bands suggests infection. The number of bands is related to complement fixation titers; the more precipitin bands, the higher the titer.

DISEASE AND NORMAL VALUES	CLINICAL SIGNIFICANCE OF ABNORMAL RESULTS
Sporotrichosis Agglutination: titers < 1:40	Titers of > 1:80 usually indicate active infection. The test commonly is negative in cutaneous infections and positive in extracutaneous infections.
Cryptococcosis Latex agglutination for cryptococcal antigen: negative	About 95% of patients with cryptococcal meningitis exhibit positive latex agglutination in cerebrospinal fluid (CSF). (Serum is less frequently positive than CSF.) Culturing is definitive because false-positives do occur. (Presence of rheumatoid factor may cause a positive reaction.) Serum antigen tests are positive in 33% of patients with pulmonary cryptococcosis; biopsy is usually required.

methods to demonstrate the presence of specific mycotic antibodies.

Purpose

■ To rapidly detect the presence of antifungal antibodies, aiding in the diagnosis of mycoses

■ To monitor effectiveness of therapy for mycoses

Cost

Expensive

Patient preparation

■ Explain to the patient that this test aids diagnosis of certain fungal infections. If appropriate, tell him that this test monitors his response to antimycotic therapy and that it may be necessary to repeat the test.

■ Tell the patient that the test requires a blood sample. Explain who will perform the venipuncture and when.

■ Explain to the patient that he may experience discomfort from the needle puncture and the tourniquet.

Normal findings

Depending on the test method, a negative finding, or normal titer, usually indicates the absence of mycosis.

Abnormal findings

The accompanying chart explains the significance of findings for specific organisms. (See *Serum test methods for fungal infections.*)

Interfering factors

■ Cross-reaction of antibodies with other antigens, such as blastomycosis and histoplasmosis antigens (possible false-positive or high titers)

■ Recent skin testing with fungal antigens (possible high titers)

■ Mycosis-caused immunosuppression (low titers or false-negative)

G

Gallium scan

The gallium scan is a total body scan used to assess certain neoplasms and inflammatory lesions that attract gallium. It's usually performed 24 to 48 hours after the I.V. injection of radioactive gallium 67 (^{67}Ga) citrate; occasionally, it's performed 72 hours after the injection or, in acute inflammatory disease, after 4 to 6 hours.

Because gallium has an affinity for benign and malignant neoplasms and inflammatory lesions, exact diagnosis requires additional confirming tests, such as ultrasonography and computerized tomography scanning. Also, be aware that many neoplasms and a few inflammatory lesions may fail to demonstrate abnormal gallium activity.

ALERT! ▼ ▼ ▼ ▼ ▼ ▼ ▼ ▼ ▼
Gallium scanning is usually contraindicated in children and during pregnancy or lactation; however, it may be performed if the potential diagnostic benefit outweighs the risks of exposure to radiation.

Purpose
■ To detect primary or metastatic neoplasms and inflammatory lesions when the site of the disease hasn't been clearly defined
■ To evaluate malignant lymphoma and identify recurrent tumors following chemotherapy or radiation therapy
■ To clarify focal defects in the liver when liver-spleen scanning and ultrasonography prove inconclusive
■ To evaluate bronchogenic carcinoma

Cost
Expensive

Patient preparation
■ Explain to the patient that this test helps detect abnormal or inflammatory tissue.
■ Tell the patient that the test requires a total body scan (usually performed 24 to 48 hours after the I.V. injection of ^{67}Ga). Explain who will perform the test and where it will take place.
■ Explain to the patient that he may experience discomfort from the injection of the ^{67}Ga. Reassure him that the dosage is only slightly radioactive and isn't harmful.
■ If a gamma scintillation camera is to be used, assure the patient that although the uptake probe and detector head may touch his skin, he'll experience no discomfort.
■ Obtain informed consent if necessary.

- Tell the patient that he may receive a laxative, an enema, or both. This test should precede barium studies because barium retention may hinder visualization of gallium activity in the bowel.

Normal findings

Gallium activity is normally demonstrated in the liver, spleen, bones, and large bowel. Activity in the bowel results from mucosal uptake of gallium and fecal excretion of gallium.

Abnormal findings

Gallium scanning may reveal inflammatory lesions — discrete abscesses or diffuse infiltration. In pancreatic or perinephric abscess, gallium activity is relatively localized; in bacterial peritonitis, gallium activity is spread diffusely within the abdomen.

Abnormally high gallium accumulation is characteristic in inflammatory bowel diseases, such as ulcerative colitis and regional ileitis (Crohn's disease), and in carcinoma of the colon. However, because gallium normally accumulates in the colon, the detection of inflammatory and neoplastic diseases is sometimes difficult.

Abnormal gallium activity may be present in various sarcomas, Wilms' tumor, and neuroblastomas; carcinoma of the kidney, uterus, vagina, and stomach; and testicular tumors, such as seminoma, embryonal carcinoma, choriocarcinoma, and teratocarcinoma, which often metastasize via the lymphatic system. In Hodgkin's disease and malignant lymphoma, gallium scanning can demonstrate abnormal activity in one or more lymph nodes or in extranodal locations. However, gallium scanning supported by lymphangiography results can gauge the extent of metastases more accurately than either test alone because neither test consistently identifies all neoplastic nodes.

After chemotherapy or radiation therapy, gallium scanning may be used to detect new or recurrent tumors. However, these forms of therapy tend to diminish tumor affinity for gallium without necessarily eliminating the tumor.

In the differential diagnosis of focal hepatic defects, abnormal gallium activity may help narrow the diagnostic possibilities. Gallium localizes in hepatomas, but not in pseudotumors; in abscesses, but not in pleural effusions; and in tumors, but not in cysts or hematomas.

In examining patients with suspected bronchogenic carcinoma, abnormal activity confirms the presence of a tumor. However, because gallium also localizes in inflammatory pulmonary diseases, such as pneumonia and sarcoidosis, a chest X-ray should be performed to distinguish a tumor from an inflammatory lesion.

Interfering factors

- Hepatic and splenic intake (possible false-negative scans due to possible obscuring of abnormal para-aortic nodes in Hodgkin's disease)
- Fecal accumulation in bowel (poor imaging of retroperitoneal space)
- Residual barium from other tests done 1 week before the scan (possible poor imaging)

Gamma-glutamyl transferase

Also called gamma-glutamyl transpeptidase, gamma glutamyl transferase (GGT) participates in the transfer of amino acids across cellular membranes and, possibly, in glutathione metabolism. The highest concentrations of GGT exist in the renal tubules, but the enzyme also appears in the liver, biliary tract epithelium, pancreas, lymphocytes, brain, and testes. The GGT test is used to measure serum GGT levels.

Purpose
■ To provide information about hepato-biliary diseases, to assess liver function, and to detect alcohol ingestion
■ To distinguish between skeletal disease and hepatic disease when the serum alkaline phosphatase level is elevated (a normal serum GGT level suggests that such elevation stems from skeletal disease)

Cost
Inexpensive

Patient preparation
■ Explain to the patient that this test is used to evaluate liver function.
■ Tell the patient that the test requires a blood sample. Explain who will perform the venipuncture and when.
■ Explain to the patient that he may experience discomfort from the needle puncture and the tourniquet.

Reference values
AGE ISSUE ✳ ✳ ✳ ✳ ✳
Normal serum GTT levels range as follows:
■ *Males: age 16 and older, 6 to 38 U/L (SI, 0.10 to 0.63 µkat/L)*
■ *Females: between ages 16 and 45, 4 to 27 U/L (SI, 0.08 to 0.46 µkat/L); age 45 and older, 6 to 37 U/L (SI, 0.10 to 0.63 µkat/L)*
■ *Children: 3 to 30 U/L (SI, 0.05 to 0.51 µkat/L)*

Abnormal findings
Serum GGT levels rise in acute hepatic diseases because enzyme production increases in response to hepatocellular injury. Moderate increases occur in acute pancreatitis, renal disease, and prostatic metastases; postoperatively; and in some patients with epilepsy or brain tumors. Levels also in-crease after alcohol ingestion because of enzyme induction. The sharpest elevations occur in patients with obstructive jaundice and hepatic metastatic infiltrations.

Serum GGT levels may also increase 5 to 10 days after acute myocardial infarction, either as a result of tissue granulation and healing or as an indication of the effects of cardiac insufficiency on the liver.

Interfering factors
■ Hemolysis due to rough handling of the sample
■ Clofibrate and hormonal contraceptives (decrease)
■ Aminoglycosides, barbiturates, glutethimide, methaqualone, and phenytoin (increase)
■ Moderate intake of alcohol (increase for at least 60 hours)

Gastric acid stimulation

The gastric acid stimulation test measures the secretion of gastric acid for 1 hour after subcutaneous injection of pentagastrin or a similar drug that stimulates gastric acid output. This test is indicated when the basal secretion test suggests abnormal gastric acid secretion and is commonly performed immediately afterward. Although this test detects abnormal gastric acid secretion, radiographic studies and endoscopy are necessary to determine the cause.
ALERT! ▼ ▼ ▼ ▼ ▼ ▼ ▼ ▼
The gastric acid stimulation test is contraindicated in patients with hypersensitivity to pentagastrin or with conditions that prohibit nasogastric intubations.

Purpose
■ To aid diagnosis of duodenal ulcer, Zollinger-Ellison syndrome, pernicious anemia, and gastric carcinoma

Cost
Expensive

Patient preparation
■ Explain to the patient that this test determines if the stomach is secreting acid properly.
■ Instruct the patient to refrain from eating, drinking, and smoking after midnight before the test.
■ Tell the patient who will perform the test, where it will take place, and that it requires passing a tube through the nose and into the stomach to collect specimens after an injection of pentagastrin.
■ Tell the patient that he may experience abdominal pain, nausea, vomiting, flushing, and transitory dizziness, faintness, and numbness of extremities and to report such symptoms immediately.
■ Check the patient's history for hypersensitivity to pentagastrin.
■ Restrict medications that may affect test results. If they must be continued, note this on the laboratory request.

Reference values
Following stimulation, gastric acid secretion ranges from 18 to 28 mEq/hour for males and from 11 to 21 mEq/hour for females.

Abnormal findings
Elevated gastric acid secretion may indicate duodenal ulcer; markedly elevated secretion suggests Zollinger-Ellison syndrome. Depressed secretion may indicate gastric carcinoma; achlorhydria may indicate pernicious anemia.

Interfering factors
■ Failure to observe pretest restrictions
■ Adrenergic blockers, cholinergics, and reserpine (increase)

■ Antacids, anticholinergics, and histamine-2 blockers and proton pump inhibitors (decrease)

Gastrin

Gastrin is a polypeptide hormone produced and stored primarily in the antrum of the stomach and to a lesser degree in the islets of Langerhans. Its main function is to facilitate digestion of food by triggering gastric acid secretion. It also stimulates the release of pancreatic enzymes and the gastric enzyme pepsin, increases gastric and intestinal motility, and stimulates bile flow from the liver. Abnormal secretion of gastrin can result from tumors (gastrinomas) and pathologic disorders that affect the stomach, pancreas, and less commonly, the esophagus and small bowel.

The gastrin test, a radioimmunoassay that provides a quantitative analysis of gastrin levels, is especially useful in patients suspected of having gastrinomas (Zollinger-Ellison syndrome). In doubtful situations, provocative testing may be necessary.

Purpose
■ To confirm the diagnosis of gastrinoma, the gastrin-secreting tumor in Zollinger-Ellison syndrome
■ To aid differential diagnosis of gastric and duodenal ulcers and pernicious anemia (serum gastrin estimation has limited value in patients with duodenal ulcer)

Cost
Inexpensive

Patient preparation
■ Explain to the patient that this test helps determine the cause of gastrointestinal symptoms

■ Instruct the patient to abstain from alcohol for at least 24 hours before the test and to fast and avoid caffeinated drinks for 12 hours before the test, although he may drink water.
■ Tell the patient that the test requires a blood sample. Explain who will perform the venipuncture and when.
■ Explain to the patient that he may experience discomfort from the needle puncture and the tourniquet.
■ Restrict drugs that may interfere with test results, especially insulin and anticholinergics, such as atropine and belladonna. If they must be continued, note this on the laboratory request.

Reference values
Normal serum gastrin levels are between 50 to 150 pg/ml (SI, 50 to 150 ng/L).

Abnormal findings
High serum gastrin levels (> 1,000 pg/ml [SI, > 1,000 ng/L]) confirm Zollinger-Ellison syndrome. (Levels as high as 450,000 pg/ml [SI, 450,000 ng/L] have been reported.)

Increased serum levels of gastrin may occur in a few patients with duodenal ulceration (< 1%) and in patients with achlorhydria (with or without pernicious anemia) or extensive stomach carcinoma (because of hyposecretion of gastric juices and hydrochloric acid).

Interfering factors
■ Failure to observe pretest restrictions
■ Acetylcholine, amino acids (especially glycine), calcium carbonate, calcium chloride, and ethanol (possible increase)
■ Anticholinergics, such as atropine and belladonna as well as hydrochloric acid and secretin, a strongly basic polypeptide (possible decrease)

■ Insulin-induced hypoglycemia (possible increase)

Glucose, fasting plasma

Commonly used to screen for diabetes mellitus, the fasting plasma glucose test (also known as the *fasting blood sugar test*) measures plasma glucose levels following a 12- to 14-hour fast.

In the fasting state, plasma glucose levels decrease, stimulating release of the hormone glucagon. Glucagon then acts to raise plasma glucose by accelerating glycogenolysis, stimulating glyconeogenesis, and inhibiting glycogen synthesis. Normally, secretion of insulin checks this rise in glucose levels. In diabetes, however, absence or deficiency of insulin allows persistently high glucose levels.

Purpose
■ To screen for diabetes mellitus
■ To monitor drug or dietary therapy in patients with diabetes mellitus

Cost
Inexpensive

Patient preparation
■ Explain to the patient that this test detects disorders of glucose metabolism and aids diagnosis of diabetes.
■ Advise the patient to fast for 12 to 14 hours before the test.
■ Tell the patient that the test requires a blood sample. Explain who will perform the venipuncture and when.
■ Explain to the patient that he may experience discomfort from the needle puncture and the tourniquet.
■ Restrict medications that may affect test results. If they must be continued, note this

on the laboratory request. Advise the patient with diabetes to resume his medication after the test.

ALERT! ▼ ▼ ▼ ▼ ▼ ▼ ▼ ▼ ▼
Alert the patient to the symptoms of hypoglycemia — weakness, restlessness, nervousness, hunger, and sweating — and tell him to report such symptoms immediately.

Reference values

The normal range for fasting plasma glucose varies according to the laboratory procedure. Generally, normal values after at least an 8-hour fast are 70 to 110 mg/dl (SI, 3.9 to 6.1 mmol/L) when measured by the glucose oxidase and hexokinase methods.

Abnormal findings

A fasting plasma glucose level of 126 mg/dl (SI, 7 mmol/L) or higher obtained on two or more occasions confirms provisional diabetes mellitus. The 2-hour postprandial plasma glucose test confirms the diagnosis of borderline or transiently elevated levels.

Although increased fasting plasma glucose levels most commonly occur with diabetes, they can also result from pancreatitis, recent acute illness (such as myocardial infarction), Cushing's syndrome, acromegaly, and pheochromocytoma. Hyperglycemia may also stem from hyperlipoproteinemia (especially type III, IV, or V), chronic hepatic disease, nephrotic syndrome, brain tumor, sepsis, or gastrectomy with dumping syndrome and is typical in eclampsia, anoxia, and seizure disorders.

Depressed plasma glucose levels can result from hyperinsulinism, insulinoma, von Gierke's disease, functional or reactive hypoglycemia, myxedema, adrenal insufficiency, congenital adrenal hyperplasia, hypopituitarism, malabsorption syndrome, and some cases of hepatic insufficiency.

Interfering factors

■ Failure to observe dietary restrictions (possible increase)
■ Acetaminophen, if using the glucose oxidase or hexokinase method (possible false-positive)
■ Arginine, benzodiazepines, chlorthalidone, corticosteroids, dextrothyroxine, diazoxide, epinephrine, furosemide, hormonal contraceptives (estrogen-progestogen combination), lithium, large doses of nicotinic acid, phenolphthalein, phenothiazines, phenytoin, recent I.V. glucose infusions, thiazide diuretics, and triamterene (possible increase)
■ Ethacrynic acid (may cause hyperglycemia); large doses in patients with uremia (may cause hypoglycemia)
■ Beta-adrenergic blockers, clofibrate, ethanol, insulin, monoamine oxidase inhibitors, and oral antidiabetic agents (possible decrease)
■ Recent illness, infection, or pregnancy (possible increase)
■ Strenuous exercise (possible decrease)

Glucose-6-phosphate dehydrogenase

An enzyme found in most body cells, glucose-6-phosphate dehydrogenase (G6PD) is involved in metabolizing glucose. The G6PD test is used to detect G6PD deficiency, a hereditary, sex-linked condition that impairs stability of the red cell membrane and allows red cells to be destroyed by strong oxidizing agents.

About 10% of black males in the United States inherit a mild G6PD deficiency; some people of Mediterranean origin inherit a severe deficiency. In some white individuals, fava beans may produce hemolytic episodes. Although a deficiency of G6PD provides partial immunity to falciparum malaria, it precipitates an adverse reaction to antimalarials.

Purpose
- To detect hemolytic anemia caused by G6PD deficiency
- To aid differential diagnosis of hemolytic anemia

Cost
Inexpensive

Patient preparation
- Explain to the patient that this test is used to detect an inherited enzyme deficiency that may affect red blood cells.
- Tell the patient that the test requires a blood sample. Explain who will perform the venipuncture and when.
- Explain to the patient that he may experience discomfort from the needle puncture and the tourniquet.

Reference values
Serum values of G6PD vary with the measurement method used but usually range from 4.3 to 11.8 U/g (SI, 0.28 to 0.76 mU/mol) of hemoglobin.

Abnormal findings
Fluorescent spot testing or staining for Heinz bodies or erythrocytes can test for G6PD deficiency. If results are positive, the kinetic quantitative assay for G6PD may be performed. Electrophoretic techniques assess genetic variants of deficiencies (which may cause lifelong, mild, or asymptomatic anemia). Some variants are symptomatic only when the patient experiences stress or illness or has been exposed to drugs or agents that elicit hemolytic episodes.

Interfering factors
- Performing the test after a hemolytic episode or a blood transfusion (possible false-negative)

- Failure to use the proper anticoagulant or to adequately mix the sample and the anticoagulant
- Aspirin, fava beans (decrease G6PD enzyme activity and precipitate hemolytic episode), nitrofurantoin, primaquine phosphate, sulfonamides, and vitamin K derivatives

Glucose tolerance, oral

The oral glucose tolerance test (OGTT), the most sensitive method of evaluating borderline cases of diabetes mellitus in selected patients, measures carbohydrate metabolism after ingestion of a challenge dose of glucose. The body absorbs this dose rapidly, causing plasma glucose levels to rise and peak within 30 minutes to 1 hour. The pancreas responds by secreting more insulin, causing plasma glucose levels to return to normal after 2 to 3 hours.

During this period, plasma and urine glucose levels are monitored to assess insulin secretion and the body's ability to metabolize glucose. Occasionally, plasma glucose levels are monitored an additional 2 to 3 hours to aid diagnosis of hypoglycemia and malabsorption syndrome. However, such extended testing is contraindicated when insulinoma is strongly suspected because prolonged fasting in such a patient can lead to fainting and coma.

In a patient with mild or diet-controlled diabetes, fasting plasma glucose levels may be in the normal range; however, insufficient secretion of insulin after ingestion of carbohydrates causes plasma glucose levels to rise sharply and return to normal slowly. This decreased tolerance for glucose helps to confirm mild diabetes.

The OGTT isn't usually used in patients with fasting plasma glucose values above 140 mg/dl (SI, > 7.7 mmol/L) or postprandial plasma glucose above 200 mg/dl (SI, > 11 mmol/L). Other tests may be used to confirm or sensitize OGTT findings, such as the I.V. glucose tolerance test or the cortisone glucose tolerance test.

Purpose
■ To confirm diabetes mellitus in selected patients
■ To aid diagnosis of hypoglycemia and malabsorption syndrome

Cost
Inexpensive

Patient preparation
■ Explain to the patient that this test evaluates glucose metabolism.
■ Instruct the patient to maintain a high-carbohydrate diet for 3 days and then to fast for 10 to 16 hours before the test.
■ Advise the patient not to smoke, drink coffee or alcohol, or exercise strenuously for 8 hours before or during the test.
■ Tell the patient that the test usually requires five blood samples and five urine specimens over several hours. Explain who will perform the venipunctures and when.
■ Explain to the patient that he may experience discomfort from the needle punctures and the tourniquet.
■ Restrict medications that may affect test results. If they must be continued, note this on the laboratory request.

ALERT! ▼ ▼ ▼ ▼ ▼ ▼ ▼ ▼ ▼
Alert the patient to the symptoms of hypoglycemia — weakness, restlessness, nervousness, hunger, and sweating — and tell him to report such symptoms immediately.

Reference values
Normal plasma glucose levels peak at 160 to 180 mg/dl (SI, 8.8 to 9.9 mmol/L) within 30 minutes to 1 hour after administration of an oral glucose test dose and return

to fasting levels or lower in 2 to 3 hours. (See *Interpreting results of the OGTT,* page 174.) Urine glucose tests remain negative throughout.

AGE ISSUE ✳ ✳ ✳ ✳ ✳
People over age 50 tend to exhibit decreasing carbohydrate tolerance, which causes an increase in glucose tolerance to upper limits of about 1 mg/dl for every year over age 50.

Abnormal findings
Depressed glucose tolerance, in which levels peak sharply before falling slowly to fasting levels, may confirm diabetes or may result from Cushing's disease, hemochromatosis, pheochromocytomas, or central nervous system lesions.

Increased glucose tolerance, in which levels may peak at less than normal, may indicate insulinoma, malabsorption syndrome, adrenocortical insufficiency (Addison's disease), hypothyroidism, or hypopituitarism.

Interfering factors
■ Carbohydrate deprivation before the test (may cause a diabetic response [abnormal increase in plasma glucose level with a delayed decrease] because the pancreas is unaccustomed to responding to high-carbohydrate load)
■ Arginine, benzodiazepines, caffeine, chlorthalidone, corticosteroids, dextrothyroxine, diazoxide, epinephrine, furosemide, hormonal contraceptives (estrogen-progestogen combination), lithium, large doses of nicotinic acid, phenolphthalein, phenothiazines, phenytoin, recent I.V. glucose infusions, thiazide diuretics, and triamterene (possible increase)
■ Amphetamines, beta-adrenergic blockers, clofibrate, ethanol, insulin, monoamine oxidase inhibitors, and oral antidiabetic drugs (possible decrease)

Because plasma glucose levels in the oral glucose tolerance test (OGTT) can be measured in various ways, inconsistent results and misinterpretation are common. Age, race, inactivity, and obesity may also affect established OGTT criteria. The American Diabetes Association recommends using the reference values obtained by the Wilkerson point system, the Fajans-Conn system, or the National Institutes of Health (NIH) system.

METHOD	HOUR	WHOLE BLOOD	PLASMA	POINTS
Wilkerson point system	Fasting	≥110 mg/dl (SI, ≥6.1 mmol/L)	≥130 mg/dl (SI, ≥7.3 mmol/L)	1
	1	≥170 mg/dl (SI, ≥9.5 mmol/L)	≥195 mg/dl (SI, ≥10.9 mmol/L)	½
	2	≥120 mg/dl (SI, ≥6.7 mmol/L)	≥140 mg/dl (SI, ≥7.7 mmol/L)	½
	3	≥110 mg/dl (SI, ≥6.1 mmol/L)	≥130 mg/dl (SI, ≥7.3 mmol/L)	1
Two or more total points confirm the diagnosis of diabetes.				
Fajans-Conn system	1	≥160 mg/dl (SI, ≥8.8 mmol/L)	≥185 mg/dl (SI, ≥10.3 mmol/L)	
	1½	≥140 mg/dl (SI, ≥7.7 mmol/L)	≥165 mg/dl (SI, ≥9.2 mmol/L)	
	2	≥120 mg/dl (SI, ≥6.7 mmol/L)	≥140 mg/dl (SI, ≥7.7 mmol/L)	
If all levels equal or exceed established values, the diagnosis of diabetes is confirmed.				
NIH system	Fasting		≥140 mg/dl (SI, ≥7.7 mmol/L)	
	2		≥200 mg/dl (SI, ≥11 mmol/L)	
If all levels exceed established values, the diagnosis of diabetes is confirmed.				

■ Failure to adhere to pretest dietary and exercise restrictions
■ Recent infection, fever, pregnancy, or acute illness such as myocardial infarction (possible increase)

Glucose, 2-hour postprandial plasma

The 2-hour postprandial plasma glucose test is a valuable screening tool for detecting diabetes mellitus. This procedure is performed on patients who have symptoms of diabetes (polydipsia and polyuria) or on patients whose fasting plasma glucose test results suggest diabetes.

The 2-hour postprandial test reliably indicates the body's insulin response to carbohydrate ingestion. It relies solely on the 2-hour postprandial plasma glucose level, avoiding the multiple venipunctures required for the oral glucose tolerance test (OGTT). If postprandial test results are borderline, the OGTT may confirm the diagnosis. (See *Preferred screening test*.)

Purpose
■ To aid diagnosis of diabetes mellitus
■ To monitor drug or diet therapy in patients with diabetes mellitus

Cost
Moderately expensive

Patient preparation

- Explain to the patient that this test evaluates glucose metabolism and helps detect diabetes.
- Tell the patient to eat a balanced meal or one containing 100 g of carbohydrate (recommended by the American Diabetes Association) before the test and then to fast for 2 hours.
- Instruct the patient to avoid smoking and strenuous exercise after the meal.
- Tell the patient that the test requires a blood sample. Explain who will perform the venipuncture and when.
- Explain to the patient that he may experience discomfort from the needle puncture and the tourniquet.

Reference values

In a person without diabetes, postprandial plasma glucose values are less than 145 mg/dl (SI, < 8 mmol/L) by the glucose oxidase or hexokinase method.

AGE ISSUE * * * * *
Plasma glucose levels are slightly elevated in people over age 50. (See Two-hour postprandial plasma glucose levels by age, *page 176.)*

Abnormal findings

Two-hour postprandial plasma glucose values of 200 mg/dl (SI, 11.1 mmol/L) or above indicate diabetes mellitus. High levels may also result from pancreatitis, Cushing's syndrome, acromegaly, or pheochromocytoma. Hyperglycemia may also be caused by hyperlipoproteinemia (especially type III, IV, or V), chronic hepatic disease, nephrotic syndrome, brain tumor, sepsis, gastrectomy with dumping syndrome, eclampsia, anoxia, or convulsive disorders.

Depressed plasma glucose levels can result from adrenal insufficiency, congenital adrenal hyperplasia, hyperinsulinism, functional or reactive hypoglycemia, hypopituitarism, insulinoma, malabsorption syndrome, myxedema, von Gierke's disease, and some cases of hepatic insufficiency.

Preferred screening test

Because the 2-hour postprandial test is a simpler procedure than the oral glucose tolerance test or the fasting plasma glucose test, it's commonly the preferred test for diabetes screening in patients with any of the following conditions:

- obesity
- family history of diabetes
- transient glycosuria or hyperglycemia (especially during pregnancy, surgery, or use of adrenal steroids) or after trauma, emotional stress, myocardial infarction, or stroke
- unexplained hypoglycemia, neuropathy, retinopathy, nephropathy, or peripheral vascular disease
- pregnancy resulting in abortion, premature labor, stillbirth, neonatal death, or a very large neonate
- recurrent infection, especially boils and abscesses.

Interfering factors

- Acetaminophen, if using the glucose oxidase or hexokinase method (possible false-positive)
- Arginine, benzodiazepines, chlorthalidone, corticosteroids, dextrothyroxine, diazoxide, epinephrine, furosemide, hormonal contraceptives (estrogen-progestogen combination), lithium, large doses of nicotinic acid, phenolphthalein, phenothiazines, phenytoin, recent I.V. glucose infusions, thiazide diuretics, and triamterene (possible increase)

Two-hour postprandial plasma glucose levels by age

The greatest difference in normal and diabetic insulin responses, and thus in plasma glucose concentration, occurs about 2 hours after a glucose challenge. Values of this test can fluctuate according to the patient's age. After age 50, for example, normal levels rise markedly and steadily, sometimes reaching 160 mg/dl (SI, 8.82 mmol/L) or higher. In younger patients, glucose concentration > 145 mg/dl (SI, > 8 mmol/L) suggests incipient diabetes and requires further evaluation.

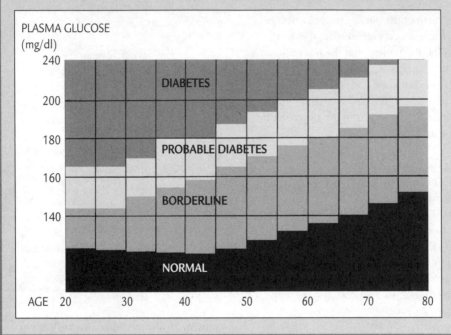

■ Ethacrynic acid (may cause hyperglycemia); large doses in patients with uremia (may cause hypoglycemia)
■ Amphetamines, beta-adrenergic blockers, clofibrate, ethanol, insulin, and monoamine oxidase inhibitors, oral antidiabetic drugs (possible decrease)
■ Recent illness, infection, or pregnancy (possible increase)
■ Strenuous exercise or stress (possible decrease)
■ Glycolysis caused by failure to refrigerate the sample or to send it to the laboratory immediately (possible decrease)

Glucose urinalysis

The glucose urinalysis test, which involves the use of commercial, plastic-coated reagent strips (Clinistix, Diastix) or glucose enzymatic test strip (Tes-Tape), is a specific, qualitative test for glycosuria. Normally, almost all glucose passes into the glomerular filtrate and is reabsorbed by the proximal renal tubule. However, if the blood glucose level exceeds the reabsorption capacity of the tubule, glucose spills into the urine.

Interpreting glucose oxidase test results

Until recently, all glucose oxidase tests used the plus (+) symbol to indicate glycosuria. However, because the plus symbol didn't reflect a standard glucose value, regulating insulin dosages was difficult, prompting some manufacturers to stop using the symbol. As the chart below shows, the reagent strip Diastix doesn't use the plus symbol, but the glucose enzymatic test strip Tes-Tape does. These tests are semiquantitative. The reagent strip Clinistix (not shown) has no quantitative value; it's strictly qualitative. Results for this test are reported as negative, light, medium, or dark.

TEST	0%	0.1%	0.25%	0.5%	1%	≥2%
DIASTIX	Negative	100 mg/dl	250 mg/dl	500 mg/dl	1,000 mg/dl	≥2,000 mg/dl
TES-TAPE	Negative	+	++	+++		++++

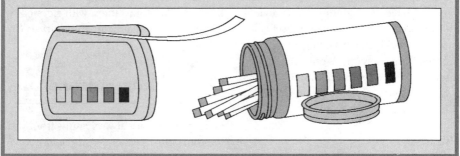

Purpose
- To detect glycosuria
- To screen for diabetes
- To monitor the degree of diabetic control for patients who can't or won't perform self-monitoring of blood glucose levels

Cost
Inexpensive

Patient preparation
- Explain to the patient that this test determines urine glucose levels.
- Tell the patient that the test requires a urine specimen, and explain when the specimen is needed.

Normal findings
Glucose shouldn't be present in urine.

Abnormal findings
Glycosuria occurs in diabetes mellitus, adrenal and thyroid disorders, hepatic and central nervous system diseases, Fanconi's syndrome, and other conditions involving low renal threshold, toxic renal tubular disease, heavy metal poisoning, glomerulonephritis, nephrosis, pregnancy, and total parenteral nutrition. It also occurs with administration of large amounts of glucose or niacin, prolonged use of phenothiazines, and use of certain other drugs, such as ammonium chloride, asparaginase, carbamazepine, corticosteroids, dextrothyroxine, lithium carbonate, and thiazide diuretics. (See *Interpreting glucose oxidase test results*.)

Interfering factors

- Ascorbic acid, levodopa, methyldopa, phenazopyridine, salicylates, tetracycline (possible false-negative)
- Diluted, stale urine
- Bacterial contamination of the specimen

Glycosylated hemoglobin

Also called *total fasting hemoglobin,* the glycosylated hemoglobin test is a tool for monitoring diabetes therapy. Measurement of glycosylated hemoglobin levels provides information about the average blood glucose level during the preceding 2 to 3 months. This test requires only one venipuncture every 6 to 8 weeks and can, therefore, be used for evaluating long-term effectiveness of diabetes therapy.

Purpose

- To assess control of diabetes mellitus

Cost

Inexpensive

Patient preparation

- Explain to the patient that this test is used to evaluate diabetes therapy.
- Tell the patient that the test requires a blood sample. Explain who will perform the venipuncture and when.
- Explain to the patient that he may experience discomfort from the needle puncture and the tourniquet.

Normal findings

Glycosylated hemoglobin values are reported as a percentage of the total hemoglobin within an erythrocyte. Glycosylated hemoglobin accounts for 4% to 7%.

Abnormal findings

In diabetes, the patient has good control of blood glucose concentrations when the glycosylated hemoglobin value is less than 8%. A glycosylated hemoglobin value greater than 10% indicates poor glucose control.

Interfering factors

- Failure to adequately mix the sample and the anticoagulant
- Hemolytic anemia (possible decrease)
- Chronic renal failure, hyperglycemia, thalassemia (possible decrease)
- Patients receiving dialysis, those that have a splenectomy, those with elevated triglycerides or fetal hemoglobin levels (increased)

Gonorrhea culture

Gonorrhea almost always results from sexual transmission of *Neisseria gonorrhoeae.* A stained smear of genital exudate can confirm gonorrhea in 90% of males with characteristic symptoms, but a culture is usually necessary, especially in asymptomatic females. Possible culture sites include the urethra (usual site in males), endocervix (usual site in females), anal canal, and oropharynx.

Purpose

- To confirm gonorrhea

Cost

Inexpensive

Patient preparation

- Describe the procedure to the patient. Explain that this test is used to confirm gonorrhea.
- Inform the patient who will perform the test and when.

■ Instruct the female patient not to douche for 24 hours before the test and that a vaginal (cervical) culture will be drawn as appropriate.

■ Tell the male patient not to void during the hour preceding the test. Warn him that males sometimes experience nausea, sweating, weakness, and fainting due to stress or discomfort when the cotton swab or wire loop is introduced into the urethra.

■ Advise the patient to avoid all sexual contact until test results are available.

■ Explain to the patient that treatment usually begins after confirmation of a positive culture, except in a person who has symptoms of gonorrhea or who has had intercourse with someone known to have gonorrhea.

■ Advise the patient that a repeat culture is required 1 week after completion of treatment to evaluate the effectiveness of therapy.

■ Inform the patient that positive culture findings must be reported to the local health department.

Normal findings

Normally, no *N. gonorrhoeae* appears in the culture.

Abnormal findings

A positive culture confirms gonorrhea.

Interfering factors

■ Pretest antimicrobial therapy
■ Contamination due to fecal material in a rectal culture
■ In males, voiding within 1 hour of specimen collection; in females, douching within 24 hours of specimen collection (fewer organisms available for culture)

Growth hormone, serum

Human growth hormone (hGH), also called *somatotropin,* is a protein secreted by acidophils of the anterior pituitary gland. It's the primary regulator of human growth. Unlike other pituitary hormones, hGH has no easily defined feedback mechanism or single target gland — it affects many body tissues. Like insulin, hGH promotes protein synthesis and stimulates amino acid uptake by cells. Hyposecretion or hypersecretion of this hormone may induce pathologic states (such as dwarfism and gigantism, respectively). This test is a quantitative analysis of serum hGH levels and may be performed as part of an anterior pituitary stimulation or suppression test.

Purpose

■ To aid differential diagnosis of dwarfism because growth retardation can result from pituitary or thyroid hypofunction
■ To confirm diagnosis of acromegaly and gigantism in adults
■ To aid diagnosis of pituitary and hypothalamic tumors
■ To help evaluate hGH therapy

Cost

Inexpensive

Patient preparation

■ Explain to the patient, or to his parents if the patient is a child, that this test measures hormone levels and helps determine the cause of abnormal growth.

■ Instruct the patient to fast and limit physical activity for 10 to 12 hours before the test.

■ Tell the patient that the test requires an early morning blood sample (between 6 a.m. and 8 a.m.). Explain who will perform the venipuncture and when.

- Explain to the patient that he may experience discomfort from the needle puncture and the tourniquet.
- Inform the patient that another sample may have to be drawn the next day for comparison.
- Restrict medications that affect serum hGH levels such as pituitary-based steroids. If they must be continued, note this on the laboratory request.
- Tell the patient to lie down and relax for 30 minutes before the test because stress and physical activity elevate serum hGH levels.

- Hemolysis due to rough handling of the sample
- Arginine, beta-adrenergic blockers such as propranolol, and estrogens (increase)
- Amphetamines, bromocriptine, dopamine, histamine, levodopa, methyldopa, and pituitary-based steroids (increase)
- Glucagon, insulin (induced hypoglycemia), and nicotinic acid (increase)
- Corticosteroids and phenothiazines such as chlorpromazine (decrease)
- Radioactive scan performed within 1 week before the test

Reference values

Normal serum hGH levels for males range from undetectable to 5 ng/ml (SI, undetectable to 5 µg/L); for females, from undetectable to 10 ng/ml (SI, undetectable to 10 µg/L). Children's values may range from undetectable to 16 ng/ml (SI, undetectable to 16 µg/L) and are usually higher.

Abnormal findings

Increased serum hGH levels may indicate a pituitary or hypothalamic tumor, usually an adenoma, which causes gigantism in children and acromegaly in adults and adolescents. Some patients with diabetes mellitus have elevated serum hGH levels without acromegaly. Suppression testing is necessary to confirm diagnosis.

Pituitary infarction, metastatic disease, and tumors may decrease serum hGH levels. Dwarfism may be due to low serum hGH levels, although only 15% of all cases of growth failure relate to endocrine dysfunction. Confirmation of diagnosis requires stimulation testing with arginine or insulin.

Interfering factors

- Failure to observe pretest restrictions

H

Haptoglobin

The haptoglobin test is used to measure serum levels of haptoglobin, a glycoprotein produced in the liver. In acute intravascular hemolysis, haptoglobin concentration decreases rapidly and may remain low for 5 to 7 days, until the liver synthesizes more glycoprotein.

Purpose
- To serve as an index of hemolysis
- To distinguish between hemoglobin and myoglobin in plasma because haptoglobin doesn't bind with myoglobin
- To investigate hemolytic transfusion reactions
- To establish proof of paternity using genetic (phenotypic) variations in haptoglobin structure

Cost
Moderately expensive

Patient preparation
- Explain to the patient that this test is used to determine the condition of red blood cells.
- Tell the patient that the test requires a blood sample. Explain who will perform the venipuncture and when.
- Explain to the patient that he may experience slight discomfort from the needle puncture and the tourniquet.
- Inform the patient that he need not restrict food and fluids.
- Restrict any medications that may affect test results. If these drugs must be continued, note this on the laboratory request.

Reference values
Normally, serum haptoglobin concentrations, measured in terms of the protein's hemoglobin-binding capacity, range from 40 to 180 mg/dl (SI, 0.4 to 1.8 g/L). Nephelometric procedures yield lower results.

Haptoglobin is absent in 90% of neonates, but in most cases, levels gradually increase to normal by age 4 months.

Abnormal findings
Markedly decreased serum haptoglobin levels are characteristic in acute and chronic hemolysis, severe hepatocellular disease, infectious mononucleosis, and transfusion reactions. Hepatocellular disease inhibits the synthesis of haptoglobin. In hemolytic transfusion reactions, haptoglobin levels begin decreasing after 6 to 8 hours and drop to 40% of pretransfusion levels after 24 hours.

If serum haptoglobin values are very low, watch for symptoms of hemolysis: chills, fever, back pain, flushing, distended neck veins, tachycardia, tachypnea, and hypotension.

In about 1% of the population, including 4% of blacks, haptoglobin is permanently absent; this disorder is known as congenital ahaptoglobinemia.

Strikingly elevated serum haptoglobin levels occur in diseases marked by chronic inflammatory reactions or tissue destruction, such as rheumatoid arthritis and malignant neoplasms.

Interfering factors
■ Hemolysis due to rough handling of the sample
■ Corticosteroids and androgens (possible increase; may mask hemolysis in patients with inflammatory disease)

Helicobacter pylori antibodies

Helicobacter pylori is a spiral, gram-negative bacterium associated with chronic gastritis and idiopathic chronic duodenal ulceration. Although a gastric sample can be obtained by endoscopy and cultured for *H. pylori*, the *H. pylori* antibodies test is a more useful noninvasive screening procedure and may be performed using the enzyme-linked immunosorbent assay.

ALERT! ▼ ▼ ▼ ▼ ▼ ▼ ▼ ▼ ▼
The Helicobacter pylori *antibodies test should be performed only on patients with GI symptoms due to the large number of healthy people who have* H. pylori *antibodies.*

Purpose
■ To help diagnose *H. pylori* antibody infection in patients with GI symptoms

Cost
Inexpensive

Patient preparation
■ Inform the patient that this test is used to diagnose the infection that may cause ulcers.
■ Tell the patient that the test requires a blood sample. Explain who will perform the venipuncture and when.
■ Explain to the patient that he may experience discomfort from the needle puncture and the tourniquet.

Normal findings
Normally, no antibodies to *H. pylori* are revealed.

Abnormal findings
A positive *H. pylori* antibody test result indicates that the patient has antibodies to the bacterium. The serologic results should be interpreted in light of the clinical findings.

Interfering factors
■ None significant

Hematocrit

A hematocrit (HCT) test may be done separately or as part of a complete blood cell count. It measures percentage by volume of packed red blood cells (RBCs) in a whole blood sample; for example, an HCT of 40% indicates that a 100-ml sample of blood contains 40 ml of packed RBCs. Packing is achieved by centrifuging anticoagulated whole blood in a capillary tube so that red cells are tightly packed without hemolysis.

Purpose
■ To aid diagnosis of polycythemia, anemia, or abnormal states of hydration

■ To aid calculation of erythrocyte indices

Cost
Inexpensive

Patient preparation
■ Explain to the patient that HCT is tested to detect anemia and other abnormal blood conditions.
■ Tell the patient that the test requires a blood sample. Explain who will perform the venipuncture and when.
■ Explain to the patient that he may experience discomfort from the needle puncture and the tourniquet.

AGE ISSUE ✻ ✻ ✻ ✻ ✻
If the patient is a child, explain to him (if he's old enough) and to his parents that a small amount of blood will be taken from his finger or earlobe.

Normal findings
HCT is usually measured electronically. The results are 3% lower than manual measurements, which trap plasma in the column of packed RBCs.

AGE ISSUE ✻ ✻ ✻ ✻ ✻
Reference values vary, depending on the type of sample, the laboratory performing the test, and the patient's age and sex, as follows:
■ *Neonates at birth: 55% to 68% (SI, 0.55 to 0.68)*
■ *Neonates age 1 week: 47% to 65% (SI, 0.47 to 0.65)*
■ *Neonates age 1 month: 37% to 49% (SI, 0.37 to 0.49)*
■ *Infants age 3 months: 30% to 36% (SI, 0.3 to 0.36)*
■ *Infants age 1: 29% to 41% (SI, 0.29 to 0.41)*
■ *Children age 10: 36% to 40% (SI, 0.36 to 0.4)*
■ *Adult males: 42% to 52% (SI, 0.42 to 0.52)*
■ *Adult females: 36% to 48% (SI, 0.36 to 0.48).*

Abnormal findings
Low HCT suggests anemia, hemodilution, or massive blood loss. High HCT indicates polycythemia or hemoconcentration due to blood loss and dehydration.

Interfering factors
■ Failure to fill the tube properly, to use the proper anticoagulant, or to adequately mix the sample and the anticoagulant
■ Hemoconcentration due to tourniquet constriction for longer than 1 minute (increase, typically 2.5% to 5%)
■ Hemodilution due to drawing the blood from arm above an I.V. infusion

Hemoglobin

The hemoglobin (Hb) test, which is usually performed as a part of a complete blood cell count, is used to measure the amount of Hb found in a deciliter (100 ml) of whole blood. Hb concentration correlates closely with the red blood cell (RBC) count and affects the Hb-RBC ratio (mean corpuscular hemoglobin [MCH] and mean corpuscular hemoglobin concentration [MCHC]).

Purpose
■ To measure the severity of anemia or polycythemia and to monitor response to therapy
■ To obtain data for calculating MCH and MCHC.

Cost
Inexpensive

Patient preparation
■ Explain to the patient that this test is used to detect anemia or polycythemia, or to assess his response to treatment.

■ Tell the patient that a blood sample will be taken. Explain who will perform the venipuncture and when.

■ Explain to the patient that he may experience discomfort from the needle puncture and the tourniquet.

AGE ISSUE ✳ ✳ ✳ ✳ ✳

If the patient is an infant or a child, explain to the parents that a small amount of blood will be taken from the finger or earlobe.

■ Inform the patient that he need not restrict food and fluids.

Reference values

AGE ISSUE ✳ ✳ ✳ ✳ ✳

Hb concentration varies depending on the type of sample drawn and the patient's age and sex:

■ Neonates at birth: *17 to 22 g/dl (SI, 170 to 220 g/L)*

■ Neonates age 1 week: *15 to 20 g/dl (SI, 150 to 200 g/L)*

■ Neonates age 1 month: *11 to 15 g/dl (SI, 110 to 150 g/L)*

■ Children: *11 to 13 g/dl (SI, 110 to 130 g/L)*

■ Adult males: *14 to 17.4 g/dl (SI, 140 to 174 g/L)*

■ Males after middle age: *12.4 to 14.9 g/dl (SI, 124 to 149 g/L)*

■ Adult females: *12 to 16 g/dl (SI, 120 to 160 g/L)*

■ Females after middle age: *11.7 to 13.8 g/dl (SI, 117 to 138 g/L)*

Those who are more physically active or who live in high altitudes may have higher values.

Abnormal findings

Low Hb concentration may indicate anemia, recent hemorrhage, or fluid retention, causing hemodilution.

Elevated Hb suggests hemoconcentration from polycythemia or dehydration.

Interfering factors

■ Failure to use the proper anticoagulant or to adequately mix the sample and the anticoagulant

■ Hemolysis due to rough handling of the sample

■ Hemoconcentration due to prolonged tourniquet constriction

■ Very high white blood cell counts, lipemia, or RBCs that are resistant to lysis (false-high)

Hemoglobin electrophoresis

Hemoglobin (Hb) electrophoresis is probably the most useful laboratory method for separating and measuring normal and some abnormal Hb. Through electrophoresis, different types of Hb are separated to form a series of distinctly pigmented bands in a medium. Results are then compared with those of a normal sample.

Hb A, A_2, S, and C, are routinely checked, but the laboratory may change the medium or its pH to expand the range of this test.

Purpose

■ To measure the amount of Hb A and to detect abnormal Hb

■ To aid diagnosis of thalassemia

Cost

Moderately expensive

Patient preparation

■ Explain to the patient that this test is used to evaluate Hb.

■ Tell the patient that a blood sample will be taken. Explain who will perform the venipuncture and when.

Variations of hemoglobin type and distribution

HEMOGLOBIN	PERCENTAGE OF TOTAL HEMOGLOBIN	CLINICAL IMPLICATIONS
Hb A	95% to 100% (SI, 0.95 to 1.0)	Normal
Hb A$_2$	4% to 5.8% (SI, 0.04 to 0.058)	ß-thalassemia minor
	1.5% to 3% (SI, 0.015 to 0.03)	Normal
	Under 1% (SI, < 0.01)	Hb H disease
Hb F	Under 1% (SI, < 0.01)	Normal
	2% to 5% (SI, 0.02 to 0.05)	ß-thalassemia minor
	10% to 90% (SI, 0.10 to 0.9)	ß-thalassemia major
	5% to 15% (SI, 0.05 to 0.15)	ß-d-thalassemia minor
	5% to 35% (SI, 0.05 to 0.35)	Heterozygous hereditary persistence of fetal hemoglobin (HPFH)
	100% (SI, 1.0)	Homozygous HPFH
Homozygous Hb S	70% to 98% (SI, 0.7 to 0.98)	Sickle cell disease
Homozygous Hb C	90% to 98% (SI, 0.9 to 0.98)	Hb C disease
Heterozygous Hb C	24% to 44% (SI, 0.24 to 0.44)	Hb C trait

■ Explain to the patient that he may feel slight discomfort from the tourniquet pressure and the needle puncture.

■ If the patient is an infant or child, explain to the parents that a small amount of blood will be taken from the finger.

■ Inform the patient that he need not restrict food and fluids.

Reference values

In adults, Hb A accounts for 95% (SI, 0.95) of all Hb; Hb A$_2$, 1.5% to 3% (SI, 0.015 to 0.030); and Hb F < 2% (SI, <0.02). In neonates, Hb F normally accounts for half the total. Hb S and Hb C are normally absent.

Abnormal findings

Hb electrophoresis allows identification of various types of Hb. Certain types may indicate a hemolytic disease. For some possible results and their associated conditions, see *Variations of hemoglobin type and distribution.*)

Interfering factors

■ Failure to fill the tube completely, to use the proper anticoagulant, or to adequately mix the sample and the anticoagulant
■ Hemolysis due to rough handling of the sample
■ Blood transfusion within the past 4 months

Hemoglobin, urine

An abnormal finding, free hemoglobin (Hb) in the urine may occur in hemolytic anemias, infection, strenuous exercise, or severe intravascular hemolysis from a transfusion reaction. Contained in red blood cells (RBCs), Hb consists of an iron-protoporphyrin complex (heme) and a polypeptide (globin). Usually, RBC destruction occurs within the reticuloendothelial system. However, when RBC destruction occurs within the circulation, free Hb enters the plasma and binds with haptoglobin. If the plasma level of Hb exceeds that of haptoglobin, the excess of unbound Hb is excreted in the urine (hemoglobinuria).

Heme proteins act like enzymes that catalyze oxidation of organic substances. This reaction produces a blue coloration; the intensity of color varies with the amount of Hb present. Microscopic examination is required to identify intact RBCs in urine (hematuria), which can occur in the presence of unbound Hb.

Purpose

■ To aid diagnosis of hemolytic anemias, infection, or severe intravascular hemolysis from a transfusion reaction

Cost

Moderately expensive

Patient preparation

■ Explain to the patient that this test detects excessive RBC destruction.
■ Tell the patient that he need not restrict food or fluid.
■ Tell the patient that the test requires a random urine specimen, and teach him the proper collection technique.
■ If the female patient is menstruating, inform her to reschedule the test as results may be altered.
■ Restrict medications that may affect test results. If they must be continued, note this on the laboratory request.

Normal findings

Normally, Hb isn't present in the urine.

Abnormal findings

Hemoglobinuria may result from severe intravascular hemolysis due to a blood transfusion reaction, burns, or a crushing injury. It may result from acquired hemolytic anemias caused by chemical or drug intoxication or malaria; congenital hemolytic anemias, such as hemoglobinopathies or enzyme defects; or paroxysmal nocturnal hemoglobinuria (another type of hemolytic anemia). Less commonly, it may signal cystitis, ureteral calculi, or urethritis.

Hemoglobinuria and hematuria occur in renal epithelial damage (which may result from acute glomerulonephritis or pyelonephritis), renal tumor, and tuberculosis.

Interfering factors

■ Failure to send the specimen to the laboratory immediately after collection
■ Nephrotoxic drugs, anticoagulants (positive results)
■ Large doses of vitamin C or drugs that contain vitamin C as a preservative (false negative)

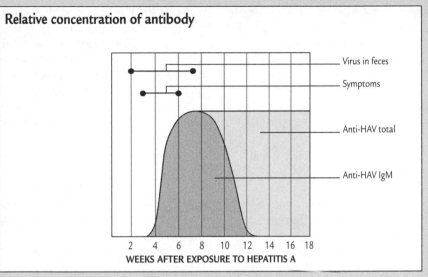

Relative concentration of antibody

Virus in feces
Symptoms
Anti-HAV total
Anti-HAV IgM

2 4 6 8 10 12 14 16 18
WEEKS AFTER EXPOSURE TO HEPATITIS A

Reprinted with permission from *Serodiagnostic Assessment of Acute Viral Hepatitis.* Abbott Park, Ill.: Abbott Laboratories, 1992.

■ Lysis of RBCs in stale or alkaline urine and contamination of the specimen by menstrual blood
■ Bacterial peroxidases in highly infected specimens (false-positive)

Hepatitis A antibodies

The hepatitis A antibodies test identifies hepatitis A antibodies that appear in the serum or body fluid of patients with hepatitis A virus (HAV). Hepatitis A is acquired through enteric transmission. The virus attacks through the GI track, and it's eliminated through the feces.

Because hepatitis A antibodies are present in blood and feces only briefly before symptoms appear, HAV may elude detection. However, anti-HAV, the antibody to HAV, appears early in the acute phase of the disease, persists for many years after recovery, and ultimately gives the patient immunity.

Purpose
■ To aid differential diagnosis of viral hepatitis

Cost
Inexpensive

Patient preparation
■ Explain to the patient that this test helps identify a type of viral hepatitis.
■ Inform the patient that he need not restrict food or fluids before the test.
■ Tell the patient that the test requires a blood sample. Explain who will perform the venipuncture and when.

- Explain to the patient that he may experience discomfort from the needle puncture and the tourniquet.
- Check the patient's history for administration of hepatitis vaccine, such as hepatitis A and hepatitis B.
- Tell the patient that confirmed viral hepatitis is reported to public health authorities in most states.

Normal findings

Serum should be negative for hepatitis A antibodies.

Abnormal findings

A single positive anti-HAV test may indicate previous exposure to the virus, but because these antibodies persist so long in the bloodstream, only evidence of rising anti-HAV titers confirms HAV as the cause of current or very recent infection. (See *Typical sequence of hepatitis A markers after exposure*, page 187.) Determining recent infection relies on identifying the antibodies as immunoglobulin M.

Interfering factors

- Hepatitis vaccine (possible positive)

Hepatitis B core antibodies

The hepatitis B core antibodies test identifies past or present hepatitis B virus (HBV) infection. HBV core antibodies are produced during or after an acute HBV infection. The core antigen is part of HBV, and the antibodies to the core antigen are usually present in chronic carriers. However, if they're present with surface protective antibodies, then they're associated with infection recovery and the patient isn't a carrier.

HBV is identified by the presence of hepatitis B antibodies, protein molecules (immunoglobulins) in serum or body fluid that either neutralize antigens or tag them for attack by other cells or chemicals. Viral transmission of HBV occurs through exposure to contaminated blood or blood products through an open wound, such as needlesticks or lacerations. Those at risk for hepatitis B include those with a history of drug abuse, individuals with sexual or household contact with infected persons, neonates born to infected mothers during delivery, hemodialysis patients, and health care employees.

Purpose

- To screen blood donors for hepatitis B
- To screen people at high risk for contracting hepatitis B such as hemodialysis nurses
- To aid differential diagnosis of viral hepatitis

Cost

Moderately expensive

Patient preparation

- Explain to the patient that this test helps identify a type of viral hepatitis.
- Inform the patient that he need not restrict food or fluids before the test.
- Tell the patient that the test requires a blood sample. Explain who will perform the venipuncture and when.
- Explain to the patient that he may experience discomfort from the needle puncture and the tourniquet.
- Check the patient's history for administration of hepatitis vaccine.
- Tell the patient that confirmed viral hepatitis is reported to public health authorities in most states.

Normal findings

Normal serum is negative for hepatitis B core antibodies.

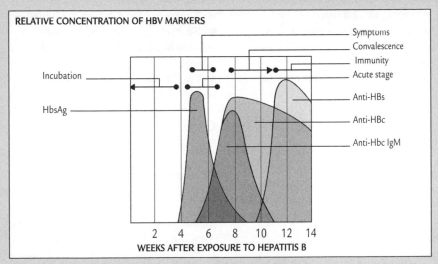

Typical sequence of hepatitis B and C markers after exposure

RELATIVE CONCENTRATION OF HBV MARKERS

Symptoms
Convalescence
Immunity
Incubation
Acute stage
Anti-HBs
HbsAg
Anti-HBc
Anti-Hbc IgM

2   4   6   8   10   12   14
WEEKS AFTER EXPOSURE TO HEPATITIS B

Reprinted with permission from *Serodiagnostic Assessment of Acute Viral Hepatitis.* Abbott Park, Ill.: Abbott Laboratories, 1992.

Abnormal findings

Positive findings may indicate that the patient is recovering from an acute HBV infection. (See *Typical sequence of hepatitis B and C markers after exposure.*)

Interfering factors

■ Hepatitis vaccine (possible positive)
■ Undetectable level of hepatitis B surface antigens (false-negative)

Hepatitis B surface antibodies

The hepatitis B virus is identified by the presence of hepatitis B antibodies, protein molecules (immunoglobulins) in serum or body fluid that either neutralize antigens or tag them for attack by other cells or chemicals. The presence of hepatitis B surface an-

tibodies indicates that a patient who has been exposed to the hepatitis B virus (HBV) is no longer contagious. These antibodies, which can also be produced by the HBV vaccine, protect the body from future HBV infection.

Purpose

■ To screen blood donors for hepatitis B
■ To screen people at high risk for contracting hepatitis B such as hemodialysis nurses
■ To aid differential diagnosis of viral hepatitis

Cost

Inexpensive

Patient preparation

■ Explain to the patient that this test helps identify a type of viral hepatitis.

- Inform the patient that he need not restrict food or fluids before the test.
- Tell the patient that the test requires a blood sample. Explain who will perform the venipuncture and when.
- Explain to the patient that he may experience discomfort from the needle puncture and the tourniquet.
- Check the patient's history for administration of the HBV vaccine.
- Tell the patient that confirmed viral hepatitis is reported to public health authorities in most states.

Normal findings

Normal serum is negative for hepatitis B surface antibodies.

Abnormal findings

A positive test result means that the patient is immune to HBV infection.

Interfering factors

- Hepatitis vaccine (possible positive)

Hepatitis B surface antigen

Hepatitis B surface antigen (HBsAg), also called *hepatitis-associated antigen* or *Australia antigen,* appears in the sera of patients with hepatitis B virus (HBV). It can be detected by radioimmunoassay or, less commonly, reverse passive hemagglutination during the extended incubation period and usually during the first 3 weeks of acute infection or if the patient is a carrier.

Because transmission of hepatitis is one of the gravest complications associated with blood transfusion, all donors must be screened for hepatitis B before their blood is stored. This screening, required by the Food and Drug Administration's Bureau of Biologics, has helped reduce the incidence

of hepatitis. This test doesn't screen for hepatitis A virus (infectious hepatitis).

Purpose

- To screen blood donors for hepatitis B
- To screen people at high risk for contracting hepatitis B such as hemodialysis nurses
- To aid differential diagnosis of viral hepatitis

Cost

Moderately expensive

Patient preparation

- Explain to the patient that this test helps identify a type of viral hepatitis.
- Inform the patient that he need not restrict food or fluids before the test.
- Tell the patient that the test requires a blood sample. Explain who will perform the venipuncture and when.
- Explain to the patient that he may experience discomfort from the needle puncture and the tourniquet.
- Check the patient's history for administration of hepatitis B vaccine.
- Tell the patient that confirmed viral hepatitis is reported to public health authorities in most states.

Normal findings

Normal serum is negative for HBsAg.

Abnormal findings

The presence of HBsAg in a patient with hepatitis confirms HBV. In chronic carriers and in people with chronic active hepatitis, HBsAg may be present in the serum several months after the onset of acute infection. It may also occur in more than 5% of patients with certain diseases other than hepatitis, such as hemophilia, Hodgkin's disease, and leukemia. If HbsAg is found in donor blood, that blood must be discarded because it carries a risk of transmitting hepatitis. Blood samples that test positive should be retested because inaccurate results do occur.

Interfering factors
- Hepatitis B vaccine (possible positive)

Hepatitis C antibodies

Hepatitis C virus (HCV), formerly known as *non-A, non-B hepatitis*, is characterized by the presence of antibodies to HCV (anti-HCV) and levels of alanine aminotransferase (ALT), which can fluctuate between normal and markedly elevated.

Levels of anti-HCV may remain positive for many years, so a reactive test indicates infection with HCV, but not the presence of immunity of infectivity. Testing for ribonucleic acid of HCV may be used to confirm infection when acute hepatitis C is suspected. Another test, using a serologic assay, can detect antibodies to the virus's nonstructural protein. This antibody has been designated anti-HCV and can appear relatively late in the infection, usually 16 to 24 weeks after the initial elevation of liver enzyme levels. The progress of infection can be monitored by periodic analysis of ALT and anti-HCV levels.

Transmitted parenterally, the clinical symptoms and epidemiology of HCV are similar to those of hepatitis B, but the rate of chronic infection is much higher because the plasma of chronically infected HCV patients remains infectious.

Purpose
- To aid differential diagnosis of viral hepatitis

Cost
Inexpensive

Patient preparation
- Explain to the patient that this test helps identify a type of viral hepatitis.
- Inform the patient that he needn't restrict food or fluids before the test.
- Tell the patient that the test requires a blood sample. Explain who will perform the venipuncture and when.
- Explain to the patient that he may experience discomfort from the needle puncture and the tourniquet.
- Check the patient's history for administration of the hepatitis B vaccine.
- Tell the patient that confirmed viral hepatitis is reported to public health authorities in most states.

Normal findings
Normal serum is negative for HCV antibodies.

Abnormal findings
The presence of anti-HCV confirms HCV.

Interfering factors
- Improper handling of sample (possible false-negative)

Hepatitis D antibodies

Hepatitis D is found primarily in patients with an acute or chronic episode of hepatitis B. Infection requires the presence of the hepatitis B surface antigen (HBsAg), while the hepatitis D virus (HDV) depends on the double-shelled type B virus to replicate. For this reason, type D infection can't outlast a type B infection, and without the HBsAg, hepatitis D can't survive. Transmission is parenteral.

Detection of the hepatitis D antigen early in the course of the infection and detection of anti-HDV antibodies in the later stages of the disease confirm the presence of serologic HDV.

Purpose
■ To aid differential diagnosis of viral hepatitis

Cost
Inexpensive

Patient preparation
■ Explain to the patient that this test helps identify a type of viral hepatitis.
■ Inform the patient that he need not restrict food or fluids before the test.
■ Tell the patient that the test requires a blood sample. Explain who will perform the venipuncture and when.
■ Explain to the patient that he may experience discomfort from the needle puncture and the tourniquet.
■ Check the patient's history for administration of hepatitis B vaccine.
■ Tell the patient that confirmed viral hepatitis is reported to public health authorities in most states.

Normal findings
Normal serum is negative for HDV antibodies.

Abnormal findings
Detection of intrahepatic delta antigens or immunoglobulin (Ig) M anti-delta antigens in acute disease (or IgM and IgG in chronic disease) confirms HDV.

Interfering factors
■ Lipemia (possible false-positive)
■ High titer rheumatoid factor (possible false-positive)

Hepatobiliary iminodiacetic scanning

Also known as *hepatobiliary imaging, cholescintigraphy,* or *gallbladder nuclear scanning,* hepatic iminodiacetic (HIDA) scanning obtains images of the hepatobiliary system to determine the patency of the cystic and common bile ducts through noninvasive scanning. The scanning is accomplished through injection of iminodiacetic acid analogues labeled with technetium 99m (^{99m}Tc). This test also evaluates gallbladder emptying.

ALERT! ▼ ▼ ▼ ▼ ▼ ▼ ▼ ▼ ▼
Hepatobiliary iminodiacetic scanning is generally contraindicated during pregnancy or lactation because it exposes the fetus or infant to radiation.

Purpose
■ To diagnose gallbladder disorders and determine degree of patency
■ To diagnose acute and chronic cholecystitis
■ To evaluate the patency of the biliary enteric bypass
■ To assess obstructive jaundice in combination with radiography or ultrasonography

Cost
Very expensive

Patient preparation
■ Explain to the patient that this test detects inflammation or obstruction of the gallbladder and its ducts.
■ Tell the patient who will perform the test and where it will take place.
■ Inform the patient that he'll receive an I.V. injection of a radionuclide.
■ Explain to the patient that he may experience some discomfort from the I.V. insertion, and that the radionuclide will be

eliminated from the body within 6 to 24 hours.

■ Inform the patient that his abdomen will be scanned after he receives the radionuclide and that repeat pictures may be taken up to 24 hours after the injection.

■ Ensure that the patient has no allergies to the media used.

■ Instruct the patient to fast for 2 to 6 hours before the scan and to comply with activity restriction during the scan.

■ Explain to the patient that sincalide may be given before the test to promote gallbladder contraction and emptying.

■ Obtain informed consent if necessary.

■ Advise the patient to drink plenty of fluids, unless contraindicated, for 24 to 48 hours after the test to eliminate the radionuclide from the body. Also, tell him to flush the toilet immediately after each voiding and to wash his hands with soap and water.

Normal findings

A normal HIDA scan shows the gallbladder to be normal in size, shape, and function; cystic and common bile ducts are patent.

Abnormal findings

Images may demonstrate acute or chronic cholecystitis, or common bile duct obstruction.

Interfering factors

■ Patient's inability to remain still during the procedure or failure to observe pretest restrictions

■ Presence of barium in GI tract (possible poor imaging)

■ Increased bilirubin levels (decreased hepatic uptake)

■ Alcoholism, fasting more than 24 hours, or total parenteral nutrition (decreased hepatic uptake)

Herpes simplex virus

Herpes simplex virus (HSV) produces a wide spectrum of clinical manifestations, including keratitis, gingivostomatitis, and encephalitis. In immunocompromised individuals, it may lead to disseminated illness.

The herpesvirus group includes Epstein-Barr virus, cytomegalovirus (CMV), varicella-zoster virus, human herpesvirus 6, herpesvirus 7, herpesvirus 8, and the two closely related serotypes of HSV — Type 1 and Type 2 herpes. Only CMV, varicella-zoster virus, and HSV replicate in the standard cell cultures used in diagnostic laboratories.

About 50% of HSV strains can be detected by characteristic cytopathic effects within 24 hours after the laboratory receives the specimen; 5 to 7 days are required to detect the remaining HSV strains. (See *Rapid monoclonal test for cytomegalovirus,* page 194.)

Alternatively, early antigens of HSV can be detected by monoclonal antibodies in shell vial cell cultures within 16 hours after receipt of the specimen with the same sensitivity and specificity as standard tube cell cultures.

Purpose

■ To confirm diagnosis of HSV infection by culturing the virus from specimens

Cost

Moderately expensive

Patient preparation

■ Explain to the patient that this test is performed to detect infection by HSV.

■ Explain to the patient that specimens will be collected from suspected lesions during the prodromal and acute stages of clinical infection.

Rapid monoclonal test for cytomegalovirus

Cytomegalovirus (CMV), a member of the herpesvirus group, can cause systemic infection in congenitally infected infants and immunocompromised patients, such as transplant recipients, patients receiving chemotherapy, and patients with acquired immunodeficiency syndrome.

Laboratory detection of CMV

In the past, CMV infections were detected in the laboratory by recognizing the distinctive cytopathic effects produced by the virus in conventional tube cell cultures. In this slow method of detecting CMV, distinctive cytopathic effects cultures grow in 9 days on average.

The faster rapid monoclonal test (*shell vial assay*) is based on centrifugal inoculation of specimens onto cell monolayers grown on round cover slips in 1-dram shell vials. The immunologic detection of early products of viral replication with specific monoclonal antibodies usually occurs after 16 hours of incubation. This assay is based on the availability of a monoclonal antibody specific for the 72-kd protein of CMV synthesized during the immediate early stage of viral replication.

Through indirect immunofluorescence, CMV-infected fibroblasts are recognized by their dense, homogeneous staining confined to the nucleus of these cells. Because of the smooth, regular shape of the nucleus and the surrounding nuclear membrane, infected cells are readily differentiated from nonspecific background fluorescence, which may be present in some specimens.

This test is used to obtain rapid laboratory diagnosis of CMV infection, especially in immunocompromised patients who have or are at risk for developing systemic infections caused by this virus.

Specimen collection

Specimens should be collected during the prodromal and acute stages of clinical infection to ensure the best chance of detecting CMV. As required by the laboratory, collect a specimen for culture. Each type of specimen requires a specific collection device, as listed below:

- *Throat:* microbiologic transport swab
- *Urine, cerebrospinal fluid:* sterile screw-capped tube or vial
- *Bronchoalveolar lavage tissue:* sterile screw-capped jar
- *Blood:* sterile tube with anticoagulant (heparin)

CMV can be detected in urine and throat specimens from asymptomatic patients. The detection of CMV from these sites indicates active, asymptomatic infection, which may herald symptomatic involvement, especially in immunocompromised patients. Detection of CMV in specimens of blood, tissue, or bronchoalveolar lavage generally indicates systemic infection and disease.

Normal findings

HSV is seldom recovered from immunocompetent patients who show no overt signs of disease.

Abnormal findings

HSV detected in specimens from dermal lesions, the eye, or cerebrospinal fluid is highly significant. Specimens from the upper respiratory tract may be associated with intermittent shedding of the virus, particularly in an immunocompromised patient.

Like other herpesviruses, HSV can be shed from immunocompromised patients intermittently in the absence of apparent disease. For epidemiologic purposes, HSV detected by characteristic cytopathic effects in standard tube cell cultures is confirmed and identified as type 1 or 2.

Interfering factors
■ Administration of antiviral drugs before specimen collection

Herpes simplex virus antibodies

Herpes simplex virus (HSV), a member of the herpesvirus group, causes various clinically severe manifestations, including genital lesions, keratitis or conjunctivitis, generalized dermal lesions, and pneumonia. Severe involvement is associated with intrauterine or neonatal infections and encephalitis; such infections are most severe in immunosuppressed patients. Of the two closely related antigenic types, Type 1 herpes usually causes infections above the waistline; Type 2 herpes infections predominantly involve the external genitalia. Primary contact with this virus occurs in early childhood as acute stomatitis or, more commonly, as an inapparent infection.

Sensitive assays, such as indirect immunofluorescence and enzyme immunoassay, are used to demonstrate immunoglobulin (Ig) M class antibodies to HSV or to detect a fourfold or greater increase in IgG class antibodies between acute- and convalescent-phase sera.

Purpose
■ To confirm infections caused by HSV
■ To detect recent or past HSV infection

Cost
Inexpensive

Patient preparation
■ Explain to the patient the purpose of the test.
■ Tell the patient that the test requires a blood sample. Explain who will perform the venipuncture and when.
■ Explain to the patient that he may experience discomfort from the needle puncture and the tourniquet.

Normal findings
Sera from patients who have never been infected with HSV will have no detectable antibodies (less than 1:5). Patients with primary HSV infection will develop both IgM and IgG class antibodies. Reportedly, over 50% of adults have IgG class antibodies to HSV because of prior infection. Reactivated infections caused by HSV can be recognized serologically only by an increase in IgG class antibodies between acute- and convalescent-phase serum.

Abnormal findings
HSV infection can be ruled out in patients whose serum shows no detectable antibodies to the virus. The presence of IgM antibodies or a fourfold or greater increase in IgG antibodies indicates active HSV infection.

Interfering factors
■ Hemolysis (may alter results)

Heterophil antibodies

Heterophil antibody tests detect and identify two immunoglobulin (Ig) M antibodies in human serum that react against foreign red blood cells (RBCs): Epstein-Barr virus (EBV) antibodies and Forssman antibodies.

In the Paul-Bunnell test — also called the *presumptive test* — EBV antibodies, found in the sera of patients with infectious mononucleosis, agglutinate with sheep RBCs in a test tube. Forssman antibodies, present in the sera of some normal persons as well as in the sera of patients with conditions such as serum sickness also agglutinate with sheep RBCs, thus rendering test results inconclusive for infectious mononucleosis.

If the Paul-Bunnell test establishes a presumptive titer, the Davidsohn differential absorption test can then distinguish between EBV antibodies and Forssman antibodies. (See *Monospot test for infectious mononucleosis.*)

Purpose
■ To aid differential diagnosis of infectious mononucleosis

Cost
Inexpensive

Patient preparation
■ Explain to the patient that this test helps detect infectious mononucleosis.
■ Tell the patient that the test requires a blood sample. Explain who will perform the venipuncture and when.
■ Tell the patient that he may experience discomfort from the needle puncture and the tourniquet.

Reference values
Normally, the titer is less than 1:56, but it may be higher in elderly people. Some laboratories refer to a normal titer as "negative" or as having "no reaction."

Abnormal findings
Although heterophil antibodies are present in the sera of about 80% of patients with infectious mononucleosis 1 month after onset, a positive finding — a titer higher than 1:56 — doesn't confirm this disorder; a high titer can also result from systemic lupus erythematosus, syphilis, cryoglobulinemia, or the presence of antibodies to

nonsyphilitic treponema (yaws, pinta, bejel).

A gradual increase in titer during week 3 or 4 followed by a gradual decrease during weeks 4 to 8 proves most conclusive for infectious mononucleosis. A negative titer doesn't always rule out this disorder; occasionally, the titer becomes reactive 2 weeks later. Therefore, if symptoms persist, the test should be repeated in 2 weeks.

Confirmation of infectious mononucleosis depends on heterophil agglutination and hematologic tests that show absolute lymphocytosis, with 10% or more atypical lymphocytes.

Interfering factors
■ Hemolysis due to rough handling of the sample
■ Narcotic use, lymphomas, hepatitis, leukemia, and phenytoin therapy (false-positive)

Holter monitoring

Also called *ambulatory electrocardiography* (ECG) or *dynamic monitoring,* Holter monitoring involves the continuous recording of heart activity over a 24-hour period as the patient follows his normal routine. During this period, the patient wears a small reel-to-reel or cassette tape recorder connected to electrodes placed on his chest and keeps a diary of his activities and any associated symptoms. After the recording period, the tape is analyzed to correlate cardiac irregularities, such as arrhythmias and ST-segment changes, with the activities noted in the patient's diary.

Purpose
■ To detect cardiac arrhythmias
■ To evaluate chest pain

■ To evaluate cardiac status after acute myocardial infarction (MI) or pacemaker implantation
■ To evaluate the effectiveness of antiarrhythmic drug therapy
■ To assess and correlate dyspnea, central nervous system symptoms (such as syncope and light-headedness), and palpitations with actual cardiac events and the patient's activities

Cost
Expensive

Patient preparation
■ Explain to the patient that this test helps determine how the heart responds to normal activity or, if appropriate, cardioactive medication.
■ Tell the patient that electrodes will be attached to his chest, that his chest may be shaved, and that he may experience discomfort during preparation of the electrode sites.
■ Explain to the patient that he'll wear a small tape recorder for 24 hours (for 5 to 7 days if a patient-activated monitor is being used).
■ Tell the patient that a shoulder strap or a special belt will be provided to carry the recorder, which weighs about 2 lb (1 kg).
■ Encourage the patient to continue his routine activities during the monitoring period. Stress the importance of logging his usual activities (such as walking, climbing stairs, urinating, sleeping, and sexual activity), emotional upsets, physical symptoms (dizziness, palpitations, fatigue, chest pain, and syncope), and ingestion of medication; show the patient a sample diary.

Normal findings
When correlated with the patient's diary, the ECG pattern shows normal sinus rhythm with no significant arrhythmias or

ST-segment changes. Changes in heart rate normally occur during various activities.

Abnormal findings

Abnormalities of the heart detected by ambulatory ECG include premature ventricular contractions (PVCs), conduction defects, tachyarrhythmias, bradyarrhythmias, and brady-tachyarrhythmia syndrome. Arrhythmias may be associated with dyspnea and central nervous system symptoms, such as dizziness and syncope.

During recovery from an MI, this test can monitor for PVCs to determine the prognosis and effectiveness of drug therapy.

ST-segment changes associated with ischemia may coincide with chest pain or increased patient activity. ST-segment changes associated with an acute MI require careful study because smoking, eating, postural changes, certain drugs, Wolff-Parkinson-White syndrome, bundle-branch block, myocarditis, myocardial hypertrophy, anemia, hypoxemia, and abnormal hemoglobin binding can produce a similar tracing on the ECG. Monitoring the MI patient for 1 to 3 days before discharge and again 4 to 6 weeks after discharge may detect ST-T wave changes associated with ischemia or arrhythmias; such information aids patient therapy and rehabilitation and refines the prognosis. Monitoring a patient with an artificial pacemaker may detect an arrhythmia, such as bradycardia, that the pacemaker fails to override.

Although ambulatory ECG correlates patient symptoms and ECG changes, it doesn't always identify the symptoms' causes. If initial monitoring proves inconclusive, the test may be repeated.

Interfering factors

■ Electrode placement over muscle mass, poor electrode contact with skin, or other failure to correctly apply the electrodes (possible muscle or movement artifact)
■ Patient's failure to carefully record daily activities and symptoms, to maintain his normal routine, or to turn on the monitor during symptoms (if using a patient-activated monitor)
■ Physiologic variation in arrhythmia frequency and severity (possible failure to detect arrhythmia during 24-hour Holter monitoring)

Homocysteine, total plasma

Homocysteine, a sulfur-containing amino acid, is a transmethylation product of methionine. It's an intermediate in the synthesis of cysteine, which is produced by the enzymatic or acid hydrolysis of proteins. The total plasma homocysteine test is useful for the biochemical diagnosis of inborn errors of methionine, folate, and vitamins B_6 and B_{12} metabolism.

Purpose

■ To diagnose inborn errors of methionine, folate, and vitamins B_6 and B_{12} metabolism
■ To detect acquired folate or cobalamin deficiency
■ To evaluate risk factors for atherosclerotic vascular disease
■ To evaluate contributing factors in the pathogenesis of neural tube defects

Cost

Moderately expensive

Patient preparation

■ Inform the patient that this test detects homocysteine levels in plasma.
■ Advise the patient to fast for 12 to 14 hours before the test.

- Tell the patient that this test requires a blood sample. Explain who will perform the venipuncture and when.
- Explain to the patient that he may experience discomfort from the needle puncture and the tourniquet.

Reference values
Normal total homocysteine levels are less than or equal to 13 μmol/L (SI, ≤ 13 μmol/L).

Abnormal findings
Low homocysteine levels are associated with inborn or acquired folate or cobalamin deficiency and inborn B_6 or B_{12} deficiency, while elevated levels are associated with a higher incidence of atherosclerotic vascular disease. In patients with type 2 diabetes mellitus, studies have shown that homocysteine levels increase with even a modest deterioration in renal function.

Interfering factors
- Failure to adhere to dietary restrictions

Human chorionic gonadotropin, serum

Human chorionic gonadotropin (hCG) is a glycoprotein hormone produced in the placenta. If conception occurs, a specific assay for hCG — commonly called the *beta-subunit assay* — may detect this hormone in the blood 9 days after ovulation. This interval coincides with the implantation of the fertilized ovum into the uterine wall. Although the precise function of hCG is still unclear, it appears that hCG, with progesterone, maintains the corpus luteum during early pregnancy.

Production of hCG increases steadily during the first trimester, peaking around 10 weeks' gestation. Levels then fall to less than 10% of first-trimester peak levels during the remainder of the pregnancy. About 2 weeks after delivery, the hormone may no longer be detectable. (See *Production of hCG during pregnancy,* page 200.)

The serum human chorionic gonadotropin test, a serum immunoassay, is a quantitative analysis of hCG beta-subunit level and is more sensitive (and costlier) than the routine pregnancy test using a urine specimen.

Purpose
- To detect early pregnancy
- To determine adequacy of hormonal production in high-risk pregnancies (for example, habitual abortion)
- To aid diagnosis of trophoblastic tumors, such as hydatidiform moles and choriocarcinoma, and tumors that ectopically secrete hCG
- To monitor treatment for induction of ovulation and conception

Cost
Inexpensive

Patient preparation
- Explain to the patient that this test determines if she's pregnant. If detection of pregnancy isn't the diagnostic objective, offer the appropriate explanation.
- Tell the patient that the test requires a blood sample. Explain who will perform the venipuncture and when.
- Explain to the patient that she may experience discomfort from the needle puncture and the tourniquet.

Reference values
Normally, hCG levels are less than 4 IU/L. During pregnancy, however, hCG levels vary widely, depending partly on the number of days after the last normal menstrual period.

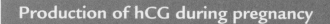
Production of hCG during pregnancy

Production of human chorionic gonadotropin (hCG) increases steadily during the first trimester, peaking around the 10th week of gestation, as shown below. Levels then fall to less than 10% of the first-trimester levels during the remainder of the pregnancy.

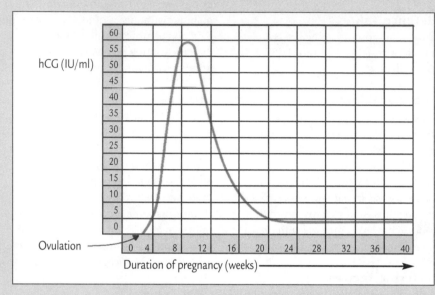

Abnormal findings

Elevated hCG beta-subunit levels indicate pregnancy; significantly higher concentrations are present in a multiple pregnancy. Increased levels may also suggest hydatidiform mole, trophoblastic neoplasms of the placenta, and nontrophoblastic carcinomas that secrete hCG (including gastric, pancreatic, and ovarian adenocarcinomas). Low hCG beta-subunit levels can occur in ectopic pregnancy or pregnancy of less than 9 days. Beta-subunit levels can't differentiate between pregnancy and tumor recurrence because they're high in both conditions.

Interfering factors

■ Heparin anticoagulants and ethylenediaminetetraacetic acid

Human chorionic gonadotropin, urine

Qualitative analysis of urine levels of human chorionic gonadotropin (hCG) allows for the detection of pregnancy as early as 14 days after ovulation. Production of hCG, a glycoprotein, which prevents degeneration of the corpus luteum at the end of the normal menstrual cycle, begins after conception. During the first trimester, hCG levels rise steadily and rapidly, peaking around the 10th week of gestation, subsequently tapering off to less than 10% of peak levels.

The most common method of evaluating hCG in urine is hemagglutination inhibition. This laboratory procedure can provide qualitative and quantitative information. The qualitative urine test is easier and less expensive than the serum hCG test (beta-subunit assay); therefore, it's used more frequently to detect pregnancy.

Purpose
- To detect and confirm pregnancy
- To aid diagnosis of hydatidiform mole or hCG-secreting tumors, threatened abortion, or dead fetus

Cost
Inexpensive

Patient preparation
- If appropriate, explain to the patient that this test determines if she's pregnant or the status of her pregnancy. Alternatively, explain how the test functions as a screen for some types of cancer.
- Tell the patient that she should restrict fluids for 8 hours before the test.
- Inform the patient that the test requires a first-voided morning specimen or urine collection over a 24-hour period, depending on whether the test is qualitative or quantitative.
- Restrict medications that may affect test results. If they must be continued, note this on the laboratory request.

Normal findings
In a qualitative immunoassay analysis, results are reported as negative (nonpregnant) or positive (pregnant) for hCG. In quantitative analysis, urine hCG levels in the first trimester of a normal pregnancy may be as high as 500,000 IU/24 hours; in the second trimester, they range from 10,000 to 25,000 IU/24 hours; and in the third trimester, from 5,000 to 15,000 IU/24 hours.

Measurable hCG levels don't normally appear in the urine of men or nonpregnant women.

Abnormal findings
During pregnancy, elevated urine hCG levels may indicate multiple pregnancy or erythroblastosis fetalis; depressed urine hCG levels may indicate threatened abortion or ectopic pregnancy.

Measurable levels of hCG in males and nonpregnant females may indicate choriocarcinoma, ovarian or testicular tumors, melanoma, multiple myeloma, or gastric, hepatic, pancreatic, or breast cancer.

Interfering factors
- Gross proteinuria (greater than 1 g/24 hours), hematuria, or an elevated erythrocyte sedimentation rate (possible false-positive, depending on the laboratory method)
- Early pregnancy, ectopic pregnancy, or threatened abortion (possible false-negative)
- Phenothiazine (possible false-negative or false-positive)

Human immunodeficiency virus antibodies

The human immunodeficiency virus (HIV) antibodies test detects antibodies to HIV in serum. HIV is the virus that causes acquired immunodeficiency syndrome (AIDS). Transmission occurs by direct exposure of a person's blood to body fluids containing the virus. The virus may be transmitted from one person to another through exchange of contaminated blood and blood products, during sexual intercourse with an infected partner, when I.V. drugs are shared, and from an infected mother to her child during pregnancy or breast-feeding.

Initial identification of HIV is usually achieved through enzyme-linked immunosorbent assay. Positive findings are confirmed by Western blot test and immunofluorescence or other tests available, which may be performed to detect antibodies.

Purpose
■ To screen for HIV in high-risk patients
■ To screen donated blood for HIV

Cost
Moderately expensive

Patient preparation
■ Explain to the patient that this test detects HIV infection.
■ Provide adequate counseling about the reasons for performing the test.
■ Tell the patient that the test requires a blood sample. Explain who will perform the venipuncture and when.
■ Explain to the patient that he may experience discomfort from the needle puncture and the tourniquet.

Normal findings
Test results are normally negative for HIV antibodies.

Abnormal findings
The test detects previous exposure to the virus. However, it doesn't identify patients who have been exposed to the virus but haven't yet made antibodies. Most patients with AIDS have antibodies to HIV. A positive test for the HIV antibody can't determine whether a patient harbors actively replicating virus or when the patient will manifest signs and symptoms of AIDS.

Many apparently healthy people have been exposed to HIV and have circulating

antibodies. The test results for such people aren't false-positives. Furthermore, patients in the later stages of AIDS may exhibit no detectable antibody in their sera because they can no longer mount an antibody response.

Interfering factors
■ None known

Human leukocyte antigen

The human leukocyte antigen (HLA) test identifies a group of antigens present on the surface of all nucleated cells but most easily detected on lymphocytes. There are four types of HLA: HLA-A, HLA-B, HLA-C, and HLA-D. These antigens are essential to immunity and determine the degree of histocompatibility between transplant recipients and donors. Numerous antigenic determinants (more than 60, for instance, at the HLA-B locus) are present for each site; one set of each antigen is inherited from each parent.

A high incidence of specific HLA types has been linked to specific diseases, such as rheumatoid arthritis and multiple sclerosis, but these findings have little diagnostic significance.

Purpose
■ To provide histocompatibility typing of transplant recipients and donors
■ To aid genetic counseling or paternity testing

Cost
Moderately expensive

Patient preparation
■ Explain to the patient that this test detects antigens on white blood cells.

- Tell the patient that the test requires a blood sample. Explain who will perform the venipuncture and when.
- Explain to the patient that he may experience discomfort from the needle puncture and the tourniquet.
- Check the patient's history for recent blood transfusions. HLA testing may need to be postponed if he has recently undergone a transfusion.

Normal findings

In HLA-A, HLA-B, and HLA-C testing, lymphocytes that react with the test antiserum undergo lysis; they're detected by phase microscopy. In HLA-D testing, leukocyte incompatibility is marked by blast formation, deoxyribonucleic acid synthesis, and proliferation.

Abnormal findings

Incompatible HLA-A, HLA-B, HLA-C, and HLA-D groups may cause unsuccessful tissue transplantation.

Many diseases have a strong association with certain types of HLAs. For example, HLA-DR5 is associated with Hashimoto's thyroiditis. HLA-B8 and HLA-Dw3 are associated with Graves' disease, whereas HLA-B8 alone is associated with chronic autoimmune hepatitis, celiac disease, and myasthenia gravis. HLA-Dw3 alone is associated with Addison's disease, Sjögren's syndrome, dermatitis herpetiformis, and systemic lupus erythematosus.

In paternity testing, a putative father who presents a phenotype (two haplotypes: one from the father and one from the mother) with no haplotype or antigen pair identical to one of the child's is excluded as the father. A putative father with one haplotype identical to one of the child's may be the father; the probability varies with the incidence of the haplotype in the population.

Interfering factors

- HLA from blood transfusion within 72 hours before sample collection

Hypersensitivity skin tests, delayed

Skin testing is one of the most important methods for evaluating the cell-mediated immune response in a patient with severe recurrent infection, infection caused by unusual organisms, or suspected disorders associated with delayed hypersensitivity. Because diminished delayed hypersensitivity may be associated with a poor prognosis in patients with certain types of cancer, this test may also be useful in determining the prognosis in such patients. A positive test reaction shows that the afferent, central, and efferent limbs of the immune response are intact and that the patient can maintain a nonspecific inflammatory response to infection.

These skin tests use new and recall antigens. New antigens, those not previously encountered by the patient, such as dinitrochlorobenzene (DNCB), evaluate the patient's primary immune response when a sensitizing dose is given, followed by a challenge dose. Recall antigens, those to which a patient has had or may have had previous exposure or sensitization, evaluate the secondary immune response; these antigens include candidin, trichophyton, streptokinase-streptodornase, purified protein derivative, staphage lysate, mumps, and mixed respiratory vaccine among others. The specific antigens chosen for this test are those to which exposure is common and which will usually provoke an immune response. In these tests, a small amount of antigen (or group of antigens) is injected intradermally or applied topically, and the test site is later examined for a

Administering test antigens

The illustration below shows the arm of a patient who is undergoing a recall antigen test, which determines whether he has previously been exposed to certain antigens. A sample panel of six test antigens has been injected into his forearm, and the test site has been marked and labeled for each antigen.

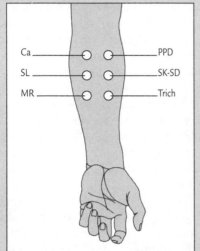

Ca — PPD
SL — SK-SD
MR — Trich

KEY:
Ca = Candidin
SL = Staphage lysate
MR = Mixed respiratory vaccine
PPD = Purified protein derivative
SK-SD = Streptokinase-streptodornase
Trich = *Trichophyton*

visible reaction. (See *Administering test antigens.*)

Another type of skin test, the patch test, is used to confirm allergic contact sensitization and to determine its cause.

AGE ISSUE ✻ ✻ ✻ ✻ ✻
Skin tests have limited value in infants because their immune systems are immature and inadequately sensitized.

Purpose
- To evaluate primary and secondary immune responses
- To assess effectiveness of immunotherapy, when the patient's immune response is augmented by adjuvants (such as bacille Calmette-Guérin [BCG] vaccine) or other means (transfer factor, levamisole).
- To diagnose fungal diseases (coccidioidomycosis, histoplasmosis), bacterial diseases (tuberculosis, brucellosis, leprosy), and viral diseases (infectious mononucleosis)
- To monitor the course of certain diseases, such as Hodgkin's disease and coccidioidomycosis

Cost
Moderately expensive

Patient preparation
- Explain to the patient that this test evaluates the immune system after application or injection of small doses of antigens.
- Tell the patient who will perform the test and where it will take place. Explain that some antigens (such as DNCB) are administered again after 2 weeks and, if the test is negative, a stronger dose of antigen may be given.
- Check the patient's history for hypersensitivity to any of the test antigens; verify if he's had a skin test previously and, if so, what his reactions were.
- Check for a history of tuberculosis or previous BCG vaccination.
- Instruct the patient to avoid washing off any marked circles on his skin until the test is completed.

Normal findings

In the DNCB test, a positive reaction (erythema, edema, induration) appears 48 to 96 hours after the second (challenge) dose; 95% of the population reacts positively to DNCB. In the recall antigen test, a positive response (5 mm or more of induration at the test site) appears 48 hours after injection.

Abnormal findings

In the DNCB test, failure to react to the challenge dose indicates diminished delayed hypersensitivity. In the recall antigen test, a positive response to less than two of the six test antigens, persistent unresponsiveness to intradermal injection of higher-strength antigens, or a generalized diminished reaction (causing less than 10 mm combined induration) indicates diminished delayed hypersensitivity.

Diminished delayed hypersensitivity can result from Hodgkin's disease (common); sarcoidosis; liver disease; congenital immunodeficiency disease, such as ataxia-telangiectasia, DiGeorge syndrome, and Wiskott-Aldrich syndrome; uremia; acute leukemia; viral diseases, such as influenza, infectious mononucleosis, measles, mumps, and rubella; fungal diseases, such as coccidioidomycosis and cryptococcosis; bacterial diseases, such as leprosy and tuberculosis; and terminal cancer. Diminished delayed hypersensitivity can also result from immunosuppressive or steroid therapy or viral vaccination.

Interfering factors

- Use of antigens that have expired or that have been exposed to heat and light or to bacterial contamination
- Hormonal contraceptives (possible false-negative)
- Strong immediate reaction to the antigen at the injection site (possible false-negative)
- Poor injection technique (possible false-negative)
- Inaccurate dilution of antigens
- Error in reading or timing test results

I J

Immune complex

When immune complexes are produced faster than they can be cleared by the lymphoreticular system, an immune complex disease, such as postinfectious syndromes, serum sickness, drug sensitivity, rheumatoid arthritis, and systemic lupus erythematosus (SLE), may occur.

Histologic examination of tissue obtained by biopsy and the use of fluorescence or peroxidase staining with antibodies specific for immunologic types generally detect immune complexes. However, tissue biopsies can't provide information about titers of complexes still in circulation; therefore, serum assays, which detect circulating immune complexes indirectly, may be required. Because of the inherent variability of these complexes, several serum test methods may be appropriate.

Most immune complex assays haven't been standardized, so more than one test may be required to achieve accurate results.

Purpose
- To demonstrate circulating immune complexes in serum
- To monitor response to therapy
- To estimate severity of disease

Cost
Moderately expensive

Patient preparation
- Explain to the patient that these tests help evaluate his immune system.
- If appropriate, tell the patient that the test will be repeated to monitor his response to therapy.
- Advise the patient that he need not restrict food or fluids before the test.
- Tell him that the test requires a blood sample. Explain who will perform the venipuncture and when.
- Tell the patient that he may experience discomfort from the needle puncture and the tourniquet.
- If the patient is scheduled for C1q assay (a component of C1), document his history of recent heparin therapy.

Normal findings
Normally, immune complexes aren't detectable in serum.

Abnormal findings
The presence of detectable immune complexes in serum has etiologic importance in many autoimmune diseases, such as SLE and rheumatoid arthritis. For definitive di-

agnosis, the presence of these complexes must be considered with the results of other studies. For example, in SLE, immune complexes are associated with high titers of antinuclear antibodies and circulating antinative deoxyribonucleic acid antibodies.

Because of their filtering function, renal glomeruli seem most vulnerable to immune complex deposition, although blood vessel walls and choroid plexuses (vascular folds in the ventricles of the brain) can be affected. Renal biopsy to detect immune complexes can provide conclusive evidence for immune complex (type III) glomerulonephritis, differentiating it from other types of glomerulonephritis.

Interfering factors
■ Failure to send the sample to the laboratory immediately
■ Presence of cryoglobulins in the serum
■ Inability to standardize rheumatoid factor inhibition tests and platelet aggregation assays

Immunoglobulins G, A, and M

Immunoglobulins, proteins that can function as specific antibodies in response to antigen stimulation, are responsible for the humoral aspects of immunity. They're classified into five groups — immunoglobulin (Ig) G, IgA, IgM, IgD, and IgE — that are normally present in serum in predictable percentages. Deviations from normal percentages are characteristic in many immune disorders, including cancer, hepatic disorders, rheumatoid arthritis, and systemic lupus erythematosus.

Immunoelectrophoresis identifies IgG, IgA, and IgM in a serum sample. The level of each is measured by radial immunodiffusion or nephelometry. Some laboratories detect immunoglobulin by indirect immunofluorescence and radioimmunoassay.

Purpose
■ To diagnose paraproteinemias, such as multiple myeloma and Waldenström's macroglobulinemia
■ To detect hypogammaglobulinemia and hypergammaglobulinemia as well as nonimmunologic diseases, such as cirrhosis and hepatitis, that are associated with abnormally high immunoglobulin levels
■ To assess the effectiveness of chemotherapy and radiation therapy

Cost
Expensive

Patient preparation
■ Explain to the patient that this test measures antibody levels.
■ If appropriate, tell the patient that the test evaluates the effectiveness of treatment.
■ Instruct the patient to restrict food and fluids, except for water, for 12 to 14 hours before the test.
■ Tell the patient that the test requires a blood sample. Explain who will perform the venipuncture and when.
■ Explain to the patient that he may experience discomfort from the needle puncture and the tourniquet.
■ Check the patient's history for drugs that may affect test results, including alcohol or narcotic abuse.

Reference values
When using nephelometry, serum immunoglobulin levels for adults range as follows:
■ *IgG:* 800 to 1800 mg/dl (SI, 8 to 18 g/L)
■ *IgA:* 100 to 400 mg/dl (SI, 1 to 4 g/L)
■ *IgM:* 55 to 150 mg/dl (SI, 0.55 to 1.5 g/L).

Serum immunoglobulin levels in various disorders

DISORDER	IgG	IgA	IgM
Immunoglobulin disorders			
Lymphoid aplasia	D	D	D
Agammaglobulinemia	D	D	D
Type I dysgammaglobulinemia (selective immunoglobulin [Ig] G and IgA deficiency)	D	D	N or I
Type II dysgammaglobulinemia (absent IgA and IgM)	N	D	D
IgA globulinemia	N	D	N
Ataxia-telangiectasia	N	D	N
Multiple myeloma, macroglobulinemia, lymphomas			
Heavy chain disease (Franklin's disease)	D	D	D
IgG myeloma	I	D	D
IgA myeloma	D	I	D
Macroglobulinemia	D	D	I
Acute lymphocytic leukemia	N	D	N
Chronic lymphocytic leukemia	D	D	D
Acute myelocytic leukemia	N	N	N
Chronic myelocytic leukemia	N	D	N
Hodgkin's disease	N	N	N
Hepatic disorders			
Hepatitis	I	I	I
Laënnec's cirrhosis	I	I	N
Biliary cirrhosis	N	N	I
Hepatoma	N	N	D
Rheumatoid arthritis	I	I	I

Serum immunoglobulin levels in various disorders *(continued)*

DISORDER	IgG	IgA	IgM
Other disorders			
Systemic lupus erythematosus	I	I	I
Nephrotic syndrome	D	D	N
Trypanosomiasis	N	N	I
Pulmonary tuberculosis	I	N	N

KEY: N = Normal; I = Increased; D = Decreased

Abnormal findings

The accompanying chart shows IgG, IgA, and IgM levels in various disorders. (See *Serum immunoglobulin levels in various disorders.*) In congenital and acquired hypogammaglobulinemias, myelomas, and macroglobulinemia, the findings confirm the diagnosis. In hepatic and autoimmune diseases, leukemias, and lymphomas, such findings are less important, but they can support the diagnosis based on other tests, such as biopsies and white blood cell differential, and on the physical examination.

Interfering factors

■ Chemotherapy or radiation therapy (possible decrease due to suppressive effects on bone marrow)
■ Anticonvulsants, asparaginase, hormonal contraceptives, hydantoin derivatives, and hydralazine (possible increase)
■ Methotrexate and severe hypersensitivity to bacille Calmette-Guérin vaccine (possible decrease)
■ Dextrans and methylprednisolone (decrease in IgM levels)

■ Dextrans and high doses of methylprednisolone and phenytoin (decrease in IgG and IgA levels)
■ Methadone (increase in IgA levels)

Insulin, serum

The serum insulin test, a radioimmunoassay, is a quantitative analysis of serum insulin levels. Insulin is usually measured concomitantly with glucose levels because glucose is the primary stimulus for insulin release.

Insulin regulates the metabolism and transport or mobilization of carbohydrates, amino acids, proteins, and lipids. Stimulated by increased plasma levels of glucose, insulin secretion reaches peak levels after meals, when metabolism and food storage are greatest.

Purpose

■ To aid diagnosis of hyperinsulinemia as well as hypoglycemia resulting from a tumor or hyperplasia of pancreatic islet cells, glucocorticoid deficiency, or severe hepatic disease

- To aid diagnosis of diabetes mellitus and insulin-resistant states

Cost
Moderately expensive

Patient preparation
- Explain to the patient that this test helps determine if the pancreas is functioning normally.
- Inform the patient that the test requires blood samples. Tell him who will perform the venipunctures and when.
- Explain that he may experience discomfort from the needle puncture and the tourniquet.
- Instruct the patient to fast for 10 to 12 hours before the test.
- Explain that questionable results may require a repeat test or a simultaneous glucose tolerance test, which requires that the patient drink a glucose solution.
- Restrict corticotropin, corticosteroids (including hormonal contraceptives), thyroid supplements, epinephrine, and other medications that may interfere with test results. If they must be continued, note this on the laboratory request.

Reference values
Serum insulin levels normally range from 0 to 35 μU/ml (SI, 144 to 243 pmol/L).

Abnormal findings
Insulin levels are interpreted in light of the prevailing glucose concentration. A normal insulin level may be inappropriate for the glucose results. High insulin and low glucose levels after a significant fast suggest the presence of an insulinoma. Prolonged fasting or stimulation testing may be required to confirm the diagnosis. In insulin-resistant diabetes mellitus, insulin levels are elevated; in non-insulin-resistant diabetes, they're low.

Interfering factors
- Failure to observe pretest restrictions
- Agitation and stress
- Hemolysis due to rough handling of the sample
- Failure to pack the insulin sample in ice
- Failure to send the sample to the laboratory promptly
- Corticosteroids (including hormonal contraceptives), corticotropin, epinephrine, and thyroid hormones (possible increase)
- Use of insulin by non-insulin-dependent patients (possible increase)
- High levels of insulin antibodies in patients with insulin-dependent diabetes mellitus

Insulin tolerance

The insulin tolerance test measures serum levels of human growth hormone (hGH) and corticotropin after administration of a loading dose of insulin and is more reliable than direct measurement of hGH and corticotropin. Insulin-induced hypoglycemia stimulates hGH and corticotropin secretion. Failure of stimulation indicates anterior pituitary or adrenal hypofunction and helps confirm an hGH or a corticotropin insufficiency.

Purpose
- To aid diagnosis of hGH and corticotropin deficiency
- To identify pituitary dysfunction
- To aid differential diagnosis of primary and secondary adrenal hypofunction

Cost
Inexpensive

Patient preparation

■ Explain to the patient, or to his parents if the patient is a child, that this test evaluates hormonal secretion.

■ Instruct the patient to fast and restrict physical activity for 10 to 12 hours before the test.

■ Explain to the patient that the test involves I.V. infusion of insulin and the collection of multiple blood samples. Tell the patient who will perform the venipunctures and when.

■ Explain to the patient that he may experience discomfort from the needle punctures and the tourniquet.

■ Warn the patient that he may experience an increased heart rate, diaphoresis, hunger, and anxiety after administration of insulin. Reassure him that these symptoms are transient, and that if they become severe, the test will be discontinued.

■ Tell the patient to lie down and relax for 90 minutes before the test.

Reference values

Normally, blood glucose falls to 50% of the fasting level 20 to 30 minutes after insulin administration. This stimulates a 10- to 20-ng/dl (SI, 10 to 20 µg/L) increase in baseline serum values for hGH and corticotropin, with peak levels occurring 60 to 90 minutes after insulin administration.

Abnormal findings

Failure of stimulation or a blunted response suggests dysfunction of the hypothalamic-pituitary-adrenal axis. An increase in serum hGH levels of less than 10 ng/dl (SI, < 10 µg/L) above baseline suggests hGH deficiency. A definitive diagnosis of hGH deficiency requires a supplementary stimulation test such as the arginine test. Additional testing is necessary to determine the site of the abnormality.

An increase in serum corticotropin levels of less than 10 ng/dl (SI, < 10 µg/L) above baseline suggests adrenal insufficiency. The metyrapone or corticotropin stimulation test then confirms the diagnosis and determines whether the insufficiency is primary or secondary.

Interfering factors

■ Failure to observe pretest restrictions of diet, medications, and physical activity

■ Hemolysis due to rough handling of the sample

■ Corticosteroids and pituitary-based drugs (increase in hGH)

■ Beta-adrenergic blockers and glucocorticoids (decrease in hGH)

■ Amphetamines, calcium gluconate, estrogens, ethanol, glucocorticoids, methamphetamines, and spironolactone (decrease in corticotropin)

Intracranial computed tomography

Intracranial computed tomography (CT) provides a series of tomograms, translated by a computer and displayed on a monitor, representing cross-sectional images of various layers of the brain. This technique can reconstruct cross-sectional, horizontal, sagittal, and coronal plane images. Hundreds of thousands of readings of radiation levels absorbed by brain tissues may be combined to depict anatomic slices of varying thickness. Specificity and accuracy are enhanced by the degree of radiation, which depends on the number of radiation density calculations made by the computer. Although magnetic resonance imaging (MRI) has surpassed CT scanning in diagnosing neurologic anatomy and pathology, the CT scan is more widely available and cost-effective and can be performed more easily in acute situations.

ALERT! ▼ ▼ ▼ ▼ ▼ ▼ ▼ ▼ ▼
Intracranial CT scanning with contrast enhancement is contraindicated in persons who are hypersensitive to iodine or contrast medium.

Purpose
■ To diagnose intracranial lesions and abnormalities
■ To monitor the effects of surgery, radiation therapy, or chemotherapy on intracranial tumors
■ To serve as a guide for cranial surgery

Cost
Very expensive

Patient preparation
■ Explain to the patient that this test permits assessment of the brain.
■ If contrast enhancement is scheduled, instruct the patient to fast for 4 hours before the test.
■ Tell the patient that a series of X-ray films will be taken of his brain. Explain who will perform the test and where it will take place.
■ Explain to the patient that there will be minimal discomfort.
■ Tell the patient that he'll be positioned on a moving CT bed, with his head immobilized and his face uncovered. The head of the table will then be moved into the scanner, which rotates around his head and makes loud clacking sounds.
■ If a contrast medium is to be used, tell the patient that he may feel flushed and warm and may experience a transient headache, a salty or metallic taste, or nausea and vomiting after the contrast medium is injected.
■ Tell the patient that if he's restless or apprehensive, a sedative may be prescribed.

■ Check the patient's history for hypersensitivity to shellfish, iodine, or contrast media as prophylactic medications may be needed.

AGE ISSUE ✳ ✳ ✳ ✳ ✳
Iodine or contrast medium may be harmful or fatal to a fetus, especially during the first trimester.

Normal findings
The density of tissue determines the amount of radiation that passes through it. Tissue densities appear as white, black, or shades of gray on the computed image obtained by intracranial CT scanning. Bone, the densest tissue, appears white; ventricular and subarachnoid cerebrospinal fluid, the least dense, appears black. Brain matter appears in shades of gray. Structures are evaluated according to their density, size, shape, and position.

Abnormal findings
Areas of altered density (they may be lighter or darker) or displaced vasculature or other structures may indicate intracranial tumor, hematoma, cerebral atrophy, infarction, edema, or congenital anomalies, such as hydrocephalus.

Intracranial tumors vary significantly in appearance and characteristics. Metastatic tumors generally cause extensive edema in early stages and can usually be defined by contrast enhancement. Primary tumors vary in density and in their capacity to cause edema, displace ventricles, and absorb contrast medium in contrast enhancement. Astrocytomas, for example, usually have low densities; meningiomas have higher densities and can generally be defined with contrast enhancement; glioblastomas, usually ill-defined, are also enhanced after injection of a contrast medium.

Because the high density of blood contrasts markedly with low-density brain tissue, it's normally easy to detect both subdural and epidural hematomas and other acute hemorrhages. Contrast enhancement helps locate subdural hematomas.

Cerebral atrophy customarily appears as enlarged ventricles with large sulci. Cerebral infarction may appear as low-density areas at the obstruction site or may not be apparent, especially within the first 24 hours if the infarction is small or doesn't cause edema. With contrast enhancement, the infarcted area may not show in the acute phase but will show clearly after resolution of the lesion. Cerebral edema usually appears as an area of marked generalized decreased density. In children, enlargement of the fourth ventricle generally indicates hydrocephalus.

Normally, the cerebral vessels don't appear on CT images. However, in patients with arteriovenous malformation, cerebral vessels may appear with slightly increased density. Contrast enhancement allows a better view of the abnormal area, but MRI is now the preferred procedure for imaging cerebral vessels.

Interfering factors
- Patient's head movement (possible poor imaging)
- Hemorrhage (possible false-negative)

Iron and total iron-binding capacity

Iron is essential to the formation and function of hemoglobin, as well as many other heme and nonheme compounds. After the intestine absorbs it, iron is distributed to various body compartments for synthesis, storage, and transport. Serum iron concentration is normally highest in the morning and declines progressively during the day, therefore, the sample should be drawn in the morning.

An iron assay is used to measure the amount of iron bound to transferrin in blood plasma. Total iron-binding capacity (TIBC) measures the amount of iron that would appear in plasma if all the transferrin were saturated with iron.

Serum iron and TIBC are of greater diagnostic usefulness when performed with the serum ferritin assay but, together, these tests may not accurately reflect the state of other iron compartments, such as myoglobin iron and the labile iron pool. Bone marrow or liver biopsy and iron absorption or excretion studies may yield more information.

Purpose
- To estimate total iron storage
- To aid diagnosis of hemochromatosis
- To help distinguish iron deficiency anemia from anemia of chronic disease (For information on another test used to differentiate anemias, see *Siderocyte stain*, page 214.)
- To help evaluate nutritional status

Cost
Inexpensive

Patient preparation
- Explain to the patient that this test evaluates the body's capacity to store iron.
- Tell the patient that the test requires a blood sample. Explain who will perform the venipuncture and when.
- Explain to the patient that he may experience discomfort from the needle puncture and the tourniquet.
- Restrict medications that may affect test results. If they must be continued, note this on the laboratory request.

Siderocyte stain

Siderocytes are red blood cells (RBCs) containing particles of nonhemoglobin iron known as *siderocytic granules.* In neonates, siderocytic granules are normally present in normoblasts and reticulocytes during hemoglobin synthesis. However, the spleen removes most of these granules from normal RBCs, and they disappear rapidly with age.

In adults, an elevated siderocyte level usually indicates abnormal erythropoiesis, which may occur in congenital spherocytic anemia, chronic hemolytic anemias (such as the thalassemias), pernicious anemia, hemochromatosis, toxicities (such as lead poisoning), infection, or severe burns. Elevated levels may also follow splenectomy because the spleen normally removes siderocytic granules.

Performing the test
The siderocyte stain test measures the number of circulating siderocytes. Venous blood is drawn into a 7-ml lavender-top tube or, for infants and children, collected in a Microtainer or a pipette and smeared directly on a 3″ × 1″ (7.5 × 2.5 cm) glass slide. When the blood smear is stained, siderocytic granules appear as purple-blue specks clustered around the periphery of mature erythrocytes. Cells containing these granules are counted as a percentage of total RBCs. The results aid differential diagnosis of the anemias and hemochromatosis and help detect toxicities.

Interpreting results
Normally, neonates have a slightly elevated siderocyte level that reaches the normal adult value of 0.5% of total RBCs in 7 to 10 days. In patients with pernicious anemia, the siderocyte level is 8% to 14%; in chronic hemolytic anemia, 20% to 100%; in lead poisoning, 10% to 30%; and in hemochromatosis, 3% to 7%. A high siderocyte level calls for additional testing (including bone marrow examination) to determine the cause of abnormal erythropoiesis.

Reference values
Normal serum iron values are as follows:
- *Males:* 60 to 170 µg/dl (SI, 10.7 to 30.4 µmol/L)
- *Females:* 50 to 130 µg/dl (SI, 9 to 23.3 µmol/L)

Normal TIBC values are 300 to 360 µg/dl (SI, 54 to 64 µmol/L) for males and females, and normal saturation is 20% to 50% (SI, 0.2 to 0.5) for males and females.

Abnormal findings
In iron deficiency, serum iron levels decrease and TIBC increases, decreasing saturation. In cases of chronic inflammation (such as in rheumatoid arthritis), serum iron may be low in the presence of adequate body stores, but TIBC may remain unchanged or may decrease to preserve normal saturation. Iron overload may not alter serum levels until relatively late but, in general, serum iron increases and TIBC remains the same, which increases the saturation.

Interfering factors
- Hemolysis due to rough handling of the sample
- Failure to send the sample to the laboratory immediately
- Chloramphenicol and hormonal contraceptives (possible false-positive)
- Corticotropin (possible false-negative)
- Iron supplements (possible false-positive serum iron values but false-negative TIBC)

K

Ketone

In the ketone test, a routine, semiquantitative screening test, a commercially prepared product is used to measure the urine level of ketone bodies. Ketone bodies are the by-products of fat metabolism; they include acetoacetic acid, acetone, and beta-hydroxybutyric acid. Excessive amounts may appear in patients with carbohydrate dehydration, which may occur in starvation or diabetic ketoacidosis (DKA).

Commercially available tests include the Acetest tablet, Chemstrip K, Ketostix, or Keto-Diastix. Each product measures a specific ketone body. For example, Acetest measures acetone and Ketostix measures acetoacetic acid.

Purpose
- To screen for ketonuria
- To identify DKA and carbohydrate deprivation
- To distinguish between a diabetic and a nondiabetic coma
- To monitor control of diabetes mellitus, ketogenic weight reduction, and treatment of DKA

Cost
Inexpensive

Patient preparation
- Explain to the patient that this test evaluates fat metabolism.
- If the patient is taking levodopa or phenazopyridine or has recently received sulfobromophthalein, Acetest tablets must be used because reagent strips may produce inaccurate results.
- Tell the patient that a urine specimen will be required.

Normal findings
Normally, no ketones are present in urine.

Abnormal findings
Ketonuria may occur in uncontrolled diabetes mellitus or starvation. It also occurs as a metabolic complication of total parenteral nutrition.

Interfering factors
- Failure to keep the reagent container tightly closed to prevent absorption of light or moisture or bacterial contamination of the specimen (false-negative)
- Levodopa, phenazopyridine, and sulfobromophthalein (false-positive results

when Ketostix or Keto-Diastix is used instead of Acetest)

Kidney-ureter-bladder radiography

Usually the first step in diagnostic testing of the urinary system, kidney-ureter-bladder (KUB) radiography surveys the abdomen to determine the position of the kidneys, ureters, and bladder, and to detect gross abnormalities.

This test doesn't require intact renal function and may aid differential diagnosis of urologic and gastrointestinal diseases, which often produce similar signs and symptoms. However, KUB radiography has many limitations and nearly always must be followed by more elaborate tests, such as excretory urography or renal computed tomography. KUB radiography shouldn't follow recent instillation of barium.

Purpose
■ To evaluate the size, structure, and position of the kidneys
■ To screen for abnormalities, such as calcifications, in the region of the kidneys, ureters, and bladder

Cost
Expensive

Patient preparation
■ Explain to the patient that this test is an X-ray and helps detect urinary system abnormalities.
■ Tell the patient who will perform the test, where it will take place, and that it will only take a few minutes.

Normal findings
The shadows of the kidneys appear bilaterally, the right slightly lower than the left. Both kidneys should be approximately the same size, with the superior poles tilted slightly toward the vertebral column, paralleling the shadows (or stripes) produced by the psoas muscles. The ureters are only visible when an abnormality such as calcification is present. Visualization of the bladder depends on the density of its muscular wall and on the amount of urine in it. Generally, the bladder's shadow can be seen but not as clearly as the kidneys' shadows.

Abnormal findings
Bilateral renal enlargement may result from polycystic disease, multiple myeloma, lymphoma, amyloidosis, diabetes, hydronephrosis, or compensatory hypertrophy. Tumor, cyst, or hydronephrosis may cause unilateral enlargement. Abnormally small kidneys may suggest end-stage glomerulonephritis or bilateral atrophic pyelonephritis. An apparent decrease in the size of one kidney suggests possible congenital hypoplasia, atrophic pyelonephritis, or ischemia. Renal displacement may be due to a retroperitoneal tumor, such as an adrenal tumor. Obliteration or bulging of a portion of the psoas muscle stripe may result from tumor, abscess, or hematoma.

Congenital anomalies, such as abnormal location or absence of a kidney, may be detected. Renal axes that parallel the vertebral column may suggest horseshoe kidney, especially if the inferior poles of the kidneys can't be clearly distinguished. A lobulated edge or border may suggest polycystic kidney disease or patchy atrophic pyelonephritis.

Opaque bodies may reflect calculi or vascular calcification due to aneurysm or atheroma; opacification may also suggest cystic tumors, fecaliths, foreign bodies, or abnormal fluid collection. Calcifications may appear anywhere in the urinary system, but positive identification requires further testing. The lone exception is staghorn calculus, which forms a perfect cast of the renal pelvis and calyces.

Interfering factors

■ Gas, stool, contrast medium, or foreign bodies in the intestine (possible poor imaging)
■ Calcified uterine fibromas or ovarian lesions
■ Obesity or ascites (possible poor imaging)

L

Lactate dehydrogenase isoenzymes

Lactate dehydrogenase (LD) catalyzes the reversible conversion of muscle lactic acid into pyruvic acid, an essential step in the metabolic processes that ultimately produce cellular energy. Because LD is present in almost all body tissues and cellular damage increases total LD levels, the diagnostic usefulness of LD is limited.

Five tissue-specific isoenzymes can be identified and measured: LD_1 and LD_2 appear primarily in the heart, red blood cells, and kidneys; LD_3 is primarily in the lungs; and LD_4 and LD_5 are in the liver, skin, and the skeletal muscles.

Purpose

- To aid in the differential diagnosis of a myocardial infarction (MI), pulmonary infarction, anemia, or liver disease
- To support creatine kinase (CK) isoenzyme test results in diagnosing an MI, or to provide diagnosis when CK-MB samples are drawn too late to show an increase
- To monitor patient response to some forms of chemotherapy

Cost

Inexpensive

Patient preparation

- Explain to the patient that this test is used primarily to detect tissue alterations.
- Tell the patient that the test requires a blood sample. Explain who will perform the venipuncture and when.
- Explain to the patient that he may experience discomfort from the needle puncture and the tourniquet.
- If an MI is suspected, tell the patient that the test will be repeated on the next two mornings to monitor progressive changes.

Reference values

Total LD levels normally range from 71 to 207 U/L (SI, 1.2 to 3.52 µkat/L). Normal distribution is as follows:
- LD_1: 14% to 26% (SI, 0.14 to 0.26) of the total
- LD_2: 29% to 39% (SI, 0.29 to 0.39) of the total
- LD_3: 20% to 26% (SI, 0.20 to 0.26) of the total
- LD_4: 8% to 16% (SI, 0.08 to 0.16) of the total
- LD_5: 6% to 16% (SI, 0.06 to 0.16) of the total.

LD isoenzyme variations in disease

DISEASE	LD$_1$	LD$_2$	LD$_3$	LD$_4$	LD$_5$
Cardiovascular					
Myocardial infarction (MI)	Diagnostic	Diagnostic	Not diagnostic	Not diagnostic	Not diagnostic
MI with hepatic congestion	Diagnostic	Diagnostic	Not diagnostic	Not diagnostic	Diagnostic
Rheumatic carditis	Diagnostic	Diagnostic	Not diagnostic	Not diagnostic	Not diagnostic
Myocarditis	Diagnostic	Diagnostic	Not diagnostic	Not diagnostic	Not diagnostic
Heart failure (decompensated)	Not diagnostic	Not diagnostic	Not diagnostic	Not diagnostic	Diagnostic
Shock	Diagnostic	Diagnostic	Diagnostic	Diagnostic	Not diagnostic
Angina pectoris	Normal	Not diagnostic	Not diagnostic	Not diagnostic	Not diagnostic
Pulmonary					
Pulmonary embolism	Normal	Not diagnostic	Not diagnostic	Not diagnostic	Not diagnostic
Pulmonary infarction	Not diagnostic	Not diagnostic	Diagnostic	Not diagnostic	Not diagnostic
Hematologic					
Pernicious anemia	Diagnostic	Diagnostic	Not diagnostic	Not diagnostic	Not diagnostic
Hemolytic anemia	Diagnostic	Diagnostic	Not diagnostic	Not diagnostic	Not diagnostic
Sickle cell anemia	Diagnostic	Diagnostic	Not diagnostic	Not diagnostic	Not diagnostic
Hepatobiliary					
Hepatitis	Not diagnostic	Not diagnostic	Not diagnostic	Not diagnostic	Diagnostic
Active cirrhosis	Not diagnostic	Not diagnostic	Not diagnostic	Not diagnostic	Diagnostic
Hepatic congestion	Not diagnostic	Not diagnostic	Not diagnostic	Not diagnostic	Diagnostic

Legend: Normal | Diagnostic | Not diagnostic

Abnormal findings

Isoenzyme electrophoresis is usually necessary for diagnosis because many common diseases increase total LD levels. With some disorders, total LD levels may be within normal limits, but abnormal proportions of each enzyme indicate specific organ tissue damage. (See *LD isoenzyme variations in disease*, page 219.)

For instance, with an acute MI, LD_1 levels are higher than LD_2 levels within 12 to 48 hours after the onset of symptoms; therefore, the LD_1-LD_2 ratio is greater than 1. This reversal of normal isoenzyme pattern is typical of myocardial damage and is known as flipped LD.

Midzone fractions (LD_2, LD_3, LD_4) may increase with granulocytic leukemia, lymphomas, and platelet disorders.

Interfering factors

■ For diagnosis of an acute MI, failure to draw the sample on schedule
■ Recent surgery or pregnancy (possible increase)
■ Prosthetic heart valve (possible increase due to chronic hemolysis)
■ Alcohol, anabolic steroids, anesthetics, narcotics, and procainamide (increase)

Lactose tolerance, oral

The oral lactose tolerance test is used to measure plasma glucose levels after ingestion of a loading dose of lactose. It's used to screen for lactose intolerance that stems from lactase deficiency.

Absence or deficiency of lactase causes undigested lactose to remain in the intestinal lumen, producing such signs and symptoms as abdominal cramps and watery diarrhea. True congenital lactase deficiency is rare. Usually, lactose intolerance is acquired because lactase levels generally decrease with age.

ALERT! ▼ ▼ ▼ ▼ ▼ ▼ ▼ ▼ ▼
Signs and symptoms of lactose intolerance include abdominal cramps, nausea, bloating, flatulence, and watery diarrhea caused by the loading dose of lactose.

Purpose
■ To detect lactose intolerance

Cost
Inexpensive

Patient preparation
■ Explain to the patient that this test is used to determine if his symptoms are due to an inability to digest lactose.
■ Instruct the patient to fast and to avoid strenuous activity for 8 hours before the test.
■ Tell the patient that the test requires a blood sample. Explain who will perform the venipuncture and when.
■ Explain to the patient that he may experience discomfort from the needle puncture and the tourniquet.
■ Restrict medications that may affect test results. If they must be continued, note this on the laboratory request.
■ Tell the patient that a stool specimen may be collected 5 hours after he receives the loading dose of lactose.

Reference values
Normally, plasma glucose levels rise more than 20 mg/dl (SI, < 1.1 mmol/L) over fasting levels within 15 to 60 minutes after ingestion of the loading dose of lactose.

Abnormal findings
A rise in plasma glucose levels of less than 20 mg/dl (SI, < 1.1 mmol/L) indicates lactose intolerance, as does stool acidity (pH of 5.5 or less) and high glucose content

(greater than 1+ on the dipstick). Accompanying symptoms provoked by the test also suggest, but don't confirm, the diagnosis because such symptoms may appear in patients with normal lactase activity. Small-bowel biopsy with lactase assay may be performed to confirm the diagnosis.

Interfering factors
■ Failure to follow diet and exercise restrictions
■ Benzodiazepines, hormonal contraceptives, insulin, propranolol, and thiazide diuretics (possible false-low)
■ Delayed emptying of stomach contents (possible decrease)
■ Glycolysis (possible false negative)

Laryngoscopy, direct

Direct laryngoscopy allows visualization of the larynx by the use of a fiber-optic endoscope or laryngoscope passed through the mouth and pharynx to the larynx. It's indicated for children, patients with strong gag reflexes due to anatomic abnormalities, and those who have had no response to short-term therapy for symptoms of pharyngeal or laryngeal disease, such as stridor and hemoptysis. Secretions or tissue may be removed during this procedure for further study.

ALERT! ▼ ▼ ▼ ▼ ▼ ▼ ▼ ▼ ▼
The test is usually contraindicated in patients with epiglottiditis; however, it may be performed on them in an operating room as long as resuscitative equipment is available.

Purpose
■ To detect lesions, strictures, or foreign bodies
■ To remove benign lesions or foreign bodies from the larynx

■ To aid in the diagnosis of laryngeal cancer
■ To examine the larynx when indirect laryngoscopy is inadequate

Cost
Expensive

Patient preparation
■ Explain to the patient that this test is used to detect laryngeal abnormalities.
■ Instruct the patient to fast for 6 to 8 hours before the test.
■ Tell the patient who will perform the procedure and where it will be done.
■ Inform the patient that he'll receive a sedative to help him relax, medication to reduce secretions and, during the procedure, a general or local anesthetic. Reassure him that this procedure won't obstruct his airway.
■ Obtain informed consent if necessary.
■ Check the patient's history for hypersensitivity to the anesthetic.
■ Tell the patient that food and fluids will be restricted after the procedure until the gag reflex returns (usually for up to 2 hours) to avoid aspiration.
■ Reassure the patient that voice loss, hoarseness, and sore throat are temporary effects.

Normal findings
A normal larynx shows no evidence of inflammation, lesions, strictures, or foreign bodies.

Abnormal findings
The combined results of direct laryngoscopy, biopsy, and radiography may indicate laryngeal cancer. Direct laryngoscopy may also show benign lesions, strictures, or foreign bodies and, with a biopsy, may distinguish laryngeal edema from a radiation re-

action or a tumor. Direct laryngoscopy can also determine vocal cord dysfunction.

Interfering factors
■ Failure to place the specimens in appropriate containers or to send them to the laboratory immediately after collection

Leucine aminopeptidase

The leucine aminopeptidase test is used to measure serum leucine aminopeptidase levels, an isoenzyme of alkaline phosphatase (ALP) that's widely distributed in body tissues. The greatest concentrations appear in the hepatobiliary tissues, pancreas, and small intestine. In patients with liver disease, serum leucine aminopeptidase levels parallel serum ALP levels.

Purpose
■ To provide information about suspected liver, pancreatic, or biliary disease
■ To differentiate skeletal disease from hepatobiliary or pancreatic disease
■ To evaluate neonatal jaundice

Cost
Inexpensive

Patient preparation
■ Explain to the patient that this test is used to evaluate liver and pancreatic function.
■ Instruct the patient to fast for at least 8 hours before the test.
■ Tell the patient that the test requires a blood sample. Explain who will perform the venipuncture and when.
■ Explain to the patient that he may experience discomfort from the needle puncture and the tourniquet.

■ Restrict medications that may affect test results. If they must be continued, note this on the laboratory request.

Reference values
Normal values are 80 to 200 U/ml (SI, 80 to 200 kU/L) in men and 75 to 185 U/ml (SI, 75 to 185 kU/L) in women.

Abnormal findings
Elevated levels can occur with biliary obstruction, tumors, strictures, or atresia; advanced pregnancy; or therapy with drugs containing estrogen or progesterone.

Interfering factors
■ Advanced pregnancy (false-high)
■ Estrogen or progesterone (false-high)

Lipase

Lipase is produced in the pancreas and secreted into the duodenum, where it converts triglycerides and other fats into fatty acids and glycerol. The destruction of pancreatic cells, which occurs with acute pancreatitis, causes large amounts of lipase to be released into the blood. The lipase test is used to measure serum lipase levels; it's most useful when performed with a serum or urine amylase test.

Purpose
■ To aid diagnosis of acute pancreatitis

Cost
Inexpensive

Patient preparation
■ Explain to the patient that this test is used to evaluate pancreatic function.
■ Instruct the patient to fast overnight before the test.

- Tell the patient that the test requires a blood sample. Explain who will perform the venipuncture and when.
- Explain to the patient that he may experience discomfort from the needle puncture and the tourniquet.
- Restrict medications that may affect test results. If they must be continued, note this on the laboratory request.

Reference values

Serum lipase levels normally are less than 160 U/L (SI, < 2.72 µkat/L).

Abnormal findings

Elevated lipase levels suggest acute pancreatitis or pancreatic duct obstruction. After an acute attack, levels remain elevated for up to 14 days. Lipase levels may also increase with other pancreatic injuries, such as perforated peptic ulcer with chemical pancreatitis due to gastric juices, and in patients with high intestinal obstruction, pancreatic cancer, or renal disease with impaired excretion.

Interfering factors

- Cholinergics, codeine, meperidine, and morphine (false-high due to spasm of the sphincter of Oddi)

Lipids, fecal

Lipids excreted in feces include monoglycerides, diglycerides, triglycerides, phospholipids, glycolipids, soaps (fatty acids and fatty acid salts), sterols, and cholesterol esters. These lipids are derived from sloughed intestinal bacterial cells and epithelial cells, unabsorbed dietary lipids, and GI secretions. Normally, dietary lipids emulsified by bile are almost completely absorbed in the small intestine, provided that biliary and pancreatic secretions are adequate.

However, excessive excretion of fecal lipids (steatorrhea) occurs with various malabsorption syndromes.

In the qualitative test, a specimen from a random stool is stained and examined microscopically for evidence of malabsorption — undigested muscle fibers and various fats. In the quantitative test, the entire 72-hour specimen is dried and weighed; the lipids therein are extracted with a solvent, evaporated, and weighed. Only the quantitative test can confirm steatorrhea.

Purpose

- To confirm steatorrhea

Cost

Inexpensive

Patient preparation

- Explain to the patient that this test evaluates the digestion of fats.
- Instruct the patient to abstain from alcohol and to maintain a high-fat diet (100 g/ day) for 3 days before the test and during the 72-hour stool collection period.
- Restrict medications that may affect test results. If they must be continued, note this on the laboratory request.
- Teach the patient how to collect a timed stool specimen.

Reference values

Fecal lipids normally make up less than 20% of excreted solids, with excretion of less than 7 g/24 hours.

Abnormal findings

Both digestive and absorptive disorders cause steatorrhea. Digestive disorders may affect the production and release of pancreatic lipase or bile; absorptive disorders, the integrity of the intestine. With pancreatic insufficiency, impaired lipid digestion may result from insufficient production of lipase. Pancreatic resection, cystic fibrosis, chronic pancreatitis, or ductal obstruction by stone or tumor may prevent the normal release or action of lipase.

With impaired liver function, faulty lipid digestion may result from inadequate production of bile salts. Biliary obstruction, which may accompany gallbladder disease, may prevent the normal release of bile salts into the duodenum. Extensive small-bowel resection or bypass may also interrupt normal enteroliver circulation of bile salts.

Diseases of the intestinal mucosa affect normal absorption of lipids; regional ileitis and atrophy resulting from malnutrition cause gross structural changes in the intestinal wall, and celiac disease and tropical sprue produce mucosal abnormalities. Scleroderma, radiation enteritis, fistulas, intestinal tuberculosis, small intestine diverticula, and altered intestinal flora may also cause steatorrhea. Whipple's disease and lymphomas cause lymphatic obstruction, which can inhibit fat absorption.

Interfering factors

■ Failure to observe pretest restrictions
■ Alcohol, aluminum hydroxide, azathioprine, bisacodyl, calcium carbonate, cholestyramine, colchicine, kanamycin, mineral oil, neomycin, and potassium chloride (possible increase or decrease due to inhibited absorption or altered chemical digestion)
■ Use of a waxed collection container, contamination of the specimen, or incomplete stool specimen collection (total weight less than 300 g)

Lipoprotein-cholesterol fractionation

Cholesterol fractionation tests are used to isolate and measure low-density-lipopro-

tein (LDL) and high-density-lipoprotein (HDL) cholesterol levels in serum. The HDL level is inversely related to the risk of coronary artery disease (CAD) — the higher the HDL level, the lower the risk of CAD. Conversely, the higher the LDL level, the higher the risk of CAD. (See *Apolipoproteins and CAD*.)

Purpose
■ To assess the risk of CAD
■ To assess efficacy of lipid-lowering drug therapy

Cost
Moderately expensive

Patient preparation
■ Tell the patient that this test is used to determine the risk of CAD.
■ Tell the patient that the test requires a blood sample. Explain who will perform the venipuncture and when.
■ Explain to the patient that he may experience discomfort from the needle puncture and the tourniquet.
■ Restrict medications that may affect test results. If they must be continued, note this on the laboratory request.
■ Instruct the patient to abstain from alcohol for 24 hours before the test, and to fast and avoid exercise for 12 to 14 hours before the test.

Reference values
Normal lipoprotein values vary by age, sex, geographic area, and ethnic group; check the laboratory for reference values. HDL levels range from 37 to 70 mg/dl (SI, 0.96 to 1.8 mmol/L) for males and from 40 to 85 mg/dl for females (SI, 1.03 to 2.2 mmol/L). LDL levels are less than 130 mg/dl (SI, <3.36 mmol/L) for individuals who don't have CAD. Borderline high

levels are greater than 160 mg/dl (SI, > 4.1 mmol/L).

The American College of Cardiology recommends an HDL level of greater than or equal to 40 mg/dl, with women maintaining an HDL cholesterol level of at least 45 mg/dl. HDL levels greater than 60 mg/dl are considered heart healthy. Optimal LDL levels are less than 100 mg/dl, with levels greater than or equal to 160mg/dl considered high.

Abnormal findings

Elevated LDL levels increase the risk of CAD; they generally reflect a healthy state but can also indicate chronic hepatitis, early stage primary biliary cirrhosis, and alcohol consumption, and can occur as a result of long-term aerobic and vigorous exercise. Rarely, a sharp rise (to as high as 100 mg/dl [SI, 2.58 mmol/L]) in a second type of HDL (alpha$_2$-HDL) may signal CAD.

Interfering factors

■ Concurrent illness, especially if accompanied by fever, recent surgery, or a myocardial infarction

■ Collecting the sample in a heparinized tube (possible false-high due to activation of the enzyme lipase, which causes release of fatty acids from triglycerides)

■ Antilipemics, such as cholestyramine, clofibrate, colestipol, dextrothyroxine, gemfibrozil, niacin, and probucol (decrease)

■ Alcohol, disulfiram, hormonal contraceptives, miconazole, and high doses of phenothiazines (possible increase)

■ Estrogens (possible increase or decrease)

■ Presence of bilirubin, hemoglobin, salicylates, iodine, and vitamins A and D

Apolipoproteins and CAD

Although measurement of apolipoproteins — the protein fractions of lipoprotein molecules — is primarily a research procedure, mounting evidence suggests that it may have important clinical applications as well. Because apolipoprotein levels can be measured directly in serum, they may indicate an individual's risk of coronary artery disease (CAD) more accurately than high-density-lipoprotein (HDL) or low-density-lipoprotein (LDL) levels, which must be measured indirectly.

Currently, eight apolipoproteins have been identified. Of these, apolipoprotein A (ApoA) — the major protein component of HDL — and apolipoprotein B (ApoB) — the major protein component of LDL — are the most clinically significant. Decreased ApoA levels (below 140 mg/dl) occur with ischemic heart disease; increased ApoB levels (above 135 mg/dl), with hyperlipidemia, angina pectoris, and myocardial infarction.

Lipoprotein phenotyping

Lipoprotein phenotyping is used to determine levels of the four major lipoproteins: chylomicrons; very-low-density lipoproteins — also called prebeta lipoproteins; low-density lipoproteins — also called beta lipoproteins; and high-density lipoproteins — also called alpha lipoproteins.

Detecting altered lipoprotein patterns is essential to identifying hyperlipoproteinemia and hypolipoproteinemia.

Familial hyperlipoproteinemias

TYPE	CAUSES AND INCIDENCE	CLINICAL SIGNS	LABORATORY FINDINGS
I	■ Deficient lipoprotein lipase, resulting in increased chylomicron levels ■ May be induced by alcoholism ■ Incidence: rare	■ Eruptive xanthomas ■ Lipemia retinalis ■ Abdominal pain	■ Increased chylomicron, total cholesterol, and triglyceride levels ■ Normal or slightly increased very-low-density-lipoprotein (VLDL) levels ■ Normal or decreased low-density-lipoprotein (LDL) and high-density-lipoprotein levels ■ Cholesterol-triglyceride ratio < 0.2
IIa	■ Deficient cell receptor, resulting in increased LDL levels and excessive cholesterol synthesis ■ May be induced by hypothyroidism ■ Incidence: common	■ Premature coronary artery disease (CAD) ■ Arcus cornea ■ Xanthelasma ■ Tendinous and tuberous xanthomas	■ Increased LDL levels ■ Normal VLDL levels ■ Cholesterol-triglyceride ratio > 2.0
IIb	■ Deficient cell receptor, resulting in increased LDL levels and excessive cholesterol synthesis ■ May be induced by dysgammaglobulinemia, hypothyroidism, uncontrolled diabetes mellitus, or nephrotic syndrome ■ Incidence: common	■ Premature CAD ■ Obesity ■ Possible xanthelasmas	■ Increased LDL, VLDL, total cholesterol, and triglyceride levels
III	■ Unknown cause, resulting in deficient VLDL-to-LDL conversion ■ May be induced by hypothyroidism, uncontrolled diabetes mellitus, or paraproteinemia ■ Incidence: rare	■ Premature CAD ■ Arcus cornea ■ Eruptive tuberous xanthomas	■ Increased total cholesterol, VLDL, and triglyceride levels ■ Normal or decreased LDL levels ■ Cholesterol-triglyceride ratio of VLDL > 0.4 ■ Broad beta band observed on electrophoresis
IV	■ Unknown cause, resulting in decreased levels of lipoprotein lipase ■ May be induced by uncontrolled diabetes mellitus, alcoholism, pregnancy, steroid or estrogen therapy, dysgammaglobulinemia, or hyperthyroidism ■ Incidence: common	■ Possibly premature CAD ■ Obesity ■ Hypertension ■ Peripheral neuropathy	■ Increased VLDL and triglyceride levels ■ Normal LDL levels ■ Cholesterol-triglyceride ratio of VLDL < 0.25

Familial hyperlipoproteinemias *(continued)*

TYPE	CAUSES AND INCIDENCE	CLINICAL SIGNS	LABORATORY FINDINGS
V	■ Unknown cause, resulting in defective triglyceride clearance ■ May be induced by alcoholism, dysgammaglobulinemia, uncontrolled diabetes mellitus, nephrotic syndrome, pancreatitis, or steroid therapy ■ Incidence: rare	■ Premature CAD ■ Abdominal pain ■ Lipemia retinalis ■ Eruptive xanthomas ■ Hepatosplenomegaly	■ Increased VLDL, total cholesterol, and triglyceride levels ■ Chylomicrons present ■ Cholesterol-triglyceride ratio < 0.6

Purpose
■ To determine classification of hyperlipoproteinemia and hypolipoproteinemia

Cost
Moderately expensive

Patient preparation
■ Explain to the patient that this test is used to determine how the body metabolizes fats.
■ Tell the patient that the test requires a blood sample. Explain who will perform the venipuncture and when.
■ Explain to the patient that he may experience discomfort from the needle puncture and the tourniquet.
■ Instruct the patient to abstain from alcohol for 24 hours before the test, to eat a low-fat meal the night before the test, and to fast after midnight before the test.
■ Check the patient's drug history for the use of heparin. If he's taking an antilipemic, such as cholestyramine, instruct him to stop taking the drug about 2 weeks before the test.
■ Notify the laboratory if the patient is receiving treatment for any other condition that might significantly alter lipoprotein metabolism, such as diabetes mellitus, nephrosis, or hypothyroidism.

Normal findings
The types of hyperlipoproteinemias and hypolipoproteinemias are identified by characteristic electrophoretic patterns.
   Familial lipoprotein disorders are classified as either hyperlipoproteinemias or hypolipoproteinemias. The six types of hyperlipoproteinemias are: I, IIa, IIb, III, IV, and V. Types IIa, IIb, and IV are relatively common. All hypolipoproteinemias are rare, including hypobetalipoproteinemia, abetalipoproteinemia, and alphalipoprotein deficiency.

Abnormal findings
See *Familial hyperlipoproteinemias.*

Interfering factors
■ Recent use of an antilipemic (decrease)
■ Failure to observe pretest restrictions
■ Administration of heparin or collection of the sample in a heparinized tube (possible false-high)

Liver biopsy

Percutaneous liver biopsy is the needle aspiration of a core of liver tissue for histologic analysis. This procedure is performed under local or general anesthesia. Findings may help to identify liver disorders after ultrasonography, computed tomography, and radionuclide studies have failed to detect them. Because many patients with liver disorders have clotting defects, testing for hemostasis should precede liver biopsy.

ALERT! ▼ ▼ ▼ ▼ ▼ ▼ ▼ ▼ ▼
Percutaneous liver biopsy is contraindicated in a patient with a platelet count below 100,000/μl; prothrombin time (PT) longer than 15 seconds; empyema of the lungs, pleurae, peritoneum, biliary tract, or liver; vascular tumor; liver angiomas; hydatid cyst; or tense ascites. If extraliver obstruction is suspected, ultrasonography or subcutaneous transliver cholangiography should rule out this condition before the biopsy is considered.

Purpose
■ To diagnose liver parenchymatous disease, malignant tumors, and granulomatous infections

Cost
Very expensive

Patient preparation
■ Explain to the patient that this test is used to diagnose liver disorders.
■ Describe the procedure to the patient. Tell him who will perform the biopsy and where it will take place.
■ Instruct the patient to restrict food and fluids for 4 to 8 hours before the test.
■ Obtain informed consent if necessary.
■ Check the patient's history for hypersensitivity to the local anesthetic.

■ Order coagulation studies (PT, partial thromboplastin time, and platelet counts) prior to the liver biopsy and review results.
■ Tell the patient that the test requires a blood sample. Explain who will perform the venipuncture and when.
■ Explain to the patient that he may experience discomfort from the needle puncture and the tourniquet.
■ Inform the patient that he'll receive a local anesthetic but that he may experience pain similar to that of a punch in his right shoulder as the biopsy needle passes the phrenic nerve.
■ Tell the patient that pressure will be applied to the puncture site and that he'll be monitored closely for bleeding after the procedure; however, he'll need to be on bed rest for 24 hours.
■ Tell the patient that he may experience pain after the procedure, which may persist for several hours, but that an analgesic may be administered.

Normal findings
The normal liver consists of sheets of hepatocytes supported by a reticulin framework.

Abnormal findings
Examination of the liver tissue may reveal diffuse liver disease, such as cirrhosis or hepatitis, or granulomatous infections such as tuberculosis. Primary malignant tumors include hepatocellular carcinoma, cholangiocellular carcinoma, and angiosarcoma, but liver metastasis is more common.

Nonmalignant findings with a known focal lesion require further studies, such as laparotomy or laparoscopy with biopsy.

Interfering factors
■ Failure to obtain a representative specimen
■ Failure to place the specimen in the proper preservative

- Failure to send the specimen to the laboratory immediately after collection
- Hemorrhage caused by inadvertent puncture of a liver blood vessel

Liver-spleen scanning

In liver-spleen scanning, a gamma camera records the distribution of radioactivity in the liver and spleen after I.V. injection of a radioactive colloid. The colloid most commonly used, technetium sulfide-99m (^{99m}Tc), concentrates in the reticuloendothelial cells through phagocytosis. About 80% to 90% of the injected colloid is taken up by Kupffer's cells in the liver, 5% to 10% by the spleen, and 3% to 5% by bone marrow. The gamma camera images either organ instantaneously without moving.

Although the test is used to detect focal disease (such as tumors, cysts, and abscesses), liver-spleen scanning demonstrates focal disease nonspecifically as a cold spot (a defect that fails to take up the colloid) and may fail to detect focal lesions smaller than $\frac{3}{4}$" (1.9 cm) in diameter. Although symptoms may aid diagnosis, liver-spleen scanning commonly requires confirmation by ultrasonography, computed tomography (CT) scan, gallium scanning, or biopsy. CT scan is the fastest method of evaluating liver or splenic injury in abdominal trauma and is preferred to other scans. (See *Flow studies.*)

ALERT! ▼ ▼ ▼ ▼ ▼ ▼ ▼ ▼ ▼
Liver-spleen scanning is usually contraindicated in children, pregnant women, and breastfeeding women.

Purpose
- To screen for liver metastases and hepatocellular disease, such as cirrhosis and hepatitis

Flow studies

In contrast to liver-spleen scanning, which provides static nuclear images, flow studies (dynamic scintigraphy) record in rapid sequence the stages of perfusion after I.V. injection of a radionuclide, such as technetium sulfide-99m. Because flow studies demonstrate the vascularity of a nonspecific focal defect, they sometimes help distinguish between metastases, tumors, cysts, and abscesses.

In flow studies, a hot defect will show early increased uptake of the radionuclide when compared to the surrounding parenchyma, and then will appear as a filling defect, or cold spot, on later routine images. Cysts and abscesses, which are avascular, fail to take up the radionuclide; hemangiomas appear characteristically hot because of their enlarged vessels.

Tumors and metastases are generally more difficult to evaluate because their vascularity is more variable. Although vascular metastases may appear hot, most metastases demonstrate poor uptake of the radionuclide. Hepatomas can also appear hot or can show perfusion similar to normal parenchyma.

- To detect focal disease (such as tumors, cysts, and abscesses) in the liver and spleen
- To demonstrate hepatomegaly or splenomegaly (in patients with palpable abdominal masses)
- To assess the liver and spleen after abdominal trauma

Cost
Very expensive

Patient preparation

■ Explain to the patient that this procedure permits examination of the liver and spleen through scintigraphs or scans taken after I.V. injection of a radioactive substance.

■ Tell the patient who will perform the test and where it will take place.

■ Explain to the patient that he may experience discomfort from the needle puncture.

■ Inform the patient not to schedule more than one radionuclide scan on the same day. Assure him that the test substance contains only trace amounts of radioactivity and allergic reactions to it are rare.

■ Explain to the patient that the detector head of the gamma camera may touch his abdomen (if appropriate), and reassure him that this isn't dangerous.

■ Tell the patient that he'll be asked to lie still and to breathe quietly during the procedure to ensure images of good quality, and that he may also be asked to hold his breath briefly. Explain to him that this technique helps to evaluate liver mobility and pliability.

■ Obtain informed consent if necessary.

■ Inform the patient that the body eliminates the radioactive substance within 6 to 24 hours. Instruct him to increase his fluid intake (unless contraindicated) to expedite this process, and to flush the toilet immediately after urinating to decrease exposure to radiation in the urine.

Normal findings

Because the liver and the spleen contain equal numbers of reticuloendothelial cells, both organs normally appear equally bright on the image. However, distribution of radioactive colloid is generally more uniform and homogeneous in the spleen than in the liver. The liver has various normal indentations and impressions, such as the gallbladder fossa and falciform ligament, that may mimic focal disease. (See *Identifying liver indentations in nuclear imaging.*)

Abnormal findings

Although it may fail to detect early hepatocellular disease, liver-spleen scanning shows characteristic, distinct patterns as such a disease progresses. The most prominent sign of hepatocellular disease is a shift of the radioactive colloid that's caused by decreased liver blood flow and impaired function of Kupffer's cells. This inhibits distribution of the colloid in the liver, causing the liver to appear uniformly decreased or patchy. The spleen and bone marrow then take up the abnormally large amounts of the colloid unabsorbed by the liver, thus concentrating more radioactivity than the liver, and appear brighter on the scan. This same distribution pattern (colloid shift) also accompanies portal hypertension due to extraliver causes.

Hepatitis and cirrhosis are both associated with hepatomegaly and a colloid shift, but certain characteristics help distinguish them. In hepatitis, distribution of the colloid is usually uniformly decreased; in cirrhosis, it's patchy. Splenomegaly is typical in cirrhosis but not in hepatitis.

Metastasis to the liver or spleen may appear on the scan as a focal defect and requires biopsy to confirm the diagnosis. Liver metastasis usually originates in the GI or genitourinary tract, the breasts, or the lungs and is more common than metastasis to the spleen. After metastasis is confirmed, serial liver-spleen studies are useful in evaluating the effectiveness of therapy.

Because cysts, abscesses, and tumors fail to take up the radioactive colloid, they ap-

Identifying liver indentations in nuclear imaging

In nuclear imaging, normal indentations and impressions may be mistaken for focal lesions. These drawings of the liver, which give both an anterior view and a posterior view, identify the contours and impressions that may be misread.

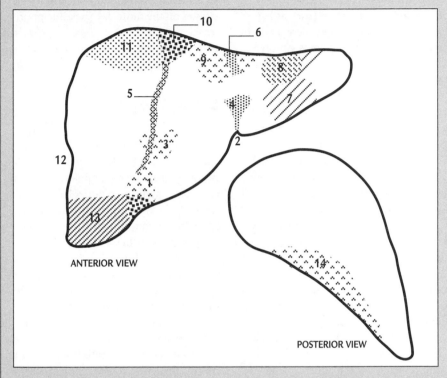

ANTERIOR VIEW

POSTERIOR VIEW

KEY:
1. Gallbladder fossa
2. Ligamentum teres and falciform ligament
3. Hilum, main branching of the portal vein
4. Pars umbilicalis portion, left portal vein
5. Variable stripe of lobar fissure between right and left lobes
6. Variable stripe of segmental fissure, left lobe
7. Thinning of left lobe
8. Impression of pectus excavatum
9. Cardiac impression
10. Hepatic veins and inferior vena cava
11. Shielding from right female breast
12. Harrison's groove or costal impression
13. Impression of hepatic flexure of colon
14. Right renal impression

pear on the scan as solitary or multiple focal defects. Liver cysts may appear as solitary defects; polycystic liver disease, as multiple defects. Splenic cysts are rarer than liver cysts and may have a parasitic or nonparasitic origin. Ultrasonography can confirm liver or splenic cysts.

Intraliver abscesses are usually pyogenic or amebic. Subphrenic abscesses, located beneath the diaphragm, may distort the dome of the right lobe. Splenic abscesses are characteristic with bacterial endocarditis. All abscesses require gallium scanning or ultrasonography to confirm diagnosis.

Benign liver tumors (such as hemangiomas, adenomas, and hamartomas) require confirming biopsy or flow studies. Primary malignant tumors (such as hepatomas) also require biopsy. Benign splenic tumors (such as hemangiomas, fibromas, myomas, and hamartomas) are rare. Primary malignant splenic tumors are also rare, except with lymphoreticular malignancies such as Hodgkin's disease. Splenic tumors also require biopsy to confirm diagnosis. Although focal disease usually inhibits uptake of radioactive colloid, both obstruction of the superior vena cava and Budd-Chiari syndrome cause markedly increased uptake.

Liver-spleen scanning can verify palpable abdominal masses and differentiate between splenomegaly and hepatomegaly.

A left upper quadrant mass may result from splenomegaly or, if the liver is grossly extended across the abdomen, from hepatomegaly. A right upper quadrant mass may result from hepatomegaly; a right lower quadrant mass may be a Riedel's lobe or a large dependent gallbladder. Splenic infarcts, commonly associated with bacterial endocarditis and massive splenomegaly, appear as peripheral defects, with decreased and irregular colloid distribution.

Scanning can assess liver injury after abdominal trauma. Intraliver hematoma appears as a focal defect; subcapsular hematoma, as a lentiform defect on the periphery of the liver; liver laceration, as a linear defect.

Scanning can also detect splenic injury after abdominal trauma. Intraliver hematoma appears as a focal defect; liver laceration, as a linear defect. Splenic hematoma appears as a focal defect in or next to the spleen and may transect it. Subcapsular hematoma appears as a lentiform defect on the periphery of the spleen.

Interfering factors

■ Radionuclides administered in other studies on the same day (possible poor imaging)
■ Patient's inability to remain still during the procedure

Lung biopsy

In lung biopsy, a specimen of pulmonary tissue is excised by closed or open technique for histologic examination. Closed technique, performed under local anesthesia, includes needle and transbronchial biopsies. Open technique, performed under general anesthesia in the operating room, includes limited and standard thoracotomies. Needle biopsy, which provides a much smaller specimen than the open technique, is appropriate when the lesion is readily accessible, originates in the lung parenchyma and is confined to it, or is affixed to the chest wall. Transbronchial biopsy, the removal of multiple tissue specimens through a fiber-optic bronchoscope, may be used in patients with diffuse infiltrative pulmonary disease or tumors or in patients with severe debilitation that contraindicates open biopsy. Open biopsy is appropriate for the study of a well-circumscribed lesion that may require resection.

Generally, a lung biopsy is recommended after chest X-rays, computed tomography scan, and bronchoscopy have failed to identify the cause of diffuse parenchymatous pulmonary disease or a pulmonary lesion. Complications of lung biopsy include bleeding, infection, and pneumothorax.

ALERT! ▼ ▼ ▼ ▼ ▼ ▼ ▼ ▼ ▼
Needle biopsy is contraindicated in patients with a lesion that's separated from the chest wall or accompanied by emphysematous bullae, cysts, or gross emphysema and in patients with coagulopathy, hypoxia, pulmonary hypertension, or cardiac disease with cor pulmonale.

Purpose
- To confirm a diagnosis of diffuse parenchymatous pulmonary disease or pulmonary lesions

Cost
Expensive

Patient preparation
- Explain to the patient that this test is used to confirm or rule out a diagnostic finding in the lung.
- Describe the procedure to the patient. Tell him who will perform the biopsy and where it will take place.
- Order a chest X-ray and blood studies (prothrombin time, partial thromboplastin time, and platelet count) before the biopsy and interpret the results.
- Instruct the patient to fast after midnight before the procedure. If the test is scheduled for the afternoon and your facility's policy permits, the patient may have clear liquids before the test.
- Obtain informed consent if necessary.
- Check the patient's history for hypersensitivity to the local anesthetic.
- Tell the patient that a mild sedative may be given before the biopsy to help him relax. Tell him that he'll receive a local anesthetic but that he may experience a sharp, transient pain when the biopsy needle touches his lung.
- Emphasize to the patient that he'll need to lie still during the procedure because

any movement or coughing can result in laceration of lung tissue from the biopsy needle.

Normal findings
Normal pulmonary tissue shows uniform texture of the alveolar ducts, alveolar walls, bronchioles, and small vessels.

Abnormal findings
Histologic examination of a pulmonary tissue specimen can reveal squamous cell or oat cell carcinoma and adenocarcinoma; such an examination may supplement the results of microbiologic cultures, deep-cough sputum specimens, chest X-rays, and bronchoscopy as well as the patient's physical history in confirming cancer or parenchymatous pulmonary disease.

Interfering factors
- Failure to obtain a representative tissue specimen or store it in the appropriate container

Lung perfusion scan

A lung perfusion scan produces an image of pulmonary blood flow after I.V. injection of a radiopharmaceutical, either human serum albumin microspheres or macroaggregated albumin bonded to technetium.

Purpose
- To assess arterial perfusion of the lungs
- To detect pulmonary emboli
- To evaluate pulmonary function before lung resection

Cost
Very expensive

Patient preparation

- Tell the patient that this test helps evaluate respiratory function.
- Describe the test for the patient. Tell him who will perform it and where it will take place.
- Tell the patient that a radiopharmaceutical will be injected into a vein in his arm and then he'll sit in front of a camera or lie under it. Explain that neither the camera nor the uptake probe emits radiation and that the amount of radioactivity in the radiopharmaceutical is minimal.
- On the laboratory request, note whether the patient has any of the following conditions: chronic obstructive pulmonary disease (COPD), parasitic disease, pulmonary edema, sickle cell disease, tumor, or vasculitis.
- Obtain informed consent if necessary.

ALERT! ▼ ▼ ▼ ▼ ▼ ▼ ▼ ▼ ▼

A lung scan is contraindicated in patients hypersensitive to the radiopharmaceutical.

Normal findings

Hot spots, which are areas with normal blood perfusion, show an elevated uptake of the radiopharmaceutical; a normal lung shows a uniform uptake pattern.

Abnormal findings

Cold spots, which are areas of low radioactive uptake, indicate poor perfusion, suggesting an embolism; however, a ventilation scan is necessary to confirm diagnosis. Decreased regional blood flow that occurs without vessel obstruction may indicate pneumonitis.

Interfering factors

- Scheduling more than one radionuclide test a day, especially if using different tracing substances (possible hindered diffusion of the tracer isotope in the second test)

- Administering all of the radiopharmaceutical while the patient is sitting (possible poor imaging due to settling of the tracer isotope in lung bases)
- Conditions such as COPD, parasitic disease, pulmonary edema, sickle cell disease, tumor, and vasculitis (possible poor imaging)

Lung ventilation scan

The lung ventilation scan is performed after the patient inhales a mixture of air and radioactive gas that delineates areas of the lung ventilated during respiration. The scan records the distribution of the gas during three phases: the buildup of radioactive gas (wash-in phase), the time after rebreathing when radioactivity reaches a steady level (equilibrium phase), and the time after the radioactive gas is removed from the lungs (wash-out phase).

Purpose

- To help diagnose pulmonary emboli
- To identify areas of the lung capable of ventilation
- To help evaluate regional respiratory function
- To locate regional hypoventilation, which may indicate atelectasis, an obstructing tumor, or chronic obstructive pulmonary disease

Cost

Very expensive

Patient preparation

- Describe the procedure to the patient. Explain to him that this test helps evaluate respiratory function.
- Tell the patient who will perform the test and where it will take place.

- Explain to the patient that he'll be asked to hold his breath for a short time after inhaling a minimal amount of radioactive gas and to remain still while a machine scans his chest.
- Obtain informed consent if necessary.

Normal findings

Normal findings include an equal distribution of gas in both lungs and normal wash-in and wash-out phases.

Abnormal findings

Unequal gas distribution in both lungs indicates poor ventilation or airway obstruction in areas with low radioactivity. With vascular obstructions such as pulmonary embolism, the perfusion to the embolized area is decreased, but the ventilation to that area is maintained; with parenchymatous disease such as pneumonia, ventilation is abnormal within the areas of consolidation.

Interfering factors

- Failure to remove jewelry and other metal objects from the scanning field (possible poor imaging)

Lupus erythematosus cell preparation

Lupus erythematosus (LE) cell preparation is an in vitro procedure used in diagnosing systemic lupus erythematosus (SLE). Although the test is less sensitive and less reliable than either the antinuclear antibodies (ANA) or the antideoxyribonucleic acid (anti-DNA) antibody tests, it's commonly used because it requires minimal equipment and reagents.

In this test, a blood sample is mixed with laboratory-treated nucleoprotein (the antigen). If the sample contains ANA, the ANA react with the nucleoprotein, causing swelling and rupture. Phagocytes from the serum then engulf the extruded nuclei, forming LE cells, which are then detected through microscopic examination of the sample.

Purpose

- To aid diagnosis of SLE
- To monitor treatment of SLE (About 60% of successfully treated patients fail to show LE cells after 4 to 6 weeks of therapy.)

Cost

Moderately expensive

Patient preparation

- Explain to the patient that this test helps detect antibodies to his own tissue or, as appropriate, to monitor his response to therapy. (See *Understanding autoantibodies in autoimmune disease,* pages 236 and 237.)
- Tell the patient that the test requires a blood sample. Explain who will perform the venipuncture and when.
- Explain to the patient that he may experience discomfort from the needle puncture and the tourniquet.
- Restrict medications that may affect test results, such as isoniazid, hydralazine, and procainamide. If they must be continued, note this on the laboratory request.

Normal findings

No LE cells are normally present in serum.

Abnormal findings

The presence of at least two LE cells may indicate SLE. Although these cells occur primarily in SLE, they may also appear with active chronic hepatitis, rheumatoid arthritis, scleroderma, and certain drug reactions. Also, up to 25% of patients with SLE show no LE cells.

Understanding autoantibodies in autoimmune disease

When the immune system produces autoantibodies against the antigenic determinants on and in cells, two types of autoimmune disease can result. *Organ-specific diseases*, such as pernicious anemia, occur when the targeted antigenic determinants are specific to an organ or tissue or to certain cells or cell types. Lymphocytes invade the target organ, tissue, or cell and destroy targeted cells. *Non–organ-specific diseases*, such as myasthenia gravis, occur when the targeted antigenic determinants are shared with other cells (self-antigens). This causes deposition of immune complexes (Type III hypersensitivity) with subsequent lesions anywhere in the body.

Various diagnostic techniques are used to detect antibodies in autoimmune disease, including radioimmunoassay, hemagglutination, complement fixation, and immunofluorescence. The chart below lists common test methods and findings in various autoimmune diseases.

DISEASE	AFFECTED AREA	ANTIGEN	ANTIBODY	DIAGNOSTIC TECHNIQUE
Autoimmune hemolytic anemia	Hematopoietic system	Red blood cells (RBCs)	Anti-RBC antibodies	Direct and indirect Coombs' test
Goodpasture's syndrome	Lungs and kidneys	Glomerular and lung basement membranes	Anti-basement membrane antibodies	Immunofluorescence of kidney biopsy specimen, radioimmunoassay
Hashimoto's thyroiditis	Thyroid gland	Thyroglobulin, second colloid antigen, cytoplasmic microsomes, cell surface antigens	Antibodies to thyroglobulin and microsomal antigens	Radioimmunoassay, hemagglutination, complement fixation, immunofluorescence
Myasthenia gravis	Neuromuscular system	Acetylcholine receptors of skeletal and heart muscle	Anti-acetylcholine antibodies	Immunoprecipitation radioimmunoassay
Pemphigus vulgaris	Skin	Desmosomes between prickle cells in the epidermis	Antibodies to intercellular substances of the skin and mucous membranes	Immunofluorescence
Pernicious anemia	Hematopoietic system	Intrinsic factor	Antibodies to gastric parietal cells and vitamin B_{12}-binding site of intrinsic factor	Immunofluorescence, radioimmunoassay
Primary biliary cirrhosis	Small bile ducts in liver	Mitochondria	Anti-mitochondrial antibodies	Immunofluorescence of mitochondrial-rich cells (kidney biopsy)

Understanding autoantibodies in autoimmune disease

DISEASE	AFFECTED AREA	ANTIGEN	ANTIBODY	DIAGNOSTIC TECHNIQUE
Rheumatoid arthritis	Joints, blood vessels, skin, muscles, and lymph nodes	Immunoglobulin (Ig) G	Anti-gamma-globulin antibodies	Sheep RBC agglutination, latex immunoglobulin agglutination, radioimmunoassay, immunofluorescence, immunodiffusion
Systemic lupus erythematosus	Skin, joints, muscles, lungs, heart, kidneys, brain, and eyes	Deoxyribonucleic acid (DNA), nucleoprotein, blood cells, clotting factors, IgG, Wassermann antigen	Antinuclear antibodies, anti-DNA antibodies, anti–double-stranded-DNA antibodies, anti–single-stranded-DNA antibodies, anti-ribonucleoprotein antibodies, anti–gamma-globulin antibodies, anti-RBC antibodies, antilymphocyte antibodies, antiplatelet antibodies, antineuronal cell antibodies, anti-Smith antibodies	Counterelectrophoresis, hemagglutination, radioimmunoassay, immunofluorescence, Coombs' test

Apart from supportive signs, a definitive diagnosis of SLE may require a confirming ANA or anti-DNA test. The ANA test commonly detects autoantibodies in the serum of SLE patients with negative LE cell test results. Anti-DNA antibodies appear in two-thirds of all SLE patients but are rare in patients with other conditions, which is why the presence of these antibodies is such a strong indicator of SLE.

Interfering factors
■ Hydralazine, isoniazid, and procainamide, chlorpromazine, clofibrate, ethosuximide, gold salts, griseofulvin, hormonal contraceptives, mephenytoin, methyldopa, methysergide, para-aminosali- cylic acid, penicillin, phenylbutazone, phenytoin, primidone, propylthiouracil, quinidine, reserpine, streptomycin, sulfonamides, tetracyclines, and trimethadione (may produce a syndrome resembling SLE)

Luteinizing hormone, plasma

The plasma luteinizing hormone (LH) test, usually ordered for anovulation and infertility studies on women, is a quantitative analysis of plasma LH or interstitial cell-stimulating hormone levels. In women, cyclic LH secretion (with follicle-stimulating hormone [FSH]) causes ovulation and transforms the ovarian follicle into the corpus luteum, which in turn secretes progesterone. (See *LH secretion peaks at ovulation*.)

In males, continuous LH secretion stimulates the interstitial (Leydig) cells of the testes to release testosterone, which stimulates and maintains spermatogenesis (with FSH).

Purpose
- To detect ovulation
- To assess female or male infertility
- To evaluate amenorrhea
- To monitor therapy designed to induce ovulation

Cost
Inexpensive

Patient preparation
- Explain to the patient that this test helps determine if her secretion of female hormones is normal.
- Tell the patient that the test requires a blood sample. Explain who will perform the venipuncture and when.
- Explain to the patient that she may experience discomfort from the needle puncture and the tourniquet.
- Restrict medications that may affect test results. If they must be continued, note this on the laboratory request.
- If the patient is taking a steroid (including estrogen and progesterone), instruct her to stop taking it 48 hours before the test.
- Note on the laboratory request which phase of the menstrual cycle the patient is in or, if applicable, that the patient is menopausal.

Reference values
Normal LH values are wide ranging.

- *Adult females, follicular phase:* 5 to 15 mIU/ml (SI, 5 to 15 IU/L)
- *Adult females, ovulatory phase:* 30 to 60 mIU/ml (SI, 30 to 60 IU/L)
- *Adult females, luteal phase:* 5 to 15 mIU/ml (SI, 5 to 15 IU/L)
- *Postmenopausal females:* 50 to 100 mIU/ml (SI, 50 to 100 IU/L)
- *Adult males:* 5 to 20 mIU/ml (SI, 5 to 20 IU/L)
- *Children:* 4 to 20 mIU/ml (SI, 4 to 20 IU/L).

Abnormal findings
In women, absence of a midcycle peak in LH secretion may indicate anovulation. Decreased or low-normal LH levels may indicate hypogonadism; these findings are commonly associated with amenorrhea. High LH levels may indicate congenital absence of ovaries or ovarian failure associated with Stein-Leventhal syndrome (polycystic ovary syndrome), Turner's syndrome (ovarian dysgenesis), menopause, or early stage acromegaly. Infertility can result from primary or secondary gonadal dysfunction.

In men, low LH values may indicate secondary gonadal dysfunction (of hypothalamic or pituitary origin); high LH values may indicate testicular failure (primary hypogonadism) or destruction or congenital absence of testes.

Interfering factors
- Failure to observe pretest restrictions of medication
- Steroids, including estrogen, progesterone, and testosterone (possible decrease)
- Radioactive scan performed within 1 week before the test

LH secretion peaks at ovulation

The menstrual cycle is divided into three distinct phases: the menstrual phase (days 1 to 5); the follicular, or proliferative, phase (days 6 to 13); and after ovulation on day 14, the luteal, or secretory, phase (days 15 to 28).

The menstrual phase
The menstrual phase of the normal cycle is characterized by endometrial sloughing, corpus luteum degeneration, and new follicle growth. During this stage, estrogen and progesterone levels are low, thus triggering an increase in follicle-stimulating hormone (FSH) secretion and luteinizing hormone (LH) secretion.

The follicular phase
During the follicular phase, the follicle stimulated by FSH reaches full size and increases its secretion of estrogen. Simultaneously, FSH secretion decreases and LH secretion increases slowly but steadily. During the late follicular phase, LH secretion increases sharply and FSH secretion increases slightly. At about the 14th day, within hours of this abrupt surge in LH, estrogen levels in the plasma drop and ovulation occurs. After ovulation, LH and FSH levels fall rapidly.

The luteal phase
During the luteal phase, the follicle reorganizes as the corpus luteum secretes progesterone and estrogen. Within 7 to 8 days after ovulation, if fertilization hasn't occurred, the corpus luteum regresses and progesterone and estrogen levels decrease. The endometrium sloughs, and the menstrual cycle begins again.

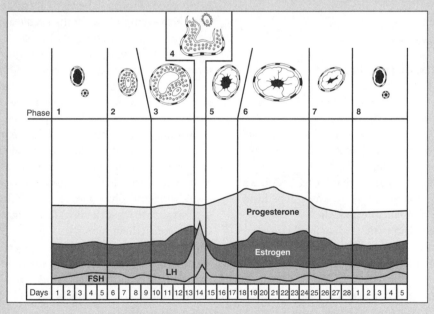

1. Menstrual phase (degeneration of corpus luteum)
2. Early follicular phase (development of follicle)
3. Late follicular phase (development of follicle)
4. Ovulation at midcycle (rupture of follicle)
5. Early luteal phase (development of corpus luteum)
6. Midluteal phase (development of corpus luteum)
7. Late luteal phase (development of corpus luteum)
8. Menstrual phase (degeneration of corpus luteum)

Lyme disease serology

Lyme disease is a multisystem disorder characterized by dermatologic, neurologic, cardiac, and rheumatic manifestations in various stages. Epidemiologic and serologic studies implicate a common tickborne spirochete, *Borrelia burgdorferi*, as the cause. Serologic tests for Lyme disease, both indirect immunofluorescent and enzyme-linked immunosorbent assays, measure antibody response to this spirochete and indicate current infection or past exposure. Serologic tests are able to identify 50% of patients with early stage Lyme disease and all patients with later complications of carditis, neuritis, and arthritis as well as patients in remission.

Purpose
■ To confirm a diagnosis of Lyme disease

Cost
Moderately expensive

Patient preparation
■ Explain to the patient that this test helps determine whether Lyme disease is the cause of his symptoms.
■ Instruct the patient to fast for 12 hours before the sample is drawn, but to drink fluids as usual.
■ Tell the patient that the test requires a blood sample. Explain who will perform the venipuncture and when.
■ Explain to the patient that he may experience discomfort from the needle puncture and the tourniquet.

Normal findings
Normal serum values are nonreactive.

Abnormal findings
A positive Lyme serology can help confirm diagnosis, but it isn't definitive. Other treponemal diseases and high rheumatoid factor titers can cause false-positive results. More than 15% of patients with Lyme disease fail to develop antibodies.

Interfering factors
■ Elevated serum lipid levels (possible inaccurate results, requiring that the test be repeated after a period of restricted fat intake)
■ Samples contaminated with other bacteria (possible false-positive)
■ Hemolysis due to rough handling of the sample

Lymph node biopsy

Lymph node biopsy is the surgical excision of an active lymph node or the needle aspiration of a nodal specimen for histologic examination. Both techniques usually use a local anesthetic and sample the superficial nodes in the cervical, supraclavicular, axillary, or inguinal region. Excision is preferred because it yields a larger specimen.

Although lymph nodes swell during infection, biopsy is indicated when nodal enlargement is prolonged and accompanied by backache, leg edema, breathing and swallowing difficulties and, later, weight loss, weakness, severe itching, fever, night sweats, cough, hemoptysis, and hoarseness. Generalized or localized lymph node enlargement is typical with such diseases as chronic lymphatic leukemia, Hodgkin's disease, infectious mononucleosis, and rheumatoid arthritis.

Complete blood cell count, liver function studies, liver and spleen scans, and X-rays should precede this test.

Purpose

■ To determine the cause of lymph node enlargement
■ To distinguish between benign and malignant lymph node processes
■ To stage metastatic cancer

Cost

Very expensive

Patient preparation

■ Explain to the patient that this test allows microscopic study of lymph node tissue.
■ Describe the procedure to the patient. Tell him who will perform the biopsy and where it will take place.
■ For excisional biopsy, instruct the patient to restrict food after midnight and to drink only clear liquids on the morning of the test (if general anesthesia is needed for deeper nodes, he must also restrict fluids). For needle biopsy, he need not restrict food or fluids.
■ Obtain informed consent if necessary.
■ Check the patient's history for hypersensitivity to the anesthetic.
■ If the patient will receive a local anesthetic, explain to him that he may experience discomfort during the injection.

Normal findings

The normal lymph node is encapsulated by collagenous connective tissue and divided into smaller lobes by tissue strands called trabeculae. It has an outer cortex, made up of lymphoid cells and nodules or follicles containing lymphocytes, and an inner medulla, made up of reticular phagocytic cells that collect and drain fluid.

Abnormal findings

Histologic examination of the tissue specimen distinguishes between malignant and nonmalignant causes of lymph node enlargement. Lymphatic cancer accounts for up to 5% of all cancers and is slightly more prevalent in males than in females. Hodgkin's disease, a lymphoma affecting the entire lymph system, is the leading cancer affecting adolescents and young adults. Lymph node cancer may also result from metastatic cancer.

When histologic results are unclear or nodular material isn't involved, mediastinoscopy or laparotomy can provide another nodal specimen. Occasionally, lymphangiography can furnish additional diagnostic information.

Interfering factors

■ Failure to obtain a representative tissue specimen or improper specimen storage
■ Inability to differentiate nodal pathology

Lymphocyte transformation

Transformation tests evaluate lymphocyte competence without the injection of antigens into the patient's skin. These in vitro tests eliminate the risk of adverse reactions but can still accurately assess the ability of lymphocytes to proliferate and to recognize and respond to antigens.

The mitogen assay, performed using nonspecific plant lectins, evaluates the miotic response of T and B lymphocytes to a foreign antigen. In the mitogen assay, a purified culture of lymphocytes from the patient's blood is incubated with a nonspecific mitogen for 72 hours — the interval during which the greatest effect on deoxyribonucleic acid (DNA) synthesis usually occurs. The culture is then pulse-labeled with tritiated thymidine, which is incorporated in the newly formed DNA of dividing cells.

The uptake of radioactive thymidine can be measured by a liquid scintillation spectrophotometer in counts per minute, which parallels the rate of mitosis. Lymphocyte responsiveness, or the extent of mitosis, is then reported as a stimulation index, determined by dividing the counts per minute of the stimulated culture by the counts per minute of a control culture. The antigen assay uses specific antigens (such as purified protein derivative, *Candida*, mumps, tetanus toxoid, and streptokinase) to stimulate lymphocyte transformation. After an incubation period of 4½ to 7 days, transformation is measured by the same method used in the mitogen assay.

The mixed lymphocyte culture (MLC) assay tests the response of lymphocytes to histocompatibility antigens determined by the D locus of the sixth chromosome. The MLC assay is useful in matching transplant recipients and donors and in testing immunocompetence. In this assay, lymphocytes from a recipient and a potential donor are cultured together for 5 days to test compatibility. Recipient and potential donor lymphocytes (if viable and unaltered) will recognize any genetic differences and undergo transformation, demonstrating incompatibility. In the one-way MLC, one group of lymphocytes is pretreated with radiation or mitomycin C so that it can't divide but can still stimulate the other group of lymphocytes.

Lymphocyte transformation is identified by an increased incorporation of radioactive thymidine labeling and is reported as the stimulation index. After the culture is labeled with radioactive thymidine, the MLC stimulation index is determined. Various lymphocyte marker assays can be performed to analyze malignant and normal cell populations. (See *Lymphocyte marker assays*.)

The ability of the neutrophils to engulf and destroy bacteria and foreign particles can also be determined.

Purpose
■ To assess and monitor genetic and acquired immunodeficiency states
■ To provide histocompatibility typing of both tissue transplant recipients and donors
■ To detect if a patient has been exposed to various pathogens, such as those that cause malaria, hepatitis, or mycoplasmal pneumonia

Cost
Expensive

Patient preparation
■ Explain to the patient that this test evaluates lymphocyte function, which is the keystone of the immune system. If appropriate, inform him that the test monitors his response to therapy. For histocompatibility typing, explain that this test helps determine the best match for a transplant.
■ Tell the patient that the test requires a blood sample. Explain who will perform the venipuncture and when.
■ Explain to the patient that he may experience discomfort from the needle puncture and the tourniquet.
■ Tell the patient that if a radioisotope scan is scheduled, the serum sample for this test is drawn first.

Normal findings
Results depend on the mitogens used. Reference ranges accompany test results. In general, a positive test result is normal; a negative test result indicates deficiency.

Lymphocyte marker assays

A normal immune response requires a balance between the regulatory activities of several interacting cell types, most notably T-helper and T-suppressor cells. By using highly specific monoclonal antibodies, levels of lymphocyte differentiation can be defined and normal and malignant cell populations analyzed. Direct and indirect immunofluorescence, microcytotoxicity, and immunoperoxidase immunoassay are the most commonly used techniques: They use an anticoagulated blood sample combined with monoclonal antibodies that react with specific T- and B-cell markers. The chart below lists some commonly ordered lymphocyte marker assays and their indications.

LYMPHOCYTE MARKER ASSAY	PURPOSE
Pan T-cell marker (CD3)	■ To measure mature T cells in immune dysfunction
T-helper/inducer subset marker (CD4)	■ To identify and characterize the proportion of T-helper cells in autoimmune or immunoregulatory disorders ■ To detect immunodeficiency disorders such as acquired immunodeficiency syndrome ■ To differentiate T-cell acute lymphoblastic leukemia from T-cell lymphomas and other lymphoproliferative disorders
T-suppressor/cytotoxic subset marker (CD8)	■ To identify and characterize the proportion of T-suppressor cells in autoimmune and immunoregulartory disorders
T-cell/E-Rosette receptor (CD2)	■ To characterize lymphoproliferative disorders
Pan-B (B-1) marker (CD20)	■ To differentiate lymphoproliferative disorders of T-cell origin, such as T-cell lymphocytic leukemia, from those of T-cell origin
Pan-B (BA-1) marker (CD19)	■ To identify B-cell lymphoproliferative disorders such as B-cell chronic lymphocytic leukemia
CALLA (common acute lymphocytic leukemia antigen) marker, CD10	■ To identify bone marrow regeneration ■ To identify non-T-cell lymphocytic leukemia
Lymphocyte subset panel (CD3/CD4/CD8/CD19)	■ To evaluate immunodeficiencies ■ To identify immunoregulation associated with autoimmune disorders ■ To characterize lymphoid neoplasms
Lymphocytic leukemia marker panel (CD3/CD4/CD8/CD19/CD10)	■ To characterize lymphocytic leukemias as T, B, non-T, or non-B, regardless of the stage of differentiation of the malignant cells

Abnormal findings

In the mitogen and antigen assays, a low stimulation index or unresponsiveness indicates a depressed or defective immune system. Serial testing can be performed to monitor the effectiveness of therapy in a patient with an immunodeficiency disease.

In the MLC test, the stimulation index is a measure of compatibility. A high index indicates poor compatibility; conversely, a low stimulation index indicates good compatibility.

A high stimulation index in response to the relevant pathogen can also demonstrate exposure to malaria, hepatitis, mycoplasmal pneumonia, periodontal disease, and certain viral infections in patients who no longer have detectable serum antibodies.

Interfering factors

- Pregnancy or the use of hormonal contraceptives (depressed lymphocyte response to phytohemagglutinin and thus a low stimulation index)
- Chemotherapy (possible inaccurate results, unless pretherapy baseline values are available for comparison)
- A radioisotope scan performed within 1 week before the test or failure to send the sample to the laboratory immediately after collection (possible inaccurate results)

Lymphangiography

Lymphangiography (or lymphography) is the radiographic examination of the lymphatic system after the injection of an oil-based contrast medium into a lymphatic vessel in each foot or, less commonly, in each hand. This test is no longer widely used.

Injection into the foot allows visualization of the lymphatics of the leg, inguinal and iliac regions, and the retroperitoneum up to the thoracic duct. Injection into the hand allows visualization of the axillary and supraclavicular nodes. Although this procedure may also be used to study the cervical region (retroauricular area), it's less useful for this purpose and is, therefore, less common.

X-ray films are taken immediately after injection to demonstrate the filling of the lymphatic system and then again 24 hours later to visualize the lymph nodes. Because the contrast medium remains in the nodes for up to 2 years, subsequent X-ray films can assess progression of disease and monitor effectiveness of treatment.

ALERT! ▼ ▼ ▼ ▼ ▼ ▼ ▼ ▼ ▼

Lymphangiography is contraindicated in patients with hypersensitivity to iodine, pulmonary insufficiency, cardiac disease, or severe renal or liver disease.

Purpose

- To detect and stage lymphomas and to identify metastatic involvement of the lymph nodes (computed tomography [CT] scan is used more frequently for staging) (See *Staging malignant lymphoma.*)
- To distinguish primary from secondary lymphedema
- To suggest surgical treatment or evaluate the effectiveness of chemotherapy and radiation therapy in controlling malignancy
- To investigate enlarged lymph nodes detected by CT scan or ultrasonography

Cost

Very expensive

Patient preparation

- Explain to the patient that this test permits examination of the lymphatic system through X-ray films taken after the injection of a contrast medium.

- Tell the patient who will perform the procedure and where it will take place. Also tell him that additional X-ray films will be taken the following day.
- Inform the patient that blue contrast medium will be injected into each foot over a period of time to outline the lymphatic vessels. Tell him that the injection causes transient discomfort and that the contrast medium discolors urine and stool for 48 hours. Also tell him that the contrast medium may give his skin and vision a bluish tinge for 48 hours.
- Tell the patient that a local anesthetic will be injected before a small incision is made in each foot.
- Advise the patient that he must remain as still as possible during injection of the contrast medium, and that he may experience some discomfort in the popliteal or inguinal areas at the beginning of the injection of the contrast medium.
- If this test is performed on an outpatient basis, advise the patient to have a friend or relative accompany him.
- Warn the patient that the incision site may be sore for several days after the procedure.
- Obtain informed consent if necessary.
- Check the patient's history to determine if he's hypersensitive to iodine, seafood, or the contrast media used in other diagnostic tests such as excretory urography.
- Tell the patient he may receive a sedative and an oral antihistamine just before the procedure (if hypersensitivity to the contrast medium is suspected).
- Fluoroscopy may be used to monitor filling of the lymphatic system.

Staging malignant lymphoma

Stage I: Involvement of a single lymph node region or of a single extralymphatic organ or site

Stage II: Involvement of two or more lymph node regions on the same side of the diaphragm or localized involvement of an extralymphatic organ or the site of one or more lymph node regions on the same side of the diaphragm

Stage III: Involvement of lymph node regions on both sides of the diaphragm, which may also be accompanied by localized involvement of an extralymphatic organ or site or of the spleen (or both)

Stage IV: Diffuse or disseminated involvement of one or more extralymphatic organs or tissues, with or without associated lymph node enlargement

Normal findings

The lymphatic system normally demonstrates homogeneous and complete filling with contrast medium on the initial films. On the 24-hour films, the lymph nodes are fully opacified and well circumscribed; the lymphatic channels are emptied a few hours after injection of the contrast medium.

Abnormal findings

Enlarged, foamy-looking nodes indicate Hodgkin's disease or malignant lymphoma. Filling defects or lack of opacification indicates metastatic involvement of the lymph nodes. The number of nodes affected, unilateral or bilateral involvement, and the extent of extranodal involvement help determine staging of lymphoma.

However, definitive staging may require additional diagnostic tests, such as a CT scan, ultrasonography, selective biopsy, or laparotomy.

In differential diagnosis of primary and secondary lymphedema, shortened lymphatic vessels and a deficient number of vessels indicate primary lymphedema. Abruptly terminating lymphatic vessels — caused by retroperitoneal tumors impinging on the vessels, inflammation, filariasis, or trauma resulting from surgery or radiation — indicate secondary lymphedema.

Interfering factors
■ Inability to cannulate the lymphatic vessels (precludes the use of the test)

M

Magnesium

The magnesium test is used to measure serum levels of magnesium, an electrolyte that's vital to neuromuscular function and also helps in intracellular metabolism, activates many essential enzymes, and affects the metabolism of nucleic acids and proteins. Magnesium also helps transport sodium and potassium across cell membranes, and influences intracellular calcium levels. Most magnesium is found in bone and intracellular fluid; a small amount is found in extracellular fluid. Magnesium is absorbed by the small intestine and excreted in the urine and stool.

Purpose
■ To evaluate electrolyte status
■ To assess neuromuscular and renal function

Cost
Inexpensive

Patient preparation
■ Explain to the patient that this test is used to determine the magnesium content of the blood.

■ Instruct the patient not to use magnesium salts (such as milk of magnesia or Epsom salt) for at least 3 days before the test, but tell him that he need not restrict food and fluids.
■ Tell the patient that the test requires a blood sample. Explain who will perform the venipuncture and when.
■ Explain to the patient that he may experience discomfort from the needle puncture and the tourniquet.

Reference values
Serum magnesium levels range from 1.3 to 2.1 mg/dl (SI, 0.65 to 1.05 mmol/L).

Abnormal findings
Elevated serum magnesium levels (hypermagnesemia) most commonly occur in patients with renal failure or with kidneys that excrete inadequate amounts of magnesium and in patients who have ingested magnesium. Adrenal insufficiency (Addison's disease) can also increase serum magnesium levels.
ALERT! ▼ ▼ ▼ ▼ ▼ ▼ ▼ ▼ ▼
Patients with elevated magnesium levels require electrocardiogram (ECG) monitoring. The practitioner should be aware of changes, such as bradycardia, prolonged PR interval,

wide QRS complex, prolonged QT interval, atrioventricular block, and asystole.

Decreased serum magnesium levels (hypomagnesemia) most commonly result from chronic alcoholism. Other causes include malabsorption syndrome, diarrhea, faulty absorption after bowel resection, prolonged bowel or gastric aspiration, acute pancreatitis, primary aldosteronism, severe burns, hypercalcemic conditions (including hyperparathyroidism), malnutrition, and therapy with certain diuretics.

ALERT! ▼ ▼ ▼ ▼ ▼ ▼ ▼ ▼ ▼

For patients with hypomagnesemia, monitor the ECG for tachycardia, widened QRS complex, prolonged QT interval, ST segment depression, and T-wave inversion.

Interfering factors

- Venous stasis due to tourniquet use
- Obtaining a sample above an I.V. site that's receiving a solution containing magnesium
- Excessive use of antacids or cathartics or excessive infusion of magnesium sulfate (increase)
- Prolonged I.V. infusions without magnesium; excessive use of diuretics (decrease)
- I.V. administration of calcium gluconate (possible false-low if measured using the Titan yellow method)
- Hemolysis (false-high)

Magnetic resonance imaging

Magnetic resonance imaging (MRI) uses a powerful magnetic field and radiofrequency waves to produce computerized images of internal organs and tissues. MRI eliminates the risks associated with exposure to X-ray beams and causes no harm to cells.

During an MRI scan, the patient is placed on a table that slides into a cylindrical magnet. The magnet causes the body's atomic protons to line up and spin in the same direction. A radiofrequency beam is then introduced into the magnetic field, causing the protons to move out of alignment. When the beam is stopped, the protons realign and release energy. The release of proton energy is detected as a signal. A receiver coil measures the signal, and these measurements provide information about the type of tissue in which the protons lie. A computer uses this information to construct an image on a video monitor, showing the proton distribution of certain atoms.

ALERT! ▼ ▼ ▼ ▼ ▼ ▼ ▼ ▼ ▼

MRIs are usually contraindicated in pregnant patients and, if I.V. contrast medium is used, in patients with hypersensitivity to iodine or with severe renal or hepatic disease. It's also contraindicated in patients with a metal implant, rod, screw, prosthetic device, or pacemaker. The scanner can't be used with patients who are extremely obese.

Purpose

- To produce tissue analysis and images not readily seen on standard X-rays

Cost

Very expensive

Patient preparation

- Describe the procedure to the patient. Inform him that he'll be placed on a narrow flat table, which is positioned inside a scanning gantry, and that the procedure takes 30 to 90 minutes.
- Tell the patient who will perform the scan and where it will take place.
- Tell the patient that he will be asked to remove any metal objects he's carrying or

wearing and that he'll need to remain still for the duration of the procedure.

■ If the patient is claustrophobic, he may be a candidate for an open MRI. (See *Open MRI.*)

■ If a contrast medium is to be used, tell the patient that an I.V. line will be started and the medium administered before the procedure.

Normal findings

Normal findings include normal anatomy without problems or disorders detected.

Abnormal findings

MRI can detect abnormalities of the bone and soft tissue of any organ or system.

Interfering factors

■ Inability of the patient to remain still during the test (possible poor imaging)

■ Use of I.V. pumps or assistive life-support equipment with metal components (possible poor imaging)

■ Playing of the radio during the MRI (possible poor imaging due to interference with the radiofrequency waves of the scanner)

Mammography

Mammography is used as a screening test for breast cancer. It helps to detect breast cysts or tumors, especially those not palpable on physical examination. Biopsy of suspicious areas may be required to confirm malignancy. Mammography may follow screening procedures such as ultrasonography or thermography. Although mammography can detect 90% to 95% of breast cancers, this test produces many false-positive results.

The American College of Radiologists and the American Cancer Society have es-

Open MRI

With an open magnetic resonance imaging (MRI) unit, the patient is only partially enclosed in a tunnel, making the unit ideal for patients with claustrophobia. Open MRI units are low-field units (0.2 to 0.5 Tesla) as opposed to closed MRI units, which are typically high-field units (1.0 to 1.5 or greater Tesla). The image quality is almost always better in a high-field unit, not only because of the field strength but also because of the gradient speed and strength, surface coils, and software.

Accurate diagnosis may be difficult unless the interpreting radiologist has experience reading low-field units. If results with an open MRI are equivocal, a repeat closed MRI should be done. For small body parts (such as the hand, wrist, foot, ankle, or elbow), a high-resolution closed MRI is recommended. Some practitioners prefer a high-resolution MRI for the cervical spine as well, because small extradural defects in the neural foramina are difficult to see even when using a high-field unit.

tablished separate guidelines for the use and potential risks of mammography. Both groups agree that despite low radiation levels, the test is contraindicated in pregnant patients. Magnetic resonance imaging, which is highly sensitive, is becoming a more popular method of breast imaging; however, it isn't very specific and leads to biopsies of many benign lesions. For those at high risk for breast cancer, a newer test, ductal lavage, may identify abnormal cells before they're large enough to form a tumor.

Purpose

- To screen for malignant breast tumors
- To investigate palpable and unpalpable breast masses, breast pain, or nipple discharge
- To help differentiate between benign breast disease and breast cancer
- To monitor patients with breast cancer who have been treated with breast-conserving surgery and radiation

Cost

Moderately expensive

Patient preparation

- Assess the patient's understanding of the test, answer her questions, and correct any misconceptions.
- Tell the patient who will perform the test and where it will take place.
- Tell the patient not to use underarm deodorant or powder on the day of the examination.
- If the patient has breast implants, tell her to inform the staff when she schedules the mammogram to ensure that a technologist familiar with imaging implants is on duty when she comes in.
- Explain to the patient that although the test takes only about 15 minutes to perform, she may be asked to wait while the films are checked to ensure they're readable.

Normal findings

A normal mammogram reveals normal duct, glandular tissue, and fat architecture. No abnormal masses or calcifications should be seen.

Abnormal findings

Well-outlined, regular, and clear spots suggest benign cysts; irregular, poorly outlined, and opaque areas suggest a malignant tumor. Malignant tumors are generally solitary and unilateral; benign cysts tend to occur bilaterally. Findings that suggest cancer require other tests, such as biopsy, for confirmation.

Interfering factors

- Powders or salves on the breasts (possible false-positive)
- Failure to remove jewelry and clothing (possible false-positive or poor imaging)
- Very glandular breasts (common in patients younger than age 30), active lactation, or previous breast surgery (possible poor imaging)
- Breast implants (possible hindrance in the detection of masses)

Mediastinoscopy

Using an exploring speculum with built-in fiber light and side slit, mediastinoscopy allows direct viewing of mediastinal structures. It also permits palpation and biopsy of paratracheal and carinal lymph nodes. This surgical procedure is indicated when other tests (such as sputum cytology, lung scans, radiography, and bronchoscopic biopsy) fail to confirm the diagnosis.

Purpose

- To detect bronchogenic carcinoma, lymphoma (including Hodgkin's disease), and sarcoidosis
- To determine stages of lung cancer (See *Staging lung cancer.*)

Cost

Very expensive

Patient preparation

- Explain to the patient that this test is used to evaluate the lymph nodes and other structures in the chest. Review the patient's history for previous mediastinos-

CLASSIFICATION	DEFINITION
Primary tumor (T)	
T0	No evidence of primary tumor
TX	Tumor proven by malignant cells in bronchopulmonary secretions but not visualized by radiography or bronchoscopy
TIS	Carcinoma in situ
T1	Tumor that is 3 cm (1⅛") or less in diameter, surrounded by normal lung or visceral pleura
T2	Tumor that is more than 3 cm in diameter or tumor of any size that invades the visceral pleura or extends to the hilar region; tumor that lies within a lobar bronchus or at least 2 cm (¾") from the carina; any associated atelectasis or obstructive pneumonitis involves less than an entire lung
T3	Tumor of any size that extends into neighboring structures, such as the chest wall, diaphragm, or mediastinum; that involves a main bronchus less than 2 cm from the carina; or that occurs with atelectasis or obstructive pneumonitis of an entire lung or with pleural effusion
Regional lymph nodes (N)	
N0	No demonstrable metastasis to regional lymph nodes
N1	Metastasis to peribronchial or ipsilateral hilar lymph nodes
N2	Metastasis to mediastinal lymph nodes
Distant metastasis (M)	
M0	No distant metastasis
M1	Distant metastasis, such as to scalene, cervical, or contralateral hilar lymph nodes as well as to brain, bones, lung, or liver
Stage grouping (T, N, and M factors may be combined into the following groups or stages)	
Occult carcinoma TX N0 M0	Bronchopulmonary secretions contain malignant cells; no other evidence of the primary tumor or of metastasis

(continued)

CLASSIFICATION	DEFINITION
Stage grouping *(continued)*	
Stage I TIS N0 M0	Carcinoma in situ
T1 N0 M0	Tumor classified as T1 without metastasis to the regional lymph nodes
T1 N1 M0	Tumor classified as T1 with metastasis to the ipsilateral hilar lymph nodes only
T2 N0 M0	Tumor classified as T2 without metastasis to nodes or distant metastasis
(Note: TX N1 M0 and T0 N1 M0 also fall under stage I but are difficult, if not impossible, to diagnose.)	
Stage II T2 N1 M0	Tumor classified as T2 with metastasis to ipsilateral hilar lymph nodes only
Stage III T3 (with any N or M)	Any tumor more extensive than T2
N3 (with any T or M)	Any tumor with metastasis to mediastinal lymph nodes
M1 (with any T or N)	Any tumor with distant metastasis

copy because scarring from a previous mediastinoscopy contraindicates the test.
■ Describe the procedure to the patient. Tell him who will perform the procedure and where it will take place.
■ Inform the patient that he'll be given general anesthesia and that he may receive a sedative the night before the test and again before the procedure.
■ Instruct the patient to fast after midnight before the test.
■ Tell the patient that he may have temporary chest pain, tenderness at the incision site, or a sore throat (from intubation). Reassure him that complications are rare with this procedure.
■ Obtain informed consent if necessary.
■ Check the patient's history for hypersensitivity to the anesthetic.

Normal findings

Lymph nodes appear as small, smooth, flat oval bodies of lymphoid tissue.

Abnormal findings

Malignant lymph nodes usually indicate inoperable, but not always untreatable, lung or esophageal cancer or lymphomas (such as Hodgkin's disease). Staging of lung cancer helps determine the therapeutic regimen. (For example, multiple nodular involvement can contraindicate surgery.)

Interfering factors

■ Previous mediastinoscopy with scarring (makes dissection of nodes difficult or impossible)

Methemoglobin

Methemoglobin (MetHb, Hb M) is a structural hemoglobin (Hb) variant, which is formed when the heme portion of deoxygenated Hb is oxidized to a ferric state. When this occurs, the heme is incapable of combining with oxygen and transporting it to the tissues, and the patient becomes cyanotic.

Purpose
■ To detect acquired methemoglobinemia, which is caused by excessive radiation or the toxic effects of chemicals or drugs
■ To detect congenital methemoglobinemia

Cost
Inexpensive

Patient preparation
■ If possible, obtain a history of the patient's hematologic status. Find out whether he has had a Hb disorder, a condition that produces nitrite, or exposure to sources of nitrites in drugs.
■ Explain to the patient that this test is used to detect abnormal Hb in the blood.
■ Tell the patient that the test requires a blood sample. Explain who will perform the venipuncture and when.
■ Explain to the patient that he may experience discomfort from the needle puncture and the tourniquet.
■ Restrict medications that may affect test results. If they must be continued, note this on the laboratory request.

Reference values
Normal MetHb levels are 0% to 1.5% (SI, 0 to 0.015) of total Hb.

Abnormal findings
Increased MetHb levels may indicate acquired or hereditary methemoglobinemia

or carbon monoxide poisoning. These levels can also result from the use of certain drugs or exposure to certain substances.

Decreased MetHb levels may occur with pancreatitis.

Interfering factors
■ Acetanilid, aniline dyes, benzocaine, chlorates, lidocaine, nitrates, nitrites, nitroglycerin, primaquine, radiation, resorcinol, and sulfonamides (possible increase)
■ Nitrite toxicity in breast-feeding infants (increase due to conversion of inorganic nitrate to nitrite ion)

Monoclonal test for cytomegalovirus, rapid

Cytomegalovirus (CMV), a member of the herpesvirus group, can cause systemic infection in congenitally infected infants and in immunocompromised patients, such as transplant recipients, patients receiving chemotherapy for neoplastic disease, and those with acquired immunodeficiency syndrome.

In the past, CMV infections were detected in the laboratory by recognizing the distinctive cytopathic effects that the virus produced in conventional tube cell cultures. In this slow method of detecting CMV, cytopathic effect cultures grow in about 9 days. The faster shell vial assay (rapid monoclonal test) is based on the availability of a monoclonal antibody specific for the 72 kd protein of CMV synthesized during the immediate early stage of viral replication.

Through indirect immunofluorescence, CMV-infected fibroblasts are recognized by their dense, homogeneous staining confined to the nucleus. Because of the smooth, regular shape of the nucleus and the surrounding nuclear membrane, infected cells are readily differentiated from nonspecific background fluorescence that may be present in some specimens.

Purpose
■ To obtain rapid laboratory diagnosis of CMV infection, especially in immunocompromised patients who have or who are at risk for developing systemic infections caused by this virus

Cost
Moderately expensive

Patient preparation
■ Explain to the patient the purpose of the test, and describe the procedure for collecting the specimen (throat, urine, cerebrospinal fluid, bronchoalveolar lavage tissue, or blood), which will depend on the laboratory used.

Normal findings
CMV shouldn't appear in a culture specimen.

Abnormal findings
CMV can be detected in urine and throat specimens from patients who are asymptomatic. However, detection from these sites indicates active, asymptomatic infection, which may herald symptomatic involvement, especially in immunocompromised patients. Detection of CMV in blood samples, tissue specimens, and specimens from bronchoalveolar lavage generally indicates systemic infection and disease.

Interfering factors
■ Administration of antiviral drugs before collection of the specimen (possible interference with detection of CMV)

Myelography

Myelography uses fluoroscopy and radiography to evaluate the spinal subarachnoid space after injection of a contrast medium. Because the contrast medium is heavier than cerebrospinal fluid (CSF), it flows through the subarachnoid space to the dependent area when the patient, lying prone on a fluoroscopic table, is tilted up or down. The fluoroscope allows visualization of the flow of the contrast medium and the outline of the subarachnoid space. X-rays are taken to provide a permanent record.

ALERT! ▼ ▼ ▼ ▼ ▼ ▼ ▼ ▼ ▼
Generally, myelography is contraindicated in patients with increased intracranial pressure, hypersensitivity to iodine or contrast media, or infection at the puncture site.

Purpose
■ To evaluate and determine the cause of neurologic symptoms (numbness, pain, weakness)
■ To identify lesions, such as tumors and herniated intervertebral disks, that partially or totally block the flow of CSF in the subarachnoid space
■ To help detect arachnoiditis, spinal nerve root injury, or tumors in the posterior fossa of the skull

Cost
Very expensive

Patient preparation
■ Explain to the patient that this test reveals obstructions in the spinal cord.
■ Describe the test for the patient, including who will administer it and where it will take place.
■ Tell the patient that his food and fluid intake will be restricted for 8 hours before the test. If the test is scheduled for the after-

noon and facility policy permits, the patient may have clear liquids before the test.

■ Explain to the patient that he may feel a transient burning sensation as the contrast medium is injected; a warm, flushed feeling; transient headache; a salty taste; or nausea and vomiting after the dye is injected. Explain that he may feel some pain caused by his positioning and the needle insertion.

■ Obtain informed consent if necessary.

■ Check the patient's history for hypersensitivity to iodine, substances that contain iodine (for example, shellfish and certain drugs), and radiographic contrast media.

■ Notify the radiologist if the patient has a history of epilepsy or phenothiazine use. If metrizamide is to be used as a contrast medium, instruct the patient to stop taking the phenothiazine 48 hours before the test.

■ Tell the patient that after the test he'll be monitored closely and that the head of his bed will be elevated. Tell him he'll remain on bed rest for an additional 6 to 8 hours.

■ If metrizamide is to be used, tell the patient that he'll need to stay in bed for 12 to 16 hours after the test. If an oil-based contrast agent is used, inform him that it will be manually removed after the test and that he'll need to remain flat in bed for 6 to 24 hours. (See *Removing contrast media after myelography*.)

■ If the puncture is to be performed in the lumbar region, tell the patient an enema may be prescribed. A sedative and anticholinergic (such as atropine sulfate) may be prescribed to reduce swallowing during the procedure. Make sure that pretest laboratory work (may include coagulation and kidney function studies) is indicated on the patient's chart.

■ Tell the patient that after the contrast medium is injected, the table may be tilted and the flow of the contrast medium observed by fluoroscope. Also tell the patient that X-rays will be taken.

Normal findings

Normally, the contrast medium flows freely through the subarachnoid space, showing no obstruction or structural abnormalities.

Abnormal findings

Myelography identifies and localizes lesions within or surrounding the spinal cord or subarachnoid space. Examples of common extradural lesions include herniated intervertebral disks and metastatic tumors. Neurofibromas and meningiomas are common lesions within the subarachnoid space, and ependymomas and astrocytomas are common within the spinal cord.

If the test confirms a spinal tumor, the patient may be taken directly to the operating room. Immediate surgery may also be necessary if the contrast medium causes a total block of the subarachnoid space.

Myelography can also help locate or confirm a ruptured or herniated disk, spinal stenosis, or abscess and, occasionally, confirm the need for surgery. This test may also detect syringomyelia (a congenital abnormality marked by fluid-filled cavities within the spinal cord and widening of the cord itself), arachnoiditis, spinal nerve root injury, and tumors in the posterior fossa of the skull. Other findings may include fractures, dislocations, thinning of bones (osteoporosis), deformities in the curvature of the spine, bone spurs, and vertebral degeneration. Test results must be correlated with the patient's history and clinical status.

Interfering factors

- Incorrect needle placement
- Lack of patient cooperation

Myocardial perfusion imaging, radiopharmaceutical

Radiopharmaceutical myocardial perfusion imaging, also known as *chemical stress imaging,* is an alternative method of assessing coronary vessel function in patients who can't tolerate exercise electrocardiography (ECG).

In this test, I.V. infusion of a selected drug — for example, adenosine, dipyridamole, or dobutamine — is used to simulate the effects of exercise by increasing blood flow in the coronary arteries. Next, a radiopharmaceutical is injected I.V. to allow imaging that assists in evaluating the cardiac vessel's response to the drug-induced stress. Both resting and stress images are obtained to evaluate coronary perfusion.

ALERT! ▼ ▼ ▼ ▼ ▼ ▼ ▼ ▼ ▼
Radiopharmaceutical myocardial perfusion imaging is usually contraindicated in women who are pregnant. Furthermore, the use of adenosine or dipyridamole is contraindicated in patients with bronchospastic lung disease or asthma. Other contraindications to the test include a myocardial infarction within 10 days of testing, acute myocarditis or pericarditis, unstable angina, arrhythmias, hypertension or hypotension, aortic or mital stenosis, hyperthyroidism, or severe infection.

Purpose

- To assess the presence and degree of coronary artery disease (CAD)
- To evaluate therapeutic procedures, such as bypass surgery or coronary angioplasty
- To evaluate myocardial perfusion

Cost

Very expensive

Patient preparation

- Describe the test, including who will perform it and where it will take place.
- Tell the patient he'll need to arrive 1 hour before the test and that an I.V. line will be initiated before the test.
- If the patient will receive adenosine or dipyridamole, instruct him to avoid taking any drug that contains theophylline for 24 to 36 hours before the test and to avoid consuming caffeinated drinks for 12 hours beforehand.
- If the patient is to receive dobutamine and he takes a beta-adrenergic blocker, instruct him to stop taking the beta-adrenergic blocker 48 hours before the test.
- If the patient takes an antihypertensive, tell him to continue taking it. If his systolic blood pressure is higher than 200 mm Hg, the dobutamine stress test can't be done until his blood pressure is under control.
- Restrict beta-adrenergic blockers, calcium channel blockers, and angiotensin-converting enzyme inhibitors 36 hours before the test.
- If the patient takes a nitrate, tell him that he should stop taking it 6 hours before the test.
- If the patient is female, confirm that she isn't pregnant before performing the test.
- Tell the patient not to eat for 3 to 4 hours before the test, although he may have water. If he needs to continue approved medications, tell him to take them with sips of water.
- Screen the patient for bronchospastic lung disease or asthma. Adenosine and dipyridamole are contraindicated in these patients; dobutamine is used instead.
- Tell the patient that a cardiologist, a nurse, an ECG technician, and a nuclear medicine technologist will be present for the infusion of the medication. Advise him that he'll be weighed first to determine the proper drug dose.

- Inform the patient that he may experience flushing, shortness of breath, dizziness, headache, chest pain, and increased heart rate during the infusion, but that these signs and symptoms will stop as soon as the infusion ends. Also, reassure him that emergency equipment will be available, if needed.
- Obtain informed consent if necessary.
- Depending on which radiopharmaceutical is used, tell the patient that he'll either undergo imaging immediately or return for imaging 45 minutes to 2 hours later. Resting imaging may be done before stress imaging or 3 to 4 hours afterward, depending on the radiopharmaceutical used.

Normal findings

Imaging should reveal characteristic distribution of the radiopharmaceutical throughout the left ventrical and show no visible defects.

Abnormal findings

Cold spots are usually due to CAD but may result from myocardial fibrosis, attenuation due to soft tissue (for example, breasts and diaphragm), or coronary spasm. The absence of cold spots in the presence of CAD may result from insignificant artifact obstruction, single-vessel disease, or collateral circulation.

Interfering factors

- Certain drugs such as digoxin (possible false-positive)
- Cold spots due to artifacts, such as implants and electrodes
- Delayed imaging (possible absence of cold spots in the presence of CAD)

Myoglobin

The myoglobin test detects the presence of myoglobin — a red pigment found in the cytoplasm of cardiac and skeletal muscle cells — in the blood. Myoglobin functions as an oxygen-binding muscle protein. It's released into the bloodstream in patients with ischemia, trauma, or inflammation of the muscle.

Purpose
■ To estimate damage to skeletal or cardiac muscle tissue (as a nonspecific test)
■ To predict flare-ups of polymyositis
■ To determine specifically whether myocardial infarction (MI) has occurred

Cost
Moderately expensive

Patient preparation
■ Explain the purpose of the test to the patient.
■ Obtain a patient history, including disorders that may be associated with increased myoglobin levels.
■ Tell the patient that the test requires a blood sample. Explain who will perform the venipuncture and when.
■ Explain to the patient that he may experience discomfort from the needle puncture and the tourniquet.
■ Inform the patient that the results need to be correlated with other tests for a definitive diagnosis.

Reference values
Normal myoglobin values are 0 to 0.09 µg/ml (SI, 5 to 70 µ/L).

Abnormal findings
Besides an MI, increased myoglobin levels may occur with acute alcohol intoxication, dermatomyositis, hypothermia (with prolonged shivering), muscular dystrophy, polymyositis, rhabdomyolysis, severe burn injuries, trauma, severe renal failure, and systemic lupus erythematosus.

Interfering factors
■ Hemolysis or radioactive scans performed within 1 week of the test
■ Recent angina, cardioversion, or improper timing of the test (possible increase)
■ I.M. injection (possible false-positive)

N

Nasopharyngeal culture

A nasopharyngeal culture is used to evaluate nasopharyngeal secretions for the presence of pathogenic organisms. It requires direct microscopic examination of a Gram-stained smear of the specimen. Preliminary identification of organisms may be used to guide clinical management and determine the need for additional testing. Cultured pathogens may then require susceptibility testing to determine appropriate antimicrobial therapy.

Purpose
■ To identify pathogens causing upper respiratory tract symptoms
■ To identify proliferation of normal nasopharyngeal flora, which may be pathogenic in debilitated and other immunocompromised patients
■ To identify *Bordetella pertussis* and *Neisseria meningitidis*, especially in very young, elderly, or debilitated patients and asymptomatic carriers
■ Infrequently, to isolate viruses, especially to identify carriers of influenza virus A and B

Cost
Inexpensive

Patient preparation
■ Explain to the patient that this test is used to isolate the cause of nasopharyngeal infection.
■ Describe the procedure to the patient. Tell him that secretions will be obtained from the back of the nose and the throat, using a cotton-tipped swab.
■ Tell the patient who will collect the specimen and when.
■ Warn the patient that he may experience slight discomfort and gagging, but reassure him that obtaining the specimen takes less than 15 seconds.
■ If the patient has recently undergone antimicrobial therapy or chemotherapy, note that on the laboratory request. Also, if the suspected organism is *Corynebacterium diphtheriae* or *B. pertussis*, note that on the request as well because these organisms need special growth media.

Normal findings
Flora commonly found in the nasopharynx include nonhemolytic streptococci, alpha-hemolytic streptococci, organisms of the *Neisseria* species (except *N. meningitidis* and

N. gonorrhoeae), coagulase-negative staphy-lococci such as *Staphylococcus epidermidis* and, occasionally, the coagulase-positive *S. aureus*.

Abnormal findings

Pathogens include group A beta-hemolytic streptococci; occasionally groups B, C, and G beta-hemolytic streptococci; *B. pertussis, C. diphtheriae, S. aureus*; large numbers of pneumococci; *Haemophilus influenzae; Myxovirus influenzae*; paramyxoviruses; *Candida albicans; Mycoplasma* species; and *Mycobacterium tuberculosis*.

Interfering factors

■ Recent antimicrobial therapy (decreased bacterial growth)
■ Failure to keep a viral specimen cold, improper technique, or failure to send the specimen to the laboratory immediately after collection

Nephrotomography

In nephrotomography, special films are exposed before and after opacification of the renal arterial network and parenchyma with contrast medium. The resulting tomographic slices clearly delineate various linear layers of the kidneys while blurring structures in front of and behind these selected planes.

Nephrotomography can be performed as a separate procedure or as an adjunct to excretory urography. It's particularly helpful in visualizing space-occupying lesions suggested by excretory urography or retrograde ureteropyelography. Additional films are exposed to define the thickness of the wall of the mass and its interior. Other tests that may resolve nephrotomographic findings include renal angiography and radionuclide renal imaging.

ALERT! ▼ ▼ ▼ ▼ ▼ ▼ ▼ ▼ ▼
Nephrotomography should be performed with extreme caution in patients with hypersensitivity to iodine-based compounds, cardiovascular disease, or multiple myeloma, and in elderly and dehydrated patients with impaired renal function, as evidenced by elevated serum creatinine levels.

Purpose

■ To differentiate between a simple renal cyst and a solid neoplasm
■ To assess renal lacerations as well as posttraumatic nonperfused areas of the kidneys
■ To localize adrenal tumors when laboratory tests indicate their presence

Cost

Very expensive

Patient preparation

■ Explain to the patient that this test provides images of sections or layers of the renal tissues and blood vessels.
■ Instruct the patient to fast for 8 hours before the test. Tell him who will perform the test and where.
■ Tell the patient that he'll be positioned on an X-ray table and that he may hear loud, clacking sounds as the films are exposed. Tell him that he may experience transient adverse reactions to the contrast medium — usually a burning or stinging sensation at the injection site, flushing, and a metallic taste.
■ Obtain informed consent if necessary.
■ Check the patient's history for hypersensitivity to iodine or iodine-containing foods or to contrast media used in other diagnostic tests. If the patient has a history of sensitivity, tell him he may need antiallergenic prophylaxis (such as diphenhydramine), or that a non–iodine-containing

Simple cyst or solid tumor: Differential diagnosis in nephrotomography

FEATURE	CYST	TUMOR
Consistency	Homogeneous	Irregular
Contact with healthy renal tissue	Sharply distinct	Poorly resolved
Density	Radiolucent	Variable radiolucent patches (or same as normal renal parenchyma)
Shape	Spherical	Variable
Wall of lesion	Thin and well defined	Thick and irregular

contrast medium may be used, as necessary.

AGE ISSUE ✱ ✱ ✱ ✱ ✱
Elderly and dehydrated patients are at increased risk for contrast-induced renal failure. I.V. fluids may be ordered before the test to keep the patient hydrated and to decrease nephrotoxic potential.

■ Tell the patient that he'll be closely monitored after the test. The patient generally receives plenty of fluids (unless contraindicated), and serum creatinine levels are monitored because of the risk of contrast-induced renal failure.

Normal findings

The size, shape, and position of the kidneys appear within normal range, with no space-occupying lesions or other abnormalities.

Abnormal findings

Among the abnormalities detectable through nephrotomography are simple cysts and solid tumors, renal sinus–related lesions, ectopic renal lobes, adrenal tumors, areas of nonperfusion, and renal lacerations following trauma. (See *Simple cyst or solid tumor: Differential diagnosis in nephrotomography.*)

Interfering factors

■ Residual barium from a recent enema or other GI studies (possible poor imaging)

Nuclear medicine scans

Nuclear medicine scans permit imaging of specific body organs or systems by a scintillating scanning camera after I.V. injection, inhalation, or oral ingestion of a radioactive tracer compound.

(For information about a specific nuclear medicine scan, see the entries for cardiac blood pool imaging, gallium scanning, liver-spleen scanning, lung perfusion scan, lung ventilation scan, Persantine-thallium imaging, radioactive iodine uptake test, radionuclide thyroid imaging, and thallium imaging.)

ALERT! ▼ ▼ ▼ ▼ ▼ ▼ ▼ ▼ ▼
Nuclear medicine scans are usually contraindicated in patients who are pregnant because of teratogenic effects. These scans are also contraindicated in patients with hyper-

sensitivity to iodine or with severe renal or hepatic disease.

Purpose
■ To produce tissue analysis and images not readily seen on standard X-rays
■ To detect or rule out malignant lesions when X-ray findings are normal or questionable

Cost
Very expensive

Patient preparation
■ Explain to the patient the purpose of the test. Tell him who will perform the test and where it will take place.
■ Tell the patient that he may have to assume various positions on a scanner table but that he'll be asked to remain still during the procedure because movement can cause artifacts, thereby prolonging the test and limiting its accuracy.
■ Note whether the patient has had prior radiologic tests using contrast media or nuclear medicine procedures.
■ Tell the patient that if a tracer isotope is used, an I.V. line will be started. Also tell him that contrast medium will be administered before the procedure and that a scintillation camera will display images on a monitor.

Findings
See specific nuclear medicine scan entry.

Interfering factors
■ Failure to observe pretest restrictions
■ Inability of the patient to remain still during the test
■ Failure to remove jewelry and other metal objects from the scanning field (obscured imaging)
■ Severe diarrhea and vomiting (impaired GI absorption of oral contrast media)

■ Renal disease (decreased uptake of contrast media)

5'-nucleotidase

The enzyme 5'-nucleotidase (5'NT) is a phosphatase formed almost entirely in the hepatobiliary tract. Unlike alkaline phosphatase (ALP), it hydrolyzes only nucleoside 5'-phosphate groups. Measurement of serum 5'NT levels helps to determine whether elevated ALP levels stem from skeletal or hepatic disease. Because 5'NT remains normal in skeletal disease and pregnancy, it's more specific for assessing hepatic dysfunction than ALP or leucine aminopeptidase.

Purpose
■ To distinguish between hepatobiliary and skeletal disease when the source of increased ALP levels is uncertain
■ To help differentiate biliary obstruction from acute hepatocellular damage
■ To detect hepatic metastasis in the absence of jaundice

Cost
Inexpensive

Patient preparation
■ Explain to the patient that this test is used to evaluate liver function.
■ Tell the patient that the test requires a blood sample. Explain who will perform the venipuncture and when.
■ Explain to the patient that he may experience discomfort from the needle puncture and the tourniquet.

Reference values
Serum 5'NT values for adults range from 2 to 17 U/L (SI, 0.034 to 0.29 μkat/L); values for children may be lower.

Abnormal findings

Extremely high levels of 5'NT occur with common bile duct obstruction (by calculi or tumors) in diseases that cause severe intrahepatic cholestasis such as neoplastic infiltrations of the liver. Slight to moderate increases may reflect acute hepatocellular damage or active cirrhosis.

Interfering factors

■ Hemolysis due to rough handling of the sample

■ Cholestatic drugs, such as codeine, meperidine, morphine, and phenothiazines as well as acetaminophen, aspirin, and phenytoin (increase)

O

One-stage factor assay: Extrinsic coagulation system

When prothrombin time (PT) and partial thromboplastin time (PTT) are prolonged, a one-stage assay is used to detect a deficiency of factor II, factor V, or factor X. If PT is abnormal but PTT is normal, factor VII may be deficient.

Purpose
- To identify a specific factor deficiency in persons with prolonged PT or PTT
- To study patients with congenital or acquired coagulation disorders
- To monitor the effects of blood component therapy in factor-deficient patients

Cost
Moderately expensive

Patient preparation
- Explain to the patient that this test is used to assess the function of the blood coagulation mechanism.
- Tell the patient that the test requires a blood sample. Explain who will perform the venipuncture and when.
- Explain to the patient that he may experience discomfort from the needle puncture and the tourniquet.
- If the patient is factor deficient and receiving blood component therapy, tell him that a series of tests may be needed to monitor therapeutic progress. (See *Factor XIII assay: The missing link.*)
- Restrict medications that may affect test results. If they must be continued, note this on the laboratory request.

Reference values
The reference ranges for most factors is 50% to 150% of normal (SI, 0.50 to 1.50).

Abnormal findings
Deficiency of factor X may also indicate disseminated intravascular coagulation (DIC). Factor V deficiency suggests severe hepatic disease, DIC, or fibrinogenolysis. Deficiencies of all four factors may be congenital; absence of factor II is lethal.

Interfering factors
- Failure to adequately mix the sample and the anticoagulant, or failure to immediately send the sample to the laboratory or place it on ice after collection

■ Hemolysis due to rough handling of the sample
■ Oral anticoagulants (possible increase in bleeding time due to inhibition of vitamin K–dependent synthesis and activation of clotting factors II, VII, and X, which form in the liver)

One-stage factor assay: Intrinsic coagulation system

When prothrombin time is normal but activated partial thromboplastin time is abnormal, a one-stage assay is used to identify a deficiency in the intrinsic coagulation system: factor VIII, factor IX, factor XI, or factor XII.

Purpose

■ To identify a specific factor deficiency
■ To study patients with congenital or acquired coagulation disorders
■ To monitor the effects of blood component therapy in factor-deficient patients

Cost

Moderately expensive

Patient preparation

■ Explain to the patient that this test is used to assess the function of the blood coagulation mechanism.
■ Tell the patient that the test requires a blood sample. Explain who will perform the venipuncture and when.

- Explain to the patient that he may experience discomfort from the needle puncture and the tourniquet.
- Restrict medications that may affect test results. If they must be continued, note this on the laboratory request.
- If the patient is factor deficient and receiving blood component therapy, tell him that a series of tests may be needed to monitor therapeutic progress.

Reference values

Reference ranges for most factors are 50% to 150% of normal activity (SI, 0.5 to 1.5).

Abnormal findings

Factor VIII deficiency may indicate hemophilia A, von Willebrand's disease, or a factor VIII inhibitor. An acquired deficiency of factor VIII may result from disseminated intravascular coagulation or fibrinolysis. Factor VIII antigen and ristocetin cofactor tests distinguish between hemophilia A (and its carrier state) and von Willebrand's disease.

Factor IX deficiency may suggest hemophilia B, or it may be acquired as a result of hepatic disease, a factor IX inhibitor, vitamin K deficiency, or warfarin therapy. Factor VIII and IX inhibitors occur after blood transfusions in patients deficient in either factor and are antibodies specific to each factor.

Factor XI deficiency may appear after the stress of trauma or surgery, or transiently in neonates. Factor XII deficiency may be inherited or acquired (such as nephrosis) and may also appear transiently in neonates.

Interfering factors

- Failure to adequately mix the sample and the anticoagulant, or failure to immediately send the sample to the laboratory or place it on ice after collection
- Hemolysis due to rough handling of the sample
- Oral anticoagulants (decrease in factor IX)
- Pregnancy (increase in factor VIII)

Orbital computed tomography scan

Orbital computed tomography (CT) scanning allows visualization of abnormalities not readily seen on standard X-rays, delineating their size, position, and relationship to adjoining structures. The scan produces a series of tomograms reconstructed by a computer and displayed as anatomic slices on a monitor. Furthermore, it can identify space-occupying lesions earlier and more accurately than other radiographic techniques and provide 3-D images of orbital structures, especially the ocular muscles and the optic nerve.

Purpose

- To evaluate pathologies of the orbit and eye — especially expanding lesions and bone destruction
- To evaluate fractures of the orbit and adjoining structures
- To determine the cause of unilateral exophthalmos

Cost

Very expensive

Patient preparation

- Describe the procedure for the patient, and explain that this test visualizes the anatomy of the eye and its surrounding structures.
- If contrast enhancement isn't scheduled, inform the patient that he doesn't need to restrict food or fluids. If contrast enhancement is scheduled, instruct the patient not

to consume any food or fluids for 4 hours before the test.

■ Tell the patient that a series of X-rays will be taken of his eye. Also tell him who will perform the test and where.

■ Tell the patient that he'll be positioned on an X-ray table and that the head of the table will be moved into the scanner, which will rotate around his head and make loud clacking sounds.

■ If a contrast medium will be used for the procedure, tell the patient that he may feel flushed and warm and experience a transient headache, a salty or metallic taste, and nausea or vomiting after the contrast medium is injected. Reassure him that these reactions to contrast media are typical.

■ Obtain informed consent if necessary.

■ Check the patient's history for hypersensitivity reactions to iodine, shellfish, or contrast media.

ALERT! ▼ ▼ ▼ ▼ ▼ ▼ ▼ ▼ ▼
Use of contrast enhancement is contraindicated in those patients with known hypersensitivity reactions to iodine, shellfish, or contrast media used in other tests.

Normal findings

Orbital structures are evaluated for size, shape, and position. Dense orbital bone provides a marked contrast to less dense periocular fat. The optic nerve and the medial and lateral rectus muscles are clearly defined. The rectus muscles appear as thin dense bands on each side, behind the eye. The optic canals should be equal in size.

Abnormal findings

Orbital CT scans can identify intraorbital and extraorbital space-occupying lesions that obscure the normal structures or cause orbital enlargement, indentation of the orbital walls, or bone destruction. This test can also help determine the type of lesion.

For example, infiltrative lesions, such as lymphomas and metastatic carcinomas, appear as irregular areas of density. However, encapsulated tumors, such as benign hemangiomas and meningiomas, appear as clearly defined masses of consistent density. CT scans can also visualize intracranial tumors that invade the orbit, thickening of the optic nerve that may occur with gliomas and meningiomas, and secondary tumors that may cause enlargement of the optic canal.

With fractures, CT scans allow a complete 3-D view of the affected structures. In determining the cause of unilateral exophthalmos, CT scans can show early erosion or expansion of the medial orbital wall, which may arise from lesions in the ethmoidal cells. These scans can also detect space-occupying lesions in the orbit or paranasal sinuses that cause exophthalmos and show thickening of the medial and lateral rectus muscles in proptosis resulting from Graves' disease.

Enhancement with a contrast medium may provide information about the circulation through abnormal ocular tissues.

Interfering factors

■ Head movement
■ Failure to remove metallic objects from examination field (possible poor imaging)

Orbital radiography

Orbital radiography evaluates the orbit, the bony cavity that houses the eye, the lacrimal glands, blood vessels, nerves, muscles, and fat. Because portions of the orbit are made up of thin bone that fractures easily, X-rays are commonly taken after facial trauma. They're also useful in diagnosing ocular and orbital pathologies. Special radiographic techniques can reveal foreign bodies in the orbit or eye that are invisible to an ophthalmoscope. Usually, a series of orbital X-rays includes a lateral view, posteroanterior view, submentovertical (base) view, stereo Waters' views (views from both sides), Towne's (half-axial) projection, and optic canal projections. If enlargement of the superior orbital fissure is suspected, apical views are obtained.

In some cases, orbital radiography is used with computed tomography scans and ultrasonography to better define an abnormality.

Purpose
■ To aid in diagnosis of orbital fractures and pathologies
■ To help locate intraorbital or intraocular foreign bodies

Cost
Moderately expensive

Patient preparation
■ Explain to the patient that this test involves taking several X-rays to assess the condition of the bones around the eye.
■ Describe the test for the patient. Tell him who will perform the test and where it will take place.
■ Tell the patient that the films will be developed and inspected before he leaves the radiography department.

Normal findings
Each orbit is made up of a roof, a floor, and medial and lateral walls. The bones of the roof and floor are very thin (the floor can be less than 1 mm thick). The medial walls, which parallel each other, are slightly thicker, except for the portion formed by the ethmoid bone. The lateral walls are the thickest part of the orbit and are strongest at the orbital rim.

The superior orbital fissure, at the back of the orbit between the lateral wall and the roof, is actually a gap between the greater and lesser wings of the sphenoid bone. The optic canal, which carries the optic nerve and ophthalmic artery, is an opening in the lesser wing of the sphenoid bone located at the apex of the orbit.

Abnormal findings
Orbital fractures associated with facial trauma are most common in the thin structures of the floor and ethmoid bone. Abnormalities are detected by comparing the size and shape of orbital structures on the affected side with those on the opposite side.

Orbital enlargement generally indicates the presence of a lesion that has caused proptosis due to increased intraorbital pressure. Any growing tumor can produce these changes. Superior orbital fissure enlargement can result from orbital meningioma, from intracranial conditions such as pituitary tumors or, more characteristically, from vascular anomalies. Optic canal enlargement may result from extraocular extension of a retinoblastoma or, in children, from an optic nerve glioma. In adults, only prolonged pathology can increase orbital size; however, in children, even a rapidly growing lesion can cause orbital enlargement because orbital bones aren't fully developed. A decrease in the size of the orbit may follow childhood enucleation of the eye or conditions such as congenital microphthalmia.

Destruction of the orbital walls may indicate a malignant neoplasm or an infection. A benign tumor or cyst produces a clear-cut local indentation of the orbital wall. Lesions of adjacent structures may also produce radiographic changes due to enlargement and erosion of the orbit.

Increased bone density may be apparent with conditions such as osteoblastic metastasis, sphenoid ridge meningioma, or Paget's disease. To confirm orbital pathology, however, radiographic findings must be supplemented with results from other appropriate tests and procedures.

Interfering factors
■ None significant

Osmolality, urine

The kidneys normally concentrate or dilute urine according to fluid intake. When intake is excessive, the kidneys excrete more water in the urine; when intake is limited, they excrete less. To make such variation possible, the distal segment of the renal tubule varies its permeability to water in response to antidiuretic hormone, which, with renal blood flow, determines urine concentration or dilution.

The urine osmolality test measures the concentrating ability of the kidneys in acute and chronic renal failure. Osmolality is a more sensitive index of renal function than dilution techniques that measure specific gravity. It measures the number of osmotically active ions or particles present per kilogram of water. Osmolality is high in concentrated urine and low in dilute urine. It's determined by the effect of solute particles on the freezing point of the fluid.

Purpose
■ To evaluate renal tubular function
■ To detect renal impairment

Cost
Inexpensive

Patient preparation
■ Explain to the patient that this test evaluates renal function.
■ Tell him that the test requires a urine specimen and collection of blood within 1 hour before or after the urine is collected.
■ Restrict diuretics, as necessary.

Reference values
For a random urine specimen, osmolality normally ranges from 50 to 1,400 mOsm/kg (SI, 50 to 1,400 mmol/kg water); for a 24-hour urine specimen, from 300 to 900 mOsm/kg (SI, 300 to 900 mmol/kg water).

Abnormal findings
Decreased renal capacity either to concentrate urine in response to fluid deprivation, or to dilute urine in response to fluid overload, may indicate tubular epithelial damage, decreased renal blood flow, loss of functional nephrons, or pituitary or cardiac dysfunction.

Interfering factors
■ Diuretics (lowered specific gravity due to increased urine volume and dilution)
■ Nephrotoxic drugs (decreased renal concentrating ability due to tubular epithelial damage)
■ Marked overhydration for several days before the test (possible depressed concentration values)
■ Dehydration or electrolyte imbalance (possible inaccurate results due to fluid retention)
■ Incomplete collection of 24-hour urine specimen (invalid results)

Osmotic fragility

Osmotic fragility measures red blood cell (RBC) resistance to hemolysis when exposed to a series of increasingly dilute saline solutions. The sooner hemolysis occurs, the greater the osmotic fragility of the cells.

Purpose
- To aid diagnosis of hereditary spherocytosis
- To confirm morphologic RBC abnormalities

Cost
Moderately expensive

Patient preparation
- Explain to the patient that this test is used to identify the cause of anemia.
- Tell the patient that the test requires a blood sample. Explain who will perform the venipuncture and when.
- Explain to the patient that he may experience discomfort from the needle puncture and the tourniquet.

Reference values
Osmotic fragility values (percentage of RBCs hemolyzed) that have been obtained photometrically are plotted against decreasing saline tonicity to produce an S-shaped curve with a slope characteristic of the disorder. Reference values differ with tonicities.

Abnormal findings
Low osmotic fragility (increased resistance to hemolysis) is characteristic of thalassemia, iron-deficiency anemia, sickle cell anemia, and other RBC disorders in which target cells are found. Low osmotic fragility also occurs after splenectomy.

High osmotic fragility (increased tendency to hemolysis) occurs with hereditary spherocytosis; spherocytosis associated with autoimmune hemolytic anemia, severe burns, or chemical poisoning; or he-

molytic disease of the newborn (erythroblastosis fetalis).

Interfering factors
- Failure to use the proper anticoagulant in the collection tube, to fill the tube completely, or to adequately mix the sample and the anticoagulant
- Presence of hemolytic organisms in the sample
- Severe anemia and other like conditions (possible invalid results because fewer RBCs are available for testing)
- Recent blood transfusion

PQ

Papanicolaou test

The Papanicolaou (Pap) test is a widely known cytologic test for early detection of cervical cancer. A physician or specially trained nurse scrapes secretions from the patient's cervix and spreads them on a slide, which is sent to the laboratory for cytologic analysis. The test relies on the ready exfoliation of malignant cells from the cervix and shows cell maturity, metabolic activity, and morphology variations.

Although cervical scrapings are the most common test specimens, the test may involve cytologic evaluation of the vaginal pool, prostatic secretions, urine, gastric secretions, cavity fluids, bronchial aspirations, sputum, or solid tumor cells obtained by fine needle aspiration. If a Pap test is positive or suggests malignancy, cervical biopsy can confirm diagnosis.

Purpose
■ To assess response to chemotherapy and radiation therapy
■ To detect inflammatory tissue changes
■ To detect malignant cells
■ To detect viral, fungal and, occasionally, parasitic invasion

Cost
Inexpensive

Patient preparation
■ Explain to the patient that the test allows the study of cervical cells.
■ Don't schedule the test during menses; the best time is mid-cycle.
■ Instruct the patient to avoid having intercourse for 24 hours, not to douche for 48 hours, and not to insert vaginal medications for 1 week before the test, because doing so can wash away cellular deposits and change the vaginal pH.
■ Tell the patient who will perform the procedure and when, that she may experience discomfort from the speculum, and that the test requires that the cervix be scraped (during which she may feel some pain).
■ Tell the patient a bimanual examination may follow removal of the speculum.

Normal findings
Normally, no malignant cells or other abnormalities are present.

Abnormal findings
Malignant cells usually have relatively large nuclei and only small amounts of cyto-

plasm. They show abnormal nuclear chromatin patterns and marked variation in size, shape, and staining properties and may have prominent nucleoli.

A Pap smear may be graded in different ways, so check your laboratory's reporting format. In the Bethesda System, the current standardized method, potentially premalignant squamous lesions fall into three categories: atypical squamous cells of undetermined significance, low-grade squamous intraepithelial lesions, and high-grade squamous intraepithelial lesions. The low-grade category includes mild dysplasia and the changes of the human papillomavirus. The high-grade category includes moderate to severe dysplasia and carcinoma in situ.

To confirm a suggestive or positive cytology report, the test may be repeated or followed by a biopsy. (See *Vaginal smears.*)

Interfering factors

■ Douching within 48 hours or having intercourse within 24 hours before the test (can wash away cellular deposits)
■ Excessive use of lubricating jelly on the speculum (false-negative)
■ Collection of the specimen during menstruation
■ Exclusive use of a specimen collected from the vaginal fornix (possible false-negative)
■ Delay in fixing the specimen (difficult cytologic interpretation due to dehydration of cells)
■ Too thin or thick a specimen

Parathyroid hormone

Parathyroid hormone (PTH) regulates plasma concentration of calcium and phosphorus. The overall effect of PTH is to raise

Clinical implications of abnormal parathyroid secretion

CONDITIONS	CAUSES	PTH LEVELS	IONIZED CALCIUM LEVELS
Primary hyperparathyroidism	▪ Parathyroid adenoma or carcinoma	High	High *to* Normal
Secondary hyperparathyroidism	▪ Chronic renal disease ▪ Severe vitamin D deficiency ▪ Calcium malabsorption ▪ Pregnancy and lactation	High	Low
Tertiary hyperparathyroidism	▪ Progressive secondary hyperparathyroidism leading to autonomous hyperparathyroidism	High	High *to* Normal
Hypoparathyroidism	▪ Usually, accidental removal of the parathyroid glands during surgery ▪ Occasionally, in association with autoimmune disease	Low	Low
Malignant tumors	▪ Squamous cell carcinoma of the lung ▪ Renal, pancreatic, or ovarian carcinoma	High *to* Normal	High

Key: High ●   Normal ●   Low ○

plasma levels of calcium while lowering phosphorus levels. Circulating PTH exists in three distinct molecular forms: the intact PTH molecule, which originates in the parathyroid glands, and two smaller circulating forms, N-terminal fragments and C-terminal fragments. Two radioimmunoassays are available to detect intact PTH and the N-terminal and C-terminal fragments. Both tests can be used to confirm diagnosis of hyperparathyroidism and hypoparathyroidism.

Each test has other specific applications as well. The C-terminal PTH assay is more useful in diagnosing chronic disturbances in PTH metabolism, such as secondary and tertiary hyperparathyroidism; it also better differentiates ectopic from primary hyperparathyroidism. The assay for intact PTH and the N-terminal fragment (both forms are measured concomitantly) more accurately reflects acute changes in PTH metabolism and thus is useful in monitoring a patient's response to PTH therapy.

The clinical and diagnostic effects of PTH excess or deficiency are directly related to the effects of PTH on bone and the renal tubules and to its interaction with ionized calcium and biologically active vitamin D. Therefore, measuring serum calcium, phosphorus, and creatinine levels with serum PTH is helpful when trying to understand the causes and effects of pathologic parathyroid function. Suppression or stimulation tests may help confirm findings.

Purpose
■ To aid the differential diagnosis of parathyroid disorders

Cost
Moderately expensive

Patient preparation
■ Explain to the patient that this test helps evaluate parathyroid function.
■ Instruct the patient to observe an overnight fast because food may affect PTH levels and interfere with the test results.
■ Tell the patient that the test requires a blood sample. Explain who will perform the venipuncture and when.
■ Explain to the patient that he may experience discomfort from the needle puncture and the tourniquet.

Reference values
Normal serum PTH levels vary, depending on the laboratory, and must be interpreted in association with serum calcium levels. Typical values for intact PTH range from 10 to 50 pg/ml (SI, 1.1 to 5.3 pmol/L); N-terminal fraction is 8 to 24 pg/ml (SI, 0.8 to 2.5 pmol/L); C-terminal fraction, 0 to 340 pg/ml (SI, 0 to 35.8 pmol/L).

Abnormal findings
Measured concomitantly with serum calcium levels, elevated serum PTH values may indicate primary, secondary, or tertiary hyperparathyroidism. Low serum PTH levels may result from hypoparathyroidism and from certain malignant diseases. (See *Clinical implications of abnormal parathyroid secretion,* page 273.)

Interfering factors
■ Failure to fast overnight before the test
■ Hemolysis due to rough handling of the sample

Partial thromboplastin time

The partial thromboplastin time test evaluates all the clotting factors of the intrinsic pathway — except platelets — by measuring the time required for formation of a fibrin clot after the addition of calcium and phospholipid emulsion to a plasma sample. Because most congenital coagulation deficiencies occur in the intrinsic pathway, the test is valuable in preoperative screening for bleeding tendencies. This is also the test of choice for monitoring heparin therapy.

Purpose
■ To screen for deficiencies of the clotting factors in the intrinsic pathways
■ To monitor response to heparin therapy

Cost
Inexpensive

Patient preparation
■ Explain to the patient that this test helps determine whether his blood clots normally.
■ Tell the patient that the test requires a blood sample. Explain who will perform the venipuncture and when.
■ Explain to the patient that he may experience discomfort from the needle puncture and the tourniquet.
■ When appropriate, tell the patient receiving heparin therapy that this test may be repeated at regular intervals to assess his response to treatment.

Normal findings
Normally, a fibrin clot forms 21 to 35 seconds (SI, 21 to 35 s) after addition of reagents. For a patient on anticoagulant therapy, monitor the desirable values for the therapy being delivered.

Abnormal findings

Prolonged values may indicate a deficiency of certain plasma clotting factors, the presence of heparin, or the presence of fibrin split products, fibrinolysins, or circulating anticoagulants that are antibodies to specific clotting factors.

Interfering factors

■ Failure to use the proper anticoagulant, fill the collection tube completely, or mix the sample and the anticoagulant adequately
■ Hemolysis due to rough handling of the sample or to excessive probing at the venipuncture site
■ Failure to send the sample to the laboratory immediately or place it on ice (may cause spurious test results)

Parvovirus B19 antibodies

Parvovirus B19, a small, single-stranded deoxyribonucleic acid virus belonging to the family Parvoviridae, destroys red blood cell (RBC) precursors and interferes with normal RBC production. It's also associated with erythema infectiosum (a self-limiting, low-grade fever and rash in young children) and aplastic crisis (in patients with chronic hemolytic anemia and immunodeficient patients with bone marrow failure). Immunoglobulin (Ig) G and IgM antibodies can be detected by enzyme-linked immunosorbent assay and immunofluorescence.

Purpose

■ To detect parvovirus B19 antibody, especially in prospective organ donors
■ To diagnose erythema infectiosum, parvovirus B19 aplastic crisis, and related parvovirus B19 diseases

Cost

Moderately expensive

Patient preparation

■ Explain to the patient the test's purpose and procedure. Explain to a potential organ donor that the test is part of a panel of tests performed before organ donation to protect the organ recipient from potential infection.
■ Tell the patient that the test requires a blood sample. Explain who will perform the venipuncture and when.
■ Explain to the patient that he may experience discomfort from the needle puncture and the tourniquet.

Normal findings

Normally, results are negative for IgM- and IgG-specific antibodies to parvovirus B19.

Abnormal findings

About 50% of adults lack immunity to parvovirus B19, with as many as 20% of susceptible adults becoming infected after exposure. Positive results have been associated with joint arthralgia, hydrops fetalis, fetal loss, transient aplastic anemia, chronic anemia in immunocompromised patients, and bone marrow failure.

Abnormal findings for the parvovirus B19 antibodies test should be confirmed using the Western blot test.

Interfering factors

■ Failure to place the sample on ice
■ Hemolysis due to rough handling of the sample

Pericardial fluid analysis

Analysis of the fluid inside the heart's pericardial sac is usually done for patients with pericardial effusion (an accumulation of excess pericardial fluid), which may result from inflammation (as in pericarditis), rupture, or penetrating trauma.

Purpose

■ To assist in identifying the cause of pericardial effusion and to help determine appropriate therapy

Cost

Expensive

Patient preparation

■ Explain to the patient that this test detects excessive fluid around the heart, determines its cause, and helps determine appropriate therapy.
■ Tell the patient who will perform the test, where it will take place, and that a local anesthetic will be injected before the aspiration needle is inserted.
■ Warn the patient that although fluid aspiration isn't painful, he may experience pressure upon insertion of the needle into the pericardial sac.
■ Advise the patient that he may be asked to briefly hold his breath to aid needle insertion and placement.
■ Tell the patient that an I.V. line will be started at a slow rate in case medications need to be administered.
■ Assure the patient that someone will remain with him during the test and that his pulse and blood pressure will be monitored after the procedure.
■ Check the patient's history for current antimicrobial usage, and record such usage on the test request form.
■ Obtain informed consent if necessary.

Normal findings

Normally, 10 to 50 ml of sterile pericardial fluid is present in the pericardium. Pericardial fluid is clear and straw-colored, with-

out evidence of pathogens, blood, or malignant cells. It normally contains fewer than 1,000/µl (SI, < 1.0 × 10⁹/L) white blood cells (WBCs). Its glucose concentration approximately equals the levels in whole blood.

Abnormal findings

Generally, pericardial effusions are classified as transudates or exudates. Transudates are protein-poor effusions that usually arise from mechanical factors altering fluid formation or resorption, such as increased hydrostatic pressure, decreased plasma oncotic pressure, or obstruction of the pericardial lymphatic drainage system by a tumor.

Most exudates result from inflammation and contain large amounts of protein. In these effusions, inflammation damages the capillary membrane, allowing protein molecules to leak into the pericardial fluid. Exudate effusions may occur in pericarditis, neoplasms, acute myocardial infarction, tuberculosis, rheumatoid disease, and systemic lupus erythematosus.

An elevated WBC count or neutrophil fraction may also accompany inflammatory conditions such as bacterial pericarditis; a high lymphocyte fraction may indicate fungal or tuberculous pericarditis. Turbid or milky effusions may result from the accumulation of lymph or pus in the pericardial sac or from tuberculosis or rheumatoid disease.

Bloody pericardial fluid may indicate hemopericardium, hemorrhagic pericarditis, or a traumatic tap. Hemopericardium, the accumulation of blood in the pericardium, may result from myocardial rupture after infarction or aortic rupture secondary to a dissecting aortic aneurysm or thoracic trauma. In hemopericardium, the fluid has a hematocrit similar to that of whole blood; in hemorrhagic pericarditis, it has a relatively low hematocrit and doesn't clot on standing.

Hemorrhagic effusions may indicate a malignant tumor, closed chest trauma, Dressler's syndrome, or postcardiotomy syndrome. A traumatic tap is easily distinguished from hemopericardium or hemorrhagic pericarditis because the fluid becomes progressively clearer.

Glucose concentrations below whole blood levels may reflect increased local metabolism due to malignancy, inflammation, or infection. Possible causes of bacterial pericarditis include *Staphylococcus aureus, Haemophilus influenzae,* and various gram-negative organisms; possible causes of granulomatous pericarditis include *Mycobacterium tuberculosis* or various fungal agents; and possible causes of viral pericarditis include coxsackieviruses, echoviruses, and others.

Interfering factors
■ Failure to use sterile collection technique (allowing skin contaminants to be mistaken for the causative organism)
■ Failure to use proper additives in test tubes
■ Antimicrobial therapy (may prevent isolation of the causative organisms)

Peritoneal fluid analysis

Peritoneal fluid analysis assesses a specimen of peritoneal fluid obtained by paracentesis. This procedure requires inserting a trocar and cannula through the abdominal wall while the patient receives a local anesthetic. If the fluid specimen is removed for therapeutic purposes, the trocar may be connected to a drainage system. However, if only a small amount of fluid is removed for diagnostic purposes, an 18G needle

may be used in place of the trocar and cannula. In a four-quadrant tap, fluid is aspirated from each quadrant of the abdomen to verify abdominal trauma and confirm the need for surgery.

Purpose
■ To determine the cause of ascites
■ To detect abdominal trauma

Cost
Expensive

Patient preparation
■ Explain to the patient that this procedure helps determine the cause of ascites or detects abdominal trauma.
■ Tell the patient that the test requires a peritoneal fluid specimen, that he'll receive a local anesthetic to minimize discomfort, and that the procedure takes about 45 minutes to perform.
■ If the patient has severe ascites, inform him that the procedure will relieve his discomfort and allow him to breathe more easily.
■ Obtain informed consent if necessary.
■ Tell the patient a blood sample may be taken for analysis and X-rays may be performed prior to peritoneal fluid analysis to ensure reliability.

Reference values
For normal peritoneal fluid values, see *Peritoneal fluid analysis,* page 278.

Abnormal findings
Milk-colored peritoneal fluid may result from chyle or lymph fluid escaping from a thoracic duct that's damaged or blocked by a malignant tumor, lymphoma, tuberculosis, parasitic infestation, adhesion, or hepatic cirrhosis; a pseudochylous condition may result from the presence of leukocytes or tumor cells. Differential diagnosis of true

Peritoneal fluid analysis

ELEMENT	NORMAL VALUE OR FINDING
Gross appearance	Sterile, odorless, clear to pale yellow color; scant amount (< 50 ml)
Red blood cells	None
White blood cells	< 300 /µl (SI, < 300 × 10^9/L)
Protein	0.3 to 4.1 g/dl (SI, 3 to 41 g/L)
Glucose	70 to 100 mg/dl (SI, 3.5 to 5 mmol/L)
Amylase	138 to 404 U/L (SI, 138 to 404 U/L)
Ammonia	< 50 µg/dl (SI, < 29 µmol/L)
Alkaline phosphatase	Males over age 18: 90 to 239 U/L (SI, 90 to 239 U/L) Females < 45: 76 to 196 U/L (SI, 76 to 196 U/L) Females > 45: 87 to 250 U/L (SI, 87 to 250 U/L)
Cytology	No malignant cells present
Bacteria	None
Fungi	None

chylous ascites depends on the presence of elevated triglyceride levels (≥ 400 mg/dl [SI ≥ 4.36 mmol/L]) and microscopic fat globules.

Cloudy or turbid fluid may indicate peritonitis due to primary bacterial infection, ruptured bowel (after trauma), pancreatitis, strangulated or infarcted intestine, or appendicitis. Bloody fluid may result from a benign or malignant tumor, hemorrhagic pancreatitis, or a traumatic tap; however, if the fluid fails to clear on continued aspiration, a traumatic tap isn't the cause. Bile-stained green fluid may indicate a ruptured gallbladder, acute pancreatitis, or a perforated intestine or duodenal ulcer.

A red blood cell count greater than 100/µl (SI, 100/L) indicates neoplasm or tuberculosis; a count greater than 100,000/µl (SI, 100,000/L) indicates intra-abdominal trauma. An elevated white blood cell count with more than 25% neutrophils occurs in 90% of patients with spontaneous bacterial peritonitis and in 50% of those with cirrhosis. A high percentage of lymphocytes suggests tuberculous peritonitis or chylous ascites. Numerous mesothelial cells indicate tuberculous peritonitis.

Protein levels rise above 3 g/dl (SI, 3 g/L) in malignancy and above 4 g/dl (SI, 4 g/L) in tuberculosis. Peritoneal fluid glucose levels fall in patients with tuberculous peritonitis and peritoneal carcinomatosis.

Amylase levels rise with pancreatic trauma, pancreatic pseudocyst, or acute pancreatitis and may also rise in intestinal necrosis or strangulation.

Peritoneal alkaline phosphatase levels rise to more than twice the normal serum levels in patients with a ruptured or strangulated small intestine. Peritoneal ammonia levels also exceed twice the normal serum levels in ruptured or strangulated large and small intestines, and in ruptured ulcer or appendix.

A protein ascitic fluid to serum ratio of 0:5 or greater may suggest a malignancy, or tuberculous or pancreatic ascites. The presence of this finding indicates a nonhepatic cause; its absence suggests uncomplicated hepatic disease. An albumin gradient between ascitic fluid and serum greater than 1 g/dl (SI > 1 g/L) indicates chronic hepatic disease; a lesser value suggests malignancy.

Cytologic examination of peritoneal fluid accurately detects malignant cells. Microbiological examination can reveal coliforms, anaerobes, and enterococci, which can enter the peritoneum from a ruptured organ or from infections accompanying appendicitis, pancreatitis, tuberculosis, or ovarian disease. Gram-positive cocci commonly indicate primary peritonitis; gram-negative organisms, secondary peritonitis. The presence of fungi may indicate histoplasmosis, candidiasis, or coccidioidomycosis.

Interfering factors
■ Contamination of the specimen with blood, bile, urine, or stool due to injury to underlying structures during paracentesis

Persantine-thallium imaging

Persantine-thallium imaging is an alternative method of assessing coronary vessel function for patients who can't tolerate exercise or stress electrocardiography (ECG). Persantine (dipyridamole) infusion simulates the effects of exercise by increasing blood flow to the collateral circulation and away from the coronary arteries, thereby inducing ischemia. Then thallium infusion allows the examiner to evaluate the cardiac vessels' response. The heart is scanned immediately after the thallium infusion and again 2 to 4 hours later. Diseased vessels can't deliver thallium to the heart, and thallium lingers in diseased areas of the myocardium.

Purpose
■ To identify exercise- or stress-induced arrhythmias
■ To assess the presence and degree of cardiac ischemia

Cost
Expensive

Patient preparation
■ Tell the patient that a painless, 5- to 10-minute baseline ECG will precede the test.
■ Explain to the patient that he'll need to restrict food and fluids before the test and avoid caffeine and other stimulants (which may cause arrhythmias).
■ Instruct the patient to continue to take his regular medications, with the possible exception of beta-adrenergic blockers.
■ Explain to the patient that an I.V. line infuses the medications for the study. Tell him who will start the I.V. and when.
■ Inform the patient that he may experience mild nausea, headache, dizziness, or flushing after Persantine administration. Reassure him that these adverse reactions are usually temporary and rarely need treatment.
■ Obtain informed consent if necessary.

Normal findings

Imaging should reveal characteristic distribution of the isotope throughout the left ventricle and no visible defects.

Abnormal findings

The presence of ST-segment depression, angina, and arrhythmias strongly suggests coronary artery disease (CAD). Persistent ST-segment depression generally indicates myocardial infarction. In contrast, transient ST-segment depression indicates ischemia from CAD.

Cold spots usually indicate CAD but may result from sarcoidosis, myocardial fibrosis, cardiac contusion, attenuation due to soft tissue (for example, breast and diaphragm), apical cleft, and coronary spasm. The absence of cold spots in the presence of CAD may result from insignificant obstruction, single-vessel disease, or collateral circulation.

Interfering factors

- Failure to observe pretest restrictions
- Artifacts such as implants and electrodes (possible false-positive)
- Absence of cold spots with CAD (possible delay in imaging)

Phenylalanine

The phenylalanine test, also called the *Guthrie screening test*, is used to screen infants for elevated serum phenylalanine levels, a possible indication of phenylketonuria (PKU). Phenylalanine is a naturally occurring amino acid essential to growth and nitrogen balance; an accumulation of this amino acid may indicate a serious enzyme deficiency. This test detects abnormal phenylalanine levels through the growth rate of *Bacillus subtilis*, an organism that needs phenylalanine to thrive. To ensure accurate results, the test must be performed after 3 full days (preferably 4 days) of milk or formula feeding.

Purpose

- To screen infants for possible PKU

Cost

Inexpensive

Patient preparation

- Explain to the parents that the test is a routine screening measure for possible PKU and is required in many states.
- Tell the parents that a small amount of blood will be drawn from the infant's heel and that collecting the sample takes only a few minutes.

Reference values

A negative test result indicates normal phenylalanine levels (< 2 mg/dl [SI, < 121 µmol/L) and no appreciable danger of PKU.

Abnormal findings

At birth, an infant with PKU usually has normal phenylalanine levels, but after milk or formula feeding begins, levels gradually increase because of a deficiency of the liver enzyme that converts phenylalanine to tyrosine. A positive test result suggests the *possibility* of PKU. A definitive diagnosis requires exact serum phenylalanine measurement and urine testing. A positive test result may also indicate hepatic disease, galactosemia, or delayed development of certain enzyme systems. (See *Confirming PKU.*)

Interfering factors

- Performing the test before the infant has received at least 3 full days of milk or formula feeding (false-negative)

Confirming PKU

If phenylalanine screening detects the possible presence of phenylketonuria (PKU), serum phenylalanine and tyrosine levels are measured to confirm the diagnosis. Phenylalanine hydroxylase is the enzyme that converts phenylalanine to tyrosine. If this enzyme is absent, increasing phenylalanine levels and falling tyrosine levels indicate PKU.

Samples are obtained by venipuncture (femoral or external jugular) and measured by fluorometry. Elevated serum phenylalanine levels (> 4 mg/dl [SI, > 242 µmol/L]) and decreased tyrosine levels — with urinary excretion of phenylpyruvic acid — confirm the diagnosis of PKU.

Phosphates

The phosphates test is used to measure serum levels of phosphates, the primary anion in intracellular fluid. Phosphates are essential in the storage and utilization of energy, calcium regulation, red blood cell function, acid-base balance, the formation of bone, and the metabolism of carbohydrates, protein, and fat. The intestines absorb most phosphates from dietary sources; the kidneys excrete phosphates and serve as a regulatory mechanism. Abnormal concentrations of serum phosphates usually result from improper excretion rather than faulty ingestion or absorption from dietary sources.

Normally, calcium and phosphates have an inverse relationship; if one is increased, the other is decreased.

Purpose
- To aid diagnosis of renal disorders and acid-base imbalance
- To detect endocrine, skeletal, and calcium disorders

Cost
Inexpensive

Patient preparation
- Explain to the patient that this test is used to measure phosphate levels in the blood.
- Tell the patient that the test requires a blood sample. Explain who will perform the venipuncture and when.
- Explain to the patient that he may experience discomfort from the needle puncture and the tourniquet.
- Restrict medications that may affect test results. If these drugs must be continued, note this on the laboratory request.

Reference values
Normally, serum phosphate levels in adults range from 2.7 to 4.5 mg/dl (SI, 0.87 to 1.45 mmol/L). In children, normal serum phosphate levels measure from 4.5 to 6.7 mg/dl (SI, 1.45 to 1.78 mmol/L).

Abnormal findings
Decreased serum phosphate levels (hypophosphatemia) may result from malnutrition, malabsorption syndromes, hyperparathyroidism, renal tubular acidosis, and treatment of diabetic ketoacidosis. In children, hypophosphatemia can suppress normal growth. Symptoms of hypophosphatemia include anemia, prolonged bleeding, bone demineralization, decreased white blood cell count, and anorexia.

Increased serum phosphate levels (hyperphosphatemia) may result from skeletal disease, healing fractures, hypoparathyroidism, acromegaly, diabetic ketoacidosis, high intestinal obstruction, lactic acidosis due to hepatic impairment, and renal failure. Hyperphosphatemia is seldom clinically significant, but it can alter bone metabolism in prolonged cases. Symptoms of hyperphosphatemia include tachycardia, muscular weakness, diarrhea, cramping, and hyperreflexia.

Interfering factors
■ Venous stasis due to tourniquet use
■ Sample obtained above an I.V. site that's receiving a solution containing phosphate
■ Excessive vitamin D intake or therapy with anabolic steroids or androgens (possible increase)
■ Use of acetazolamide, epinephrine, insulin, or phosphate-binding antacids; excessive excretion due to prolonged vomiting or diarrhea; vitamin D deficiency; extended I.V. infusion of dextrose 5% in water (possible decrease)
■ Hemolysis of the sample (false-high)

Phospholipids

The phospholipids test is a quantitative analysis of phospholipids, the major form of lipids in cell membranes. Phospholipids are involved in cellular membrane composition and permeability and help control enzyme activity within the membrane. They aid transport of fatty acids and lipids across the intestinal barrier and from the liver and other fat depots to other body tissues. Phospholipids are essential for pulmonary gas exchange.

Purpose
■ To aid in the evaluation of fat metabolism
■ To aid diagnosis of chronic pancreatitis, diabetes mellitus, hypolipoproteinemia,

hypothyroidism, nephrotic syndrome, and obstructive jaundice

Cost
Inexpensive

Patient preparation
■ Explain to the patient that this test is used to determine how the body metabolizes fats.
■ Tell the patient that the test requires a blood sample. Explain who will perform the venipuncture and when.
■ Explain to the patient that he may experience discomfort from the needle puncture and the tourniquet.
■ Instruct the patient to abstain from drinking alcohol for 24 hours before the test and not to eat or drink anything after midnight before the test.
■ Restrict medications that may affect test results. If they must be continued, note this on the laboratory request.

Reference values
Normal phospholipid levels range from 180 to 320 mg/dl (SI, 1.80 to 3.20 g/L). Although men usually have higher levels than women, values in pregnant women exceed those of men.

Abnormal findings
Elevated phospholipid levels may indicate chronic pancreatitis, diabetes mellitus, hypothyroidism, nephrotic syndrome, or obstructive jaundice. Decreased levels may indicate primary hypolipoproteinemia.

Interfering factors
■ Failure to observe pretest restrictions
■ Clofibrate and other antilipemics (possible decrease)
■ Epinephrine, estrogens, and some phenothiazines (increase)

Placental estriol

The placental estriol test, also referred to as *maternal urine estriol*, monitors fetal viability by measuring urine levels of placental estriol, the predominant estrogen excreted in urine during pregnancy. A steady rise in estriol reflects a properly functioning placenta and, in most cases, a healthy, growing fetus. Normally, estriol is secreted in much smaller amounts by the ovaries in nonpregnant females, by the testes in males, and by the adrenal cortex in both sexes.

The usual clinical indication for this test is high-risk pregnancy. Serial testing is necessary to plot the expected rise in estriol levels or to show the absence of such a rise. The specimen of choice for this test is a 24-hour urine specimen because estriol levels fluctuate diurnally. Radioimmunoassay is the usual test method. Generally, serum estriol levels are considered more reliable than urine levels.

Purpose
■ To assess fetoplacental status, especially in high-risk pregnancy

Cost
Moderately expensive

Patient preparation
■ Explain to the patient that this test helps determine whether the placenta is functioning properly, which is essential to the health of the fetus.
■ Advise the patient that this test requires urine collection over a 24-hour period, and instruct her on how to collect the specimen and keep it on ice during the collection period.
■ Restrict medications that may affect test results. If they must be continued, note this on the laboratory request.

Normal findings
Normal urine estriol values vary considerably, but serial measures of urine estriol levels, when plotted on a graph, should share a steadily rising curve. (See *Urine estriol levels in a typical pregnancy*, page 284.)

Abnormal findings
A 40% drop from baseline values that occurs on 2 consecutive days strongly suggests placental insufficiency and impending fetal distress. A 20% drop over 2 weeks or failure of consecutive estriol levels to rise in a normal curve similarly indicates inadequate placental function and undesirable fetal status. These developments may necessitate cesarean delivery, depending on the patient's condition and other apparent signs of fetal distress.

A chronically low urine estriol curve may result from fetal adrenal insufficiency, congenital anomalies (such as anencephaly), Rh isoimmunization, or placental sulfatase deficiency.

A high-risk pregnancy in which the maternal glomerular filtration rate decreases may cause a low-normal estriol curve. Such a pregnancy may occur in a patient with hypertension or diabetes mellitus, for example. The pregnancy may continue as long as no complications develop and estriol levels continue to rise. However, falling estriol levels or a sudden drop from baseline values indicates severe fetal distress.

High urine estriol levels may occur in multiple pregnancy.

Interfering factors
■ Failure to collect all urine during the 24-hour period and to properly store the specimen during the collection period
■ Failure to refrigerate the specimen or keep it on ice

Urine estriol levels in a typical pregnancy

Because urine estriol levels rise as normal gestation proceeds (as shown below), any significant changes in serial urine determinations suggest abnormal conditions that may require prompt medical intervention.

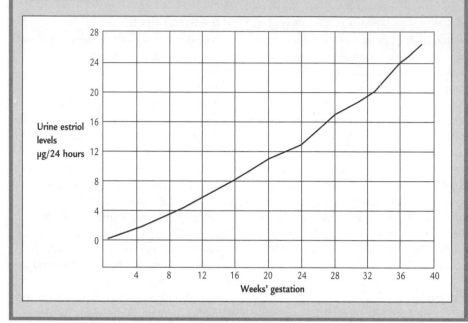

- Failure to maintain the specimen's prescribed pH level
- Ampicillin, cascara sagrada, hydrochlorothiazide, meprobamate, methenamine mandelate, phenazopyridine, phenothiazines, senna, steroid hormones, and tetracyclines (decrease)
- Anemia, hepatic or intestinal diseases, malnutrition, and maternal hemoglobinopathy (decrease)

Platelet aggregation

After vascular injury, platelets gather at the injury site and clump together to form an aggregate or plug that helps maintain hemostasis and promotes healing. The platelet aggregation test, an in vitro procedure, is used to measure the rate at which the platelets in a plasma sample form a clump after the addition of an aggregating reagent.

Purpose
- To assess platelet aggregation
- To detect congenital and acquired platelet bleeding disorders

Cost
Moderately expensive

Patient preparation
- Explain to the patient that this test is used to determine whether blood clots properly.

■ Tell the patient that the test requires a blood sample. Explain who will perform the venipuncture and when.

■ Explain to the patient that he may experience discomfort from the needle puncture and the tourniquet.

■ Instruct the patient to fast or to maintain a nonfat diet for 8 hours before the test because lipemia can affect the test results.

■ Restrict medications that may affect test results. If they must be continued, note this on the laboratory request.

■ Because the list of medications known to alter the results of this test is long and continually growing, the patient should be as free from drugs as possible before the test.

■ If the patient has taken aspirin within the past 14 days and the test can't be postponed, ask the laboratory to verify the presence of aspirin in the plasma. If test results are abnormal for such a sample, the use of aspirin must be discontinued and the test repeated in 2 weeks.

Normal findings

Normal platelet aggregation occurs in 3 to 5 minutes (SI, 3 to 5 m), but findings are temperature-dependent and vary with the laboratory. Platelet aggregation curves obtained by using different reagents help to distinguish various qualitative platelet defects.

Abnormal findings

Abnormal findings may indicate Bernard-Soulier syndrome, Glanzmann's thrombasthenia, polycythemia vera, severe liver disease, storage pool disease, uremia, or von Willebrand's disease.

Interfering factors

■ Failure to observe pretest restrictions

■ Hemolysis due to rough handling of the sample or to excessive probing at the venipuncture site

■ Aspirin and aspirin compounds, antihistamines, anti-inflammatory drugs, phenothiazines, phenylbutazone, sulfinpyrazone, and tricyclic antidepressants (decrease)

■ Ingestion of large amounts of garlic (inhibits platelet aggregation)

Platelet count

Platelets, or thrombocytes, are the smallest formed elements in blood. They promote coagulation and the formation of a hemostatic plug in vascular injury. The platelet count test is one of the most important screening tests of platelet function because it assesses bleeding disorders associated with disease processes such a malignancies and liver disease. Accurate counts are vital.

Purpose

■ To evaluate platelet production

■ To assess effects of chemotherapy or radiation therapy on platelet production

■ To diagnose and monitor severe thrombocytosis or thrombocytopenia

■ To confirm a visual estimate of platelet number and morphology from a stained blood film

Cost

Inexpensive

Patient preparation

■ Explain to the patient that this test is used to determine whether his blood clots normally.

■ Tell the patient that the test requires a blood sample. Explain who will perform the venipuncture and when.

- Explain to the patient that he may experience discomfort from the needle puncture and the tourniquet.
- Restrict medications that may affect test results. If they must be continued, note this on the laboratory request.

Reference values

Normal platelet counts range from 140,000 to 400,000/μl (SI, 140 to 400 × 10⁹/L) in adults and from 150,000 to 450,000/μl (SI, 150 to 450 × 10⁹/L) in children.

Abnormal findings

A decreased platelet count (thrombocytopenia) can result from aplastic or hypoplastic bone marrow; infiltrative bone marrow disease such as leukemia, or disseminated infection; megakaryocytic hypoplasia; ineffective thrombopoiesis due to folic acid or vitamin B_{12} deficiency; pooling of platelets in an enlarged spleen; increased platelet destruction due to drugs or immune disorders; disseminated intravascular coagulation; Bernard-Soulier syndrome; or mechanical injury to platelets.

An increased platelet count (thrombocytosis) can result from hemorrhage, infectious disorders, iron deficiency anemia, recent surgery, pregnancy, splenectomy, or inflammatory disorders. In such cases, the platelet count returns to normal after the patient recovers from the primary disorder. However, the count remains elevated in primary thrombocythemia, myelofibrosis with myeloid metaplasia, polycythemia vera, and chronic myelogenous leukemia.

When the platelet count is abnormal, diagnosis usually requires further studies, such as complete blood cell count, bone marrow biopsy, direct antiglobulin test (direct Coombs' test), and serum protein electrophoresis.

Interfering factors

- Hemolysis due to rough handling of the sample or to excessive probing at the venipuncture site
- Heparin (decrease)
- Acetazolamide, acetohexamide, antineoplastics, brompheniramine, carbamazepine, chloramphenicol, ethacrynic acid, furosemide, gold salts, hydroxychloroquine, indomethacin, isoniazid, mefenamic acid, mephenytoin, methazolamide, methimazole, methyldopa, oral diazoxide, oxyphenbutazone, penicillamine, penicillin, phenylbutazone, phenytoin, pyrimethamine, quinidine, quinine, salicylates, streptomycin, sulfonamides, thiazide and thiazide-like diuretics, and tricyclic antidepressants (possible decrease)
- Excitement, high altitudes, persistent cold temperatures, or strenuous exercise (increase)

Plethysmography

Plethysmography, also called *occlusive impedance phlebography*, is a reliable, widely used, noninvasive test that measures venous flow in the limbs. Electrodes from a plethysmograph are applied to the patient's leg to record changes in electrical resistance (*impedance*) caused by blood volume variations that may result from respiration or venous occlusion.

Purpose

- To detect deep vein thrombosis (DVT) in the proximal deep veins of the leg
- To screen patients at high risk for thrombophlebitis
- To evaluate patients with suspected pulmonary embolism (because most pulmonary emboli are complications of DVT in the leg)

Cost
Expensive

Patient preparation
■ Explain to the patient that this test helps detect DVT.
■ Inform the patient that he need not restrict food, fluid, or medications before the test.
■ Explain to the patient that the test requires that both legs be tested and that three to five tracings may be made for each leg.
■ Tell the patient who will perform the test and where it will take place.
■ Assure the patient that the test is painless and safe.
■ Emphasize to the patient that accurate testing requires that leg muscles be relaxed and breathing be normal. Tell the patient that if he experiences pain that interferes with leg relaxation, a mild analgesic may be ordered.

Normal findings
Temporary venous occlusion normally produces a sharp rise in venous volume; release of the occlusion produces rapid venous outflow.

Abnormal findings
When clots in a major deep vein obstruct venous outflow, the pressure in the distal leg (calf) veins rises and these veins become distended. Such veins can't expand further when additional pressure is applied with an occlusive thigh cuff. Blockage of major deep veins also decreases the rate at which blood flows from the leg. If significant thrombi are present in a major deep vein of the lower leg (popliteal, femoral, or iliac), calf vein filling and venous outflow rate are reduced. In such cases, evaluate the need for further treatment, such as anticoagulant therapy, taking the patient's overall condition into consideration.

Interfering factors
■ Decreased peripheral arterial blood flow due to shock, increased vasoconstriction, low cardiac output, or arterial occlusive disease
■ Extrinsic venous compression, as from pelvic tumors, large hematomas, constricting clothing, or bandages
■ Failure to breathe normally or to completely relax leg muscles due to pain
■ Cold extremities due to cold room temperature

Pleural biopsy

Pleural biopsy is the removal of pleural tissue by needle biopsy or open biopsy for histologic examination. Needle pleural biopsy is performed under local anesthesia. It generally follows or is done in conjunction with thoracentesis (aspiration of pleural fluid), which is performed when the cause of an effusion is unknown, but it can be performed separately.

Open pleural biopsy, which is performed in the absence of pleural effusion, permits direct visualization of the pleura and the underlying lung. It's performed in the operating room.

ALERT! ▼ ▼ ▼ ▼ ▼ ▼ ▼ ▼ ▼
Pleural biopsy is contraindicated in patients with severe bleeding disorders.

Purpose
■ To differentiate between nonmalignant and malignant disease
■ To diagnose viral, fungal, or parasitic disease and collagen vascular disease of the pleura

Cost

Expensive

Patient preparation

- Describe the procedure to the patient, and answer any questions he may have.
- Explain to the patient that this test permits microscopic examination of pleural tissue.
- Tell the patient who will perform the biopsy and where it will take place.
- Explain to the patient that blood studies will precede the biopsy and that chest X-rays will be taken before and after the biopsy.
- Obtain informed consent if necessary.
- Check the patient's history for hypersensitivity to the local anesthetic.
- Tell the patient that he'll receive a local anesthetic and should experience minor pain during the procedure.

Normal findings

The normal pleura consists primarily of mesothelial cells that are flattened in a uniform layer. Layers of areolar connective tissue that contain blood vessels, nerves, and lymphatics lie below.

Abnormal findings

Histologic examination of the tissue specimen can reveal malignant disease, tuberculosis, and viral, fungal, parasitic, or collagen vascular disease. Primary neoplasms of the pleura are generally fibrous and epithelial.

Interfering factors

- Failure to use the proper fixative or to obtain an adequate specimen
- Patient's inability to remain still, keep from coughing, or follow instructions during the procedure

Pleural fluid analysis

The pleura, a two-layer membrane that covers the lungs and lines the thoracic cavity, maintains a small amount of lubricating fluid between its layers to minimize friction during respiration. Increased fluid in this space may result from such diseases as cancer or tuberculosis or from blood or lymphatic disorders, and can cause respiratory difficulty.

In pleural fluid analysis, also called *thoracentesis*, the thoracic wall is punctured to obtain a specimen of pleural fluid for analysis or to relieve pulmonary (and possibly cardiac) compression and resultant respiratory distress.

Purpose

- To determine the cause and nature of pleural effusion
- To permit better radiographic visualization of a lung with large effusions

Cost

Expensive

Patient preparation

- Explain to the patient that the test assesses the space around the lungs for fluid.
- Tell the patient who will perform the test, where it will take place, and that chest X-rays or an ultrasound study may precede the test to help locate the fluid.
- Check the patient's history for hypersensitivity to local anesthetics and note as an allergy.
- Warn the patient that he may feel a stinging sensation on injection of the anesthetic and some pressure during withdrawal of the fluid.
- Tell the patient not to cough, breathe deeply, or move during the test to minimize the risk of injury to the lung.

Characteristics of pulmonary transudate and exudate

The following characteristics help classify pleural fluid as either a transudate or an exudate.

CHARACTERISTIC	TRANSUDATE	EXUDATE
Appearance	Clear	Cloudy, turbid
Specific gravity	< 1.016	> 1.016
Clot (fibrinogen)	Absent	Present
Protein	< 3 g/dl	> 3 g/dl
White blood cells	Few lymphocytes	Many lymphocytes; may be purulent
Red blood cells	Few	Variable
Glucose level	Equal to serum level	May be less than serum level
Lactate dehydrogenase	Low	High

Normal findings

Normally, the pleural cavity maintains negative pressure and contains less than 20 ml of serous fluid.

Abnormal findings

Pleural effusion results from the abnormal formation or reabsorption of pleural fluid. Certain characteristics classify pleural fluid as either a transudate (a low-protein fluid that has leaked from normal blood vessels) or an exudate (a protein-rich fluid that has leaked from blood vessels with increased permeability).

Pleural fluid may contain blood (hemothorax), chyle (chylothorax), or pus (empyema) and necrotic tissue. Blood-tinged fluid may indicate a traumatic tap; if so, the fluid should clear as aspiration progresses.

Transudative effusion generally results from diminished colloidal pressure, increased negative pressure within the pleural cavity, ascites, systemic and pulmonary venous hypertension, heart failure, hepatic cirrhosis, and nephritis. (See *Characteristics of pulmonary transudate and exudate*.)

Exudative effusion results from disorders that increase pleural capillary permeability (possibly with changes in hydrostatic or colloid osmotic pressures), lymphatic drainage interference, infections, pulmonary infarctions, and neoplasms. Exudative effusion associated with depressed glucose levels, elevated lactate dehydrogenase (LD) isoenzymes, rheumatoid arthritis cells, and negative smears, cultures, and cytologic examination may indicate pleurisy associated with rheumatoid arthritis.

The most common pathogens that appear in culture studies of pleural fluid are *Mycobacterium tuberculosis, Staphylococcus aureus, Streptococcus pneumoniae* and other streptococci, *Haemophilus influenzae* and, in the case of a ruptured pulmonary abscess, anaerobes such as *Bacteroides*. Cultures are usually positive during the early stages of infection; however, antibiotic therapy may produce a negative culture despite a positive Gram stain and grossly purulent fluid. Empyema may result from complications of pneumonia, pulmonary abscess, perforation of the esophagus, or penetration from mediastinitis. A high percentage of neutrophils suggests septic inflammation; predominating lymphocytes suggest tuberculosis, or fungal or viral effusions.

Serosanguineous fluid may indicate pleural extension of a malignant tumor. Elevated LD in a nonpurulent, nonhemolyzed, nonbloody effusion may also suggest malignancy. Pleural fluid glucose levels that are 30 to 40 mg/dl lower than blood glucose levels may indicate a malignant tumor, a bacterial infection, nonseptic inflammation, or metastasis. Increased amylase levels occur in pleural effusions associated with pancreatitis.

Interfering factors
■ Antimicrobial therapy before aspiration of fluid for culture (possible decrease in numbers of bacteria, making it difficult to isolate the infecting organism)

Porphyrins, urine

The urine porphyrins test is a quantitative analysis of urine porphyrins (most notably, uroporphyrins and coproporphyrins) and their precursors (porphyrinogens such as porphobilinogen [PBG]). Porphyrins are red-orange fluorescent compounds, consisting of four pyrrole rings that are produced during heme biosynthesis. They're present in all protoplasm, figure in energy storage and utilization, and are normally excreted in urine in small amounts. Elevated urine levels of porphyrins or porphyrinogens, therefore, reflect impaired heme biosynthesis. Such impairment may result from inherited enzyme deficiencies (congenital porphyrias) or from defects due to such disorders as hemolytic anemias and hepatic disease (acquired porphyrias).

Determination of the specific porphyrins and porphyrinogens found in a urine specimen can help identify the impaired metabolic step in heme biosynthesis. Occasionally, a preliminary qualitative screening is performed on a random specimen. However, a positive finding on the screening test must be confirmed by the quantitative analysis of a 24-hour specimen. For correct diagnosis of a specific porphyria, urine porphyrin levels should be correlated with plasma and fecal porphyrin levels.

Purpose
■ To aid diagnosis of congenital or acquired porphyrias

Cost
Moderately expensive

Patient preparation
■ Explain to the patient that this test detects abnormal hemoglobin formation.
■ Tell the patient the test requires urine collection over a 24-hour period, discarding the first specimen and retaining the last.
■ Restrict medications that may affect test results. If they must be continued, note this on the laboratory request.

Reference values
Normal urine porphyrin and precursor values fall in the following ranges:
■ *uroporphyrins:* 27 to 52 µg/24 hours (SI, 32 to 63 nmol/day)
■ *coproporphyrins:* 34 to 230 µg/24 hours (SI, 52 to 351 nmol/day).

Urine porphyrin levels in porphyria

In porphyria, defective heme biosynthesis increases urine porphyrins and their corresponding precursors.

PORPHYRIA	PORPHYRINS		PORPHYRIN PRECURSORS	
	Uroporphyrins	Coproporphyrins	∂-amino-levulinic acid	Porphobilinogen
Erythropoietic porphyria	Highly increased	Increased	Normal	Normal
Erythropoietic protoporphyria	Normal	Normal	Normal	Normal
Acute intermittent porphyria	Variable	Variable	Highly increased	Highly increased
Variegate porphyria	Normal or slightly increased; may be highly increased during acute attack	Normal or slightly increased; may be highly increased during acute attack	Highly increased during acute attack	Normal or slightly increased; highly increased during acute attack
Coproporphyria	Not applicable	May be highly increased during acute attack	Increased during acute attack	Increased during acute attack
Porphyria cutanea tarda	Highly increased	Increased	Variable	Variable

Abnormal findings

Increased urine levels of porphyrins and porphyrin precursors are characteristic of porphyria. (See *Urine porphyrin levels in porphyria.*) Infectious hepatitis, Hodgkin's disease, central nervous system disorders, cirrhosis, and heavy metal, benzene, or carbon tetrachloride toxicity may also increase porphyrin levels.

Interfering factors

■ Failure to properly store the specimen during the collection period or to protect it from exposure to light

■ Failure to send the specimen to the laboratory immediately after the collection is completed

■ Barbiturates, chloral hydrate, chlordiazepoxide, chlorpropamide, meprobamate, or sulfonamides induce porphyria or porphyrinuria; they should be discontinued 12 days before the test if possible (increase)

■ Griseofulvin, hormonal contraceptives (increase)

■ Pregnancy or menstruation (possible increase or decrease)

■ Rifampin (elevated urine urobilinogen)

Potassium, serum

The serum potassium test is used to measure serum levels of potassium, the major intracellular cation. Potassium helps to maintain cellular osmotic equilibrium and to regulate muscle activity, enzyme activity, and acid-base balance. It also influences renal function.

The body has no efficient method for conserving potassium; the kidneys excrete nearly all ingested potassium, even when the body's supply is depleted. Potassium deficiency can develop rapidly and is quite common. Dietary intake of at least 40 mEq/day is essential.

Purpose
■ To evaluate clinical signs of potassium excess (hyperkalemia) or potassium depletion (hypokalemia)
■ To monitor renal function, acid-base balance, and glucose metabolism
■ To evaluate neuromuscular and endocrine disorders
■ To detect the origin of arrhythmias

Cost
Inexpensive

Patient preparation
■ Explain to the patient that this test is used to determine the potassium content of blood.
■ Tell the patient that the test requires a blood sample. Explain who will perform the venipuncture and when.
■ Explain to the patient that he may experience discomfort from the needle puncture and the tourniquet.
■ Restrict medications that may affect test results. If they must be continued, note this on the laboratory request.

Reference values
Normally, serum potassium levels range from 3.5 to 5 mEq/L (SI, 3.5 to 5 mmol/L).

Abnormal findings
Abnormally high serum potassium levels are common in conditions in which excess cellular potassium enters the blood, such as burn injuries, crush injuries, diabetic ketoacidosis, transfusions of large amounts of blood, and myocardial infarction. Hyperkalemia may also indicate reduced sodium excretion, possibly due to renal failure (preventing normal exchange of sodium and potassium) or Addison's disease (due to potassium buildup and sodium depletion).

ALERT! ▼ ▼ ▼ ▼ ▼ ▼ ▼ ▼ ▼
In patients with hyperkalemia, electrocardiography (ECG) reveals flattened P waves, a prolonged PR interval, a wide QRS complex, a tall, tented T wave, and ST-segment depression.

Below-normal serum potassium values commonly result from aldosteronism or Cushing's syndrome, loss of body fluids (such as long-term diuretic therapy, vomiting, or diarrhea), and excessive licorice ingestion. Although serum values and clinical symptoms can indicate a potassium imbalance, an ECG allows a definitive diagnosis.

ALERT! ▼ ▼ ▼ ▼ ▼ ▼ ▼ ▼ ▼
In patients with hypokalemia, ECG reveals flattened T waves, ST-segment depression, and U-wave elevation.

Interfering factors
■ Repeated clenching of the fist before venipuncture, delay in drawing blood after applying a tourniquet, or excessive hemolysis of the sample (increase)
■ Excessive or rapid potassium infusion; renal toxicity from administration of amphotericin B, methicillin, or tetracycline;

and spironolactone or penicillin G potassium therapy (increase)

■ Diuretic therapy (especially with thiazides but not with triamterene, amiloride, or spironolactone); insulin and glucose administration; and I.V. infusions without potassium (decrease)

Potassium, urine

The urine potassium test is a quantitative test that measures urine levels of potassium, a major intracellular cation that helps regulate acid-base balance and neuromuscular function. Potassium imbalance may cause such signs and symptoms as muscle weakness, nausea, diarrhea, confusion, hypotension, and electrocardiogram changes; severe imbalance may lead to cardiac arrest.

Most commonly, a serum potassium test is performed to detect hyperkalemia (abnormally high levels) or hypokalemia (abnormally low levels). A urine potassium test may be performed to evaluate hypokalemia when a history and physical examination fail to uncover the cause. If results suggest a renal disorder, additional renal function tests may be ordered.

Purpose
■ To determine whether hypokalemia is caused by renal or extrarenal disorders

Cost
Inexpensive

Patient preparation
■ Explain to the patient that this test evaluates his kidney function.
■ Tell the patient that the test requires urine collection over a 24-hour period, discarding the first specimen and retaining the last.

■ Restrict medications that may affect test results. If they must be continued, note this on the laboratory request.

Reference values
Normal urine potassium excretion in adults is 25 to 125 mmol/24 hours (SI, 25 to 125 mmol/d) and varies with diet. In children, normal urine potassium excretion is 22 to 57 mmol/24 hours (SI, 22 to 57 mmol/d).

Abnormal findings
In a patient with hypokalemia, urine potassium concentration less than 10 mmol/24 hours (SI, 10 mmol/d) suggests normal renal function, indicating that potassium loss is most likely the result of a GI disorder such as malabsorption syndrome.

In a patient with hypokalemia lasting more than 3 days, urine potassium concentration above 10 mmol/24 hours indicates renal loss of potassium. These losses may result from such disorders as aldosteronism, renal tubular acidosis, or chronic renal failure. However, extrarenal disorders, such as dehydration, starvation, Cushing's disease, or salicylate intoxication, may also elevate urine potassium levels.

Interfering factors
■ Excess dietary potassium (increase)
■ Failure to collect all the urine, to put the specimen on ice
■ Failure to send the specimen to the laboratory immediately after collection
■ Potassium-wasting medications, such as acetazolamide, ammonium chloride, and thiazide diuretics (increase)
■ Excess vomiting or stomach suctioning

Pregnanediol, urine

Using gas chromatography or radioimmunoassay, the urine pregnanediol test measures urine levels of pregnanediol, the chief metabolite of progesterone. Although biologically inert, pregnanediol has diagnostic significance because it reflects about 10% of the endogenous production of its parent hormone.

Progesterone is produced in nonpregnant females by the corpus luteum during the latter half of each menstrual cycle, preparing the uterus for implantation of a fertilized ovum. If implantation doesn't occur, progesterone secretion drops sharply; if implantation does occur, the corpus luteum secretes more progesterone to further prepare the uterus for pregnancy and to begin development of the placenta. Toward the end of the first trimester, the placenta becomes the primary source of progesterone secretion, producing the progressively larger amounts needed to maintain pregnancy.

Normally, urine levels of pregnanediol reflect variations in progesterone secretion during the menstrual cycle and during pregnancy. Direct measurement of plasma progesterone levels by radioimmunoassay may also be done.

Purpose
■ To evaluate placental function in pregnant females
■ To evaluate ovarian function in nonpregnant females
■ To aid in the diagnosis of menstrual disorder

Cost
Moderately expensive

Patient preparation
■ Explain to the patient that this test evaluates placental or ovarian function.
■ Tell the patient that the test requires collection of urine over a 24-hour period, discarding the first specimen and retaining the last.
■ Advise the pregnant patient that this test may be repeated several times to obtain serial measurements.
■ Restrict medications that may affect test results. If they must be continued, note this on the laboratory request.

Reference values
In nonpregnant females, urine pregnanediol values normally range from 0.5 to 1.5 mg/24 hours during the follicular phase of the menstrual cycle. In pregnant females, the values range as follows:
■ *first trimester:* 10 to 30 mg/24 hours
■ *second trimester:* 35 to 70 mg/24 hours
■ *third trimester:* 70 to 100 mg/24 hours.

In postmenopausal females, urine pregnanediol levels range from 0.2 to 1 mg/24 hours. In males, urine pregnanediol levels are 0 to 1 mg/24 hours.

Abnormal findings
During pregnancy, a marked decrease in urine pregnanediol levels based on a single 24-hour urine specimen or a steady decrease in pregnanediol levels in serial measurements may indicate placental insufficiency and requires immediate investigation. A precipitous drop in urine pregnanediol values may suggest fetal distress — for example, threatened abortion or preeclampsia — or fetal death. However, pregnanediol measurements aren't reliable indicators of fetal viability because levels can remain normal even after fetal death, as long as maternal circulation to the placenta remains adequate.

In nonpregnant females, abnormally low urine pregnanediol levels may occur with anovulation, amenorrhea, or other menstrual abnormalities. Low to normal urine pregnanediol levels may be associated with hydatidiform mole. Elevations may indicate luteinized granulosa or theca cell tumors, diffuse thecal luteinization, or metastatic ovarian cancer.

Adrenal hyperplasia or biliary tract obstruction may elevate urine pregnanediol values in males or females. Some forms of primary hepatic disease produce abnormally low levels in both sexes.

Interfering factors
■ Failure to properly store the specimen during the collection period
■ Combination hormonal contraceptives, drugs containing corticotropin, methenamine hippurate, methenamine mandelate, and progestogens (possible increase or decrease)

Proctosigmoidoscopy

Proctosigmoidoscopy uses a proctoscope, sigmoidoscope, and digital examination to evaluate the lining of the distal sigmoid colon, rectum, and anal canal. It's indicated in patients with recent changes in bowel habits, lower abdominal and perineal pain, prolapse on defecation, pruritus, and passage of mucus, blood, or pus in the stool. Specimens may be obtained from suspicious areas of the mucosa by biopsy, lavage or cytology brush, or culture swab. Possible complications of this procedure include rectal bleeding and, rarely, bowel perforation.

Purpose
■ To aid diagnosis of inflammatory, infectious, and ulcerative bowel disease

■ To detect hemorrhoids, hypertrophic anal papilla, polyps, fissures, fistulas, and abscesses in the rectum and anal canal

Cost
Expensive

Patient preparation
■ Explain to the patient that this procedure allows visual examination of the lining of the distal sigmoid colon, rectum, and anal canal.
■ Tell the patient that the test requires passage of two special instruments through the anus. Tell him who will perform the procedure and where it will be done.
■ Check the patient's history for allergies, medications, and information pertinent to the current complaint. Find out whether he has had a barium test within the past week because barium in the colon hinders accurate examination.
■ If a special bowel preparation is necessary, explain to the patient that this clears the intestine to ensure a better view.
■ Instruct the patient to maintain a clear liquid diet for 24 to 48 hours before the test, to avoid eating fruits and vegetables before the procedure, and to fast the morning of the procedure.
■ Tell the patient he may receive a warm tap-water or sodium biphosphate enema 3 to 4 hours before the procedure.
■ Tell the patient that he may be secured to a tilting table that rotates into horizontal and vertical positions.
■ Inform the patient that an I.V. line may be started if an I.V. sedative is to be used. If the procedure is being done on an outpatient basis, advise him to arrange for someone to drive him home and to avoid alcohol for 24 hours.
■ Obtain informed consent if necessary.

Normal findings

The mucosa of the sigmoid colon appears light pink-orange and is marked by semilunar folds and deep tubular pits. The rectal mucosa is redder due to its rich vascular network, deepens to a purple hue at the pectinate line (the anatomic division between the rectum and anus), and has three distinct valves. The lower two-thirds of the anus (anoderm) is lined with smooth gray-tan skin and joins with the hair-fringed perianal skin.

Abnormal findings

Visual examination and palpation demonstrate abnormalities of the anal canal and rectum, including internal and external hemorrhoids, hypertrophic anal papilla, anal fissures, anal fistulas, and anorectal abscesses. The examination may also reveal inflammatory bowel diseases, polyps, cancer, and other tumors. Biopsy, culture, and other laboratory tests are typically necessary to detect various disorders.

Interfering factors

■ Barium in the intestine from previous diagnostic studies (hinders visualization)
■ Large amounts of stool in the intestine (hinders visual examination and advancement of the endoscope)
■ Failure to place histologic or cytologic specimens in the appropriate preservative
■ Failure to send the specimens to the laboratory immediately

Progesterone, plasma

Progesterone, an ovarian steroid hormone secreted by the corpus luteum, causes thickening and secretory development of the endometrium in preparation for implantation of the fertilized ovum. Progesterone levels, therefore, peak during the midluteal phase of the menstrual cycle. Progesterone may prolong the surge of luteinizing hormone after ovulation. If implantation doesn't occur, progesterone (and estrogen) levels drop sharply and menstruation begins about 2 days later. (See *The endometrial cycle*.)

During pregnancy, the placenta releases about 10 times the normal monthly amount of progesterone to maintain the pregnancy. Increased secretion begins toward the end of the first trimester and continues until delivery. Progesterone causes thickening of the endometrium, which contains large amounts of stored nutrients for the developing ovum (blastocyst). In addition, progesterone prevents abortion by decreasing uterine contractions and, with estrogen, prepares the breasts for lactation.

The plasma progesterone test, a radioimmunoassay, is a quantitative analysis of plasma progesterone levels. It provides reliable information about corpus luteum function in fertility studies or placental function in pregnancy. Serial determinations are recommended. Although plasma levels provide accurate information, progesterone can also be monitored by measuring urine pregnanediol, a catabolite of progesterone.

Purpose

■ To assess corpus luteum function as part of infertility studies
■ To evaluate placental function during pregnancy
■ To aid in confirming ovulation (test results support basal body temperature readings)

Cost

Inexpensive

The endometrial cycle

Each month, progesterone, released by the corpus luteum, stimulates endometrial thickening in preparation for implantation of a fertilized ovum. The endometrial layer contains nutrients necessary for growth of the blastocyst. Immediately after menstruation, in the proliferative phase, the endometrium is thin and relatively homogenous. It continuously thickens until the end of the secretory phase, just before the menstrual phase begins again.

MENSTRUAL	PROLIFERATIVE	SECRETORY	MENSTRUAL

1 2 3 4 5 6 7 8 9 10 11 12 13 14 15 16 17 18 19 20 21 22 23 24 25 26 27 28 1 2 3 4 5

Days →

Patient preparation

■ Explain to the patient that this test helps determine whether her female sex hormone secretion is normal.

■ Tell the patient that the test requires a blood sample. Explain who will perform the venipuncture and when.

■ Explain to the patient that she may experience discomfort from the needle puncture and the tourniquet.

■ Inform the patient that the test may be repeated at specific times coinciding with phases of her menstrual cycle or at each prenatal visit.

Reference values

Normal values during menstruation are as follows:

■ *follicular phase:* < 150 ng/dl (SI, < 5 nmol/L)

■ *luteal phase:* 300 to 1,200 ng/dl (SI, 10 to 40 nmol/L).

Normal values during pregnancy are as follows:

■ *first trimester:* 1,500 to 5,000 ng/dl (SI, 50 to 160 nmol/L)

■ *second and third trimesters:* 8,000 to 20,000 ng/dl (SI, 250 to 650 nmol/L).

Normal values in menopausal women are 10 to 22 ng/dl (SI, 0.33 to 0.73 nmol/L).

Abnormal findings

Elevated progesterone levels may indicate ovulation, luteinizing tumors, ovarian cysts that produce progesterone, or adrenocortical hyperplasias and tumors that produce progesterone along with other steroidal hormones.

Low progesterone levels are associated with amenorrhea associated with several causes (such as panhypopituitarism or gonadal dysfunction), toxemia of pregnancy, threatened abortion, and fetal death.

Interfering factors
■ Progesterone or estrogen therapy
■ Use of radioisotopes or scans within 1 week of the test
■ Hemolysis due to rough handling of the sample

Prolactin

Prolactin is essential for the development of the mammary glands for lactation during pregnancy and for stimulating and maintaining lactation postpartum. Like human growth hormone, prolactin acts directly on tissues, and its levels rise in response to sleep and physical or emotional stress.

The prolactin test, a radioimmunoassay, is a quantitative analysis of serum prolactin levels, which normally rise 10- to 20-fold during pregnancy, corresponding to concomitant elevations in human placental lactogen levels. After delivery, prolactin secretion falls to basal levels in mothers who don't breast-feed. However, prolactin secretion increases during breast-feeding, apparently as a result of a stimulus triggered by suckling that curtails the release of prolactin-inhibiting factor by the hypothalamus. This in turn allows transient elevations of prolactin secretion by the pituitary gland.

This test is considered useful in patients suspected of having pituitary tumors, which are known to secrete prolactin in excessive amounts. Another test used to eval-uate hypothalamic dysfunction is the thyrotropin-releasing hormone (TRH) stimulation test. (See *TRH stimulation test.*)

Purpose
■ To facilitate diagnosis of pituitary dysfunction, possibly due to pituitary adenoma
■ To aid in the diagnosis of hypothalamic dysfunction regardless of cause
■ To evaluate secondary amenorrhea and galactorrhea

Cost
Moderately expensive

Patient preparation
■ Tell the patient that this test helps evaluate hormonal secretion.
■ Advise the patient to restrict food and fluids and limit physical activity for 12 hours before the test and to relax for about 30 minutes before the test.
■ Tell the patient that the test requires a blood sample. Explain who will perform the venipuncture and when.
■ Explain to the patient that she may experience discomfort from the needle puncture and the tourniquet.
■ Restrict medications that may affect test results. If they must be continued, note this on the laboratory request.

Reference values
Normal values range from undetectable to 23 ng/ml (SI, undetectable to 23 µg/L) in nonlactating females. Levels normally rise 10- to 20-fold during pregnancy and, after delivery, fall to basal levels in mothers who don't breast-feed. Prolactin secretion increases during breast-feeding.

Abnormal findings
Abnormally high prolactin levels (100 to 300 ng/ml [SI, 100 to 300 µg/L]) suggest

autonomous prolactin production by a pituitary adenoma, especially when amenorrhea or galactorrhea is present (Forbes-Albright syndrome). Rarely, hyperprolactinemia may also result from severe endocrine disorders such as hypothyroidism. Idiopathic hyperprolactinemia may be associated with anovulatory infertility. Confirm slight elevations with repeat measurements on two other occasions.

Decreased prolactin levels in a lactating mother cause failure of lactation and may be associated with postpartum pituitary infarction (Sheehan's syndrome). Abnormally low prolactin levels have also been found in some patients with empty sella syndrome. In these patients, a flattened pituitary gland makes the pituitary fossa look empty.

Interfering factors

■ Failure to take into account physiologic variations related to sleep or stress
■ Estrogens, ethanol, methyldopa, and morphine (increase)
■ Ergot alkaloids and levodopa (decrease)
■ Radioactive scan performed within 1 week before the test or recent surgery
■ Breast stimulation

Prostate-specific antigen

Prostate-specific antigen (PSA) appears in normal, benign hyperplastic, and malignant prostatic tissue as well as metastatic prostatic carcinoma. Serum PSA levels are used to monitor the spread of recurrence of prostate cancer and to evaluate the patient's response to treatment. Measurement of serum PSA levels along with a digital rectal examination is now recommended as a screening test for prostate cancer in men over age 50. It's also useful in assess-

TRH stimulation test

The thyrotropin-releasing hormone (TRH) stimulation test evaluates hypothalamic dysfunction and pituitary tumors by stimulating the release of prolactin. A venipuncture is performed to obtain a baseline prolactin level and then the patient is assisted into the supine position. An I.V. bolus of synthetic TRH in a dose of 500 µg/ml over 15 to 30 seconds is administered, and blood samples are obtained at 15- and 30-minute intervals to measure prolactin.

A baseline prolactin reading greater than 200 ng/ml (SI, > 200 IU/L) indicates a pituitary tumor, although levels between 30 and 200 ng/ml (SI, 30 to 200 IU/L) are also consistent with this condition. Normally, patients show at least a twofold increase in prolactin after injection of TRH. If the prolactin level fails to rise, hypothalamic dysfunction or adenoma of the pituitary gland is likely.

ing response to treatment in patients with stage B3 to D1 prostate cancer and in detecting tumor spread or recurrence.

Purpose

■ To screen for prostate cancer in men over age 50
■ To monitor the course of prostate cancer and aid evaluation of treatment

Cost

Moderately expensive

Patient preparation

■ Explain to the patient that this test is used to screen for prostate cancer, or, if appropriate, to monitor the course of treatment.

- Tell the patient that the test requires a blood sample. Explain who will perform the venipuncture and when.
- Explain to the patient that he may experience discomfort from the needle puncture and the tourniquet.

ALERT! ▼ ▼ ▼ ▼ ▼ ▼ ▼ ▼ ▼
Collect the sample either before digital prostate examination or at least 48 hours after examination to avoid falsely elevated PSA levels.

Reference values

Normal values are as follows:

- *ages 40 to 50:* 2 to 2.8 ng/ml (SI, 2 to 2.8 µg/L)
- *ages 51 to 60:* 2.9 to 3.8 ng/ml (SI, 2.9 to 3.8 µg/L)
- *ages 61 to 70:* 4 to 5.3 ng/ml (SI, 4 to 5.3 µg/L)
- *ages 71 and older:* 5.6 to 7.2 ng/ml (SI, 5.6 to 7.2 µg/L).

Abnormal findings

About 80% of patients with prostate cancer have pretreatment PSA values greater than 4 ng/ml. However, PSA results alone don't confirm a diagnosis of prostate cancer. (See

Controversy over PSA screening.) About 20% of patients with benign prostatic hyperplasia also have levels greater than 4 ng/ml. Further assessment and testing, including tissue biopsy, are needed to confirm cancer.

Interfering factors
■ Excessive doses of chemotherapeutic drugs, such as cyclophosphamide, diethylstilbestrol, and methotrexate (possible increase or decrease)

Protein C

Vitamin K-dependent, protein C is produced in the liver and circulates in the plasma. It acts as a potent anticoagulant by suppressing activated factors V and VIII. Deficiencies of protein C may be acquired or congenital.

If a deficiency of protein C is identified, further immunologic tests may be needed to determine the type of deficiency. Identifying the role of protein C deficiency in idiopathic venous thrombosis may help prevent thromboembolism.

Purpose
■ To investigate the mechanism of idiopathic venous thrombosis

Cost
Moderately expensive

Patient preparation
■ Explain to the patient that this test evaluates blood clotting.
■ Tell the patient that the test requires a blood sample. Explain who will perform the venipuncture and when.
■ Explain to the patient that he may experience discomfort from the needle puncture and the tourniquet.

■ Restrict medications that may affect test results. If they must be continued, note this on the laboratory request.

Reference values
The normal range of protein C is 70% to 140% (SI, 0.70 to 1.40).

Abnormal findings
Rare, homozygous protein C deficiency is characterized by rapidly fatal thrombosis in the perinatal period, a condition known as purpura fulminans.

The more common heterozygous deficiency is associated with genetic susceptibility to venous thromboembolism before age 30 and continuing throughout life. The patient may require long-term treatment with warfarin therapy or protein C supplements from plasma fractions.

Protein C deficiency is also seen in patients with liver cirrhosis and vitamin K deficiency and in those taking warfarin.

Interfering factors
■ Hemolysis due to rough handling of the sample or to excessive probing at the venipuncture site
■ Anticoagulant therapy

Protein electrophoresis

Protein electrophoresis separates serum albumin and globulins by using an electric field to differentiate the proteins according to their size, shape, and electric charge at pH 8.6 into five distinct fractions: albumin, alpha$_1$, alpha$_2$, beta, and gamma proteins. Because each moves at a different rate, the fractions have recognizable, measurable patterns.

How hepatic diseases affect protein fractions

Because the liver synthesizes albumin as well as alpha and beta globulins, changes in the concentration of these major plasma proteins can indicate hepatic malfunction or hepatocellular damage. Although total protein levels — the sum of albumin and globulin fractions — may remain normal, hepatic disease will alter one, several, or all of the protein fractions.

	NORMAL	HEPATITIS	CIRRHOSIS	OBSTRUCTIVE JAUNDICE	METASTATIC LIVER CANCER
Total protein	100%	0	–	0	0
Albumin	53%	0	–	0/–	–
Alpha$_1$-globulin	14%	–	0	0	+
Alpha$_2$-globulin	14%	–	0	0/+	+
Beta globulin	12%	+	+	0/+	0/+
Gamma globulin	20%	+	+	0	0/+

KEY: 0 = normal   + = increased   – = decreased

Purpose
■ To aid diagnosis of hepatic disease, protein deficiency, renal disorders, and GI and neoplastic diseases

Cost
Moderately expensive

Patient preparation
■ Explain to the patient that this test is used to determine the protein content of blood.
■ Tell the patient that the test requires a blood sample. Explain who will perform the venipuncture and when.
■ Explain to the patient that he may experience discomfort from the needle puncture and the tourniquet.
■ Restrict medications that may affect test results. If they must be continued, note this on the laboratory request.

ALERT! ▼ ▼ ▼ ▼ ▼ ▼ ▼ ▼ ▼
This test must be performed on a serum sample to avoid measuring the fibrinogen fraction.

Reference values
Normally, total serum protein levels range from 6.4 to 8.3 g/dl (SI, 64 to 83 g/L), and the albumin fraction ranges from 3.5 to 5 g/dl (SI, 35 to 50 g/L). The alpha$_1$-globulin fraction ranges from 0.1 to 0.3 g/dl (SI, 1 to 3 g/L); alpha$_2$-globulin ranges from 0.6 to 1 g/dl (SI, 6 to 10 g/L). Beta globulin ranges from 0.7 to 1.1 g/dl (SI, 7 to 11 g/L); gamma globulin ranges from 0.8 to 1.6 g/dl (SI, 8 to 16 g/L).

Abnormal findings
See *How hepatic diseases affect protein fractions,* and *Clinical implications of abnormal protein levels.*

Clinical implications of abnormal protein levels

	TOTAL PROTEINS	ALBUMIN	GLOBULINS
INCREASED LEVELS	■ Chronic inflammatory disease (such as rheumatoid arthritis or early-stage Laënnec's cirrhosis) ■ Dehydration ■ Diabetic ketoacidosis ■ Fulminating and chronic infections ■ Multiple myeloma ■ Monocytic leukemia ■ Vomiting, diarrhea	■ Multiple myeloma	■ Chronic syphilis ■ Collagen diseases ■ Diabetes mellitus ■ Hodgkin's disease ■ Levels variable in neoplastic and renal diseases, hepatic dysfunction, and blood dyscrasias ■ Multiple myeloma ■ Rheumatoid arthritis ■ Subacute bacterial endocarditis ■ Systemic lupus erythematosus ■ Tuberculosis
DECREASED LEVELS	■ Benzene and carbon tetrachloride poisoning ■ Blood dyscrasias ■ Essential hypertension ■ GI disease ■ Heart failure ■ Hepatic dysfunction ■ Hemorrhage ■ Hodgkin's disease ■ Hyperthyroidism ■ Malabsorption ■ Malnutrition ■ Nephrosis ■ Severe burns ■ Surgical and traumatic shock ■ Toxemia of pregnancy ■ Uncontrolled diabetes mellitus	■ Acute cholecystitis ■ Collagen diseases ■ Diarrhea ■ Essential hypertension ■ Hepatic disease ■ Hyperthyroidism ■ Hypogammaglobulinemia ■ Malnutrition ■ Metastatic carcinoma ■ Nephritis, nephrosis ■ Peptic ulcer ■ Plasma loss from burns ■ Rheumatoid arthritis ■ Sarcoidosis ■ Systemic lupus erythematosus	■ Levels variable in neoplastic and renal diseases, hepatic dysfunction, and blood dyscrasias

Interfering factors

■ Pretest administration of a contrast agent, such as sulfobromophthalein (false-high total protein)

■ Pregnancy or cytotoxic drugs (possible decrease in serum albumin)

■ Use of plasma instead of serum

Protein, urine

The urine protein test is a quantitative test for proteinuria. Normally, the glomerular membrane allows only proteins of low molecular weight to enter the filtrate. The renal tubules then reabsorb most of these proteins, normally excreting a small amount that's undetectable by a screening test. A damaged glomerular capillary membrane and impaired tubular reabsorption allow excretion of proteins in the urine.

A qualitative screening typically precedes this test. A positive result requires quantitative analysis of a 24-hour urine specimen by acid precipitation tests. Electrophoresis can detect albumin, Bence Jones protein, hemoglobins, or myoglobins.

Purpose

■ To aid diagnosis of pathologic states characterized by proteinuria, primarily renal disease

Cost

Inexpensive

Patient preparation

■ Explain to the patient that this test detects proteins in the urine.

■ Tell the patient that the test usually requires urine collection over a 24-hour period; random collection can be done.

■ Restrict medications that may affect test results. If they must be continued, note this on the laboratory request.

Reference values

At rest, normal urine protein values range from 50 to 80 mg/24 hours (SI, 50 to 80 mg/d).

Abnormal findings

Proteinuria is a chief characteristic of renal disease. When proteinuria is present in a single specimen, a 24-hour urine collection is required to identify specific renal abnormalities.

Proteinuria can result from glomerular leakage of plasma proteins (a major cause of protein excretion), from overflow of filtered proteins of low molecular weight (when these are present in excessive concentrations), from impaired tubular reabsorption of filtered proteins, and from the presence of renal proteins derived from the breakdown of kidney tissue.

Persistent proteinuria indicates renal disease resulting from increased glomerular permeability. Minimal proteinuria (< 0.5 g/24 hours), however, is most commonly associated with renal diseases in which glomerular involvement isn't a major factor, as in chronic pyelonephritis.

Moderate proteinuria (0.5 to 4 g/24 hours) occurs in several types of renal disease — acute or chronic glomerulonephritis, amyloidosis, toxic nephropathies — or in diseases in which renal failure typically develops as a late complication (diabetes or heart failure, for example). Heavy proteinuria (> 4 g/24 hours) is commonly associated with nephrotic syndrome.

When accompanied by an elevated white blood cell count, proteinuria indicates urinary tract infection. When accompanied by hematuria, proteinuria indicates local or diffuse urinary tract disorders. Other pathologic states (infections and lesions of the central nervous system, for example) can also result in detectable amounts of proteins in the urine.

Many drugs (such as amphotericin B, gold preparations, aminoglycosides, and trimethadione) inflict renal damage, causing true proteinuria. This makes the routine evaluation of urine proteins essential during such treatment. In all forms of proteinuria, fractionation results obtained by electrophoresis provide more precise information than the screening test. For example, excessive hemoglobin in the urine indicates intravascular hemolysis, elevated myoglobin suggests muscle damage, albumin suggests increased glomerular permeability, and Bence Jones protein suggests multiple myeloma.

Not all forms of proteinuria have pathologic significance. Benign proteinuria can result from changes in body position. Functional proteinuria is associated with exercise as well as emotional or physiologic stress and is usually transient.

Interfering factors
■ Contamination of the specimen with toilet tissue or stool
■ Acetazolamide, cephalosporins, iodine-containing contrast media, para-aminosalicylic acid, penicillin, sodium bicarbonate, sulfonamides, and tolbutamide (possible false-positive or false-negative)
■ Very dilute urine, such as from forcing fluids (may depress protein values and cause a false-negative result)

Prothrombin time

Prothrombin time (PT) measures the time required for a fibrin clot to form in a citrat-ed plasma sample after addition of calcium ions and tissue thromboplastin (factor III).

Purpose
■ To evaluate extrinsic coagulation system (factors V, VII, and X, and prothrombin and fibrinogen)
■ To monitor response to oral anticoagulant therapy

Cost
Inexpensive

Patient preparation
■ Explain to the patient that this test is used to determine whether the blood clots normally.
■ Restrict medications that may affect test results. If they must be continued, note this on the laboratory request.
■ Tell the patient that the test requires a blood sample. Explain who will perform the venipuncture and when.
■ Explain to the patient that he may experience discomfort from the needle puncture and the tourniquet.
■ When appropriate, explain that this test is used to monitor the effects of oral anticoagulants; the test will be performed daily when therapy begins and will be repeated at longer intervals when medication levels stabilize.

Normal findings
Normally, PT values range from 10 to 14 seconds (SI, 10 to 14 s). Values vary, however, depending on the source of tissue thromboplastin and the type of sensing devices used to measure clot formation. In a patient receiving oral anticoagulants, PT is usually maintained between 1 and 2.5 times the normal control value. (See *International Normalized Ratio*, page 306.)

Abnormal findings

Prolonged PT may indicate deficiencies in fibrinogen; prothrombin; factors V, VII, or X (specific assays can pinpoint such deficiencies); or vitamin K. It may also result from ongoing oral anticoagulant therapy.

Prolonged PT that exceeds 2.5 times the control value is commonly associated with abnormal bleeding.

Interfering factors
- Failure to fill the collection tube completely (possible false-high)
- Salicylates, more than 1 g/day (increase)
- Fibrin or fibrin split products in the sample or plasma fibrinogen levels less than 100 mg/dl (possible prolonged PT)
- Antihistamines, cardiac glycosides, chloral hydrate, corticosteroids, diuretics, glutethimide, griseofulvin, progestin-estrogen combinations, pyrazinamide, vitamin K, and xanthines, such as caffeine and theophylline (possible decrease)
- Alcohol in excess, anabolic steroids, cholestyramine resin, corticotropin, heparin I.V. (within 5 hours of sample collection), indomethacin, mefenamic acid, methimazole, phenylbutazone, phenytoin, propylthiouracil, quinidine, quinine, thyroid hormones, or vitamin A (prolonged PT)
- Antibiotics, barbiturates, clofibrate, hydroxyzine, mineral oil, or sulfonamides (possible increase or decrease)

Pulmonary angiography

Pulmonary angiography, also called *pulmonary arteriography*, is the radiographic examination of the pulmonary circulation following injection of a radiopaque iodine contrast agent into the pulmonary artery or one of its branches.

Possible complications include arterial occlusion, myocardial perforation or rupture, ventricular arrhythmias from myocardial irritation, and acute renal failure from hypersensitivity to the contrast agent.

ALERT! ▼ ▼ ▼ ▼ ▼ ▼ ▼ ▼ ▼
Pulmonary angiography is contraindicated during pregnancy.

Purpose
■ To detect pulmonary embolism in a patient who's equivocal
■ To evaluate pulmonary circulation abnormalities
■ To evaluate pulmonary circulation preoperatively in the patient with congenital heart disease
■ To locate a large embolus before surgical removal

Cost
Expensive

Patient preparation
■ Describe the procedure to the patient. Explain that this test permits evaluation of the blood vessels to help identify the cause of his symptoms.
■ Instruct the patient to fast for 8 hours before the test or as prescribed. Tell him who will perform the test, where it will take place, and that laboratory work for kidney function and coagulation may precede the test.
■ Tell the patient a small puncture will be made in the blood vessel of the right arm where blood samples are usually drawn, or in the right groin at the femoral vein, and that a local anesthetic will be used to numb the area. Inform him that a small catheter will then be inserted into the blood vessel and passed into the right side of the heart and then to the pulmonary artery.
■ Tell the patient the contrast agent will then be injected into this artery. Warn him that he may feel flushed, experience an urge to cough, or experience a salty taste

for approximately 3 to 5 minutes after the injection.
■ Inform the patient that his heart rate will be monitored continuously during the procedure.
■ Obtain informed consent if necessary.
■ Check the patient's history for hypersensitivity to anesthetics, iodine, seafood, or radiographic contrast agents and note as an allergy.
■ Order laboratory tests (including prothrombin time, partial thromboplastin time, platelet count, and blood urea nitrogen and serum creatinine levels), and notify the radiologist conducting the study of any abnormal results.
■ Tell the patient that afterward he'll need to maintain bed rest for about 6 hours and will be monitored closely.

Normal findings
Normally, the contrast agent flows symmetrically and without interruption through the pulmonary circulatory system.

Abnormal findings
Interruption of blood flow may result from emboli and from other types of pulmonary vascular abnormalities or tumors.

Interfering factors
■ None significant

Pulmonary function

Pulmonary function tests (volume, capacity, and flow rate tests) are a series of measurements that evaluate ventilatory function through spirometric measurements; they're performed on patients with suspected pulmonary dysfunction.

Of the seven tests used to determine volume, tidal volume (V_T) and expiratory reserve volume (ERV) are direct spirographic measurements; minute volume, carbon dioxide response, inspiratory reserve volume, and residual volume are calculated from the results of other pulmonary function tests; and thoracic gas volume is calculated from body plethysmography.

Of the pulmonary capacity tests, vital capacity (VC), inspiratory capacity (IC), functional residual capacity, total lung capacity, and forced expiratory flow may be measured directly or calculated from the results of other tests. Forced vital capacity, flow-volume curve, forced expiratory volume (FEV), peak expiratory flow rate, and maximal voluntary ventilation are direct spirographic measurements. Diffusing capacity for carbon monoxide is calculated from the amount of carbon monoxide exhaled.

ALERT! ▼ ▼ ▼ ▼ ▼ ▼ ▼ ▼ ▼
Pulmonary function tests are contraindicated in patients with acute coronary insufficiency, angina, or recent myocardial infarction.

Purpose
■ To determine the cause of dyspnea and whether a functional abnormality is obstructive or restrictive
■ To assess the effectiveness of specific therapeutic regimens
■ To measure pulmonary dysfunction
■ To evaluate a patient before surgery or as part of a job screening (firefighting, for example)

Cost
Moderately expensive

Patient preparation
■ Explain to the patient that these tests evaluate pulmonary function. Instruct him to eat only a light meal before the tests and not to smoke for 12 hours before the tests.

■ Describe the tests and equipment. Explain who will perform the tests, where they will take place, and how long they will last.
■ Describe the operation of a spirometer, and explain that the accuracy of the tests depends on the patient's cooperation.
■ Inform the laboratory if the patient is taking an analgesic that depresses respiration; restrict bronchodilators for 8 hours before the test.

Reference values
Normal values are predicted for each patient based on age, height, weight, and sex and are expressed as a percentage. Usually, results are considered abnormal if they're less than 80% of these values.

The following reference values can be calculated at bedside with a portable spirometer: V_T, 5 to 7 ml/kg of body weight; ERV, 25% of VC; IC, 75% of VC; FEV_1, 83% of VC (after 1 second); FEV_2, 94% of VC (after 2 seconds); and FEV_3, 97% of VC (after 3 seconds).

Abnormal findings
See *Interpreting pulmonary function tests.*

Interfering factors
■ Hypoxia, metabolic disturbances, or lack of patient cooperation
■ Pregnancy or gastric distention (possible displacement of lung volume)
■ Narcotic analgesic or sedative (possible decrease in inspiratory and expiratory forces)
■ Bronchodilators (possible temporary improvement in pulmonary function)

PULMONARY FUNCTION TEST	METHOD OF CALCULATION	IMPLICATIONS
Tidal volume (V_T): amount of air inhaled or exhaled during normal breathing	Determine the spirographic measurement for 10 breaths, and then divide by 10.	Decreased V_T may indicate restrictive disease and requires further testing, such as full pulmonary function studies or chest X-rays.
Minute volume (MV): total amount of air expired per minute	Multiply V_T by the respiratory rate.	Normal MV can occur in emphysema; decreased MV may indicate other diseases such as pulmonary edema. Increased MV can occur with acidosis, increased carbon dioxide (CO_2), decreased partial pressure of arterial oxygen, exercise, and low compliance states.
CO_2 response: increase or decrease in MV after breathing various CO_2 concentrations	Calculate by plotting changes in MV against increasing inspired CO_2 concentrations.	Reduced CO_2 response may occur in emphysema, myxedema, obesity, hypoventilation syndrome, and sleep apnea.
Inspiratory reserve volume (IRV): amount of air inspired over above-normal inspiration	Subtract V_T from inspiratory capacity.	Abnormal IRV alone doesn't indicate respiratory dysfunction; IRV decreases during normal exercise.
Expiratory reserve volume (ERV): amount of air exhaled after normal expiration	Direct spirographic measurement	ERV varies, even in healthy people, but usually decreases in obese patients.
Residual volume (RV): amount of air remaining in the lungs after forced expiration	Subtract ERV from functional residual capacity (FRC).	RV $\geq 35\%$ of total lung capacity after maximal expiratory effort may indicate obstructive disease.
Vital capacity (VC): total volume of air that can be exhaled after maximum inspiration	Direct spirographic measurement or add V_T, IRV, and ERV	Normal or increased VC with decreased flow rates may indicate any condition that causes a reduction in functional pulmonary tissue, such as pulmonary edema. Decreased VC with normal or increased flow rates may indicate decreased respiratory effort resulting from neuromuscular disease, drug overdose, or head injury; decreased thoracic expansion; or limited movement of the diaphragm.

(continued)

PULMONARY FUNCTION TEST	METHOD OF CALCULATION	IMPLICATIONS
Inspiratory capacity (IC): amount of air that can be inhaled after normal expiration	Direct spirographic measurement or add IRV and V_T	Decreased IC indicates restrictive disease.
Thoracic gas volume (TGV): total volume of gas in lungs from both ventilated and nonventilated airways	Body plethysmography	Increased TGV indicates air trapping, which may result from obstructive disease.
Functional residual capacity (FRC): amount of air remaining in lungs after normal expiration	Nitrogen washout, helium dilution technique, or add ERV and RV	Increased FRC indicates overdistention of lungs, which may result from obstructive pulmonary disease.
Total lung capacity (TLC): total volume of the lungs when maximally inflated	Add V_T, IRV, ERV, and RV; or FRC and IC; or VC and RV.	Low TLC indicates restrictive disease; high TLC indicates overdistended lungs caused by obstructive disease.
Forced vital capacity (FVC): amount of air exhaled forcefully and quickly after maximum inspiration	Direct spirographic measurement; expressed as a percentage of the total volume of gas exhaled	Decreased FVC indicates flow resistance in the respiratory system from obstructive disease such as chronic bronchitis, or from restrictive disease such as pulmonary fibrosis.
Flow-volume curve, also called flow-volume loop: greatest rate of flow (V_{max}) during FVC maneuvers versus lung volume change	Direct spirographic measurement at 1-second intervals; calculated from flow rates (expressed in L/second) and lung volume changes (expressed in liters) during maximal inspiratory and expiratory maneuvers	Decreased flow rates at all volumes during expiration indicate obstructive disease of the small airways, such as emphysema. A plateau of expiratory flow near TLC, a plateau of inspiratory flow at mid-VC, and a square wave pattern through most of VC indicate obstructive disease of large airways. Normal or increased peak expiratory flow rate, decreased flow with decreasing lung volumes, and markedly decreased VC indicate restrictive disease.
Forced expiratory volume (FEV): volume of air expired in the 1st, 2nd, or 3rd second of an FVC maneuver	Direct spirographic measurement; expressed as a percentage of FVC	Decreased FEV_1 and increased FEV_2 and FEV_3 may indicate obstructive disease; decreased or normal FEV_1 may indicate restrictive disease.

PULMONARY FUNCTION TEST	METHOD OF CALCULATION	IMPLICATIONS
Forced expiratory flow (FEF): average rate of flow during the middle half of FVC	Calculated from the flow rate and the time needed for expiration of middle 50% of FVC	Low FEF (25% to 75%) indicates obstructive disease of the small and medium-sized airways.
Peak expiratory flow rate (PEFR): V_{max} during forced expiration	Calculated from the flow-volume curve or by direct spirographic measurement, using a pneumotachometer or electronic tachometer with a transducer to convert flow to electrical output display	Decreased PEFR may indicate a mechanical problem, such as upper airway obstruction or obstructive disease. PEFR is usually normal in restrictive disease but decreases in severe cases. Because PEFR is effort dependent, it's also low in a person who has poor expiratory effort or doesn't understand the procedure.
Maximal voluntary ventilation (MVV), also called maximum breathing capacity: greatest volume of air breathed per unit of time	Direct spirographic measurement	Decreased MVV may indicate obstructive disease; normal or decreased MVV may indicate restrictive disease such as myasthenia gravis.
Diffusing capacity for carbon monoxide (DL_{CO}): milliliters of carbon monoxide diffused per minute across the alveolocapillary membrane	Calculated from analysis of amount of carbon monoxide exhaled compared with amount inhaled	Decreased DL_{CO} due to a thickened alveolocapillary membrane occurs in interstitial pulmonary diseases, such as pulmonary fibrosis, asbestosis, and sarcoidosis; DL_{CO} is reduced in emphysema because of the loss of alveolocapillary membrane.

Pulse oximetry

Pulse oximetry is a continuous noninvasive study of arterial blood oxygen saturation (Sao_2) using a clip or probe attached to a sensor site (usually the earlobe or fingertip). The percentage expressed is the ratio of oxygen to hemoglobin.

Purpose
- To monitor oxygenation of the tissues and organs perioperatively and during an acute illness
- To monitor oxygenation in patients with higher oxygen needs (such as those on a ventilator or those receiving a high percentage of oxygen) or when weaning from an oxygen source
- To monitor oxygen saturation during activities to determine patient tolerance

- To determine effectiveness of bronchodilators
- To monitor oxygenation during testing for sleep apnea

Cost
Inexpensive

Patient preparation
- Explain to the patient that this test assesses oxygen content in the hemoglobin. Describe the procedure and answer questions.
- Explain who will perform the test, where it will take place, and how long it will last.
- Instruct the patient to remove false fingernails or nail polish prior to the test.
- Explain to the patient that the area where the clip or probe is attached must be massaged to increase blood flow.

Reference values
Sao_2 levels are normally greater than 95%.

Abnormal findings
Hypoxemia with levels less than 95% indicates impaired cardiopulmonary function or abnormal gas exchange.

Interfering factors
- Movement of the finger, ear, or alternate sensor site
- Improper placement of the probe or clip
- Administrations of lipid emulsions, anemic conditions, certain medications (such as vasopressors), elevated carboxyhemoglobin (carbon monoxide) levels in the blood, hypotension, nail polish or false fingernails, vasoconstriction, or vessel obstruction

Pyruvate kinase

An erythrocyte enzyme, pyruvate kinase (PK) takes part in the anaerobic metabolism of glucose. An abnormally low PK level is an inherited autosomal recessive trait that may cause a red cell membrane defect associated with congenital hemolytic anemia. PK assay confirms PK deficiency when red cell enzyme deficiency is the suspected cause of anemia.

Purpose
- To differentiate PK-deficient hemolytic anemia from other congenital hemolytic anemias or from acquired hemolytic anemia
- To detect PK deficiency in asymptomatic, heterozygous inheritance

Cost
Inexpensive

Patient preparation
- Explain to the patient that this test is used to detect inherited enzyme deficiencies.
- Tell the patient that the test requires a blood sample. Explain who will perform the venipuncture and when.
- Explain to the patient that he may experience discomfort from the needle puncture and the tourniquet.
- Check the patient's history for a recent blood transfusion, and note it on the laboratory request.

Reference values
Serum PK levels range from 9 to 22 U/g of hemoglobin; in the low substrate assay, they range from 1.7 to 6.8 U/g of hemoglobin.

Abnormal findings

Low serum PK levels confirm a diagnosis of PK deficiency and allow differentiation between PK-deficient hemolytic anemia and other inherited disorders.

Interfering factors

■ Failure to remove white cells from sample (possible false results)
■ Recent blood transfusion or recent hemolytic event

R

Radioactive iodine uptake

The radioactive iodine uptake (RAIU) test evaluates thyroid function by measuring the amount of orally ingested radioactive isotopes of iodine, ^{123}I or ^{131}I, that accumulates in the thyroid gland after 6 and 24 hours. An external single counting probe measures the radioactivity in the thyroid as a percentage of the original dose, thus indicating its ability to trap and retain iodine. The RAIU test accurately diagnoses hyperthyroidism but is less accurate for hypothyroidism. Indications for this test include abnormal results of chemical tests used to evaluate thyroid functioning.

Purpose
■ To evaluate thyroid function
■ To help diagnose hyperthyroidism or hypothyroidism
■ To help distinguish between primary and secondary disorders
■ To help differentiate Graves' disease from hyperfunctioning toxic adenoma (performed concurrently with radionuclide thyroid imaging and the T_3 resin uptake test)

Cost
Expensive

Patient preparation
■ Tell the patient that RAIU testing assesses thyroid function.
■ Instruct the patient to fast beginning at midnight the night before the test.
■ Explain to the patient that he'll receive radioactive iodine and then be scanned after 6 hours and again after 24 hours.
■ Assure the patient that the test is painless and that the small amount of radioactivity used is harmless.
■ Tell the patient that test results will be available within 24 hours.
■ Check the patient's history for iodine exposure, which may interfere with test results. Note any prior radiologic tests using contrast media, nuclear medicine procedures, or thyroid medications on the film request. Iodine hypersensitivity isn't considered a contraindication because the amount of iodine used is similar to the amount consumed in a normal diet.
■ Inform the patient that the RAIU test is contraindicated during pregnancy and lactation because of possible teratogenic effects.

Normal findings

At 6 hours, 5% to 20% of the radioactive iodine should accumulate in the thyroid; at 24 hours, accumulation should be 15% to 40%. The balance of the radioactive iodine is excreted in the urine. Local variations in the normal range of iodine uptake may occur due to regional differences in dietary iodine intake and procedural differences among laboratories.

Abnormal findings

Below-normal iodine uptake may indicate hypothyroidism, subacute thyroiditis, or iodine overload. Above-normal uptake may indicate hyperthyroidism, early Hashimoto's thyroiditis, hypoalbuminemia, lithium ingestion, or iodine-deficient goiter. However, in hyperthyroidism, the rate of turnover may be so rapid that a false-normal measurement occurs at 24 hours.

Interfering factors

■ Cough syrups, diuresis, ingestion of iodine preparations including iodized salt, renal failure, severe diarrhea, some multivitamins, and X-ray contrast media studies (decrease)
■ Anticoagulants, antihistamines, corticosteroids, penicillins, phenylbutazone, salicylates, thyroid hormones, and thyroid hormone antagonists (decrease)
■ Iodine-deficient diet or phenothiazines (increase)

Radionuclide thyroid imaging

In radionuclide thyroid imaging, the thyroid is studied by gamma camera after the patient receives a radioisotope (^{123}I, ^{99m}Tc pertechnetate, or ^{131}I). Thyroid imaging typically follows the discovery of a palpable mass, an enlarged gland, or an asymmetrical goiter and is performed concurrently with thyroid uptake tests and measurements of serum triiodothyronine (T_3), thyroid-stimulating hormone, and serum thyroxine levels. Later, thyroid ultrasonography may be performed.

ALERT! ▼ ▼ ▼ ▼ ▼ ▼ ▼ ▼ ▼
Radionuclide thyroid imaging is contraindicated in patients who are pregnant or lactating and in patients with a previous allergy to iodine, shellfish, or radioactive tracers.

Purpose

■ To assess the size, structure, and position of the thyroid gland
■ To evaluate thyroid function (in conjunction with other thyroid tests)

Cost

Expensive

Patient preparation

■ Tell the patient that this test helps determine the cause of thyroid dysfunction.
■ If ^{123}I or ^{131}I will be used, tell the patient to fast after midnight the night before the test. Fasting isn't required if an I.V. injection of ^{99m}Tc pertechnetate is used.
■ Explain to the patient that after he receives the radiopharmaceutical, a gamma camera will be used to produce an image of his thyroid. Tell him that the imaging procedure will take about 30 minutes, and assure him that his exposure to radiation is minimal.
■ Ask the patient whether he has undergone tests that used radiographic contrast media within the past 60 days. Note previous radiographic contrast media exposure on the X-ray request.
■ Discontinue such medications as thyroid hormones, thyroid hormone antago-

Results of thyroid imaging in thyroid disorders

CONDITION	FINDINGS	CAUSES
Hypothyroidism	▪ Glandular damage or absent gland	▪ Surgical removal of gland ▪ Inflammation ▪ Radiation ▪ Neoplasm (rare)
Hypothyroid goiter	▪ Enlarged gland ▪ Decreased uptake (of radioactive iodine) if glandular destruction is present ▪ Increased uptake possible from congenital error in thyroxine synthesis	▪ Insufficient iodine intake ▪ Hypersecretion of thyroid-stimulating hormone (TSH) caused by thyroid hormone deficiency
Myxedema (cretinism in children)	▪ Normal or slightly reduced gland size ▪ Uniform pattern ▪ Decreased uptake	▪ Defective embryonic development, resulting in congenital absence or underdevelopment of thyroid gland ▪ Maternal iodine deficiency
Hyperthyroidism (Graves' disease)	▪ Enlarged gland ▪ Uniform pattern ▪ Increased uptake	▪ Unknown, but may be hereditary ▪ Production of thyroid-stimulating immunoglobulins
Toxic nodular goiter	▪ Multiple hot spots	▪ Long-standing simple goiter
Hyperfunctioning adenomas	▪ Solitary hot spot	▪ Adenomatous production of tri-iodothyronine and thyroxine, suppressing TSH secretion and producing atrophy of other thyroid tissue
Hypofunctioning adenomas	▪ Solitary cold spot	▪ Cyst or nonfunctioning nodule
Benign multinodular goiter	▪ Multiple nodules with variable or no function	▪ Local inflammation ▪ Degeneration
Thyroid carcinoma	▪ Usually a solitary cold spot with occasional or no function	▪ Neoplasm

nists, and iodine preparations (Lugol's solution, some multivitamins, and cough syrups) 2 to 2 weeks before the test; and discontinue phenothiazines, corticosteroids, salicylates, anticoagulants, and antihistamines 1 week before the test. Instruct the patient to stop consuming iodized salt, iodinated salt substitutes, and seafood for 14 to 21 days. Discontinue liothyronine, propylthiouracil, and methimazole 3 days before the test, and thyroxine, 10 days before the test.

- The patient receiving an oral radioisotope should fast for another 2 hours after administration.
- Obtain an informed consent form if necessary.

Normal findings

Normally, radionuclide thyroid imaging reveals a thyroid gland that's about 2" (5.1 cm) long and 1" (2.5 cm) wide, with a uniform uptake of the radioisotope and without tumors. The gland is butterfly-shaped, with the isthmus located at the midline. Occasionally, a third lobe called the pyramidal lobe may be present; this is a normal variant.

Abnormal findings

During radionuclide thyroid imaging, hyperfunctioning nodules (areas of excessive iodine uptake) appear as black regions called hot spots. The presence of hot spots requires a follow-up T_3 thyroid suppression test to determine whether the hyperfunctioning areas are autonomous. Hypofunctioning nodules (areas of little or no iodine uptake) appear as white or light gray regions called cold spots. If a cold spot appears, subsequent thyroid ultrasonography may be performed to rule out cysts; in addition, fine-needle aspiration and biopsy of such nodules may be performed to rule out malignancy. (See *Results of thyroid imaging in thyroid disorders*.)

Interfering factors

- Iodine-deficient diet, phenothiazines (increase)
- Decreased uptake of radioactive iodine due to renal disease; ingestion of iodinated salt substitutes, iodine preparations, iodized salt, or seafood; and use of aminosalicylic acid, corticosteroids, cough syrups containing inorganic iodine, multivitamins, thyroid hormone antagonists, or thyroid hormones (decrease)
- Severe diarrhea and vomiting, impairing GI absorption of radioiodine (decrease)

Raji cell assay

Raji cell assay, which is performed to detect the presence of circulating immune complexes, studies the Raji lymphoblastoid cell line. Identifying these cells, which have receptors for immunoglobulin G complement, helps to evaluate autoimmune disease.

Purpose

- To detect circulating immune complexes
- To aid the study of autoimmune disease

Cost

Moderately expensive

Patient preparation

- Explain to the patient the purpose of the test.
- Tell the patient that the test requires a blood sample. Explain who will perform the venipuncture and when.
- Explain to the patient that he may experience discomfort from the needle puncture and the tourniquet.

Normal findings

Normally, Raji cells aren't present in the blood sample.

Abnormal findings

A positive Raji cell assay can detect immune complexes, including those found in viral, microbial, and parasitic infections; metastasis; autoimmune disorders; and drug reactions. This test may also detect immune complexes associated with celiac disease, cirrhosis of the liver, Crohn's disease, cryoglobulinemia, dermatitis herpetiformis, sickle cell anemia, and ulcerative colitis.

Interfering factors
■ Hemolysis due to rough handling of the sample

Red blood cell count

The red blood cell (RBC) count, also called an *erythrocyte count*, is part of a complete blood cell count. It is used to detect the number of RBCs in a microliter (μl), or cubic millimeter (mm³), of whole blood.

Purpose
■ To provide data for calculating mean corpuscular volume and mean corpuscular hemoglobin, which reveal RBC size and hemoglobin content
■ To support other hematologic tests for diagnosing anemia or polycythemia

Patient preparation
■ Explain to the patient that this test is used to evaluate the number of RBCs and to detect possible blood disorders.
■ Tell the patient that the test requires a blood sample. Explain who will perform the venipuncture and when.
■ Explain to the patient that he may experience discomfort from the needle puncture and the tourniquet.
AGE ISSUE ✳ ✳ ✳ ✳ ✳
If the patient is a child, explain to him (if he's old enough) and his parents that a small amount of blood will be taken from the finger or earlobe.

Reference values
Normal RBC values vary, depending on the type of sample and on the patient's age and sex, as follows:
■ *adult males:* 4.5 to 5.5 million RBCs/μl (SI, 4.5 to 5.5 × 10^{12}/L) of venous blood
■ *adult females:* 4 to 5 million RBCs/μl (SI, 4 to 5 × 10^{12}/L) of venous blood
■ *children:* 4.6 to 4.8 million RBCs/μl (SI, 4.6 to 4.8 × 10^{12}/L) of venous blood
■ *full-term neonates:* 4.4 to 5.8 million RBCs/μl (SI, 4.4 to 5.8 × 10^{12}/L) of capillary blood at birth, decreasing to 3 to 3.8 million RBCs/μl (SI, 3 to 3.8 × 10^{12}/L) at age 2 months and increasing slowly thereafter.

Normal values may exceed these levels in patients living at high altitudes or those who are very active.

Abnormal findings
An elevated RBC count may indicate absolute or relative polycythemia. A depressed count may indicate anemia, fluid overload, or hemorrhage beyond 24 hours. Further tests, such as stained cell examination, hematocrit, hemoglobin, red cell indices, and white cell studies, are needed to confirm the diagnosis.

Interfering factors
■ Hemoconcentration due to prolonged tourniquet constriction
■ Hemodilution due to drawing the sample from the same arm used for I.V. infusion of fluids
■ High white blood cell count (false-high test results in semiautomated and automated counters)
■ Diseases that cause RBCs to agglutinate or form rouleaux (false decrease)
■ Hemolysis due to rough handling of the sample or drawing the blood through a small-gauge needle for venipuncture

Comparative red cell indices in anemias

	NORMAL VALUES (Normocytic, normochromic)	IRON DEFICIENCY ANEMIA (Microcytic, hypochromic)	PERNICIOUS ANEMIA (Macrocytic, normochromic)
MCV	82 to 99 μm^3	60 to 80 μm^3	96 to 150 μm^3
MCH	26 to 32 pg/cell	5 to 25 pg/cell	33 to 53 pg/cell
MCHC	30 to 36 g/dl	20 to 30 g/dl	33 to 38 g/dl

Key:
MCV = Mean corpuscular volume
MCH = Mean corpuscular hemoglobin
MCHC = Mean corpuscular hemoglobin concentration

Red cell indices

Using the results of the red blood cell (RBC) count, hematocrit, and total hemoglobin tests, red cell indices (erythrocyte indices) provide important information about the size, hemoglobin concentration, and hemoglobin weight of an average RBC.

Purpose
■ To aid diagnosis and classification of anemias

Cost
Inexpensive

Patient preparation
■ Explain to the patient that this test helps determine whether he has anemia.
■ Tell the patient that the test requires a blood sample. Explain who will perform the venipuncture and when.
■ Explain to the patient that he may experience discomfort from the needle puncture and the tourniquet.

Reference values
The indices tested include mean corpuscular volume (MCV), mean corpuscular hemoglobin (MCH), and mean corpuscular hemoglobin concentration (MCHC).

MCV, the ratio of hematocrit (packed cell volume) to the RBC count, expresses the average size of the erythrocytes and indicates whether they're undersized (microcytic), oversized (macrocytic), or normal (normocytic). MCH, the hemoglobin-RBC ratio, gives the weight of hemoglobin in an average red cell. MCHC, the ratio of hemoglobin weight to hematocrit, defines the concentration of hemoglobin in 100 ml of packed RBCs. It helps to distinguish normally colored (normochromic) RBCs from paler (hypochromic) RBCs.

The range of normal red cell indices is as follows:
■ *MCV:* 84 to 99 μm^3
■ *MCH:* 26 to 32 pg/cell
■ *MCHC:* 30 to 36 g/dl.

Abnormal findings

Low MCV and MCHC indicate microcytic, hypochromic anemias caused by iron deficiency anemia, pyridoxine-responsive anemia, or thalassemia. A high MCV suggests macrocytic anemias caused by megaloblastic anemias, folic acid or vitamin B_{12} deficiency, inherited disorders of deoxyribonucleic acid synthesis, or reticulocytosis. Because MCV reflects the average volume of many cells, a value within the normal range can encompass RBCs of varying size, from microcytic to macrocytic. (See *Comparative red cell indices in anemias*, page 319.)

Interfering factors

■ Failure to use the proper anticoagulant or to adequately mix the sample and the anticoagulant
■ Hemolysis due to rough handling of the sample or use of a small-gauge needle for blood aspiration
■ Hemoconcentration due to prolonged tourniquet constriction
■ High white blood cell count (false-high RBC count in semiautomated and automated counters, invalidating MCV and MCHC results)
■ Falsely elevated hemoglobin values (invalidate MCH and MCHC results)
■ Diseases that cause RBCs to agglutinate or form rouleaux (false-low RBC count)

Renal angiography

Renal angiography is radiographic examination of the renal vasculature and parenchyma; it requires arterial injection of a contrast medium and permits radiographic examination of the renal vasculature and parenchyma. As the contrast pervades the renal vasculature, rapid-sequence radiographs show the vessels during three phases of filling: arterial, nephrographic, and venous.

This procedure virtually always follows standard bolus aortography, which shows individual variations in number, size, and condition of the main renal arteries, aberrant vessels, and the relationship of the renal arteries to the aorta.

ALERT! ▼ ▼ ▼ ▼ ▼ ▼ ▼ ▼ ▼
Renal angiography is contraindicated in patients who are pregnant and in patients with bleeding tendencies, allergy to contrast media, and renal failure due to end-stage renal disease.

Purpose

■ To demonstrate the configuration of total renal vasculature before surgical procedures
■ To determine the cause of renovascular hypertension, such as from stenosis, thrombotic occlusions, emboli, and aneurysms
■ To evaluate chronic renal disease or renal failure
■ To investigate renal masses and renal trauma
■ To detect complications following renal transplantation, such as a nonfunctioning shunt or rejection of the donor organ
■ To differentiate highly vascular tumors from avascular cysts

Cost

Expensive

Patient preparation

■ Explain to the patient that this test permits visualization of the kidneys, blood vessels, and functional units and aids in diagnosing renal disease or masses.
■ Instruct the patient to fast for 8 hours before the test and to drink extra fluids the day before the test and the day after the test

to maintain adequate hydration. Oral medication may be continued.

■ Order a laxative or an enema the evening before the test.

■ Tell the patient who will perform the test and where it will take place.

■ Describe the procedure to the patient, and inform him that he may experience transient discomfort (flushing, burning sensation, and nausea) during injection of the contrast medium.

■ Obtain informed consent if necessary.

■ Document the patient's history for hypersensitivity to iodine-based contrast media or iodine-containing foods such as shellfish. Order prophylactic antiallergenics (diphenhydramine or corticosteroids) as appropriate.

■ Ensure that recent laboratory test results (blood urea nitrogen and serum creatinine levels and bleeding studies) are documented on the patient's chart.

■ Verify adequate renal function and adequate clotting ability.

■ Tell the patient that he'll be monitored closely, bed rest will be maintained, and his leg will need to be kept straight for at least 6 hours after the test.

Normal findings

Renal arteriographs show normal arborization of the vascular tree and normal architecture of the renal parenchyma.

Abnormal findings

Renal tumors usually show hypervascularity; renal cysts typically appear as clearly delineated, radiolucent masses. Renal artery stenosis caused by arteriosclerosis produces a noticeable constriction in the blood vessels, usually within the proximal portion of its length; this is a crucial finding in confirming renovascular hypertension. Renal artery dysplasia, unlike renal artery stenosis, usually affects the middle and distal portions of the vessel. Alternating aneurysms and stenotic regions give this rare disorder a characteristic beads-on-a-string appearance.

In renal infarction, blood vessels may appear to be absent or cut off, with the normal tissue replaced by scar tissue. Another typical finding is the appearance of triangular areas of infarcted tissue near the periphery of the affected kidney. The kidney itself may appear shrunken because of tissue scarring.

Renal angiography may also detect renal artery aneurysms (saccular or fusiform) and renal arteriovenous fistula with abnormal widening of and direct passage between the renal artery and renal vein. Destruction, distortion, and fibrosis of renal tissue with areas of reduced and tortuous vascularity may be noted in severe or chronic pyelonephritis, and an increase in capsular vessels with abnormal intrarenal circulation may indicate renal abscesses or inflammatory masses.

When angiography is used to evaluate renal trauma, it may detect intrarenal hematoma, parenchymal laceration, shattered kidneys, and areas of infarction. Renal angiography may also be useful in distinguishing pseudotumors from tumors or cysts, in evaluating the volume of residual functioning renal tissue in hydronephrosis, and in evaluating donors and recipients before and after renal transplantation.

Interfering factors

■ Recent contrast studies, such as barium enema or an upper GI series (possible poor imaging)

■ Presence of stool or gas in the GI tract (possible poor imaging)

Renal computed tomography

Renal computed tomography (CT) provides a useful image of the kidneys made from a series of tomograms or cross-sectional slices, which are then translated by a computer and displayed on a monitor. The image density reflects the amount of radiation absorbed by renal tissue and permits identification of masses and other lesions. An I.V. contrast medium may be injected to accentuate the renal parenchyma's density and help differentiate renal masses. This highly accurate test is usually performed to investigate diseases found by other diagnostic procedures such as excretory urography.

Purpose
■ To detect and evaluate renal abnormalities, such as tumor, obstruction, calculi, polycystic kidney disease, congenital anomalies, and abnormal fluid accumulation around the kidneys
■ To evaluate the retroperitoneum

Cost
Very expensive

Patient preparation
■ Explain to the patient that this test permits examination of the kidneys.
■ If contrast enhancement isn't ordered, inform the patient that he need not restrict food or fluids. If contrast enhancement is ordered, instruct him to fast for 4 hours before the test.
■ Tell the patient who will perform the test and where it will take place.
■ Inform the patient that he'll be positioned on an X-ray table and that a scanner will take films of his kidneys. Warn him that the scanner may make loud, clacking sounds as it rotates around his body.

■ Tell the patient that he may experience transient adverse effects, such as flushing, metallic taste, and headache, after injection of the contrast medium.
■ Obtain informed consent if necessary.
■ Document the patient's history for hypersensitivity to shellfish, iodine, or contrast media.
■ Tell the patient that he may receive sedatives before the procedure.

Normal findings
Normally, the density of the renal parenchyma is slightly higher than that of the liver but is much less dense than bone, which appears white on a CT scan. The density of the collecting system is generally low (black), unless a contrast medium is used to enhance it to a higher (whiter) density. The position of the kidneys is evaluated according to the surrounding structures; the size and shape of the kidneys are determined by counting cuts between the superior and inferior poles and following the contour of the renal outline.

Abnormal findings
Renal masses appear as areas of different density than normal parenchyma, possibly altering the kidneys' shape or projecting beyond their margins. Renal cysts, for example, appear as smooth, sharply defined masses, with thin walls and a lower density than normal parenchyma. Tumors such as renal cell carcinoma, however, are usually not as well delineated; they tend to have thick walls and nonuniform density. With contrast enhancement, solid tumors show a higher density than renal cysts but a lower density than normal parenchyma. Tumors with hemorrhage, calcification, or necrosis show higher densities. Vascular tumors are more clearly defined with contrast enhancement. Adrenal tumors are confined

masses, usually detached from the kidneys and from other retroperitoneal organs.

Renal CT scanning may also identify other abnormalities, including obstructions, calculi, polycystic kidney disease, congenital anomalies, and abnormal accumulations of fluid around the kidneys, such as hematomas, lymphoceles, and abscesses. After nephrectomy, CT scanning can detect abnormal masses such as recurrent tumors in a renal fossa that should be empty.

Interfering factors
■ Presence of contrast media from other recent tests or presence of foreign bodies, such as catheters or surgical clips (possible poor imaging)

Renal imaging, radionuclide

Radionuclide renal imaging, which involves I.V. injection of a radionuclide followed by scintigraphy, provides a wealth of information for evaluating the kidneys. Observing the uptake concentration and transit of the radionuclide during this test allows assessment of renal blood flow, renal structure, and nephron and collecting system function. Depending on the patient's clinical presentation, this procedure may include dynamic scans to assess renal perfusion and function or static scans to assess structure.

The radioisotope injected depends on the specific information required and the examiner's preference. However, this procedure usually includes double isotope technique to obtain a sequence of perfusion and function studies, followed by static images. This test may also be substituted for excretory urography in patients with hypersensitivity to contrast agents.

Purpose
■ To detect and assess functional and structural renal abnormalities (such as lesions)
■ To detect renovascular hypertension and acute and chronic renal disease (such as pyelonephritis and glomerulonephritis)
■ To assess renal transplantation or renal injury due to trauma and obstruction of the urinary tract

Cost
Expensive

Patient preparation
■ Explain to the patient that this test permits evaluation of the structure, blood flow, and function of the kidneys.
■ Tell the patient who will perform the test, where it will take place, and that it takes about 90 minutes.
■ Inform the patient that he'll receive an injection of a radionuclide and that he may experience transient flushing and nausea.
■ Emphasize to the patient that only a small amount of radionuclide is administered and that it's usually excreted within 24 hours.
■ Tell the patient that several series of films will be taken of his bladder.
■ Restrict antihypertensive medication if appropriate.
■ Patients who are pregnant and young children may receive supersaturated solution of potassium iodide 1 to 3 hours before the test to block thyroid uptake of iodine.

Normal findings
Because 25% of cardiac output goes directly to the kidneys, renal perfusion should be evident immediately following uptake of the technetium and diethylenetriamine penta-acetic acid (used for the perfusion study) in the abdominal aorta. Within 1 to

2 minutes, a normal pattern of renal circulation should appear. The radionuclide should delineate the kidneys simultaneously, symmetrically, and with equal intensity.

The Hippuran radiation dose administered for the function study rapidly outlines the kidneys—which should be normal in size, shape, and position—and also defines the collecting system and bladder. Maximum counts for the radionuclide in the kidneys occur within 5 minutes after injection (and within 1 minute of each other) and should fall to approximately one-third or less of the maximum counts in the same kidney within 25 minutes. Within this time, the function of both kidneys can be compared as the concentration of radionuclide shifts from the cortex to the pelvis, and finally to the bladder.

Renal function is best evaluated comparing these images to the renogram curves. Total function is considered normal when the effective renal plasma flow is 429 ml/minute or greater and the percentage of the dose excreted in the urine at 30 to 35 minutes is greater than 66%.

Abnormal findings

Images from the perfusion study can identify impeded renal circulation, such as that caused by trauma and renal artery stenosis or renal infarction. These conditions may occur in patients with renovascular hypertension and abdominal aortic disease. Because malignant renal tumors are usually vascular, these images can help differentiate tumors from cysts.

In evaluating a kidney transplant, abnormal perfusion may indicate obstruction of the vascular grafts. The function study can detect abnormalities of the collecting system and extravasation of the urine. Markedly decreased tubular function causes reduced radionuclide activity in the collecting system; outflow obstruction causes decreased radionuclide activity in the tubules, with increased activity in the collecting system. This test can also define the level of ureteral obstruction. Static images can demonstrate lesion, congenital abnormalities, and traumatic injury. These images also detect space-occupying lesions within or surrounding the kidney, such as tumors, infarcts, and inflammatory masses; they can also identify congenital disorders, such as horseshoe kidney and polycystic kidney disease. They can define regions of infarction, rupture, or hemorrhage after trauma.

A lower than normal total concentration of the radionuclide, as opposed to focal defects, suggests a diffuse renal disorder, such as acute tubular necrosis, severe infection, or ischemia. In a patient who has had a kidney transplant, decreased radionuclide uptake generally indicates organ rejection. Failure of visualization may indicate congenital ectopia or aplasia.

Definitive diagnosis usually requires the combined analysis of static images, perfusion studies, and function studies.

Interfering factors
■ Antihypertensives (possible masking of abnormalities)
■ Scans of different organs performed on the same day (possible poor imaging)

Renal ultrasonography

In renal ultrasonography, high-frequency sound waves are transmitted from a transducer to the kidneys and perirenal structures. The resulting echoes are displayed on a monitor as anatomic images.

Renal ultrasonography can be used to detect abnormalities or clarify those detected by other tests. It's especially useful in cases in which excretory urography is ruled out. Unlike excretory urography, this test isn't dependent on renal function and therefore may be useful in patients with renal failure. Ultrasonography of the ureter, bladder, and gonads also may be used to evaluate urologic disorders.

Purpose
- To determine the size, shape, and position of the kidneys, their internal structures, and perirenal tissues
- To evaluate and localize urinary obstruction and abnormal fluid accumulation
- To assess and diagnose complications after kidney transplantation
- To detect renal or perirenal masses
- To differentiate between renal cysts and solid masses
- To verify placement of a nephrostomy tube

Cost
Expensive

Patient preparation
- Explain to the patient that this test is used to detect kidney abnormalities.
- Tell the patient who will perform the test, where it will take place, and that he may be asked to breathe deeply to visualize upper portions of the kidney.

Normal findings
The kidneys are located between the superior iliac crests and the diaphragm. The renal capsule should be outlined sharply; the cortex should produce more echoes than the medulla. In the center of each kidney, the renal collecting systems appear as irregular areas of higher density than surrounding tissue. The renal veins and, depending on the scanner, some internal structures can be visualized. If the bladder is also being evaluated, its size, shape, position, and urine content can be determined.

Abnormal findings
Cysts are usually fluid-filled, circular structures that don't reflect sound waves. Tumors produce multiple echoes and appear as irregular shapes. Abscesses found within or around the kidneys usually echo sound waves poorly; their boundaries are slightly more irregular than those of cysts. A perirenal abscess may displace the kidney anteriorly.

Generally, acute pyelonephritis and glomerulonephritis aren't detectable unless the renal parenchyma is significantly scarred and atrophied. In such patients, the renal capsule appears irregular and the kidney may appear smaller than normal; also, an increased number of echoes may arise from the parenchyma due to fibrosis.

In patients with hydronephrosis, renal ultrasonography may show a large, echo-free, central mass that compresses the renal cortex. Calyceal echoes are usually circularly diffused and the pelvis significantly enlarged. This test can also be used to detect congenital anomalies, such as horseshoe, ectopic, or duplicated kidneys. Ultrasonography clearly detects renal hypertrophy.

Following renal transplantation, compensatory hypertrophy of the transplanted kidney is normal, but an acute increase in size indicates rejection.

This test allows identification of abnormal accumulations of fluid within or around the kidneys that sometimes arise from an obstruction. It also allows evaluation of perirenal structures and can identify abnormalities of the adrenal glands, such as tumors, cysts, and adrenal dysfunction. However, a normal adrenal gland is difficult to define ultrasonically because of its small size.

Renal ultrasonography can be used to detect changes in the shape of the bladder that result from masses and can assess urine volume. Increased urine volume or residual urine post-voiding may indicate bladder outlet obstruction.

Interfering factors
■ Retained barium from a previous test (possible poor imaging)
■ Obese patient (possible poor imaging)

Renal venography

Renal venography is a relatively simple procedure allowing radiographic examination of the main renal veins and their tributaries. In this test, contrast medium is injected by percutaneous catheter passed through the femoral vein and inferior vena cava into the renal vein. Indications for renal venography include renal vein thrombosis, tumor, and venous anomalies.

ALERT! ▼ ▼ ▼ ▼ ▼ ▼ ▼ ▼ ▼
Renal venography is contraindicated in severe thrombosis of the inferior vena cava.

Purpose
■ To detect renal vein thrombosis
■ To evaluate renal vein compression due to extrinsic tumors or retroperitoneal fibrosis
■ To assess renal tumors and detect invasion of the renal vein or inferior vena cava
■ To detect venous anomalies and defects
■ To differentiate renal agenesis from a small kidney
■ To collect renal venous blood samples for evaluation of renovascular hypertension

Cost
Expensive

Patient preparation
■ Explain to the patient that this test permits radiographic study of the renal veins.
■ If needed, instruct the patient to fast for 4 hours before the test.
■ Tell the patient who will perform the test and where it will take place.
■ Inform the patient that a catheter will be inserted into a vein in the groin area after he's given a sedative and a local anesthetic.
■ Tell the patient that he may feel mild discomfort during injection of the local anesthetic and contrast medium and that he may feel transient burning and flushing from the contrast medium.
■ Warn the patient that the X-ray equipment may make loud, clacking noises as the films are taken.
■ Document the patient's history for hypersensitivity to contrast media, iodine, or iodine-containing foods such as shellfish. Also document his history and any coagulation studies for indications of bleeding disorders, and make sure that pretest blood urea nitrogen and urine creatinine levels are adequate because the kidneys clear contrast media.
■ If renin assays will be done, restrict salt intake and medications, such as antihypertensive drugs, diuretics, estrogen, and hormonal contraceptives.
■ Obtain informed consent if necessary.
■ Tell the patient that he may receive a sedative before testing.
■ Tell the patient that after the procedure, he should increase his fluid intake (unless contraindicated) to help clear contrast media.

Normal findings
After injection of the contrast medium, opacification of the renal vein and tributaries should occur immediately. Normal renin content of venous blood in an adult

in a supine position is 1.5 to 1.6 ng/ml/ hour.

Abnormal findings

Occlusion of the renal vein near the inferior vena cava or the kidney indicates renal vein thrombosis. If the clot is outlined by contrast medium, it may look like a filling defect. However, a clot can usually be identified because it's within the lumen and less sharply outlined than a filling defect. Collateral venous channels, which opacify with retrograde filling during contrast injection, typically surround the occlusion. Complete occlusion prolongs transit of the contrast medium through the renal veins.

A filling defect of the renal vein may indicate obstruction or compression by extrinsic tumor or retroperitoneal fibrosis. A renal tumor that invades the renal vein or inferior vena cava usually produces a filling defect with a sharply defined border.

Venous anomalies are indicated by opacification of abnormally positioned or clustered vessels. Absence of a renal vein differentiates renal agenesis from a small kidney.

Elevated renin content in renal venous blood usually indicates essential renovascular hypertension when assay results correspond for both kidneys. Elevated renin levels in one kidney indicate a unilateral lesion and usually require further evaluation by arteriography.

Interfering factors

■ Recent contrast studies or stool or gas in the bowel
■ Failure to restrict salt, antihypertensive drugs, diuretics, estrogen, or hormonal contraceptives

Renin activity, plasma

Renin secretion from the kidneys is the first stage of the renin-angiotensin-aldosterone cycle, which controls the body's sodium-potassium balance, fluid volume, and blood pressure. Renin is released into the renal veins in response to sodium depletion and blood loss. The plasma renin activity test is a screening procedure for renovascular hypertension but doesn't unequivocally confirm it.

Purpose

■ To screen for renal origin of hypertension
■ To help plan treatment of essential hypertension, a genetic disease commonly aggravated by excess sodium intake
■ To help identify hypertension linked to unilateral (sometimes bilateral) renovascular disease by renal vein catheterization
■ To help identify primary aldosteronism (Conn's syndrome) resulting from aldosterone-secreting adrenal adenoma
■ To confirm primary aldosteronism (sodium-depleted plasma renin test)

Cost

Moderately expensive

Patient preparation

■ Explain to the patient that this test is used to determine the cause of hypertension.
■ Restrict medications that may affect test results. If they must be continued, note this on the laboratory request.
■ Tell the patient to maintain a normal sodium diet (3 g/day) during this period.
■ For the sodium-depleted plasma renin test, order furosemide (or, if he has angina or cerebrovascular insufficiency, chlorthiazide) and tell him to follow a low-sodium diet for 3 days.

- The patient shouldn't receive radioactive treatments for several days before the test.
- Tell the patient that the test requires a blood sample. Explain who will perform the venipuncture and when.
- Explain to the patient that he may experience discomfort from the needle puncture and the tourniquet.
- If a recumbent sample is ordered, tell the patient that he'll need to remain in bed at least 2 hours before the sample is obtained. (Posture influences renin secretion.) If an upright sample is ordered, tell him that he'll need to stand or sit upright for 2 hours before the test is performed.
- Tell the patient that the procedure will be done in the X-ray department and that he'll receive a local anesthetic.
- Obtain informed consent if necessary.

Reference values

Levels of plasma renin activity and aldosterone vary with dietary sodium intake, as follows:
- *normal sodium diet:* 1.1 to 4.1 ng/ml/hour (SI, 0.30 to 1.14 ng LS)
- *restricted sodium diet:* 6.2 to 12.4 ng/ml/hour (SI, 1.72 to 3.44 ng LS).

Abnormal findings

Elevated plasma renin levels may occur in essential hypertension (uncommon), malignant and renovascular hypertension, cirrhosis, hypokalemia, hypovolemia due to hemorrhage, renin-producing renal tumors (Bartter's syndrome), and adrenal hypofunction (Addison's disease). Elevated plasma renin levels may also be found in chronic renal failure with parenchymal disease, end-stage renal disease, and transplant rejection.

Decreased plasma renin levels may indicate hypervolemia due to a high-sodium diet, salt-retaining steroids, primary aldosteronism, Cushing's syndrome, licorice ingestion syndrome, or essential hypertension with low plasma renin levels.

High serum and urine aldosterone levels with low plasma renin activity help identify primary aldosteronism. In the sodium-depleted renin test, low plasma renin confirms this and differentiates it from secondary aldosteronism (characterized by increased plasma renin).

Interfering factors

- Failure to observe pretest restrictions
- Improper patient positioning during test
- Failure to chill the collection tube, syringe, and sample or to send the sample to the laboratory immediately
- Antihypertensives, hormonal contraceptives, ingestion of licorice, pregnancy, salt intake, severe blood loss, and therapy with diuretics or vasodilators (increase)
- Antidiuretic therapy and salt-retaining corticosteroid therapy (decrease)
- Radioisotope use within 2 days before the test

Respiratory syncytial virus antibodies

Respiratory syncytial virus (RSV), a member of the paramyxovirus group, is the major viral cause of severe lower respiratory tract disease in infants but may cause infections in people of any age. RSV infections are most common and produce the most severe disease during the first 6 months of life. Initial infection involves viral replication in epithelial cells of the upper respiratory tract, but in younger children especially, the infection spreads to the bronchi, the bronchioles, and even the parenchyma of the lungs.

In the RSV antibodies test, immunoglobulin (Ig) G and IgM class antibodies are quantified using indirect immunofluorescence.

Purpose
■ To diagnose infections caused by RSV

Cost
Moderately expensive

Patient preparation
■ Explain to the patient (or to his parents) the purpose of the test.
■ Tell the patient or parents that the test requires a blood sample. Explain who will perform the venipuncture and when.
■ Explain to the patient or parents that the patient may experience discomfort from the needle puncture and the tourniquet.

Normal findings
Sera from patients who have never been infected with RSV have no detectable antibodies to the virus (less than 1:5).

Abnormal findings
The qualitative presence of IgM or a fourfold or greater increase in IgG antibodies indicates active RSV infection. Note that in infants, serologic diagnosis of RSV infections is difficult because of the presence of maternal IgG antibodies. Thus, the presence of IgM antibodies is most significant.

Interfering factors
■ Hemolysis due to rough handling of the sample

Reticulocyte count

Reticulocytes are nonnucleated, immature red blood cells (RBCs) that remain in the peripheral blood for 24 to 48 hours while maturing. They're generally larger than mature RBCs. In the reticulocyte count test, reticulocytes in a whole blood sample are counted and expressed as a percentage of the total RBC count. Because the manual method of reticulocyte counting uses only a small sample, values may be imprecise and should be compared with the RBC count or hematocrit.

Purpose
■ To aid in distinguishing between hypoproliferative and hyperproliferative anemias
■ To help assess blood loss, bone marrow response to anemia, and therapy for anemia

Cost
Inexpensive

Patient preparation
■ Explain to the patient that this test is used to detect anemia or to monitor its treatment.
■ Tell the patient that the test requires a blood sample. Explain who will perform the venipuncture and when.
■ Explain to the patient that he may experience discomfort from the needle puncture and the tourniquet.
AGE ISSUE ✻ ✻ ✻ ✻ ✻
If the patient is an infant or child, explain to the parents that a small amount of blood will be taken from the finger or earlobe.
■ Restrict medications that may affect test results. If they must be continued, note this on the laboratory request.

Reference values
Reticulocytes compose 0.5% to 2.5% (SI, 0.005 to 0.025) of the total RBC count. In infants, the normal reticulocyte count ranges from 2% to 6% (SI, 0.02 to 0.06) at birth, decreasing to adult levels in 1 to 2 weeks.

Abnormal findings

A low reticulocyte count indicates hypoproliferative bone marrow (hypoplastic anemia) or ineffective erythropoiesis (pernicious anemia).

A high reticulocyte count indicates a bone marrow response to anemia caused by hemolysis or blood loss. The reticulocyte count may also increase after therapy for iron deficiency anemia or pernicious anemia.

Interfering factors

- Prolonged tourniquet constriction
- Azathioprine, chloramphenicol, dactinomycin, and methotrexate (possible false-low)
- Antimalarials, antipyretics, corticotropin, furazolidone (in infants), and levodopa (possible false-high)
- Sulfonamides (possible false-low or false-high)
- Recent blood transfusion
- Hemolysis due to rough handling of the sample or use of a small-gauge needle for blood aspiration

Rheumatoid factor

The rheumatoid factor (RF) test is the most useful immunologic test for confirming rheumatoid arthritis (RA). In this disease, "renegade" immunoglobulin (Ig) G antibodies, produced by lymphocytes in the synovial joints, react with IgM antibody to produce immune complexes, complement activation, and tissue destruction. How IgG molecules become antigenic is unknown, but they may be altered by aggregating with viruses or other antigens. Techniques for detecting RF include the sheep cell agglutination test and the latex fixation test. Although the presence of this autoantibody is diagnostically useful, it may not be etiologically related to RA.

Purpose

- To confirm RA, especially when clinical diagnosis is doubtful

Cost

Inexpensive

Patient preparation

- Explain to the patient that this test helps confirm RA.
- Tell the patient that the test requires a blood sample. Explain who will perform the venipuncture and when.
- Explain to the patient that he may experience discomfort from the needle puncture and the tourniquet.

Reference values

Normal RF titer is less than 1:20. A normal rheumatoid screening test is nonreactive.

Abnormal findings

Non-RA and RA populations aren't clearly separated with regard to the presence of RF: 25% of patients with RA have a nonreactive titer; 8% of non-RA patients are reactive at greater than 39 IU/ml, and only 3% of non-RA patients are reactive at greater than 80 IU/ml.

Patients with various non-RA diseases characterized by chronic inflammation may test positive for RF. These diseases include systemic lupus erythematosus, polymyositis, tuberculosis, infectious mononucleosis, syphilis, viral hepatic disease, and influenza.

Interfering factors

- Inadequately activated complement (possible false-positive)

- Serum with high lipid or cryoglobulin levels (possible false-positive, requiring repetition of the test after restricting fat intake)
- Serum with high IgG levels (possible false-negative due to competition with IgG on the surface of latex particles or sheep red blood cells used as substrate)

Rh typing

The Rhesus (Rh) system classifies blood by the presence or absence of antigen D, formerly known as Rh_O, on the surface of red blood cells (RBCs). In Rh typing, a patient's RBCs are mixed with serum containing anti-Rh_O(D) antibodies and observed for agglutination. If agglutination occurs, the Rh_O(D) antigen is present and the patient's blood is typed Rh-positive; if agglutination doesn't occur, the antigen is absent and the patient's blood is typed Rh-negative.

Prospective blood donors are fully tested to exclude the D^u variant, a weak variant of the D antigen, before being classified as having Rh-negative blood. People who have this antigen are considered Rh-positive donors but are generally transfused as Rh-negative recipients.

Purpose
- To establish blood type according to the Rh system
- To help determine the donor's compatibility before transfusion
- To determine whether the patient will require an Rh_O(D) immune globulin injection

Cost
Inexpensive

Patient preparation
- Explain to the patient that the test determines or verifies blood group to ensure safe transfusion.
- Tell the patient that the test requires a blood sample. Explain who will perform the venipuncture and when.
- Explain to the patient that he may experience discomfort from the needle puncture and the tourniquet.
- Check the patient's history for recent administration of dextran, I.V. contrast media, or drugs that may alter results.
- Tell the pregnant patient that after testing the laboratory may give her a card identifying that she may need to receive Rh_O(D).

Findings
Classified as Rh-positive or Rh-negative, donor blood may be transfused only if it's compatible with the recipient's blood. (See *Implications of Rh_O(D) typing test results*, page 332.)

If an Rh-negative woman delivers an Rh-positive baby or aborts a fetus whose Rh type is unknown, she should receive an Rh_O(D) injection within 72 hours to prevent hemolytic disease of the neonate in future births.

Interfering factors
- Recent administration of dextran or I.V. contrast media (cellular aggregation resembling antibody-mediated agglutination)
- Methyldopa, cephalosporins, and levodopa (possible false-positive for the D^u antigen due to positive direct antiglobulin [Coombs'] test)

Implications of Rh₀(D) typing test results

Classified as Rh$_o$(D)-positive, Rh$_o$(D)-negative, or Rh(D^u)-positive, donor blood may be transfused only if it's compatible with the recipient's blood, as shown below.

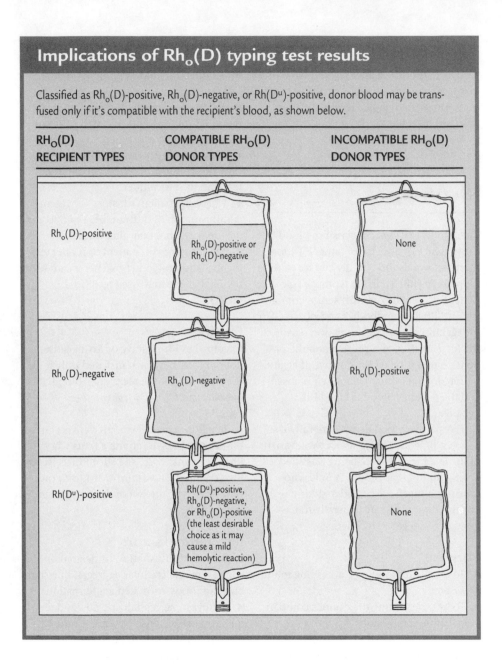

RH$_O$(D) RECIPIENT TYPES	COMPATIBLE RH$_O$(D) DONOR TYPES	INCOMPATIBLE RH$_O$(D) DONOR TYPES
Rh$_o$(D)-positive	Rh$_o$(D)-positive or Rh$_o$(D)-negative	None
Rh$_o$(D)-negative	Rh$_o$(D)-negative	Rh$_o$(D)-positive
Rh(D^u)-positive	Rh(D^u)-positive, Rh$_o$(D)-negative, or Rh$_o$(D)-positive (the least desirable choice as it may cause a mild hemolytic reaction)	None

Rubella antibodies

Although rubella (German measles) is generally a mild viral infection in children and young adults, it can produce severe infection in the fetus, resulting in spontaneous abortion, stillbirth, or congenital rubella syndrome. Because rubella infection normally induces immunoglobulin (Ig) G and IgM antibody production, measuring rubella antibodies can determine present infection as well as immunity resulting from past infection. The hemagglutination inhibition test is the most commonly used serologic test for rubella antibodies.

Purpose
■ To diagnose rubella infection, especially congenital infection
■ To determine susceptibility to rubella in children and in women of childbearing age

Cost
Inexpensive

Patient preparation
■ Explain to the patient that this test diagnoses or evaluates susceptibility to rubella.
■ Tell the patient that the test requires a blood sample and that if a current infection is suspected, a second blood sample will be needed in 2 to 3 weeks to identify a rise in the titer. Explain who will perform the venipuncture and when.
■ Explain to the patient that he may experience discomfort from the needle puncture and the tourniquet.

Normal findings
Titer of 1:8 or less indicates little or no immunity against rubella; titer of more than 1:10 indicates adequate protection against rubella.

IgM results are reported as positive or negative. The presence of rubella specific IgM class antibody indicates congenital or recent infection.

Abnormal findings
Hemagglutination inhibition antibodies normally appear 2 to 4 days after the onset of the rash, peak in 3 to 4 weeks, and then slowly decline but remain detectable for life. A fourfold or greater rise from the acute to the convalescent titer indicates a recent rubella infection.

The presence of rubella-specific IgM antibodies indicates recent infection in an adult and congenital rubella in an infant.

Interfering factors
■ Hemolysis due to rough handling of the sample

S

Schirmer test

The Schirmer tearing test assesses the function of the major lacrimal glands, which are responsible for reflex tearing in response to stressful situations such as the presence of a foreign body. Reflex tearing is stimulated by the insertion of a strip of filter paper into the lower conjunctival sac, followed by measurement of the amount of moisture absorbed by the paper. (See *Proper filter placement in the Schirmer test.*) Both eyes are tested simultaneously.

A variation of this test evaluates the function of the accessory lacrimal Krause's glands and glands of Wolfring by instillation of a topical anesthetic before insertion of the filter papers. The anesthetic inhibits reflex tearing by the major lacrimal glands, ensuring measurement of only the basic tear film that's normally produced by the accessory glands. This tear film usually maintains adequate corneal moisture under normal circumstances.

Purpose
■ To measure tear secretion in persons with a suspected tearing deficiency

Cost
Inexpensive

Patient preparation
■ Explain to the patient that this test measures secretion of tears.
■ Tell the patient that the test requires a strip of filter paper to be placed in the lower part of each eye for 5 minutes. Ensure him that the procedure is painless.
■ If the patient wears contact lenses, tell him that he'll have to remove them before the test. If an anesthetic is to be instilled, tell him he won't be able to reinsert the lenses for 2 hours after the test.
■ If a topical anesthetic is to be instilled, advise the patient not to rub his eyes for at least 30 minutes after instillation because this can cause a corneal abrasion.

Reference values
A Schirmer test strip should show at least 15 mm of moisture after 5 minutes. However, because tear production decreases with age, normal test results in patients over age 40 may range from 10 to 15 mm. Both eyes usually secrete the same amount of tears.

Abnormal findings

Although the Schirmer tearing test is a simple and efficient method of measuring the rate of tear secretion, up to 15% of the patients tested have false-positive or false-negative results. Because the test is rapid and simple, it may be repeated and findings compared. Additional testing, such as a slit-lamp examination with fluorescein or rose bengal stain, is necessary to corroborate results.

A positive result confirmed by additional testing indicates a definite tearing deficiency, which may result from aging or, more seriously, from Sjögren's syndrome, a systemic disease of unknown origin that's most common among postmenopausal women. Tearing deficiency may also arise secondarily to systemic diseases, such as lymphoma, leukemia, and rheumatoid arthritis.

Interfering factors

■ Patient closing his eyes too tightly during the test (increased tearing)
■ Contact of the test strip with the cornea (causes reflex tearing, which affects test results)

Semen analysis

Semen analysis is a simple, inexpensive, and reasonably definitive test that's used in a broad range of applications, including evaluation of a man's fertility. Fertility analysis usually includes measuring the volume of seminal fluid, performing sperm counts, and microscopically examining spermatozoa. Sperm are counted in much the same way that white blood cells, red blood cells, and platelets are counted in a blood sample. Motility and morphology are studied microscopically after staining a drop of semen.

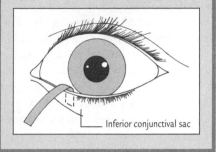

Proper filter placement in the Schirmer test

This illustration shows the proper placement of the filter paper for the Schirmer test. The filter paper should be inserted into the inferior conjunctival sac of each eye.

Inferior conjunctival sac

If analysis detects an abnormality, additional tests (for example, liver, thyroid, pituitary, or adrenal function tests) may be performed to identify the underlying cause and to screen for metabolic abnormalities (such as diabetes mellitus). Significant abnormalities — such as greatly decreased sperm count or motility, or marked increase in morphologically abnormal forms — may require testicular biopsy.

Purpose

■ To evaluate male fertility in an infertile couple
■ To substantiate the effectiveness of vasectomy
■ To rule out paternity on grounds of complete sterility
■ To detect semen on the body or clothing of a suspected rape victim or elsewhere at the crime scene
■ To identify blood group substances to exonerate or incriminate a criminal suspect

Cost

Moderately expensive

Patient preparation

■ Provide written instructions, and inform the patient that, to evaluate fertility, the most desirable specimen requires masturbation, ideally in a physician's office or a laboratory.

■ Tell the patient to follow the instructions given to him regarding the period of sexual continence (usually a fixed number of days between 2 and 5) before the test because this may increase his sperm count.

■ If the patient prefers to collect the specimen at home, emphasize the importance of delivering the specimen to the laboratory within 1 hour after collection. Warn him not to expose the specimen to extreme temperatures or to direct sunlight (which can also increase its temperature). Ideally, the specimen should remain at body temperature until liquefaction is complete (about 20 minutes). To deliver a semen specimen during cold weather, suggest that the patient keep the specimen container in a coat pocket on the way to the laboratory to protect the specimen from exposure to cold.

■ Alternatives to collection by masturbation include coitus interruptus or the use of a condom. For collection by coitus interruptus, instruct the patient to withdraw immediately before ejaculation and to deposit the ejaculate in a suitable specimen container. For collection by condom, tell the patient to first wash the condom with soap and water, rinse it thoroughly, and allow it to dry completely. (Powders or lubricants applied to the condom may be spermicidal.) Special sheaths that don't contain spermicide are also available for semen collection. After collection, instruct him to tie the condom, place it in a glass jar, and promptly deliver it to the laboratory.

■ Fertility may also be determined by collecting semen from the woman after coitus to assess the ability of the spermatozoa to penetrate the cervical mucus and remain active. For the postcoital cervical mucus test, instruct the patient to report for examination 1 to 2 days before ovulation as determined by basal temperature records. A urine luteinizing hormone-releasing hormone test may help predict ovulation in patients with irregular cycles. Instruct the couple to abstain from intercourse for 2 days and then to have intercourse 2 to 8 hours before the examination. Remind them to avoid using lubricants. Explain to the patient scheduled for this test that the procedure takes only a few minutes. Tell her that she'll be placed in the lithotomy position and that a speculum will be inserted into the vagina to collect the specimen. Also tell her that she may feel some pressure but no pain during this procedure.

Normal findings

Normal semen volume ranges from 0.7 to 6.5 ml. Paradoxically, the semen volume of many men in infertile couples is increased. Abstinence for 1 week or more results in progressively increased semen volume. (With abstinence of up to 10 days, sperm counts increase, sperm motility progressively decreases, and sperm morphology stays the same.) Liquefied semen is generally highly viscid, translucent, and gray-white, with a musty or acrid odor. After liquefaction, specimens of normal viscosity can be poured in drops. Normally, semen is slightly alkaline, with a pH of 7.3 to 7.9.

Other normal characteristics of semen: It coagulates immediately and liquefies within 20 minutes; the normal sperm count is 20 to 150 million/ml and can be greater; 40% of spermatozoa have normal morphology; and 20% or more of spermatozoa show progressive motility within 4 hours of collection.

The normal postcoital cervical mucus test shows 10 to 20 motile spermatozoa per microscopic high-power field and spinnbarkeit (a measurement of the tenacity of the mucus) of at least 4″ (10.2 cm). These findings indicate adequate spermatozoa and receptivity of the cervical mucus. Shaking or dead sperm may indicate antisperm antibodies.

Abnormal findings

Abnormal semen is *not* synonymous with infertility. Only one viable spermatozoon is needed to fertilize an ovum. Although a normal sperm count is 20 million/ml or more, many men with sperm counts below 1 million/ml have fathered normal children. Only men who can't deliver *any* viable spermatozoa in their ejaculate during sexual intercourse are absolutely sterile. Nevertheless, subnormal sperm counts, decreased sperm motility, and abnormal morphology are usually associated with decreased fertility.

Other tests may be necessary to evaluate the patient's general health, metabolic status, or the function of specific endocrine glands (pituitary, thyroid, adrenal, or gonadal).

Interfering factors

■ Poor timing of test within the menstrual cycle (abnormal postcoital test results)
■ Prior cervical conization or cryotherapy and some medications such as clomiphene (possible abnormal postcoital test results due to changes in cervical mucus)
■ Delayed transport of the specimen, exposure to extreme temperatures or direct sunlight, or the presence of toxic chemicals in the container or the condom (possible decrease in number of viable sperm)

■ An incomplete specimen — for example, from coitus interruptus or improper collection technique (decrease in specimen volume)

Sex chromatin

Although sex chromatin tests can screen for abnormalities in the number of sex chromosomes, the faster, simpler, and more accurate full karyotype (chromosome analysis) has all but replaced them. Sex chromatin tests are usually indicated for abnormal sexual development, ambiguous genitalia, amenorrhea, and suspected chromosomal abnormalities. (See *Understanding sex chromosome anomalies*, pages 338 and 339.)

Purpose

■ To quickly screen for abnormal sexual development (both X and Y chromatin tests)
■ To aid assessment of an infant with ambiguous genitalia (X chromatin test only)
■ To determine the number of Y chromosomes in an individual (Y chromatin test only)

Cost

Moderately expensive

Patient preparation

■ Explain to the patient or his parents, if appropriate, why the test is being performed.
■ Tell the patient or parents that the test requires the inside of his cheek to be scraped to obtain a specimen. Explain who will perform the test.
■ Assure the patient or parents that the test takes only a few minutes but may require a follow-up chromosome analysis.

Understanding sex chromosome anomalies

DISORDER AND CHROMOSOMAL ANEUPLOIDY	CAUSES AND INCIDENCE	PHENOTYPIC FEATURES
Klinefelter's syndrome ■ 47,XXY ■ 48,XXXY ■ 49,XXXXY ■ 48,XX,YY ■ 49,XXX,YY ■ Mosaics: XXY, XXXY, or XXXXY/XX or XY	Nondisjunction or improper chromatid separation during anaphase I or II of oogenesis or spermatogenesis results in abnormal gamete. 1 in 1,000 male births	■ Syndrome usually inapparent until puberty ■ Small penis and testes ■ Sparse facial and abdominal hair; feminine distribution of pubic hair ■ Somewhat enlarged breasts (gynecomastia) ■ Sexual dysfunction ■ Truncal obesity ■ Sterility ■ Possible mental retardation (greater incidence with increased X chromosomes)
Polysomy Y ■ 47,XYY	Nondisjunction during anaphase II of spermatogenesis causes both Y chromosomes to pass to the same pole and results in Y sperm. 1 in 1,000 male births	■ Above-average stature (often over 72″ [182.9 cm]) ■ Increased incidence of severe acne ■ May display aggressive, psychopathic, or criminal behavior ■ Normal fertility ■ Learning disabilities
Turner's syndrome (gonadal dysgenesis) ■ 45,XO ■ Mosaics: XO/XX or XO/XXX ■ Aberrations of X chromosomes, including deletion of short arm of one X chromosome, presence of a ring chromosome, or presence of an isochromosome on the long arm of an X chromosome	Nondisjunction during anaphase I or II of spermatogenesis results in sperm without any sex chromosomes. 1 in 3,500 female births (most common chromosome complement in first-trimester spontaneous abortions)	■ Short stature (usually under 57″ [144.8 cm]) ■ Webbed neck ■ Low posterior hairline ■ Broad chest with widely spaced nipples ■ Underdeveloped breasts ■ Juvenile external genitalia ■ Primary amenorrhea common ■ Congenital heart disease (30% with coarctation of the aorta) ■ Renal abnormalities ■ Sterility caused by underdeveloped internal reproductive organs (ovaries are merely strands of connective tissue) ■ No mental retardation, but possible problems with space perception and orientation
Other X polysomes	Nondisjunction at anaphase I or II of oogenesis	
■ 47,XXX	1 in 1,400 female births	■ In many cases, no obvious anatomic abnormalities ■ Normal fertility

DISORDER AND CHROMOSOMAL ANEUPLOIDY	CAUSES AND INCIDENCE	PHENOTYPIC FEATURES
Other X polysomes *(continued)*		
■ 48,XXXX	Rare	■ Mental retardation ■ Ocular hypertelorism ■ Reduced fertility
■ 49,XXXXX	Rare	■ Severe mental retardation ■ Ocular hypertelorism with uncoordinated eye movement ■ Abnormal development of sexual organs ■ Various skeletal anomalies

■ Inform the patient or parents that the laboratory generally requires as long as 4 weeks to complete the analysis.

Normal findings

A normal female (XX) has only one X chromatin mass (the number of X chromatin masses discernible is one fewer than the number of X chromosomes in the cells examined). For various reasons, an X chromatin mass is ordinarily discernible in only 20% to 50% of the buccal mucosal cells of a normal woman.

A normal male (XY) has only one Y chromatin mass (the number of Y chromatin masses equals the number of Y chromosomes in the cells examined).

Abnormal findings

In most laboratories, if less than 20% of the cells in a buccal smear contain an X chromatin mass, some cells are presumed to contain only one X chromosome, necessitating full karyotyping. Persons with female phenotypes and positive Y chromatin masses run a high risk of developing malignancies in their intra-abdominal gonads.

In such persons, removal of these gonads is indicated and should generally be performed before age 5.

The patient or his parents require genetic counseling after the cause of chromosomal abnormal sexual development has been identified. A medical team comprised of physicians, psychologists, psychiatrists, and educators must decide the child's sex if a child is phenotypically of one sex and genotypically of the other. This careful evaluation should be made early to prevent developmental problems related to incorrect gender identification.

Interfering factors

■ Obtaining saliva instead of buccal cells (false specimen)
■ Cell deterioration due to failure to apply cell fixative to the slide
■ Presence of bacteria or wrinkles in the cell membrane, analysis of degenerative cells, or use of an outdated stain

Sickle cells

The sickle cell test, also known as the *hemoglobin S (Hb S) test*, is used to detect sickle cells, which are severely deformed, rigid erythrocytes that may slow blood flow. Sickle cell trait (characterized by heterozygous Hb S) is found almost exclusively in blacks: 0.2% of the blacks born in the United States have sickle cell disease.

Although the sickle cell test is useful as a rapid screening procedure, it may produce erroneous results. Hb electrophoresis should be performed to confirm the diagnosis if sickle cell disease is strongly suspected.

Purpose
■ To identify sickle cell disease and sickle cell trait

Cost
Moderately expensive

Patient preparation
■ Explain to the patient that this test is used to detect sickle cell disease.
■ Tell the patient that the test requires a blood sample. Explain who will perform the venipuncture and when.
■ Explain to the patient that he may experience discomfort from the needle puncture and the tourniquet.
AGE ISSUE * * * * *
If the patient is an infant or child, explain to his parents that a small amount of blood will be taken from the finger or earlobe.
■ Check the patient's history for a blood transfusion within the past 3 months.

Normal findings
Results of this test are reported as positive or negative. A negative result suggests the absence of Hb S.

Abnormal findings
A positive result may indicate the presence of sickle cells, but Hb electrophoresis is needed to further diagnose the sickling tendency of cells. Rarely, in the absence of Hb S, other abnormal Hb may cause sickling.

Interfering factors
■ Failure to fill the tube completely, to use the proper anticoagulant in the collection tube, or to adequately mix the sample and the anticoagulant
■ Hemolysis due to rough handling of the sample or use of a small-gauge needle for blood aspiration
■ Hb concentration less than 10%, elevated Hb S levels in infants under age 6 months, or transfusion within 3 months of the test (possible false-negative)

Skeletal magnetic resonance imaging

A noninvasive technique, skeletal magnetic resonance imaging (MRI) produces clear and sensitive tomographic images of bone and soft tissue. The scan provides superior contrast of body tissues and allows imaging of multiple planes, including direct sagittal and coronal views in regions that can't be easily visualized with X-rays or computed tomography scans. MRI eliminates any risks associated with exposure to X-ray beams and causes no known harm to cells.
ALERT! ▼ ▼ ▼ ▼ ▼ ▼ ▼ ▼ ▼
MRI can't be performed on patients with pacemakers, intracranial aneurysm clips, or other ferrous metal implants.

Purpose
■ To evaluate bony and soft-tissue tumors
■ To identify changes in bone marrow composition
■ To identify spinal disorders

Cost

Very expensive

Patient preparation

■ Explain to the patient that this test assesses bone and soft tissue. Tell him who will perform the test and where it will take place.

■ Explain that although MRI is painless and involves no exposure to radiation from the scanner, a contrast medium may be used, depending on the type of tissue being studied.

■ Explain to the patient that if he's claustrophobic or if extensive time is required for scanning, a mild sedative may be administered to reduce anxiety. Open scanners have been developed for use on patients with extreme claustrophobia or morbid obesity, but tests using such machines take longer.

■ Explain to the patient the need to lie flat; then describe the test procedure.

■ Explain to the patient that he'll hear the scanner clicking, whirring, and thumping as it moves inside its housing.

■ Ask the patient whether he has any surgically implanted joints, pins, clips, valves, pumps, or pacemakers containing metal that could be attracted to the strong MRI magnet. If he does, he can't have the test.

■ Obtain informed consent if necessary.

Normal findings

MRI should reveal no pathology in bone, muscles, and joints.

Abnormal findings

MRI may reveal primary and metastatic bone tumors and diseases of the spinal canal and cord.

Interfering factors

■ Excessive patient movement
■ Patient can't fit into scanner

Skin biopsy

Skin biopsy is the removal of a small piece of tissue under local anesthesia from a lesion suspected of being malignant or from other dermatoses. One of three techniques may be used: shave biopsy, punch biopsy, or excisional biopsy. Shave biopsy uses a scalpel to slice a superficial specimen from the site. Punch biopsy removes an oval core from the center of a lesion down to the dermis or subcutaneous tissue. Excisional biopsy removes the entire lesion with a small border of normal skin.

Lesions suspected of being malignant usually have changed color, size, or appearance or have failed to heal properly after injury. Fully developed lesions should be selected for biopsy whenever possible because they provide more diagnostic information than lesions that are resolving or in early developing stages.

Purpose

■ To provide differential diagnosis among basal cell carcinoma, squamous cell carcinoma, malignant melanoma, and benign growths

■ To diagnose chronic bacterial or fungal skin infections

Cost

Moderately expensive

Patient preparation

■ Explain to the patient that skin biopsy provides a specimen for microscopic study.

■ Describe the procedure to the patient, and answer any questions he may have.

■ Tell the patient who will perform the procedure and where it will take place.

■ Tell the patient that he may receive a local anesthetic to minimize pain during the procedure.

■ Obtain informed consent if necessary.

■ Check the patient's history for hypersensitivity to the local anesthetic.

Normal findings
Normal skin consists of squamous epithelium (epidermis) and fibrous connective tissue (dermis).

Abnormal findings
Histologic examination of the tissue specimen may reveal a benign or malignant lesion. Benign growths include cysts, seborrheic keratoses, warts, pigmented nevi (moles), keloids, dermatofibromas, and multiple neurofibromas.

Malignant tumors include basal cell carcinoma, squamous cell carcinoma, and malignant melanoma. Basal cell carcinoma occurs on hair-bearing skin; the most common location is the face, including the nose and its folds. Squamous cell carcinoma most commonly appears on the lips, mouth, and genitalia. Malignant melanoma, the deadliest skin cancer, can spread through the body by way of the lymphatic system and blood vessels.

Cultures can be used to detect chronic bacterial and fungal infections in which flora are relatively sparse.

Interfering factors
■ Improper selection of the biopsy site
■ Failure to use the appropriate fixative or a sterile container

Skull radiography

Although skull radiography is of limited value in assessing patients with head injuries, skull X-rays are extremely valuable for studying abnormalities of the base of the skull and the cranial vault, congenital and perinatal anomalies, and systemic diseases that produce bone defects of the skull. For more accurate assessment of head injuries as well as of skull and head abnormalities, nonenhanced computed tomography studies of the head are done.

Skull radiography evaluates the three groups of bones that comprise the skull: the calvaria (vault), the mandible (jaw bone), and the facial bones. The calvaria and the facial bones are closely connected by immovable joints with irregular serrated edges called sutures. The bones of the skull form an anatomic structure so complex that a complete skull examination requires several radiologic views of each area.

Purpose
■ To detect fractures in patients with head trauma
■ To aid diagnosis of pituitary tumors
■ To detect congenital anomalies
■ To detect metabolic and endocrinologic disorders

Cost
Moderately expensive

Patient preparation
■ Explain to the patient that his head will be immobilized and that several X-rays of his skull will be taken from various angles.
■ Tell the patient that this test helps determine the presence of anomalies and helps establish a diagnosis.
■ Tell the patient who will perform the test and where it will take place.

Normal findings
A radiologist interprets the X-rays, evaluating the size, shape, thickness, and position of the cranial bones as well as the vascular markings, sinuses, and sutures. All should be normal for the patient's age.

Abnormal findings
Skull radiography is commonly used to diagnose fractures of the vault or base, although basilar fractures may not show on

the film if the bone is dense. This test may confirm congenital anomalies and may show erosion, enlargement, or decalcification of the sella turcica that results from increased intracranial pressure (ICP). A marked rise in ICP may cause the brain to expand and press against the inner bony table of the skull, yielding visible marks or impressions.

In conditions such as osteomyelitis (with possible calcification of the skull itself) and chronic subdural hematomas, X-rays may show abnormal areas of calcification. The X-rays can detect neoplasms within brain substance that contains calcium (such as oligodendrogliomas or meningiomas) or the midline shifting of a calcified pineal gland caused by a space-occupying lesion.

Radiography may also detect other changes in bone structure, for example, those that arise from metabolic disorders, such as acromegaly or Paget's disease.

Interfering factors
■ Improper positioning of the patient and excessive head movement (possible poor imaging)

Sleep studies

Also known as *polysomnography*, sleep studies are tests used to help in the differential diagnosis of sleep-disordered breathing. Several parameters are evaluated for the patient being tested for sleep disorder; these include cardiac rate and rhythm, chest and abdominal wall movement, nasal and oral airflow, oxygen saturation, muscle activity, retinal function, and brain activity during the sleep phase.

Purpose
■ To diagnose breathing disorders in persons with a history of excessive snoring,

narcolepsy, excessive daytime sleepiness, insomnia, cardiac rhythm disorders, and restless leg spasms

Cost
Expensive

Patient preparation
■ Explain the purpose of the test to the patient, and tell him to maintain normal sleep schedules so that he's neither deprived of sleep nor overrested.
■ Inform the patient that sleep studies are usually scheduled for the evening and night hours, usually 10 p.m. to 6 a.m., and take place in a designated sleep laboratory.
■ Explain to the patient that he should abstain from caffeinated products and naps for 2 to 3 days before the test.
■ Tell the patient electrodes are secured to his skin (depending on the type of monitoring being used) and that lights are turned off and the EEG monitored for a baseline reading before the patient falls asleep.
■ If you order split–night studies, tell the patient with known sleep apnea that he will be monitored during normal sleep the first half of the night. Then tell him that during the second half of the night, he'll be monitored while continuous positive airway pressure or nasal ventilation to open the obstructed airway is applied.

Normal findings
A normal sleep study shows a respiratory disturbance index (or apnea-hypopnea index) of fewer than 5 to 10 episodes per study period and normal electrocardiogram (cardiac rate and rhythm), impedance (chest and abdominal wall motion), airway (nasal and oral airflow), arterial oxygen saturation (oximetry), leg electromyogram (for muscle activity), electrooculogram (for retinal function), and EEG (for brain activity).

Abnormal findings

Abnormal recordings reveal obstructive sleep apnea syndrome. Abnormal movement during sleep indicates a seizure or movement disorder.

Interfering factors

- Defective electrodes, diaphoresis, environmental noises, electrophysiologic artifacts
- Patient's inability to fall asleep

Small-bowel biopsy

Small-bowel biopsy is used to evaluate diseases of the intestinal mucosa, which may cause malabsorption or diarrhea. It produces larger specimens than those produced by endoscopic biopsy and allows removal of tissue from areas beyond an endoscope's reach. (See *Endoscopic biopsy of the GI tract*.)

Several similar types of capsules are available for tissue collection. In each, a mercury-weighted bag is attached to one end of the capsule; a thin polyethylene tube about 5' (1.5 m) long is attached to the other end. When the bag, capsule, and tube are in place in the small bowel, suction on the tube draws the mucosa into the capsule and closes it, cutting off the piece of tissue within. Although this is an invasive procedure, it causes little pain and rarely causes complications.

Small-bowel biopsy verifies diagnosis of some diseases such as Whipple's disease and may help confirm others such as tropical sprue. Capsule biopsy is an invasive procedure, but it causes little pain and complications are rare.

ALERT! ▼ ▼ ▼ ▼ ▼ ▼ ▼ ▼ ▼

Biopsy is contraindicated in uncooperative patients, those taking aspirin or anticoagulants, *and those with uncontrolled coagulation disorders.*

Purpose

- To help diagnose diseases of the intestinal mucosa

Cost

Very expensive

Patient preparation

- Explain to the patient that this test is used to identify intestinal disorders.
- Describe the procedure to the patient and answer questions.
- Instruct the patient to restrict food and fluids for at least 8 hours before the test.
- Tell the patient who will perform the biopsy and where it will take place.
- Tell the patient that he may receive a local anesthetic to suppress the gag reflex, that a capsule will be placed in his pharynx, and that he'll be asked to flex his neck and swallow as the tube is advanced and monitored with fluoroscopy.
- Obtain informed consent if necessary.
- Ensure that coagulation tests have been performed and that the results are recorded on the patient's chart. Restrict aspirin and anticoagulants; if these drugs must be continued, note this on the laboratory request.

ALERT! ▼ ▼ ▼ ▼ ▼ ▼ ▼ ▼ ▼

Tell the patient to report abdominal pain or bleeding.

Normal findings

A normal small-bowel biopsy specimen consists of fingerlike villi, crypts, columnar epithelial cells, and round cells.

Abnormal findings

Small-bowel tissue that reveals histologic changes in cell structure may indicate Whipple's disease, abetalipoproteinemia, lymphoma, lymphangiectasia, eosinophilic

Endoscopy allows direct visualization of the GI tract and any site that requires biopsy of tissue specimens for histologic analysis. This relatively painless procedure can detect cancer, lymphoma, amyloidosis, candidiasis, and gastric ulcers; can support a diagnosis of Crohn's disease, chronic ulcerative colitis, gastritis, esophagitis, and melanosis coli in laxative abuse; and can monitor progression of Barrett's esophagus, multiple gastric polyps, colon cancer and polyps, and chronic ulcerative colitis. Its complications, notably hemorrhage, perforation, and aspiration, are rare.

Preparation

Careful patient preparation is vital for this procedure. Describe the procedure to the patient, and reassure him that he'll be able to breathe with the endoscope in place. Instruct him to fast for at least 8 hours before the procedure. Obtain informed consent if necessary. Order an enema if appropriate.

Tell the patient that just before the procedure he'll be sedated and that the back of his throat will be sprayed with a local anesthetic to suppress his gag reflex. Assure him that suction equipment and bipolar cauterizing electrodes will be on hand to prevent aspiration and excessive bleeding.

To facilitate patient understanding of the procedure, explain the process of obtaining the specimen:
- An endoscope is passed into the upper or lower GI tract to visualize the lesion, node, or other abnormal area.
- A biopsy forceps is pushed through the channel in the endoscope until it, too, can be seen.
- The forceps is opened, positioned at the biopsy site, and closed on the tissue; the closed forceps and tissue specimen are then removed from the endoscope, and the tissue is taken from the forceps.
- The specimen is placed mucosal side up on fine-mesh gauze or filter paper and inserted into a labeled specimen bottle containing fixative.
- When all specimens have been collected, the endoscope is removed and the specimens are sent to the laboratory immediately.

enteritis, and such parasitic infections as giardiasis and coccidiosis. Abnormal specimens may also suggest celiac sprue, tropical sprue, infectious gastroenteritis, intraluminal bacterial overgrowth, folate and vitamin B_{12} deficiency, radiation enteritis, and malnutrition, but such disorders require further studies.

Interfering factors

- Failure to fast before biopsy (possible poor specimen or vomiting and aspiration)

- Mechanical failure of the biopsy capsule or hole in the tubing (possible difficulty in removing tissue specimen)
- Incorrect handling or positioning of the specimen or failure to place it in a fixative

Sodium

The sodium test is used to measure serum levels of sodium in relation to the amount of water in the body. Sodium, the major extracellular cation, affects body water distribution, maintains osmotic pressure of ex-

Fluid imbalances

This chart lists the causes, signs and symptoms, and diagnostic test findings associated with hypervolemia (increased fluid volume) and hypovolemia (decreased fluid volume).

CAUSES	SIGNS AND SYMPTOMS	LABORATORY FINDINGS
Hypervolemia		
■ Increased water intake ■ Decreased water output caused by renal disease ■ Heart failure ■ Excessive ingestion or infusion of sodium chloride ■ Long-term administration of adrenocortical hormones ■ Excessive infusion of isotonic solutions	■ Increased blood pressure, pulse rate, body weight, and respiratory rate ■ Bounding peripheral pulses ■ Moist pulmonary crackles ■ Moist mucous membranes ■ Moist respiratory secretions ■ Edema ■ Weakness ■ Seizure and coma caused by swelling of brain cells	■ Decreased red blood cell (RBC) count, hemoglobin concentration, packed cell volume, serum sodium concentration (dilutional decrease), and urine specific gravity
Hypovolemia		
■ Decreased water intake ■ Fluid loss caused by fever, diarrhea, and vomiting ■ Systemic infection ■ Impaired renal concentrating ability ■ Fistulous drainage ■ Severe burns ■ Hidden fluid in body cavities	■ Increased pulse and respiratory rates ■ Decreased blood pressure and body weight ■ Weak and thready peripheral pulses ■ Thick, slurred speech ■ Thirst ■ Oliguria ■ Anuria ■ Dry skin	■ Increased RBC count, hemoglobin concentration, packed cell volume, serum sodium concentration, and urine specific gravity

tracellular fluid, and helps promote neuromuscular function. It also helps maintain acid-base balance and influences chloride and potassium levels.

Purpose

■ To evaluate fluid-electrolyte and acid-base balance and related neuromuscular, renal, and adrenal functions

Cost

Inexpensive

Patient preparation

■ Explain to the patient that this test is used to determine the sodium content of blood.

■ Tell the patient that the test requires a blood sample. Explain who will perform the venipuncture and when.

■ Explain to the patient that he may experience discomfort from the needle puncture and the tourniquet.

■ Restrict medications that may affect test results. If they must be continued, note this on the laboratory request.

Reference values

Normally, serum sodium levels range from 135 to 145 mEq/L (SI, 135 to 145 mmol/L).

Abnormal findings

Sodium imbalance can result from a loss or gain of sodium or from a change in the patient's state of hydration. Increased serum sodium levels (hypernatremia) may be due to inadequate water intake, water loss in excess of sodium (such as diabetes insipidus, impaired renal function, prolonged hyperventilation and, occasionally, severe vomiting or diarrhea), and sodium retention (such as aldosteronism). Hypernatremia can also result from excessive sodium intake.

ALERT! ▼ ▼ ▼ ▼ ▼ ▼ ▼ ▼ ▼

The patient with hypernatremia and associated loss of water should be observed for signs of thirst, restlessness, irritability, confusion, muscle twitching, dry and sticky mucous membranes, flushed skin, oliguria, and diminished reflexes. If increased total body sodium causes water retention, note that the patient should be observed for hypertension, tachycardia, dyspnea, edema, and heart failure.

Abnormally low serum sodium levels (hyponatremia) may result from inadequate sodium intake or excessive sodium loss due to profuse sweating, GI suctioning, diuretic therapy, diarrhea, vomiting, adrenal insufficiency, burns, and chronic renal insufficiency with acidosis. Urine sodium determinations are usually more sensitive to early changes in sodium balance and should be evaluated simultaneously with serum sodium findings.

ALERT! ▼ ▼ ▼ ▼ ▼ ▼ ▼ ▼ ▼

The patient with hyponatremia should be watched for apprehension, lassitude, headache, decreased skin turgor, abdominal cramps, and tremors that may progress to seizures. (See Fluid imbalances.*)*

Interfering factors

■ Hemolysis due to rough handling of the sample

■ Most diuretics (decrease by promoting sodium excretion)

■ Chlorpropamide, lithium, and vasopressin (decrease by inhibiting water excretion)

■ Corticosteroids (increase by promoting sodium retention)

■ Antihypertensives, such as hydralazine, methyldopa, and reserpine (possible increase due to sodium and water retention)

Spinal computed tomography

Much more versatile than conventional radiography, computed tomography (CT) of the spine provides detailed high-resolution images in the cross-sectional, longitudinal, sagittal, and lateral planes. Multiple X-ray beams from a computerized body scanner are directed at the spine from different angles; these pass through the body and strike radiation detectors, producing electrical impulses. A computer then converts these impulses into digital information, which is displayed as a three-dimensional image on a monitor. Storage of the digital information allows electronic re-creation and manipulation of the image, creating a permanent record of the images to enable reexamination without repeating the procedure.

CT scans are helpful in defining the lesions causing spinal cord compression. Metastatic disease and discogenic disease with osteophyte formation and calcification are examples of pathologic processes diagnosed by CT scans. Since the advent of magnetic resonance imaging, CT scans are used less frequently to diagnose infection, abscesses, hematomas, and some disk herniations.

ALERT! ▼ ▼ ▼ ▼ ▼ ▼ ▼ ▼ ▼
CT scan of the spine with contrast enhancement is contraindicated in patients who are hypersensitive to iodine, shellfish, or contrast media used in radiographic studies.

Purpose
■ To diagnose spinal lesions and abnormalities
■ To monitor the effects of spinal surgery or therapy

Cost
Very expensive

Patient preparation
■ Explain to the patient that this procedure allows visualization of his spine.
■ If contrast enhancement isn't ordered, tell the patient that he need not restrict food or fluids. If contrast is ordered, instruct him to fast for 4 hours before the test.
■ Tell the patient that a series of scans will be taken of his spine. Explain who will perform the procedure and where it will take place.
■ Reassure the patient that the procedure is painless, but inform him that he may find having to remain still for a prolonged period uncomfortable.
■ Explain to the patient that he'll be positioned on an X-ray table inside a CT body-scanning unit and be told to lie still. The computer-controlled scanner will revolve around him taking multiple scans.
■ If a contrast medium is used, tell the patient that he may feel flushed and warm and may experience a transient headache, a salty taste, and nausea or vomiting after injection of the contrast medium. Reassure him that these reactions are normal.
■ Check the patient's history for hypersensitivity reactions to iodine, shellfish, or contrast media. If such reactions have occurred, prophylactic medications may be needed or contrast enhancement may not be used.
■ If the patient appears restless or apprehensive about the procedure, tell him that a mild sedative can be given.
■ Obtain informed consent if necessary.

Normal findings
In the CT image, spinal tissue appears white, black, or gray, depending on its density. Vertebrae, the densest tissues, are white; cerebrospinal fluid is black; soft tissues appear in shades of gray.

Abnormal findings
By highlighting areas of altered density and depicting structural malformation, CT scanning can reveal all types of spinal lesions and abnormalities. It's particularly useful in detecting and localizing tumors, which appear as masses varying in density. Measuring this density and noting the configuration and location relative to the spinal cord can usually identify the type of tumor. For example, a neurinoma (schwannoma) appears as a spherical mass dorsal to the cord. A darker, wider mass lying more laterally or ventrally to the cord may be a meningioma.

CT scans also reveal degenerative processes and structural changes in detail. Herniated nucleus pulposus shows as an obvious herniation of disk material with unilateral or bilateral nerve root compression; if the herniation is midline, spinal cord compression will be evident. Cervical spondylosis shows as cervical cord compression due to bony hypertrophy of the cervical spine; lumbar stenosis as hypertrophy of the lumbar vertebrae, causing cord compression by decreasing space within the spinal column. Facet disorders show as soft-tissue changes, bony overgrowth, and spurring of the vertebrae, which result in nerve root compression. Fluid-filled arachnoidal and other paraspinal cysts show as dark masses displacing the spinal cord. Vascular malformations, evident after contrast enhancement, show as masses or clusters, usually on the dorsal aspect of the spinal cord.

Congenital spinal malformations, such as meningocele, myelocele, and spina bifida, show as abnormally large, dark gaps between the white vertebrae.

Interfering factors
■ Excessive patient movement
■ Failure to remove metallic objects from the scan area (possible poor imaging)

Sputum culture

Bacteriologic examination of sputum (material raised from the lungs and bronchi) is an important aid to the management of lung disease. The usual method of specimen collection is deep coughing and expectoration, which may require ultrasonic nebulization, hydration, or chest physiotherapy; other methods include tracheal suctioning and bronchoscopy.

Purpose
■ To isolate and identify the cause of pulmonary infection, thus aiding diagnosis of respiratory diseases (most commonly bronchitis, tuberculosis, lung abscess, and pneumonia)

Cost
Inexpensive

Patient preparation
■ Explain to the patient that this test is used to identify the organism causing respiratory tract infection.
■ Tell the patient that the test requires a sputum specimen, and inform him who will collect the specimen and how it will be obtained.
■ If the suspected organism is *Mycobacterium tuberculosis,* tell the patient that as many as three consecutive morning specimens may be required.
■ If the specimen is to be collected by expectoration, tell the patient that deep breaths and a forced, deep cough are needed. Tell him to brush his teeth and gargle with water before the specimen collection to reduce contaminating oropharyngeal bacteria.
■ If the specimen is to be collected by tracheal suctioning, tell the patient that he'll experience discomfort as the catheter passes into the trachea.
■ If the specimen is to be collected by bronchoscopy, instruct the patient to fast for 6 hours before the procedure.
■ Tell the patient that he'll receive a local anesthetic just before the test to minimize discomfort during passage of the tube.
■ Obtain informed consent if necessary.
ALERT! ▼ ▼ ▼ ▼ ▼ ▼ ▼ ▼ ▼
Tracheal suctioning is contraindicated in patients with esophageal varices.

Normal findings
Flora commonly found in the respiratory tract include alpha-hemolytic streptococci, *Neisseria* species, and diphtheroids. The presence of normal flora doesn't rule out infection.

Abnormal findings
Because sputum is invariably contaminated with normal oropharyngeal flora, a culture isolate must be interpreted in light of the

patient's overall clinical condition. Isolation of M. *tuberculosis* is always a significant finding.

Interfering factors

■ Failure to report current or recent antimicrobial therapy on the laboratory request (possible false-negative)
■ Collection over an extended period, which may cause pathogens to deteriorate or become overgrown by commensals (not accepted as a valid specimen by laboratories)

Stool examination for ova and parasites

Normal bacterial flora in stool include several potentially pathogenic organisms. Stool examination is valuable for identifying pathogens that cause overt GI disease, such as typhoid and dysentery, and carrier states. A sensitivity test may follow isolation of the pathogen. Stool examination may also be used to detect certain viruses such as enterovirus, which can cause aseptic meningitis.

Purpose

■ To identify GI disease caused by pathogenic organisms
■ To identify carrier states

Cost

Moderately expensive

Patient preparation

■ Explain to the patient that this test is used to determine the cause of GI distress or to determine whether he's a carrier of infectious organisms.
■ Tell the patient that the test requires the collection of a stool specimen on 3 consecutive days.

■ Check the patient's history for dietary patterns, recent antimicrobial therapy, and recent travel that might suggest endemic infections or infestations.
ALERT! ▼ ▼ ▼ ▼ ▼ ▼ ▼ ▼ ▼
Specimens should be collected before antimicrobial therapy begins.

Normal findings

A large percentage of normal fecal flora consists of anaerobes, including non-spore-forming bacilli, clostridia, and anaerobic streptococci. The remaining percentage consists of aerobes, including gram-negative bacilli (predominantly *Escherichia coli* and other Enterobacteriaceae, plus small amounts of *Pseudomonas*), gram-positive cocci (mostly enterococci), and a few yeasts.

Abnormal findings

The most common pathogenic organisms of the GI tract are Shigella, Salmonella, and *Campylobacter jejuni*. Less common pathogenic organisms include *Vibrio cholerae, V. parahaemolyticus, Clostridium botulinum, C. difficile, C. perfringens, Staphylococcus aureus,* enterotoxigenic *E. coli,* and *Yersinia enterocolitica.* Isolation of some pathogens indicates bacterial infection in patients with acute diarrhea and may require antimicrobial sensitivity tests. Normal fecal flora may include *C. difficile, E. coli,* and other organisms. Therefore, isolation of these organisms may require further tests to demonstrate invasiveness or toxin production.

Isolation of pathogens such as *C. botulinum* indicates food poisoning; the pathogens must also be isolated from the contaminated food. In a patient undergoing long-term antimicrobial therapy, isolation of large numbers of *S. aureus* or yeast may indicate infection. (Asymptomatic carrier states are also indicated by these enteric pathogens.) Isolation of enteroviruses may indicate aseptic meningitis.

If a stool culture shows no unusual growth, detection of viruses by immunoassay or electron microscopy may be used to diagnose nonbacterial gastroenteritis. Highly increased polymorphonuclear leukocytes in fecal material may indicate an invasive pathogen. (See *Pathogens of the GI tract.*)

Interfering factors

■ Contamination of the specimen by urine (possible injury to or destruction of enteric pathogens)

■ Antimicrobial therapy (possible decrease in bacterial growth)

■ Failure to transport the specimen promptly or, if delivery is delayed, to use a transport medium, such as buffered glycerol, that stabilizes pH (possible loss of enteric pathogens or overgrowth of nonpathogenic organisms)

Stress test

Also referred to as an *exercise electrocardiogram* (ECG), a stress test evaluates the heart's response to physical stress, providing important diagnostic information that can't be obtained from a resting ECG alone.

An ECG and blood pressure readings are taken while the patient walks on a treadmill or pedals a stationary bicycle, and his response to a constant or an increasing workload is observed. Unless complications develop, the test continues until the patient reaches the target heart rate (determined by an established protocol) or experiences chest pain or fatigue. The patient who has recently had a myocardial infarction (MI) or coronary artery surgery may walk the treadmill at a slow pace to determine his activity tolerance before discharge.

Pathogens of the GI tract

The presence of the following pathogens in a stool culture may indicate certain disorders:

Aeromonas hydrophila: gastroenteritis, which causes diarrhea, especially in children

Bacillus cereus: food poisoning, acute gastroenteritis (rare)

Campylobacter jejuni: gastroenteritis

Clostridium botulinum: food poisoning and infant botulism (a possible cause of sudden infant death syndrome)

Toxin-producing *Clostridium difficile:* pseudomembranous enterocolitis

Clostridium perfringens: food poisoning

Enterotoxigenic *Escherichia coli:* gastroenteritis (resembles cholera or shigellosis)

Salmonella: gastroenteritis, typhoid fever, nontyphoidal salmonellosis, paratyphoid fever, enteric fever

Shigella: shigellosis, bacillary dysentery

Staphylococcus aureus: food poisoning, suppression of normal bowel flora from antimicrobial therapy

Vibrio cholerae: cholera

Vibrio parahaemolyticus: food poisoning, especially seafood

Yersinia enterocolitica: gastroenteritis, enterocolitis (resembles appendicitis), mesenteric lymphadenitis, ileitis.

ALERT! ▼ ▼ ▼ ▼ ▼ ▼ ▼ ▼ ▼
Because an exercise ECG places considerable stress on the heart, it may be contraindicated in patients with ventricular aneurysm, dissecting aortic aneurysm, uncontrolled arrhythmias, pericarditis, myocarditis, severe anemia, uncontrolled hypertension, unstable angina, or heart failure.

Purpose

■ To help diagnose the cause of chest pain or other possible cardiac pain
■ To determine the functional capacity of the heart after surgery or MI
■ To screen for asymptomatic coronary artery disease (CAD), particularly in men over age 35
■ To help set limitations for an exercise program
■ To identify arrhythmias that develop during physical exercise
■ To evaluate the effectiveness of antiarrhythmic or antianginal therapy
■ To evaluate myocardial perfusion

Cost

Expensive

Patient preparation

■ Explain to the patient that this test records the heart's electrical activity and performance under stress.
■ Instruct the patient not to eat, smoke, or drink alcoholic or caffeinated beverages for 3 hours before the test but to continue his prescribed drug regimen unless directed otherwise.
■ Tell the patient who will perform the test, where it will take place, and how long it will last.
■ Tell the patient that the test will cause fatigue and that he'll be slightly breathless and sweaty, but assure him that the test poses few risks. He may, in fact, stop the test if he experiences fatigue or chest pain.
■ Advise the patient to wear comfortable socks and shoes and loose, lightweight shorts or slacks. Men usually don't wear a shirt during the test, and women generally wear a bra and a lightweight short-sleeved blouse or a patient gown with a front closure.
■ Explain that electrodes will be attached to several areas on the patient's chest and,

possibly, his back after the skin areas are cleaned and abraded. Reassure him that he won't feel any current from the electrodes; however, they may itch slightly.
■ Tell the patient that his blood pressure will be checked periodically throughout the procedure, and assure him that his heart rate will be monitored continuously.
■ If the patient needs a multistage treadmill test, explain that the speed and incline of the treadmill will increase at predetermined intervals and that he'll be informed of each adjustment.
■ If the patient needs a bicycle ergometer test, explain that the resistance he experiences in pedaling increases gradually as he tries to maintain a specific speed.
■ Encourage the patient to report his feelings during the test to the technician who's conducting the test. Tell him that his blood pressure and ECG will be monitored for 10 to 15 minutes after the test.
■ Obtain informed consent if necessary.

Normal findings

In a normal exercise ECG, the P and T waves, the QRS complex, and the ST-segment change minimally; a slight ST-segment depression occurs in some patients, especially women. The heart rate rises in direct proportion to the workload and metabolic oxygen demand; blood pressure also rises as workload increases. The patient attains the endurance levels predicted by his age and the appropriate exercise protocol. (See *Exercise ECG tracings*.)

Abnormal findings

Although criteria for judging test results vary, two findings strongly suggest an abnormality: a flat or downsloping ST-segment depression of 1 mm or more for at least 0.08 second after the junction of the QRS and ST segments (J point) and a markedly depressed J point with an

Exercise ECG tracings

These tracings are from an abnormal exercise electrocardiogram (ECG) obtained during a tread-mill test performed on a patient who had just undergone a triple coronary artery bypass graft. The first tracing shows the heart at rest, with a blood pressure of 124/80 mm Hg. In the second tracing, the patient worked up to a 10% grade at 1.7 mph before experiencing angina at 2 minutes, 25 seconds. The tracing shows a depressed ST segment; heart rate was 85 beats/minute, and blood pressure was 140/70 mm Hg. The third tracing shows the heart at rest 6 minutes after the test; blood pressure was 140/90 mm Hg.

RESTING

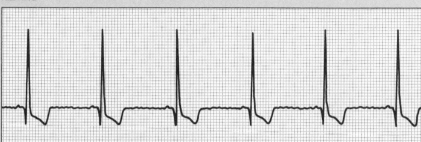

ANGINA

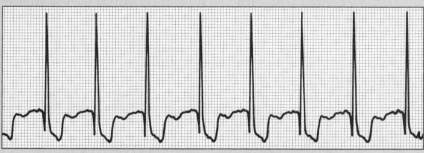

RECOVERY

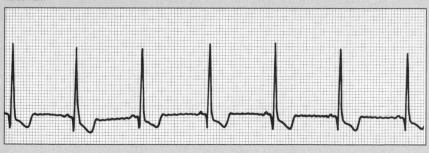

upsloping but depressed ST segment of 1.5 mm below the baseline 0.08 second after the J point. T-wave inversion also signifies ischemia. Initial ST-segment depression on the resting ECG must be further depressed by 1 mm during exercise to be considered abnormal.

Hypotension resulting from exercise, ST-segment depression of 3 mm or more, downsloping ST segments, and ischemic ST segments appearing within the first 3 minutes of exercise and lasting 8 minutes into the posttest recovery period may indicate multivessel or left CAD. ST-segment elevation may indicate dyskinetic left ventricular wall motion or severe transmural ischemia.

The predictive value of this test for CAD varies with the patient's history and sex; false-negative and false-positive test results are common. This is typically related to the effects of drugs, such as digoxin, or caffeine ingestion before testing. To detect CAD accurately, thallium imaging and stress testing, exercise multiple-gated acquisition scanning, or coronary angiography may be necessary.

Interfering factors
- Failure to observe pretest restrictions
- Inability to exercise to the target heart rate due to fatigue or failure to cooperate
- Electrolyte imbalance, Wolff-Parkinson-White syndrome (anomalous atrioventricular excitation), or use of a cardiac glycoside (possible false-positive)
- Conditions that affect left ventricular hypertrophy, such as congenital abnormalities and hypertension (possible interference with testing for ischemia)
- Beta-adrenergic blockers (may make test results difficult to interpret)

Synovial fluid analysis

In synovial fluid analysis, or *arthrocentesis*, a sterile needle is inserted into a joint space — most commonly the knee — to obtain a fluid specimen for analysis. This procedure is indicated for patients with undiagnosed articular disease and symptomatic joint effusion, a condition marked by the excessive accumulation of synovial fluid. Although rare, complications associated with synovial fluid aspiration include joint infection and hemorrhage leading to hemarthrosis (accumulation of blood within the joint).

Purpose
- To aid differential diagnosis of arthritis, particularly septic or crystal-induced arthritis
- To identify the cause and nature of joint effusion
- To relieve the pain and distention resulting from accumulation of fluid within the joint
- To administer a drug locally (usually corticosteroids)

Cost
Expensive

Patient preparation
- Describe the procedure to the patient, and answer any questions he may have.
- Explain to the patient that this test helps determine the cause of joint inflammation and swelling and also helps relieve the associated pain.
- Instruct the patient to fast for 6 to 12 hours before the test if glucose testing of synovial fluid is ordered; otherwise, inform him that he need not restrict food or fluids before the test.
- Tell the patient who will perform the test and where it will take place.

Normal findings in synovial fluid

FEATURE	RESULTS
Gross	
Color	Colorless to pale yellow
Clarity	Clear
Quantity (in knee)	0.3 to 3.5 ml
Viscosity	5.7 to 1,160
pH	7.2 to 7.4
Mucin clot	Good
Microscopic	
White blood cell (WBC) count	0 to 200/µl
WBC differential:	
▪ Lymphocytes	▪ 0 to 78/µl
▪ Monocytes	▪ 0 to 71/µl
▪ Clasmatocytes	▪ 0 to 26/µl
▪ Polymorphonuclear lymphocytes	▪ 0 to 25/µl
▪ Other phagocytes	▪ 0 to 21/µl
▪ Synovial lining cells	▪ 0 to 12/µl
Microbiological	
Formed elements	Absence of crystals and cartilage debris
Bacteria	None
Serologic	
Complement:	
▪ For 10 mg protein/dl	3.7 to 33.7 U/ml
▪ For 20 mg protein/dl	7.7 to 37.7 U/ml
Rheumatoid arthritis cells	None
Lupus erythematosus cells	None
Chemical	
Total protein	10.7 to 21.3 mg/dl
Fibrinogen	None
Glucose	70 to 100 mg/dl
Uric acid	2 to 8 mg/dl (men), 2 to 6 mg/dl (women)
Hyaluronate	0.3 to 0.4 g/dl
Partial pressure of arterial carbon dioxide	40 to 60 mm Hg
Partial pressure of arterial oxygen	40 to 80 mm Hg

Synovial fluid findings in various disorders

DISEASE	COLOR	CLARITY	VISCOSITY	MUCIN CLOT
Group 1 noninflammatory				
Traumatic arthritis	Straw to bloody to yellow	Transparent to cloudy	Variable	Good to fair
Osteoarthritis	Yellow	Transparent	Variable	Good to fair
Group II inflammatory				
Systemic lupus erythematosus	Straw	Clear to slightly cloudy	Variable	Good to fair
Rheumatic fever	Yellow	Slightly cloudy	Variable	Good to fair
Pseudogout	Yellow	Slightly cloudy (if acute)	Low (if acute)	Fair to poor
Gout	Yellow to milky	Cloudy	Low	Fair to poor
Rheumatoid arthritis	Yellow to green	Cloudy	Low	Fair to poor
Group III septic				
Tuberculous arthritis	Yellow	Cloudy	Low	Poor
Septic arthritis	Gray or bloody	Turbid, purulent	Low	Poor

■ Warn the patient that although he'll receive a local anesthetic, he may still feel transient pain when the needle penetrates the joint capsule.

■ Obtain informed consent if necessary.

■ Check the patient's history for hypersensitivity to iodine compounds (such as povidone-iodine), lidocaine, procaine, or other local anesthetics.

■ Tell the patient that he may receive a sedative as needed.

■ Tell the patient that he may receive a corticosteroid as indicated.

■ If synovial fluid glucose levels are being measured, tell the patient that a venipuncture to obtain a sample for blood glucose analysis may be done.

■ Tell the patient that after the test, ice or cold packs may be applied to the affected joint for 24 to 36 hours after aspiration to decrease pain and swelling and that pillows may be used for support. If a large quantity of fluid was aspirated, tell him than an elastic bandage may be applied to stabilize the joint.

■ Tell the patient that depending on his condition, he may be able to resume normal activity immediately after the procedure. However, warn him to avoid excessive

% NEUTROPHILS	WBC COUNT/ DEBRIS	CARTILAGE CRYSTALS	ARTHRITIS CELLS	RHEUMATOID BACTERIA
1,000; 25%	None	None	None	None
700; 15%	Usually present	None	None	None
2,000; 30%	None	None	Lupus erythematosus (LE) cells	None
14,000; 50%	None	None	Possibly LE cells	None
15,000; 70%	Usually present	Calcium pyrophosphate	None	None
20,000; 70%	None	Urate	None	None
20,000; 70%	None	Occasionally, cholesterol	Usually present	None
20,000; 60%	None	None	None	Usually present
90,000; 90%	None	None	None	Usually present

use of the affected joint for a few days after the test even if pain and swelling subside.

Normal findings

Routine examination includes gross analysis for color, clarity, quantity, viscosity, pH, and the presence of a mucin clot as well as microscopic analysis for white blood cell (WBC) count and differential. Special examination includes microbiological analysis for formed elements (including crystals) and bacteria, serologic analysis, and chemical analysis for such components as glucose, protein, and enzymes. (See *Normal findings in synovial fluid,* page 355.)

Abnormal findings

Examination of synovial fluid may reveal various joint diseases, including noninflammatory disease (traumatic arthritis and osteoarthritis), inflammatory disease (systemic lupus erythematosus, rheumatic fever, pseudogout, gout, and rheumatoid arthritis), and septic disease (tuberculous and septic arthritis). (See *Synovial fluid findings in various disorders.*)

Interfering factors

■ Failure to adhere to dietary restrictions
■ Acid diluents added to the specimen for WBC count (alteration in cell count)

■ Failure to adequately mix the specimen and the anticoagulant or to send the specimen to the laboratory immediately after collection

Synovial membrane biopsy

Biopsy of the synovial membrane is needle excision of a tissue specimen for histologic examination of the thin epithelium lining the diarthrodial joint capsules. In a large joint such as the knee, preliminary arthroscopy can aid selection of the biopsy site. Synovial membrane biopsy is performed when analysis of synovial fluid — a viscous, lubricating fluid contained within the synovial membrane — proves nondiagnostic or when the fluid is absent.

Purpose
■ To diagnose gout, pseudogout, bacterial infections and lesions, and granulomatous infections
■ To aid diagnosis of systemic lupus erythematosus (SLE), rheumatoid arthritis, or Reiter's syndrome
■ To monitor joint pathology

Cost
Expensive

Patient preparation
■ Explain to the patient that this test provides a tissue specimen from the membrane that lines the affected joint.
■ Describe the procedure to the patient, and answer any questions he may have.
■ Tell the patient who will perform the procedure and where it will take place.
■ Inform the patient that complications include infection and bleeding into the joint, but they're rare.
■ Advise the patient that he'll receive a local anesthetic to minimize discomfort but

that he'll experience pain when the needle enters the joint.
■ Obtain informed consent if necessary.
■ Check the patient's history for hypersensitivity to the local anesthetic.
■ Inform the patient which site — knee (most common), elbow, wrist, ankle, or shoulder — has been chosen for this biopsy (usually, the most symptomatic joint is selected).
■ Tell the patient that he may be given a sedative to help him relax.
■ Tell the patient that after the test he'll need to rest the joint for 1 day before resuming normal activity.

Normal findings
The synovial membrane contains cells that are identical to those found in other connective tissue. The membrane surface is relatively smooth, except for villi, folds, and fat pads that project into the joint cavity. The membrane tissue produces synovial fluid and contains a capillary network, lymphatic vessels, and a few nerve fibers. A pathologic condition of the synovial membrane also affects the synovial fluid's cellular composition.

Abnormal findings
Histologic examination of synovial tissue can diagnose coccidioidomycosis, gout, pseudogout, hemochromatosis, tuberculosis, sarcoidosis, amyloidosis, pigmented villonodular synovitis, synovial tumors, and synovial cancer (rare). Such examination can also aid diagnosis of rheumatoid arthritis, SLE, and Reiter's disease.

Interfering factors
■ Failure to obtain several biopsy specimens
■ Failure to obtain the specimens away from the anesthetic's infiltration site

T

Tensilon test

The Tensilon test involves careful observation of the patient after I.V. administration of Tensilon (edrophonium chloride), a rapid, short-acting anticholinesterase that improves muscle strength by increasing muscle response to nerve impulses. If the patient demonstrates myasthenic crisis, neostigmine is administered immediately; with cholinergic crisis, administer atropine. Patients with respiratory ailments such as asthma should receive atropine during the test to minimize adverse reactions to Tensilon.

ALERT! ▼ ▼ ▼ ▼ ▼ ▼ ▼ ▼ ▼
Because of the systemic adverse reactions that Tensilon may produce, this test may be contraindicated in patients with hypotension, bradycardia, apnea, or mechanical obstruction of the intestine or urinary tract.

Purpose
■ To aid in the diagnosis of myasthenia gravis
■ To aid in the differentiation between myasthenic and cholinergic crises
■ To monitor oral anticholinesterase therapy

Cost
Very expensive

Patient preparation
■ Explain to the patient that this test helps determine the cause of muscle weakness.
■ Describe the test for the patient. Tell him who will perform it, where it will take place, and its expected duration. Don't describe the exact response that will be evaluated; foreknowledge can affect the test's objectivity.
■ Explain to the patient that a small tube will be inserted into a vein in his arm and that a drug will be administered periodically. Tell him that he'll be asked to make repetitive muscle movements and that his reactions will be observed. Also tell him that the test may be repeated several times to ensure accuracy.
■ Inform the patient that Tensilon has some unpleasant adverse effects, but reassure him that someone will be with him at all times and that any reactions will quickly disappear.
■ Check the patient's history for drug hypersensitivity and respiratory disease. Also check for drugs that affect muscle function, including anticholinesterases, because

these drugs should be withheld. If they must be continued, note this on the laboratory request, including the time of the most recent dose.

■ Obtain informed consent if necessary.

Normal findings

Patients who don't have myasthenia gravis usually develop fasciculation in response to Tensilon. The physician must interpret the responses carefully to distinguish patients who have myasthenia gravis from those who don't.

Abnormal findings

If the patient has myasthenia gravis, muscle strength should improve promptly after the administration of Tensilon. The degree of improvement depends on the muscle group being tested; improvement is usually obvious within 30 seconds. Although the maximum benefit lasts only several minutes, lingering effects may persist — up to 2 hours in a patient receiving prednisone, for example. All patients with myasthenia gravis show improved muscle strength with this test; however, if the patient only responds slightly the test may need to be repeated to confirm the diagnosis. Additionally, the test may yield inconsistent results if the myasthenia gravis is affecting only the ocular muscles, as in mild or early forms of the disorder.

Tensilon may produce a positive response in patients with motor neuron disease and in those with certain neuropathies or myopathies. However, the response is usually less dramatic and less consistent than with myasthenia gravis.

Patients in myasthenic crisis show brief improvement in muscle strength after Tensilon is administered. Patients in cholinergic crisis (from anticholinesterase overdose) may experience exaggerated muscle

weakness. If Tensilon increases the patient's muscle strength without increasing the occurrence of adverse reactions, the oral anticholinesterase dosage can be increased. If Tensilon decreases the patient's muscle strength with severe adverse reactions, the dosage should be reduced. If the test shows no change in muscle strength and only mild adverse effects occur, the dosage should remain the same.

Interfering factors

■ Prednisone (possible delay of Tensilon's effect on muscle strength)

■ Quinidine and anticholinergics (inhibit the action of Tensilon)

■ Procainamide and muscle relaxants (inhibit normal muscle response)

Terminal deoxynucleotidyl transferase

Using indirect immunofluorescence, the terminal deoxynucleotidyl transferase (TdT) test measures levels of TdT. The test differentiates certain types of leukemia and lymphomas marked by primitive cells that can't be identified by histology alone.

Purpose

■ To help differentiate acute lymphocytic leukemia (ALL) from acute nonlymphocytic leukemia

■ To help differentiate lymphoblastic lymphoma from malignant lymphoma

■ To monitor the patient's response to therapy, to help determine his prognosis, or to obtain an early diagnosis of a relapse

Cost

Expensive

Patient preparation

- Explain to the patient that this test detects an enzyme that can help classify tissue origin.

If the patient is scheduled for a blood test, prepare him in the following way:

- Tell the patient that the test requires a blood sample. Explain who will perform the venipuncture and when.
- Explain to the patient that he may experience discomfort from the needle puncture and the tourniquet.
- Tell the patient to fast for 12 to 14 hours before the test.

If the patient is scheduled for bone marrow aspiration, prepare him in the following way:

- Describe the test for the patient. Tell him who will perform it, where it will take place, and its expected duration. Then answer the patient's questions.
- Check the patient's history for hypersensitivity to the local anesthetic. Inform him that he'll receive a local anesthetic and that he'll feel pressure on insertion of the biopsy needle and a brief, pulling pain when the marrow is withdrawn.
- Obtain informed consent if necessary.
- Tell the patient that he may receive a mild sedative 1 hour before the test.

Normal findings

TdT is present in less than 2% of marrow cells and is undetectable in normal peripheral blood.

Abnormal findings

TdT-positive cells are present in more than 90% of patients with ALL, in 33% of patients with chronic myelogenous leukemia in blast crisis, and in 5% of patients with nonlymphocytic leukemia. TdT-positive cells are absent in patients with ALL who are in remission.

Interfering factors

- Failure to obtain a representative specimen during bone marrow aspiration
- Bone marrow regeneration, idiopathic thrombocytopenic purpura, and neuroblastoma, causing TdT-positive bone marrow (possible false-positive)

AGE ISSUE ✱ ✱ ✱ ✱ ✱

The performance of bone marrow aspiration on a child may produce a false-positive result because of the presence of TdT-positive bone marrow in children during the proliferation of prelymphocytes.

Testosterone

The principal androgen secreted by the interstitial cells of the testes (Leydig cells), testosterone induces puberty in the male and maintains secondary male sex characteristics. Prepubertal levels of testosterone are low. Increased testosterone secretion during puberty stimulates growth of the seminiferous tubules and sperm production. It also contributes to the enlargement of external genitalia, accessory sex organs (such as prostate glands), and voluntary muscles and to the growth of facial, pubic, and axillary hair. Testosterone production begins to increase at the onset of puberty and continues to rise during adulthood. Production begins to taper off at about age 40 and eventually drops to about one-fifth the peak level by age 80. In women, the adrenal glands and ovaries secrete small amounts of testosterone.

This competitive protein-binding test measures plasma or serum testosterone levels. When combined with the measurement of plasma gonadotropin levels (follicle-stimulating hormone and luteinizing hormone), it's a reliable aid in the evaluation of gonadal dysfunction in men and women.

Purpose

■ To facilitate the differential diagnosis of male sexual precocity in boys younger than age 10 (True precocious puberty must be distinguished from pseudoprecocious puberty.)
■ To aid in the differential diagnosis of hypogonadism (Primary hypogonadism must be distinguished from secondary hypogonadism.)
■ To evaluate male infertility or other sexual dysfunction
■ To evaluate hirsutism and virilization in women

Cost

Moderately expensive

Patient preparation

■ Explain to the patient that this test helps determine if male sex hormone secretion is adequate.
■ Tell the patient that the test requires a blood sample. Explain who will perform the venipuncture and when.
■ Explain to the patient that he may experience discomfort from the needle puncture and the tourniquet.

Reference values

Normal testosterone levels are (laboratory values vary slightly):
■ *males:* 300 to 1,200 ng/dl (SI, 10.4 to 41.6 nmol/L)
■ *females:* 20 to 80 ng/dl (SI, 0.7 to 2.8 nmol/L)
■ *prepubertal children:* values lower than adult levels

Abnormal findings

Elevated testosterone levels in prepubertal boys may indicate true sexual precocity due to excessive gonadotropin secretion or pseudoprecocious puberty due to male hormone production by a testicular tumor.

They can also indicate congenital adrenal hyperplasia, which results in precocious puberty in boys (from ages 2 to 3) and pseudohermaphroditism and milder virilization in girls.

Increased testosterone levels can occur with a benign or malignant adrenal tumor, hyperthyroidism, or incipient puberty. In women with ovarian tumors or polycystic ovary syndrome, testosterone levels may rise, leading to hirsutism.

Low testosterone levels can indicate primary hypogonadism (as in Klinefelter's syndrome) or secondary hypogonadism (hypogonadotropic eunuchoidism) from hypothalamic-pituitary dysfunction. Low levels can also follow orchiectomy, testicular or prostate cancer, delayed male puberty, estrogen therapy, and cirrhosis of the liver.

Interfering factors

■ Exogenous sources of estrogens and androgens, thyroid and growth hormones, and other pituitary-based hormones
■ Estrogens (decrease free testosterone levels by increasing sex hormone–binding globulin, which binds testosterone)
■ Androgens (possible increase)

Thallium imaging

Also called *cold spot myocardial imaging* or *thallium scintigraphy,* thallium imaging evaluates myocardial blood flow after I.V. injection of the radioisotope thallium 201 or Cardiolite. The main difference between these two tracers is that Cardiolite has a better energy spectrum for imaging. Cardiolite requires living myocardial cells for uptake and allows for imaging the myocardial blood flow before and after reperfusion. This allows for better estimation of myocardial salvage. Because thallium, the physiologic analogue of potassium, concentrates in healthy myocardial tissue but not in necrotic or ischemic tissue, areas of the heart with a normal blood supply and intact cells rapidly take it up. Areas with poor blood flow and ischemic cells fail to take up the isotope and appear as cold spots on a scan.

This test is performed while the patient is in a resting state or after induced stress. Resting imaging can detect acute myocardial infarction (MI) within the first few hours of symptoms but doesn't distinguish an old from a new infarct. Stress imaging, performed after the patient exercises on a treadmill until he experiences angina or rate-limiting fatigue, can assess known or suspected coronary artery disease (CAD) and can evaluate the effectiveness of antianginal therapy or balloon angioplasty and the patency of grafts after coronary artery bypass surgery. Possible complications of stress testing include arrhythmias, angina pectoris, and MI.

ALERT! ▼ ▼ ▼ ▼ ▼ ▼ ▼ ▼ ▼

Contraindications include impaired neuromuscular function, pregnancy, locomotor disturbances, an acute MI or myocarditis, aortic stenosis, acute infection, unstable metabolic conditions (such as diabetes), digoxin toxicity, and recent pulmonary infarction.

Purpose

■ To assess myocardial scarring and perfusion

■ To demonstrate the location and extent of an acute or chronic MI, including transmural and postoperative infarction (resting imaging)

■ To diagnose CAD (stress imaging)

■ To evaluate the patency of grafts after coronary artery bypass surgery

■ To evaluate the effectiveness of antianginal therapy or balloon angioplasty (stress imaging)

Cost

Very expensive

Patient preparation

■ Explain to the patient that these tests help determine if any areas of the heart muscle aren't receiving an adequate supply of blood.

■ If the patient will be undergoing stress imaging, instruct him to restrict alcohol, tobacco, and nonprescribed drugs for 24 hours before the test and to have nothing by mouth for 3 hours before the test. Tell him to wear walking shoes during the treadmill exercise and to immediately report fatigue, pain, or shortness of breath.

■ Describe the test for the patient. Tell him who will perform it, where it will take place, and how long it will take. Explain that additional scans may be required.

■ Tell the patient that he'll receive a radioactive tracer I.V. and that multiple images of his heart will be scanned. Tell him it's important to lie still when the images are taken.

■ Warn the patient that he may experience discomfort from skin abrasion during preparation for electrode placement. Assure him that the test involves minimal radiation exposure.

■ Obtain informed consent if necessary.

ALERT! ▼ ▼ ▼ ▼ ▼ ▼ ▼ ▼ ▼

If the patient develops chest pain, dyspnea, fatigue, syncope, hypotension, ischemic electrocardiogram changes, significant arrhythmias, or critical signs and symptoms (pale, clammy skin; confusion; or staggering), stress imaging should be stopped immediately.

Normal findings

Imaging should show normal distribution of the isotope throughout the left ventricle and no defects (cold spots). The results may be normal if the patient has narrowed coronary arteries but adequate collateral circulation.

Abnormal findings

Persistent defects indicate an MI; transient defects (those that disappear after 3 to 6 hours of rest) indicate ischemia from CAD. After coronary artery bypass surgery, improved regional perfusion suggests patency of the graft. Increased perfusion after ingestion of an antianginal suggests relief from ischemia. Improved perfusion after balloon angioplasty indicates increased coronary flow.

Interfering factors

■ Cold spots (possibly due to sarcoidosis, myocardial fibrosis, cardiac contusion, attenuation due to soft tissue, apical cleft, coronary spasm, and artifacts, such as implants and electrodes)
■ Absence of cold spots in the presence of CAD (possibly due to insignificant obstruction, inadequate stress, delayed imaging, collateral circulation, or single-vessel disease, particularly of the right or left circumflex coronary arteries)

Throat culture

A throat culture is used primarily to isolate and identify pathogens. Culture results are considered in relation to the patient's clinical status, recent antimicrobial therapy, and amount of normal flora.

Purpose

■ To isolate and identify group A beta-hemolytic streptococci
■ To screen asymptomatic carriers of pathogens, especially *Neisseria meningitidis*

Cost

Inexpensive

Patient preparation

■ Explain to the patient that this test is used to identify microorganisms that may be causing his symptoms or to screen for asymptomatic carriers.
■ Inform the patient that a specimen will be collected from his throat. Tell him who will collect the specimen and when.
■ Describe the procedure for the patient. Warn him that he may gag during the swabbing.
■ Check the patient's history for recent antimicrobial therapy. Determine immunization history if pertinent to preliminary diagnosis. Tell the patient that the throat specimen must be procured before beginning antimicrobial therapy.

ALERT! ▼ ▼ ▼ ▼ ▼ ▼ ▼ ▼ ▼
If the patient has epiglottiditis or diphtheria, laryngospasm may occur after the culture is obtained.

Normal findings

Normal throat flora include nonhemolytic and alpha-hemolytic streptococci, *Neisseria* species, staphylococci, diphtheroids, some hemophilus, pneumococci, yeasts, enteric gram-negative rods, spirochetes, *Veillonella* species, and *Micrococcus* species.

Abnormal findings

Pathogens that may be cultured include group A beta-hemolytic streptococci *(Streptococcus pyogenes)*, which can cause scarlet fever and pharyngitis; *Candida albicans*, which can cause thrush; *Corynebacterium diphtheriae*, which can cause diphtheria; and *Bordetella pertussis*, which can cause whooping cough. The laboratory report should indicate the prevalent organisms and the quantity of pathogens cultured.

Antithrombin III test

The antithrombin III (AT III) test helps detect the cause of impaired coagulation, especially hypercoagulation, by measuring levels of AT III. This protein inactivates thrombin and inhibits coagulation. Normally, a balance exists between AT III and thrombin; an AT III deficiency increases coagulation.

AT III may be evaluated by a functional clotting assay or by synthetic substrates. Exogenous heparin is added to a fresh, citrated blood sample to accelerate AT III activity. Then, excess thrombin (factor Xa) is added to the plasma. The amount of factor Xa not activated by AT III is quantitated by clotting time or spectrophotometry and is compared to a normal control. Although reference values may vary for each laboratory, they should be between 80% and 120% of normal activity.

Decreased AT III levels may indicate disseminated intravascular coagulation, thromboembolic hypercoagulation, or a hepatic disorder. Slightly decreased levels can result from the use of hormonal contraceptives.

Elevated levels can result from kidney transplantation or the use of an oral anticoagulant or anabolic steroid.

Interfering factors

■ Failure to report recent or current antimicrobial therapy on the laboratory request (possible false-negative)
■ Failure to use the proper transport medium

Thrombin time, plasma

The plasma thrombin time test measures how quickly a clot forms when a standard amount of bovine thrombin is added to a platelet-poor plasma sample from the patient and to a normal plasma control sample. After thrombin is added, the clotting time for each sample is compared and recorded. Because thrombin rapidly converts fibrinogen to a fibrin clot, this test (also known as the *thrombin clotting time test*) allows a quick but imprecise estimation of plasma fibrinogen levels, which are a function of clotting time. (See *Antithrombin III test*.)

Purpose

■ To detect a fibrinogen deficiency or defect
■ To aid in the diagnosis of disseminated intravascular coagulation (DIC) and hepatic disease
■ To monitor the effectiveness of treatment with heparin or a thrombolytic

Cost

Inexpensive

Patient preparation

■ Explain to the patient that this test helps determine if his blood clots normally.
■ Tell the patient that the test requires a blood sample. Explain who will perform the venipuncture and when.
■ Explain to the patient that he may experience discomfort from the needle puncture and the tourniquet.
■ Restrict medications that may affect test results. If they must be continued, note this on the laboratory request.

Reference values

Normal thrombin times range from 10 to 15 seconds (SI, 10 to 15 s). Test results are usually reported with a normal control value.

Abnormal findings

A prolonged thrombin time may indicate heparin therapy, hepatic disease, DIC, hypofibrinogenemia, or dysfibrinogenemia. Patients with prolonged thrombin times may require quantitation of fibrinogen levels. If DIC is suspected, the test for fibrin split products is also necessary.

Interfering factors

■ Presence of inhibitory substances such as heparin, fibrinogen, or fibrin degradation products (prolonged clotting time)
■ Hemolysis caused by excessive probing during venipuncture or rough handling of the sample (possible inaccurate results)
■ Failure to use the proper anticoagulant in the collection tube, to mix the sample and the anticoagulant adequately, or to send the sample to the laboratory immediately after collection (possible inaccurate results)

Thyroid biopsy

Thyroid biopsy is the excision of a thyroid tissue specimen for histologic examination. This procedure is indicated in patients with thyroid enlargement or nodules, breathing and swallowing difficulties, vocal cord paralysis, unexplained weight loss, hemoptysis, and a sensation of fullness in the neck. It's commonly performed when noninvasive tests, such as thyroid ultrasonography and scans, are abnormal or inconclusive. Coagulation studies should always precede thyroid biopsy.

Thyroid tissue may be obtained with a hollow needle and the patient under local anesthesia or during open (surgical) biopsy and the patient under general anesthesia. Fine-needle aspiration with a cytologic smear examination can aid in diagnosis and replace an open biopsy. Open biopsy, performed in the operating room, provides more information than needle biopsy; it also permits direct examination and immediate excision of suspicious tissue.

ALERT! ▼ ▼ ▼ ▼ ▼ ▼ ▼ ▼ ▼
Thyroid biopsy should be used cautiously in patients with coagulation defects, as indicated by prolonged prothrombin time or partial thromboplastin time.

Purpose

■ To differentiate between benign and malignant thyroid disease
■ To help diagnose Hashimoto's disease, hyperthyroidism, and nontoxic nodular goiter

Cost

Very expensive

Patient preparation

■ Explain to the patient that this test permits microscopic examination of a thyroid tissue specimen.
■ Describe the test for the patient. Tell him who will perform it, where it will take place, and how long it will take. Then answer the patient's questions.
■ Inform the patient that he doesn't need to restrict food or fluids, unless he's to receive general anesthesia.
■ Check the patient's history for hypersensitivity to anesthetics or analgesics. Tell the patient that he'll receive a local anesthetic to minimize pain during the biopsy but that he may experience some pressure when the tissue specimen is obtained.

- Check the results of the patient's coagulation studies, and make sure that they're on his chart.
- Advise the patient that he may have a sore throat the day after the test.
- Tell the patient that he may receive a sedative before the biopsy.
- Obtain informed consent if necessary.

Normal findings

Histologic examination of normal tissue shows fibrous networks dividing the gland into pseudolobules that are made up of follicles and capillaries. Cuboidal epithelia line the follicle walls and contain the protein thyroglobulin, which stores thyroxine and triiodothyronine.

Abnormal findings

Malignant tumors appear as well-encapsulated, solitary nodules of uniform but abnormal structure. Papillary carcinoma is the most common thyroid cancer. Follicular carcinoma, a less common form, strongly resembles normal cells.

Benign tumors, such as nontoxic nodular goiter, demonstrate hypertrophy, hyperplasia, and hypervascularity. Distinct histologic patterns characterize subacute granulomatous thyroiditis, Hashimoto's thyroiditis, and hyperthyroidism.

Because thyroid tumors are usually multicentric and small, a normal histologic report doesn't rule out cancer.

Interfering factors

- Failure to obtain a representative tissue specimen

Thyroid-stimulating hormone

Thyroid-stimulating hormone (TSH), or thyrotropin, promotes increases in the size, number, and activity of thyroid cells and stimulates the release of triiodothyronine and thyroxine. These hormones affect the body's metabolism and are essential for normal growth and development.

This test measures serum TSH levels by radioimmunoassay. It can detect primary hypothyroidism and determine whether the hypothyroidism results from thyroid gland failure or from pituitary or hypothalamic dysfunction. Normal serum TSH levels rule out primary hypothyroidism. This test may not distinguish between low-normal and subnormal levels, especially in secondary hypothyroidism.

Purpose

- To confirm or rule out primary hypothyroidism and distinguish it from secondary hypothyroidism
- To monitor drug therapy in patients with primary hypothyroidism

Cost

Moderately expensive

Patient preparation

- Explain to the patient that this test helps to assess thyroid gland function.
- Tell the patient that the test requires a blood sample. Explain who will perform the venipuncture and when.
- Explain to the patient that he may experience discomfort from the needle puncture and the tourniquet.
- If the patient is taking a steroid, thyroid hormone, aspirin, or other drug that may influence the test results, instruct him not to take the drug before the test. If the drug must be continued, note this on the laboratory request.
- Tell the patient that he should lie down and relax for 30 minutes before the test.

Reference values

Normal TSH values range from undetectable to 15 µIU/ml (SI, 15 mU/L).

Abnormal findings

TSH levels may be slightly elevated in euthyroid patients with thyroid cancer. Levels that exceed 20 µIU/ml (SI, 20 mU/L) suggest primary hypothyroidism or, possibly, endemic goiter.

Low or undetectable TSH levels may be normal, but they occasionally indicate secondary hypothyroidism (with inadequate secretion of TSH or thyrotropin-releasing hormone [TRH]). Low TSH levels may also result from hyperthyroidism (Graves' disease) or thyroiditis; both are marked by hypersecretion of thyroid hormones, which suppresses TSH release. Provocative testing with TRH is necessary to confirm the diagnosis. (See *TRH challenge test.*)

Interfering factors

■ Failure to observe pretest restrictions

Thyroid-stimulating hormone, neonatal

The neonatal thyroid-stimulating hormone (TSH) test is an immunoassay that confirms congenital hypothyroidism after an initial screening test detects low thyroxine (T$_4$) levels. Normally, TSH levels surge after birth, triggering a rise in thyroid hormone that's essential for neurologic development. In primary congenital hypothyroidism, the thyroid gland doesn't respond to TSH stimulation, resulting in decreased thyroid hormone levels and increased TSH levels.

AGE ISSUE ✳ ✳ ✳ ✳ ✳
Early detection and treatment of congenital hypothyroidism is critical to prevent mental retardation and cretinism. Diagnosis should be made as soon as possible.

Purpose

■ To confirm diagnosis of congenital hypothyroidism

Cost

Inexpensive

Patient preparation

■ Explain to the infant's parents that this test helps confirm the diagnosis of congenital hypothyroidism. Emphasize the importance of detecting the disorder early so that prompt therapy can prevent irreversible brain damage.

■ Tell the infant's parents that a heel stick will be performed to collect the sample. Also tell them when it will be done.

Reference values

At age 1 to 2 days, TSH levels are normally 25 to 30 µIU/ml (SI, 25 to 30 mU/L). Thereafter, levels are normally less than 25 µIU/ml (SI, < 25 mU/L).

Abnormal findings

Neonatal TSH levels must be interpreted in light of T_4 levels. Increased TSH levels accompanied by decreased T_4 levels indicate primary congenital hypothyroidism (thyroid gland dysfunction). Low TSH and T_4 levels may be present in patients with secondary congenital hypothyroidism (pituitary or hypothalamic dysfunction). Normal TSH levels accompanied by low T_4 levels may indicate hypothyroidism due to a congenital defect in T_4-binding globulin or transient congenital hypothyroidism due to prematurity or prenatal hypoxia. A complete thyroid workup must be done to confirm the cause of hypothyroidism before treatment can begin.

Interfering factors

■ Failure to let a filter paper sample dry completely

■ Corticosteroids, T_4, and triiodothyronine (decrease)

■ Excessive topical resorcinol, lithium carbonate, potassium iodide, and TSH injection (increase)

Thyroid-stimulating immunoglobulin

Thyroid-stimulating immunoglobulin (TSI), formerly called long-acting thyroid stimulator, appears in the blood of most patients with Graves' disease. It stimulates the thyroid gland to produce and excrete excessive amounts of thyroid hormone.

Reportedly, 90% of patients with Graves' disease have elevated TSI levels. An abnormal test result strongly suggests Graves' disease, despite normal routine thyroid tests in patients suspected of having Graves' disease or progressive exophthalmos.

Purpose

■ To aid in the evaluation of suspected thyroid disease

■ To aid in the diagnosis of suspected thyrotoxicosis, especially in patients with exophthalmos

■ To monitor the treatment of thyrotoxicosis

Cost

Expensive

Patient preparation

■ Explain to the patient that this test evaluates thyroid function.

■ Tell the patient that the test requires a blood sample. Explain who will perform the venipuncture and when.

■ Explain to the patient that he may experience discomfort from the needle puncture and the tourniquet.

Reference values

TSI doesn't normally appear in serum. However, it's considered normal at levels equal to or greater than 1.3 index.

Abnormal findings

Increased TSI levels are associated with exophthalmos, Graves' disease (thyrotoxicosis), and recurrence of hyperthyroidism.

Interfering factors

■ Administration of radioactive iodine within 48 hours of the test

Thyroxine, total

Thyroxine (T_4) is an amine secreted by the thyroid gland in response to thyroid-stimulating hormone (TSH) and, indirectly, thyrotropin-releasing hormone. The rate of secretion is normally regulated by a complex system of negative and positive feedback mechanisms.

Only a fraction of T_4 (about 0.05%) circulates freely in the blood; the rest binds strongly to plasma proteins, primarily thyroxine-binding globulin (TBG). This minute fraction is responsible for the clinical effects of thyroid hormone. TBG binds so tenaciously that T_4 survives in the plasma for a relatively long time, with a half-life of about 6 days. This immunoassay, one of the most common thyroid diagnostic tools, measures the total circulating T_4 level when TBG is normal. An alternative test is the Murphy-Pattee, or T_4 (D), based on competitive protein binding.

Purpose

■ To evaluate thyroid function
■ To aid in the diagnosis of hyperthyroidism and hypothyroidism
■ To monitor patient response to antithyroid drug therapy in hyperthyroidism or to thyroid replacement therapy in hypothyroidism (TSH estimates are needed to confirm hypothyroidism.)

Cost

Moderately expensive

Patient preparation

■ Explain to the patient that this test helps evaluate thyroid gland function.

■ Tell the patient that the test requires a blood sample. Explain who will perform the venipuncture and when.
■ Explain to the patient that he may experience discomfort from the needle puncture and the tourniquet.
■ Restrict medications that may affect test results. If they must be continued, note this on the laboratory request. If this test is being performed to monitor thyroid therapy, the patient should continue to receive daily thyroid supplements.

Reference values

Normally, total T_4 levels range from 5 to 13.5 µg/dl (SI, 60 to 165 mmol/L).

Abnormal findings

Abnormally elevated T_4 levels are consistent with primary and secondary hyperthyroidism, including excessive T_4 (levothyroxine) replacement therapy (factitious or iatrogenic hyperthyroidism). Subnormal levels suggest primary or secondary hypothyroidism, or T_4 suppression by normal, elevated, or replacement levels of triiodothyronine (T_3). In doubtful cases of hypothyroidism, TSH levels may be indicated.

Normal T_4 levels don't guarantee euthyroidism — for example, normal readings occur with T_3 toxicosis. Overt signs of hyperthyroidism require further testing.

Interfering factors

■ Hereditary factors and hepatic disease (possible increase or decrease in TBG)
■ Protein-wasting disease (such as nephrotic syndrome) and androgens (possible decrease in TBG)
■ Estrogens, levothyroxine, methadone, and progestins (increase)
■ Free fatty acids, heparin, iodides, liothyronine sodium, lithium, methylthiouracil, phenylbutazone, phenytoin, propylthio-

uracil, salicylates (high doses), steroids, sulfonamides, and sulfonylureas (decrease)
- Clofibrate (possible increase or decrease)

Thyroxine and triiodothyronine, free

The free thyroxine (FT_4) and free triiodothyronine (FT_3) tests, commonly done simultaneously, measure serum levels of FT_4 and FT_3, the minute portions of T_4 and T_3 not bound to thyroxine-binding globulin (TBG) and other serum proteins. FT_4 and FT_3 are unbound hormones and are responsible for the thyroid's effects on cellular metabolism. Measurement of free hormone serum levels is the best indicator of thyroid function.

Purpose
- To measure the metabolically active form of the thyroid hormones
- To aid in the diagnosis of hyperthyroidism and hypothyroidism when TBG levels are abnormal

Cost
Inexpensive

Patient preparation
- Explain to the patient that this test helps evaluate thyroid function.
- Tell the patient that the test requires a blood sample. Explain who will perform the venipuncture and when.
- Explain to the patient that he may experience discomfort from the needle puncture and the tourniquet.

Reference values
Normal range for FT_4 is 0.9 to 2.3 ng/dl (SI, 10 to 30 nmol/L); for FT_3, 0.2 to 0.6 ng/dl (SI, 0.003 to 0.009 nmol/L). Values vary, depending on the laboratory.

Abnormal findings
Elevated FT_4 and FT_3 levels indicate hyperthyroidism, unless peripheral resistance to thyroid hormone is present. T_3 toxicosis, a distinct form of hyperthyroidism, yields high FT_3 levels with normal or low FT_4 values. Low FT_4 levels usually indicate hypothyroidism, except in patients receiving replacement therapy with T_3. Patients receiving thyroid therapy may have varying levels of FT_4 and FT_3, depending on the preparation used and the time of sample collection.

Interfering factors
- Hemolysis due to rough handling of the sample
- Thyroid therapy, depending on dosage (possible increase)

TORCH test

The TORCH test helps detect exposure to pathogens involved in congenital and neonatal infections. TORCH is an acronym for *t*oxoplasmosis, *o*ther agents (viruses), *r*ubella, *c*ytomegalovirus, and *h*erpes simplex. These pathogens are commonly associated with congenital and neonatal infections that aren't clinically apparent and may cause severe central nervous system impairment. This test detects specific immunoglobulin M–associated antibodies in neonatal blood.

Purpose
- To aid in the diagnosis of acute, congenital, and intrapartum infections

Cost
Expensive

Patient preparation

- Explain the purpose of the test to the infant's parents.
- Tell the parents that the test requires a blood sample. Explain who will perform the venipuncture or cord blood sample, as appropriate, and when.
- Explain to the parents that the infant may experience discomfort from the needle puncture or the tourniquet.

Normal findings

Normal test results are negative for TORCH agents.

Abnormal findings

Toxoplasmosis is diagnosed by sequential examination that shows rising antibody titers, changing titers, and serologic conversion from negative to positive; a titer of 1:256 suggests recent *Toxoplasma* infection.

AGE ISSUE ✳ ✳ ✳ ✳ ✳

In infants younger than age 6 months, rubella infection is associated with a marked and persistent rise (over time) in complement-fixing antibody titer. Persistence of rubella antibody in an infant older than age 6 months strongly suggests congenital infection. Congenital rubella is associated with cardiac anomalies, neurosensory deafness, growth retardation, and encephalitic symptoms.

Detection of herpes antibodies in cerebrospinal fluid with signs of herpetic encephalitis and persistent herpes simplex virus type 2 antibody levels confirms herpes simplex infection in a neonate without obvious herpetic lesions.

Interfering factors

- Hemolysis due to rough handling of the sample

Transesophageal echocardiography

Transesophageal echocardiography (TEE) combines ultrasound with endoscopy to give a better view of the heart's structures. In this procedure, a small transducer is attached to the end of a gastroscope and inserted into the esophagus, allowing images to be taken from the posterior aspect of the heart. This causes less tissue penetration and interference from chest wall structures and produces high-quality images of the thoracic aorta, except for the superior ascending aorta, which is shadowed by the trachea.

This test is appropriate for both inpatients and outpatients, for patients under general anesthesia, and for critically ill, intubated patients.

Purpose

To visualize and evaluate:
- thoracic and aortic disorders, such as dissection and aneurysm
- valvular disease, especially in the mitral valve and in prosthetic devices
- endocarditis
- congenital heart disease
- intracardiac thrombi
- cardiac tumors
- valvular repairs

Cost

Very expensive

Patient preparation

- Explain to the patient that this test allows visual examination of heart function and structures.
- Describe the test for the patient. Tell him who will perform it, where it will take place, and how long it will take.
- Tell the patient to fast for 6 hours before the test.

- Review the patient's medical history for possible contraindications to the test, such as esophageal obstruction or varices, GI bleeding, previous mediastinal radiation therapy, or severe cervical arthritis.
- Ask the patient if he has any allergies, and note his response on the chart.
- Explain to the patient that his throat will be sprayed with a topical anesthetic and that he may gag when the tube is inserted.
- Tell the patient that an I.V. line will be inserted to administer sedation before the procedure and that he may experience discomfort from the needle puncture or the tourniquet. Reassure him that he'll be made as comfortable as possible during the procedure and that his blood pressure and heart rate will be monitored continuously.
- Tell the patient that ultrasound images are recorded during the procedure and then reviewed afterward.
- Obtain informed consent if necessary.
- Tell the patient that he won't be given food or water until his gag response returns.
- If the procedure is done on an outpatient basis, tell the patient that someone must drive him home.

ALERT! ▼ ▼ ▼ ▼ ▼ ▼ ▼ ▼ ▼
Vasovagal responses may occur with gagging, so observe the cardiac monitor closely. Laryngospasm, arrhythmias, or bleeding increase the risk of complications; if any of these occur, postpone the test.

Normal findings

Transesophageal echocardiography should reveal no cardiac problems.

Abnormal findings

This test can reveal thoracic and aortic disorders, endocarditis, congenital heart disease, intracardiac thrombi, or tumors, and it can evaluate valvular disease or repairs.

Possible findings include aortic dissection or aneurysm, mitral valve disease, and congenital defects such as patent ductus arteriosus.

Interfering factors

- Transesophageal approach (restricted visualization of the left atrial appendage and ascending or descending aorta)
- Hyperinflation of lungs due to such causes as chronic obstructive pulmonary disease or mechanical ventilation (possible poor imaging)

Transferrin

A quantitative analysis of serum transferrin (siderophilin) levels is used to evaluate iron metabolism. Transferrin is a glycoprotein that's formed in the liver. It transports circulating iron (obtained from dietary sources or the breakdown of red blood cells by reticuloendothelial cells) to the bone marrow for use in hemoglobin synthesis or to the liver, spleen, and bone marrow for storage. A serum iron level is usually obtained simultaneously.

Purpose

- To determine the iron-transporting capacity of the blood
- To evaluate iron metabolism in iron deficiency anemia

Cost

Inexpensive

Patient preparation

- Explain to the patient that this test is used to determine the cause of anemia.
- Tell the patient that the test requires a blood sample. Explain who will perform the venipuncture and when.

- Explain to the patient that he may experience discomfort from the needle puncture and the tourniquet.
- Restrict medications that may affect test results. If they must be continued, note this on the laboratory request.

Reference values
Normal serum transferrin values range from 200 to 400 mg/dl (SI, 2 to 4 g/L).

Abnormal findings
Inadequate transferrin levels may lead to impaired hemoglobin synthesis and, possibly, anemia. Low serum levels may indicate inadequate production of transferrin due to hepatic damage or excessive protein loss from renal disease. Decreased transferrin levels may also result from acute or chronic infection or cancer.

Increased serum transferrin levels may indicate severe iron deficiency.

Interfering factors
- Hormonal contraceptives and late pregnancy (possible increase)

Trichomonads, urogenital secretions in

Microscopic examination of urine or vaginal, urethral, or prostatic secretions can detect urogenital infection by *Trichomonas vaginalis*, a parasitic, flagellate protozoan that's usually transmitted sexually. This test is more commonly performed on women than on men because women are more likely to experience symptoms of trichomoniasis; men may experience symptoms of urethritis or prostatitis.

Purpose
- To confirm trichomoniasis

Cost
Moderately expensive

Patient preparation
- Explain to the patient that this test can identify the cause of urogenital infection.
- If the patient is a woman, tell her that the test requires a sample of vaginal secretions or urethral discharge, and ask her not to douche before the test.
- If the patient is a man, tell him that the test requires a sample of urethral or prostatic secretions.
- Inform the patient who will perform the procedure and when.

Normal findings
Trichomonads are normally absent from the urogenital tract.

Abnormal findings
Trichomonads confirm trichomoniasis. In about 25% of women and in most infected men, trichomonads may be present without associated pathology.

Interfering factors
- Failure to send the specimen to the laboratory immediately after collection
- Collection of the specimen after trichomonacide therapy begins (fewer trichomonads in the specimen)

Triglycerides

Serum triglyceride analysis provides quantitative analysis of triglycerides — the main storage form of lipids — that constitute about 95% of fatty tissue. Although not in itself diagnostic, the triglyceride test permits early identification of hyperlipidemia and the risk of coronary artery disease (CAD).

Purpose

■ To screen for hyperlipidemia or pancreatitis
■ To help identify nephrotic syndrome and poorly controlled diabetes mellitus
■ To determine the risk of CAD
■ To calculate low-density lipoprotein cholesterol level using the Freidewald equation

Cost

Inexpensive

Patient preparation

■ Explain to the patient that this test is used to detect disorders of fat metabolism.
■ Tell the patient that the test requires a blood sample. Explain who will perform the venipuncture and when.
■ Explain to the patient that he may experience discomfort from the needle puncture and the tourniquet.
■ Instruct the patient to fast for at least 12 hours before the test and to abstain from alcohol for 24 hours. Tell the patient that he can drink water.
■ Restrict medications that may affect test results. If they must be continued, note this on the laboratory request.

Reference values

Triglyceride values vary with age and sex. Although there's controversy about the most appropriate normal ranges, values of 40 to 180 mg/dl (SI, 0.44 to 2.01 mmol/L) for adult men and 10 to 190 mg/dl (SI, 0.11 to 2.21 mmol/L) for adult women are widely accepted.

Abnormal findings

Increased or decreased serum triglyceride levels suggest a clinical abnormality; additional tests are required for a definitive diagnosis.

A mild to moderate increase in serum triglyceride levels indicates biliary obstruction, diabetes mellitus, nephrotic syndrome, endocrinopathy, or overconsumption of alcohol. Markedly increased levels without an identifiable cause reflect congenital hyperlipoproteinemia and necessitate lipoprotein phenotyping to confirm the diagnosis.

Decreased serum triglyceride levels are rare and occur mainly in patients with malnutrition or abetalipoproteinemia.

Interfering factors

■ Failure to observe pretest restrictions
■ Use of glycol-lubricated collection tube
■ Antilipemics (decrease serum lipid levels)
■ Cholestyramine and colestipol (decrease cholesterol levels but increase or have no effect on triglyceride levels)
■ Corticosteroids (long-term use), estrogen, ethyl alcohol, furosemide, hormonal contraceptives, and miconazole (increase)
■ Clofibrate, dextrothyroxine, gemfibrozil, and niacin (decrease cholesterol and triglyceride levels)
■ Probucol (decreases cholesterol levels but has variable effect on triglyceride levels)

Triiodothyronine, total

The total triiodothyronine (T_3) test is a highly specific radioimmunoassay that measures the total (bound and free) serum content of T_3 to investigate clinical indications of thyroid dysfunction. Like thyroxine (T_4) secretion, T_3 secretion occurs primarily in response to thyroid-stimulating hormone (TSH) and, secondarily, to thyrotropin-releasing hormone.

Although T_3 is present in the bloodstream in minute quantities and is meta-

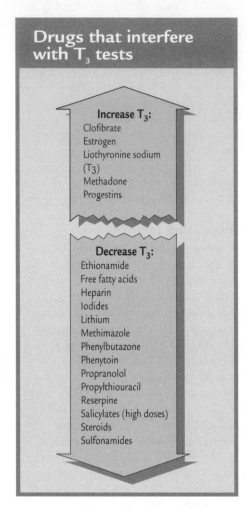

Drugs that interfere with T_3 tests

Increase T_3:
Clofibrate
Estrogen
Liothyronine sodium (T_3)
Methadone
Progestins

Decrease T_3:
Ethionamide
Free fatty acids
Heparin
Iodides
Lithium
Methimazole
Phenylbutazone
Phenytoin
Propranolol
Propylthiouracil
Reserpine
Salicylates (high doses)
Steroids
Sulfonamides

■ To aid in the diagnosis of hypothyroidism and hyperthyroidism
■ To monitor clinical response to thyroid replacement therapy in patients with hypothyroidism

Cost
Moderately expensive

Patient preparation
■ Explain to the patient that this test helps to evaluate thyroid gland function and will help in determining the cause of his symptoms.
■ If the patient is taking a steroid, propranolol, cholestyramine, clofibrate, or another drug that may influence his test results, instruct him not to take the drug before the test. If the drug must be continued, note this on the laboratory request.
■ Tell the patient that the test requires a blood sample. Explain who will perform the venipuncture and when.
■ Explain to the patient that he may experience discomfort from the needle puncture and the tourniquet.
■ If the patient must receive thyroid preparations such as T_3 (liothyronine), the administration time must be noted on the laboratory request. Otherwise, T_3 levels aren't reliable.

Reference values
Normal serum T_3 levels range from 80 to 200 ng/dl (SI, 1.2 to 3 nmol/L).

Abnormal findings
Serum T_3 and T_4 levels usually rise and fall in tandem. However, in T_3 toxicosis, T_3 levels rise, whereas total and free T_4 levels remain normal. T_3 toxicosis occurs in patients with Graves' disease, toxic adenoma, or toxic nodular goiter. T_3 levels also surpass T_4 levels in patients receiving thyroid replacement therapy containing more T_3

bolically active for only a short time, its impact on body metabolism dominates that of T_4. A significant difference between the two major thyroid hormones is that T_3 binds less firmly to thyroxine-binding globulin (TBG). Consequently, T_3 persists in the bloodstream for a short time; half disappears in about 1 day, whereas half of T_4 disappears in 6 days.

Purpose
■ To aid in the diagnosis of T_3 toxicosis

than T_4. In iodine-deficient areas, the thyroid may produce larger amounts of the more cellularly active T_3 than of T_4 in an effort to maintain the euthyroid state.

Generally, T_3 levels appear to be a more accurate diagnostic indicator of hyperthyroidism. Although T_3 and T_4 levels are increased in about 90% of patients with hyperthyroidism, there's a disproportionate increase in T_3. In some patients with hypothyroidism, T_3 levels may fall within the normal range and not be diagnostically significant.

A rise in serum T_3 levels normally occurs during pregnancy. Low T_3 levels may appear in euthyroid patients with systemic illness (especially hepatic or renal disease), during severe acute illness, and after trauma or major surgery. In such patients, TSH levels are within normal limits. Low serum T_3 levels are also found in some euthyroid patients with malnutrition.

Interfering factors
■ Markedly increased or decreased TBG levels, regardless of the cause
■ Failure to take into account medications that affect T_3 levels, such as steroids, clofibrate, cholestyramine, and propranolol (See *Drugs that interfere with T_3 tests*.)

Troponin I and cardiac troponin T

Troponin I (cTn I) and cardiac troponin T (cTn T) are proteins in the striated cells, part of the calcium-binding complex of the thin myofilaments of myocardial tissue. Troponins are extremely specific markers of cardiac damage. When injury occurs to the myocardial tissue, these proteins are released into the bloodstream, increasing from normally undetectable blood levels to levels of more than 50 µg/ml. Elevations in troponin levels can be seen within 1 hour of a myocardial infarction (MI) and will persist for a week or longer, making this a useful diagnostic tool.

Purpose
■ To detect and diagnose an acute MI or reinfarction
■ To evaluate possible causes of chest pain

Cost
Moderately expensive

Patient preparation
■ Explain to the patient that this test helps assess myocardial injury.
■ Tell the patient that the test requires multiple blood samples to detect fluctuations in serum levels. Explain who will perform the venipuncture and when.
■ Explain to the patient that he may experience discomfort from the needle puncture and the tourniquet.

Reference values
Laboratories may give varying results, with some calling a result abnormal if it shows any detectable levels and others giving a range for abnormal results.

Normally, cTn I levels are less than 0.4 µg/ml. cTn T levels are less than 0.1 µg/ml. cTn I levels below 0.4 µg/ml aren't suggestive of cardiac injury, and levels of 0.5 to 1.9 µg/ml are indeterminate for cardiac injury. cTn I levels greater than 2.0 µg/ml suggest cardiac injury. Results of a qualitative cTn T rapid immunoassay that are greater than 0.2 µg/ml are considered positive for cardiac injury. When quantitative serum assays for cTn T are done, the upper limit for normal is 0.1 µg/ml. As long as tissue injury continues, the troponin levels will remain high.

Abnormal findings

Troponin levels rise rapidly and are detectable within 1 hour of myocardial cell injury. cTn I levels aren't detectable in people without cardiac injury.

Interfering factors

■ Sustained vigorous exercise (possible increase in cTn T in the absence of significant cardiac damage associated with the presence of non-cardiac specific cTn T found in these skeletal muscles)
■ Cardiotoxic drugs such as doxorubicin (possible increase)
■ Renal disease and certain surgical procedures (possible increase in cTn T)
■ Myocardial injury (increase in cTn I)

Tuberculin skin tests

Tuberculin skin tests are used to screen for previous infection by the tubercle bacillus. They're routinely performed in children, young adults, and patients with radiographic findings that suggest this infection. In the old tuberculin (OT) and purified protein derivative (PPD) tests, intradermal injection of the tuberculin antigen causes a delayed hypersensitivity reaction in patients with active or dormant tuberculosis.

The Mantoux test uses a single-needle intradermal injection of PPD, permitting precise measurement of the dose. Multipuncture tests, such as the tine test, MonoVacc tests, and Aplitest, use intradermal injections with tines impregnated with OT or PPD. Because they require less skill and are more rapidly administered, multipuncture tests are generally used for screening. An abnormal multipuncture test result usually requires a Mantoux test for confirmation.

ALERT! ▼ ▼ ▼ ▼ ▼ ▼ ▼ ▼ ▼
Tuberculin skin tests are contraindicated in patients with a current reaction to a smallpox vaccination, a rash, a skin disorder, or active TB.

Purpose

■ To distinguish tuberculosis (TB) from blastomycosis, coccidioidomycosis, and histoplasmosis
■ To identify people who need diagnostic investigation for TB because of possible exposure

Cost

Inexpensive

Patient preparation

■ Explain to the patient that this test helps detect TB.
■ Tell the patient that the test requires an intradermal injection, which may cause him transient discomfort.
■ Check the patient's history for active TB, the results of previous skin tests, and hypersensitivities.

ALERT! ▼ ▼ ▼ ▼ ▼ ▼ ▼ ▼ ▼
If the patient has had TB, don't order a skin test. If he has had a positive reaction to previous skin tests, consult facility policy or the health department. If he has had an allergic reaction to acacia, don't order an OT test because this product contains acacia.

■ If the tuberculin test is performed on an outpatient basis, tell the patient that he'll have to return at a specified time so that the test results can be read. Inform him that a positive reaction to a skin test appears as a red, hard, raised area at the injection site. Instruct him not to scratch the area, even though it may itch.
■ Stress that a positive reaction doesn't always indicate active TB.

Normal findings

In tuberculin skin tests, normal findings show no, or only minimal, reactions. In the Mantoux test, no induration may appear, or the patient may develop induration less than 5 mm in diameter.

In the tine and Aplitest tests, no vesiculation or induration may appear, or the patient may develop induration less than 2 mm in diameter. In the MonoVacc tests, no induration appears.

Abnormal findings

A positive tuberculin reaction indicates previous infection by tubercle bacilli. It doesn't distinguish between an active and a dormant infection or provide a definitive diagnosis. If a positive reaction occurs, sputum smear and culture and chest radiography are necessary for further information.

In the Mantoux test, induration 5 to 9 mm in diameter indicates a borderline reaction; larger induration, a positive reaction. Because patients infected with atypical mycobacteria other than tubercle bacilli may have borderline reactions, repeat testing is necessary.

In the tine or Aplitest tests, vesiculation indicates a positive reaction; induration 2 mm in diameter without vesiculation requires confirmation by the Mantoux test. Any induration in the MonoVacc test indicates a positive reaction; however, it requires confirmation by the Mantoux test.

Interfering factors

■ Subcutaneous injection, usually indicated by erythema greater than 10 mm in diameter without induration
■ Corticosteroids, other immunosuppressants, and live vaccine viruses (such as those for measles, mumps, rubella, or polio) within 4 to 6 weeks before the test (possible suppression of skin reaction)

■ Viral infection, malnutrition, febrile illness, uremia, immunosuppressive disorders, or miliary TB in elderly people (possible suppression of skin reaction)
■ Less than 10-week period since infection (possible suppression of skin reaction)
■ Improper dilution, dosage, or storage of the tuberculin

Tumor markers (CA 15-3 [27,29]; CA 19-9; CA-125; and CA-50)

Tumor markers are substances produced and secreted by tumor cells, indicating tumor activity. They can be found in the serum of cancer patients. Specific tests are ordered depending on the type of cancer the patient has. The CA 15-3 antigen (breast-cystic fluid protein or BCFP) may be used in conjunction with the carcinoembryonic antigen and is particularly helpful in breast cancer patients (CA-27, metastatic breast cancer, breast-cystic fluid protein 29, BCFP). CA 19-9 carbohydrate antigen may be ordered for patients with pancreas, hepatobiliary, or lung cancer. The CA-125 glycoprotein antigen and serum carbohydrate antigen is commonly associated with types of ovarian cancers. The CA-50 may be ordered for patients with GI or pancreatic cancer.

A combination of markers may be used due to low sensitivity and specificity of the markers. Few tumor markers meet Food and Drug Administration approval because of the controversy surrounding their role in cancer diagnosis and treatment.

Purpose

■ To assist tumor staging and identify metastasis

- To monitor and detect disease recurrence
- To assess therapeutic response to therapy

Cost
Expensive

Patient preparation
- Explain the purpose of the test to the patient, as appropriate.
- Tell the patient that he should follow directions given to him by the laboratory or the cancer center. Let him know that fasting may be involved and other factors may be identified that may interfere with test results. Note interfering factors on the appropriate laboratory request.
- Tell the patient that the test requires a blood sample. Explain who will perform the venipuncture and when.
- Explain to the patient that he may experience discomfort from the needle puncture and the tourniquet.

Reference values
Normal values for these tumor markers are:
- CA 15-3 (27,29): less than 30 U/ml
- CA 19-9: less than 70 U/ml
- CA-125: less than 34 U/ml
- CA-50: less than 17 U/ml.

Abnormal findings
CA 15-3 (27,29) is greatly increased in patients with metastatic breast cancer; it's also increased in those with pancreatic, lung, colorectal, ovarian, or liver cancer. It decreases with therapy; an increase after therapy suggests progressive disease.

CA 19-9 is increased in patients with pancreatic, hepatobiliary, or lung cancer. It may be mildly increased in those with gastric or colorectal cancer.

CA-125 is increased in patients with epithelial ovarian, fallopian tube, endometrial, endocervical, pancreatic, or liver cancer. It's slightly increased in those with colon, breast, lung, or GI cancer.

CA-50 is increased in patients with GI or pancreatic cancers.

Interfering factors
- Benign breast or ovarian disease (increase in CA 15-3 [27,29])
- Cholecystitis, cirrhosis, cystic fibrosis, gallstones, and pancreatitis (slight increase in CA 19-9)
- Acute and chronic hepatitis, ascites, endometriosis, GI disease, Meigs' syndrome, menstruation, pancreatitis, pelvic inflammatory disease, peritonitis, pleural effusion, pregnancy, and pulmonary disease (increase in CA-125)

U

Ultrasonography of the abdominal aorta

In ultrasonography of the abdominal aorta, a transducer directs high-frequency sound waves into the abdomen over a wide area from the xiphoid process to the umbilical region. The echoing sound waves are displayed on a monitor to indicate internal organs, the vertebral column, and the size and course of the abdominal aorta and other major vessels.

Purpose
■ To detect and measure a suspected abdominal aortic aneurysm (findings may be supported and refined by angiography or computed tomography angiography)
■ To detect and measure the expansion of a known abdominal aortic aneurysm

Cost
Very expensive

Patient preparation
■ Explain to the patient that this procedure allows examination of the abdominal aorta.

■ Describe the procedure to the patient. Tell him that a transducer will pass smoothly over his abdomen in direct contact with his skin, directing sound waves into the abdominal vessels and organs. Assure him that he'll feel only mild pressure.
■ Tell the patient who will perform the procedure, where it will take place, and its expected duration. Also tell him that the lights may be lowered and that he'll feel only slight pressure.
■ If the patient has an aneurysm, reassure him that the sound waves from the ultrasonography won't cause the aneurysm to rupture.
■ Instruct the patient to fast for 8 to 12 hours before the procedure to minimize bowel gas and motility. Tell him that he may receive simethicone to reduce bowel gas, if needed.
■ Tell the patient that he'll need to remain still during the procedure and to hold his breath when requested, to aid visualization.

Normal findings
In adults, the normal abdominal aorta tapers from about 1" to ⅝" (2.5 to 1.6 cm) in diameter along its length from the dia-

phragm to the bifurcation. It descends through the retroperitoneal space, anterior to the vertebral column, and slightly left of the midline. Four of its major branches are usually well visualized: the celiac trunk, the renal arteries, the superior mesenteric artery, and the common iliac arteries.

Abnormal findings

A luminal diameter of the abdominal aorta greater than 1½" (3.8 cm) suggests an aneurysm; greater than 2¾" (7 cm) suggests an aneurysm with a high risk of rupture.

Interfering factors

■ Bowel gas and motility, excessive body movement, surgical wounds, and severe dyspnea
■ Residual barium from GI contrast studies within past 24 hours
■ Air introduced during endoscopy within past 12 to 24 hours
■ Mesenteric fat in obese patients

Ultrasonography of the gallbladder and biliary system

With ultrasonography of the gallbladder and biliary system, a focused beam of high-frequency sound waves passes into the right upper quadrant of the abdomen, creating echoes that vary with changes in tissue density. These echoes are converted to images on a screen, indicating the size, shape, and position of the gallbladder and biliary system.

Purpose

■ To confirm a diagnosis of cholelithiasis
■ To diagnose acute cholecystitis
■ To distinguish between obstructive and nonobstructive jaundice

Cost

Very expensive

Patient preparation

■ Explain to the patient that this procedure allows examination of the gallbladder and the biliary system.
■ Describe the procedure to the patient. Tell him that a transducer will pass smoothly over his abdomen in direct contact with his skin, but assure him that he'll feel only mild pressure.
■ Tell the patient who will perform the procedure, where it will take place, and its expected duration. Also tell him that the lights may be lowered and that he'll feel only slight pressure.
■ Tell the patient that he'll need to remain still during the procedure and to hold his breath when requested in order to aid visualization and ensure that the gallbladder is in the same place for each scan.
■ Instruct the patient to eat a fat-free meal in the evening and then to fast for 8 to 12 hours before the procedure, if possible; this promotes accumulation of bile in the gallbladder and enhances ultrasonic visualization.

Normal findings

The normal gallbladder is sonolucent; it appears circular on transverse scans and pear shaped on longitudinal scans. Although the size of the gallbladder varies, its outer walls normally appear sharp and smooth. Intrahepatic radicles seldom appear because the flow of sonolucent bile is very fine. The cystic duct may also be indistinct — the result of folds known as Heister's valves that line the cystic duct lumen. When visualized, the cystic duct has a serpentine appearance. The common bile duct, in contrast, has a linear appearance but is sometimes obscured by overlying bowel gas.

Abnormal findings

Gallstones within the gallbladder lumen or the biliary system typically appear as mobile, echogenic areas, usually associated with an acoustic shadow. The size of gallstones generally parallel the size of their shadows; gallstones 5 mm or larger usually produce shadows. However, if the gallbladder is distended with bile, gallstones as small as 1 mm can be detected because of the acoustic contrast between liquid bile and solid gallstones. Detecting stones in the biliary ducts, which contain little bile, may be difficult. When the gallbladder is shrunken or fully impacted with gallstones, inadequate bile may likewise make gallstone detection difficult, and the gallbladder itself may not be detectable. In this case, an acoustic shadow in the gallbladder fossa indicates cholelithiasis; the presence of such a shadow in the cystic and common bile ducts can also indicate cholelithiasis.

Polyps and carcinoma within the gallbladder lumen are distinguished from gallstones by their fixity. Polyps usually appear as sharply defined, echogenic areas; carcinoma, as a poorly defined mass, commonly associated with a thickened gallbladder wall.

Biliary sludge within the gallbladder lumen appears as a fine layer of echoes that slowly gravitates to the dependent portion of the gallbladder as the patient changes position. Although biliary sludge may arise without accompanying pathology, it may also result from obstruction and can predispose the patient to gallstone formation.

Acute cholecystitis is indicated by an enlarged gallbladder with thickened, double-rimmed walls, usually with gallstones within the lumen. Precholecystic fluid may also be present. In chronic cholecystitis, the walls of the gallbladder appear thickened; the organ itself, however, is generally contracted. In obstructive jaundice, ultrasonography readily demonstrates a dilated biliary system and, usually, a dilated gallbladder. Dilated intrahepatic radicles appear tortuous and irregular; a dilated gallbladder usually loses its characteristic pear shape, becoming spherical.

Biliary obstruction may result from intrinsic factors, such as a gallstone or small carcinoma within the biliary system. (Ultrasonography can't distinguish between these two echogenic masses.) Alternatively, it may result from extrinsic factors such as a mass in the hepatic portal that compresses the cystic duct and interferes with bile drainage from the intrahepatic radicles or from pathology in the head of the pancreas that obstructs the common bile duct. Such pathology includes carcinoma and pancreatitis, although ultrasonography can't distinguish between the two. When ultrasonography fails to clearly define the site of biliary obstruction, percutaneous transhepatic cholangiography or endoscopic retrograde cholangiopancreatography should be performed.

Interfering factors

■ Failure to observe pretest dietary restrictions

■ Overlying bowel gas or retained barium from a previous test (possible poor imaging)

■ Deficiency of body fluids in a dehydrated patient, obscuring boundaries between organs and tissue structures (possible poor imaging)

Ultrasonography of the liver

Ultrasonography of the liver produces images by channeling high-frequency sound waves into the right upper quadrant of the abdomen. Resultant echoes are converted to cross-sectional images on a monitor; different shades of gray depict various tissue densities. Ultrasonography can show intrahepatic structures and the organ's size, shape, and position.

This procedure is indicated for patients with jaundice of unknown cause, unexplained hepatomegaly and abnormal biochemical test results, suspected metastatic tumors and elevated serum alkaline phosphatase levels, or recent abdominal trauma.

When used with liver-spleen scanning, ultrasonography can define cold spots (focal defects that fail to pick up the radionuclide) as tumors, abscesses, or cysts; it also provides better views of the periportal and perihepatic spaces than liver-spleen scanning. If ultrasonography fails to provide definitive diagnosis, computed tomography, gallium scanning, or liver biopsy may yield more information.

Purpose
■ To distinguish between obstructive and nonobstructive jaundice
■ To screen for hepatocellular disease
■ To detect hepatic metastasis and hematoma
■ To define cold spots as tumors, abscesses, or cysts

Cost
Very expensive

Patient preparation
■ Explain to the patient that this procedure allows examination of the liver.
■ Describe the procedure to the patient. Tell him that a transducer will pass smoothly over his abdomen in direct contact with his skin, but assure him that he'll feel only mild pressure.

■ Tell the patient who will perform the procedure, where it will take place, and its expected duration. Also tell him that the lights may be lowered and that he'll feel only slight pressure.
■ Instruct the patient to fast for 8 to 12 hours before the procedure to minimize bowel gas and motility. Tell him that he may receive simethicone to reduce bowel gas, if needed.
■ Tell the patient that he'll need to remain still during the procedure and to hold his breath when requested, to aid visualization.

Normal findings
The liver normally demonstrates a homogeneous, low-level echo pattern, interrupted only by the different echo patterns of its portal and hepatic veins, the aorta, and the inferior vena cava. Hepatic veins appear completely sonolucent; portal veins have margins that are highly echogenic.

Abnormal findings
With obstructive jaundice, ultrasonography shows dilated intrahepatic biliary radicles and extrahepatic ducts. Conversely, with nonobstructive jaundice, ultrasonography shows a biliary tree of normal diameter.

Ultrasonographic characteristics of hepatocellular disease are generally nonspecific, and disorders in early stages can escape detection; liver-spleen scanning is a more sensitive diagnostic tool. With cirrhosis, ultrasonography may demonstrate variable liver size; dilated, tortuous portal branches associated with portal hypertension; and an irregular echo pattern with increased echo amplitude, causing overall increased attenuation. Demonstration of splenomegaly by spleen ultrasonography or liver-spleen scanning aids in its diagnosis. With fatty infiltration of the liver, ultrasonography may show hepatomegaly and a regular echo pattern that, although greater in echo amplitude than that of normal parenchyma, doesn't alter attenuation.

Ultrasonographic characteristics of metastasis in the liver vary widely; metastasis may appear either hypoechoic or echogenic, poorly defined or well defined. For example, metastatic lymphomas and sarcomas are generally hypoechoic; mucin-secreting adenocarcinoma of the colon is highly echogenic. Liver biopsy is necessary to confirm tumor type. Serial ultrasonography may be used to monitor the effectiveness of therapy.

Primary hepatic tumors also present a varied appearance and may mimic metastases, requiring angiography and liver biopsy for definitive diagnosis. Hepatomas are the most common malignant tumors in adults; hepatoblastomas are most common in children. Benign tumors are far less common than malignant ones.

Abscesses usually appear as sonolucent masses with ill-defined, slightly thickened borders and accentuated posterior wall transmission; scattered internal echoes, caused by necrotic debris, may also be present. Because they produce similar echo patterns, intrahepatic abscesses are occasionally mistaken for hematomas, necrotic metastases, or hemorrhagic cysts. Gas-containing intrahepatic abscesses, which may be echogenic, are sometimes confused with solid intrahepatic lesions. Subphrenic abscesses occur between the diaphragm and the liver; subhepatic abscesses appear inferior to the liver and anterior to the upper pole of the right kidney. Ascitic fluid resembles a subhepatic abscess, but lacks internal echoes and has a more regular border.

Cysts usually appear as spherical, sonolucent areas with well-defined borders and accentuated posterior wall transmission. When a cyst can't be distinguished from an abscess or necrotic metastases, gallium scanning, computed tomography, and angiography should be performed.

Hematomas — either intrahepatic or subcapsular — usually result from trauma. Intrahepatic hematomas appear as poorly defined, relatively sonolucent masses and may have scattered internal echoes due to clotting; serial ultrasonography can differentiate between a hematoma and a cyst or tumor as the hematoma becomes smaller. A subcapsular hematoma may appear as a focal, sonolucent mass on the periphery of the liver or as a diffuse, sonolucent area surrounding part of the liver.

Interfering factors

■ Overlying ribs and gas or residual barium in the stomach or colon (possible inaccurate results)
■ Deficiency of body fluids in a dehydrated patient, obscuring boundaries between organs and tissue structures (possible inaccurate results)

Ultrasonography of the pancreas

In ultrasonography of the pancreas, cross-sectional images of the pancreas are produced by channeling high-frequency sound waves into the epigastric region and converting the resultant echoes to real-time images, which are displayed on a monitor. The pattern varies with tissue density and indicates the size, shape, and position of the pancreas and surrounding viscera.

Purpose

■ To aid in the diagnosis of pancreatitis, pseudocysts, and pancreatic carcinoma

Cost

Very expensive

Patient preparation

■ Explain to the patient that this procedure permits examination of the pancreas.
■ Describe the procedure to the patient. Tell him that a transducer will pass smoothly over his epigastric region in direct contact with his skin, channeling sound waves into the pancreas. Assure him that he'll feel only mild pressure.
■ Tell the patient who will perform the procedure, where it will take place, and its expected duration. Also tell him that the lights may be lowered and that he'll feel only slight pressure.
■ Instruct the patient to fast for 8 to 12 hours before the procedure to minimize bowel gas and motility. Tell him that he may receive simethicone to reduce bowel gas, if needed.
■ If the patient is a smoker, ask him to abstain before the test; this eliminates the risk of swallowing air while inhaling, which interferes with test results.
■ Tell the patient that he'll need to remain still during the procedure and to hold his breath when requested in order to aid visualization.

Normal findings

The pancreas normally demonstrates a coarse, uniform echo pattern and usually appears more echogenic than the adjacent liver.

Abnormal findings

Alterations in the size, contour, and parenchymal texture of the pancreas characterize pancreatic disease. An enlarged pancreas with decreased echogenicity and distinct borders suggests pancreatitis; a well-defined mass with an essentially echo-free interior indicates pseudocyst; and an ill-defined mass with scattered internal echoes or a mass in the head of the pancreas (obstructing the common bile duct)

and a large noncontracting gallbladder suggest pancreatic carcinoma.

A subsequent computed tomography scan and biopsy of the pancreas may be necessary to confirm a diagnosis.

Interfering factors

■ Gas or residual barium in the stomach and intestine (possible poor imaging)
■ Deficiency of body fluids in a dehydrated patient, obscuring boundaries between organs and tissue structures (possible poor imaging)
■ Obesity (possible poor imaging)
■ Fatty infiltration of pancreas (possible poor imaging)

Ultrasonography of the pelvis

In pelvic ultrasonography, high-frequency sound waves are reflected to a transducer to provide images of the interior pelvic area on a monitor. Techniques of sound imaging include A-mode (amplitude modulation, recorded as spikes), B-mode (brightness modulation), gray scale (a representation of organ texture in shades of gray), and real-time imaging (instantaneous images of the tissues in motion, similar to fluoroscopic examination). Selected views may be photographed for later examination and a permanent record of the test.

Purpose

■ To detect foreign bodies and distinguish between cystic and solid masses (tumors)
■ To measure organ size
■ To evaluate fetal viability, position, gestational age, and growth rate
■ To detect multiple pregnancy
■ To confirm fetal abnormalities and maternal abnormalities

■ To guide amniocentesis by determining placental location and fetal position

Cost
Very expensive

Patient preparation
■ Describe the test to the patient, and tell her the reason it's being performed.
■ Assure the patient that this procedure is safe, noninvasive, and painless.
■ Because this test requires a full bladder as a landmark to define pelvic organs, instruct the patient to drink liquids and not to void before the test.
■ Tell the patient who will perform the procedure and where it will take place.
■ Explain that a water enema may be necessary to produce a better outline of the large intestine.
■ Reassure the patient that the test won't harm the fetus.

Normal findings
The uterus is normal in size and shape. The ovaries' size, shape, and sonographic density are normal. The body of the uterus lies on the superior surface of the bladder; the uterine tubes are attached laterally. The ovaries are located on the lateral pelvic walls, with the external iliac vessels above the ureter posteroinferiorly and covered medially by the fimbriae of the uterine tubes. No other masses are visible. If the patient is pregnant, the gestational sac and fetus are of normal size in relation to gestational age.

Abnormal findings
Cystic and solid masses have homogeneous densities; however, solid masses (such as fibroids) appear denser. Inappropriate fetal size may indicate a miscalculated conception or delivery date, fetal anomalies, or a dead fetus. Abnormal echo patterns may indicate foreign bodies (such as an intrauterine device), multiple pregnancy, maternal abnormalities (such as placenta previa or abruptio placentae), fetal abnormalities (such as molar pregnancy or abnormalities of the arms and legs, spine, heart, head, kidneys, and abdomen), fetal malpresentation (such as breech or shoulder presentation), and cephalopelvic disproportion.

Interfering factors
■ Failure to fill the bladder, obesity, or fetal head deep in the pelvis (possible poor imaging)

Ultrasonography of the spleen

With ultrasonography of the spleen, a focused beam of high-frequency sound waves passes into the left upper quadrant of the abdomen, creating echoes that vary with changes in tissue density. These are displayed on a monitor as real-time images that indicate the size, shape, and position of the spleen and surrounding viscera.

Ultrasonography is indicated in patients with an upper left quadrant mass of unknown origin; with known splenomegaly, to evaluate changes in splenic size; with left upper quadrant pain and local tenderness; or with recent abdominal trauma.

Purpose
■ To demonstrate splenomegaly
■ To monitor the progression of primary and secondary splenic disease and to evaluate the effectiveness of therapy
■ To evaluate the spleen after abdominal trauma
■ To help detect splenic cysts and subphrenic abscesses

Cost

Very expensive

Patient preparation

■ Explain to the patient that this procedure allows examination of the spleen.

■ Tell the patient who will perform the procedure, where it will take place, and its expected duration. Also tell him that the lights may be lowered and that he'll feel only slight pressure.

■ Instruct the patient to fast for 8 to 12 hours before the procedure to minimize bowel gas and motility. Tell him that he may receive simethicone to reduce bowel gas, if needed.

■ Describe the procedure to the patient. Tell him that a transducer will pass smoothly over his abdomen in direct contact with his skin. Assure him that he'll feel only mild pressure.

■ Tell the patient that he'll need to remain still during the procedure and to hold his breath when requested in order to aid visualization.

Normal findings

The splenic parenchyma normally demonstrates a homogeneous, low-level echo pattern; its individual vascular channels aren't usually apparent. The superior and lateral splenic borders are clearly defined, each having a convex margin. The undersurface and medial borders, in contrast, show indentations from surrounding organs (stomach, left kidney, and pancreas). The hilar region, where the vascular pedicle enters the spleen, commonly produces an area of highly reflective echoes. The medial surface is generally concave, which helps differentiate between left upper quadrant masses and an enlarged spleen. Even when splenomegaly is present, the spleen generally remains concave medially unless a space-occupying lesion distorts this contour.

Abnormal findings

Ultrasonography can show splenomegaly, but it usually doesn't indicate the cause; a computed tomography (CT) scan can provide more specific information. Splenomegaly is generally accompanied by increased echogenicity. Enlarged vascular channels are commonly visible, especially in the hilar region. If space-occupying lesions distort the splenic contour, liver-spleen scanning should be performed to confirm splenomegaly.

Abdominal trauma may result in splenic rupture or subcapsular hematoma. With splenic rupture, ultrasonography demonstrates splenomegaly and an irregular, sonolucent area (the presence of free intraperitoneal fluid); however, these findings must be confirmed by arteriography. With subcapsular hematoma, ultrasonography shows splenomegaly as well as a double contour, altered splenic position, and a relatively sonolucent area on the periphery of the spleen. The double contour results from blood accumulation between the splenic parenchyma and the intact splenic capsule. As the spleen enlarges, a transverse section shows its anterior margin extending more anteriorly than the aorta. Ultrasonography may be difficult and painful after abdominal trauma because the transducer may have to pass across fractured ribs and contusions; CT scanning, which differentiates blood and fluid in the peritoneal space, should be used instead.

With a subphrenic abscess, ultrasonography shows a sonolucent area beneath the diaphragm. Clinical findings may differentiate between an abscess and blood or fluid accumulation.

Used with liver-spleen scanning, ultrasonography differentiates cold spots as cystic or solid lesions. It shows cysts as spherical, sonolucent areas with well-defined, regular margins with acoustic enhancement behind them. When ultrasonography fails to identify a cyst as splenic or extrasplenic — especially if the cyst is located in the upper pole of the left kidney and the adrenal gland, or in the tail of the pancreas — a CT scan and arteriography are used. Ultrasonography can readily clarify cystic cold spots, but using a CT scan with a contrast medium is superior for evaluating primary and metastatic tumors. Ultrasonography usually fails to identify tumors associated with lymphoma and chronic leukemia because these resemble tumors of the splenic parenchyma.

Interfering factors
■ Overlying ribs, aerated left lung, gas or residual barium in the colon or the stomach (possible poor imaging)
■ Deficiency of body fluids in a dehydrated patient, obscuring boundaries between organs and tissue structures (possible poor imaging)
■ Body physique affecting the spleen's shape or adjacent masses displacing the spleen (possible poor imaging, may be mistaken for splenomegaly)
■ Patient with splenic trauma (possible difficulty in tolerating the procedure)

Ultrasonography of the vagina

With vaginal ultrasonography, a probe inserted into the vagina reflects high-frequency sound waves to a transducer, forming an image of the pelvic structures. This study allows better evaluation of pelvic anatomy and an earlier diagnosis of pregnancy. It also circumvents the poor visualization encountered with obese patients.

Purpose
■ To establish pregnancy with fetal heart motion as early as the 5th to 6th week of gestation
■ To determine an ectopic pregnancy
■ To evaluate an abnormal pregnancy
■ To diagnose fetal abnormalities and placental location
■ To visualize retained products of conception
■ To evaluate adnexal pathology, such as tubo-ovarian abscess, hydrosalpinx, and ovarian masses
■ To evaluate the uterine lining (in cases of dysfunctional uterine bleeding and postmenopausal bleeding)
■ To monitor follicular growth during infertility treatment

Cost
Very expensive

Patient preparation
■ Describe the procedure to the patient, and explain the reason for the test.
■ Assure the patient that the procedure is safe.
■ Tell the patient that a protective sheath is placed over the transducer and sound waves help produce images on the screen.

Normal findings
If the patient isn't pregnant, the uterus and ovaries are normal in size and shape. The body of the uterus lies on the superior surface of the bladder; the uterine tubes are attached laterally. The ovaries are located on the lateral pelvic walls, with the external iliac vessels above the ureter posteroinferiorly and covered medially by the fimbriae of the uterine tubes. If the patient is pregnant, the gestational sac and fetus are of normal size for the gestational dates.

Abnormal findings

Vaginal ultrasonography may reveal an empty uterus if the patient was pregnant. Free peritoneal fluid may be visible in the pelvic cavity, indicating possible peritonitis. Ectopic pregnancies may also be visible in the pelvic cavity.

Interfering factors

- Mistaking the bowel for the ovaries
- Small tubal mass (possible difficulty in detecting ectopic pregnancies)

Upper GI and small-bowel series

The upper GI and small-bowel series is the fluoroscopic examination of the esophagus, stomach, and small intestine after the patient ingests barium sulfate, a contrast agent. As the barium passes through the digestive tract, fluoroscopy outlines peristalsis and the mucosal contours of the respective organs, and spot films record significant findings. This test is indicated for patients who have upper GI symptoms (difficulty in swallowing, regurgitation, burning or gnawing epigastric pain), signs of small-bowel disease (diarrhea, weight loss), and signs of GI bleeding (hematemesis, melena).

Although this test can detect various mucosal abnormalities, subsequent biopsy is commonly needed to rule out malignancy or distinguish specific inflammatory diseases. Oral cholecystography, barium enema, and routine X-rays should always precede this test because retained barium clouds anatomic detail on X-ray films.

ALERT! ▼ ▼ ▼ ▼ ▼ ▼ ▼ ▼ ▼ ▼
The upper GI and small-bowel series may be contraindicated in patients with obstruction or perforation of the digestive tract. Barium may intensify the obstruction or seep into the

abdominal cavity. Sometimes a small-bowel series is performed to find a "transition zone." If a perforation is suspected, Gastrografin (a water-soluble contrast medium) rather than barium may be used. The test is also contraindicated in pregnant patients because of the radiation's possible teratogenic effects.

Purpose

- To detect hiatus hernia, diverticula, and varices
- To aid in the diagnosis of strictures, blockages, ulcers, tumors, regional enteritis, and malabsorption syndrome
- To help detect motility disorders

Cost

Very expensive

Patient preparation

- Explain to the patient that this procedure uses ingested barium and X-ray films to examine the esophagus, stomach, and small intestine.
- Tell the patient to consume a low-residue diet for 2 to 3 days before the test and then to fast and avoid smoking after midnight the night before the test.
- Describe the procedure to the patient. Tell him who will perform the procedure, where it will take place, and its expected duration.
- Inform the patient that he'll be placed on an X-ray table that rotates into vertical, semivertical, and horizontal positions and that he'll be adequately secured and assisted to supine, prone, and side-lying positions.
- Describe the milk shake consistency and chalky taste of the barium mixture. Tell him that he'll have to drink 16 to 20 oz (473 to 591 ml) for a complete examination.
- Inform the patient that his abdomen may be compressed to ensure proper coat-

ing of the stomach or intestinal walls with barium or to separate overlapping bowel loops.

■ If the patient is taking an oral medication, tell him not to take it after midnight the night before the test. If he's taking an anticholinergic or a narcotic, tell him not to take it for 24 hours before the test because these drugs affect the motility of the small intestine. Antacids, histamine-2-receptor antagonists, and proton pump inhibitors are also sometimes withheld for several hours if gastric reflux is suspected.

■ Tell him he may receive a cathartic or enema afterward and to expect his stool to be light colored for 24 to 72 hours.

Normal findings

After the barium suspension is swallowed, it pours over the base of the tongue into the pharynx and is propelled by a peristaltic wave through the entire length of the esophagus in about 2 seconds. The bolus evenly fills and distends the lumen of the pharynx and esophagus, and the mucosa appears smooth and regular. When the peristaltic wave reaches the base of the esophagus, the cardiac sphincter opens, allowing the bolus to enter the stomach. After passage of the bolus, the cardiac sphincter closes.

As barium enters the stomach, it outlines the characteristic longitudinal folds called rugae, which are best observed using the double-contrast technique. When the stomach is completely filled with barium, its outer contour appears smooth and regular without evidence of flattened, rigid areas suggestive of intrinsic or extrinsic lesions.

After barium enters the stomach, it quickly empties into the duodenal bulb through relaxation of the pyloric sphincter. Although the mucosa of the duodenal bulb is relatively smooth, circular folds become

apparent as barium enters the duodenal loop. These folds deepen and become more numerous in the jejunum. The barium temporarily lodges between these folds, producing a speckled pattern on the X-ray film. As barium enters the ileum, the circular folds become less prominent and, except for their broadness, resemble those in the duodenum. The film also shows that the diameter of the small intestine tapers gradually from the duodenum to the ileum.

Abnormal findings

X-ray studies of the esophagus may reveal strictures, tumors, hiatal hernia, diverticula, varices, and ulcers (particularly in the distal esophagus). Benign strictures usually dilate the esophagus, whereas malignant ones cause erosive changes in the mucosa. Tumors produce filling defects in the column of barium, but only malignant ones change the mucosal contour. Nevertheless, biopsy is necessary for definitive diagnosis of both esophageal strictures and tumors.

Motility disorders, such as esophageal spasm, are usually difficult to detect because spasms are erratic and transient; manometry, which measures the length and pressure of peristaltic contractions and evaluates the function of the cardiac sphincter, is generally performed to detect such disorders. However, achalasia (cardiospasm) is strongly suggested when the distal esophagus has a beaking appearance. Gastric reflux appears as a backflow of barium from the stomach into the esophagus.

X-ray studies of the stomach may reveal tumors and ulcers. Malignant tumors, usually adenocarcinomas, appear as filling defects on the X-ray film and usually disrupt peristalsis. Benign tumors, such as adenomatous polyps and leiomyomas, appear as outpouchings of the gastric mucosa and generally don't affect peristalsis. Ulcers occur most commonly in the stomach and duodenum (particularly in the duodenal bulb), and these two areas are thus examined together. Benign ulcers usually demonstrate evidence of partial or complete healing and are characterized by radiating folds extending to the edge of the ulcer crater. Malignant ulcers, usually associated with a suspicious mass, generally have radiating folds that extend beyond the ulcer crater to the edge of the mass. However, biopsy is necessary for definitive diagnosis of tumors and ulcers.

Occasionally, this test detects signs that suggest pancreatitis or pancreatic carcinoma. Such signs include edematous changes in the mucosa of the antrum or duodenal loop or dilation of the duodenal loop. These findings mandate further studies for pancreatic disease, such as endoscopic retrograde cholangiopancreatography, abdominal ultrasonography, or computed tomography scanning.

X-ray studies of the small intestine may reveal regional enteritis, malabsorption syndrome, and tumors. Although regional enteritis may not be detected in its early stages, small ulcerations and edematous changes develop in the mucosa as the disease progresses. Edematous changes, segmentation of the barium column, and flocculation characterize malabsorption syndrome. Filling defects occur with Hodgkin's disease and lymphosarcoma.

Interfering factors
■ Failure to observe diet, smoking, and medication restrictions (possible inaccurate results)
■ Excess air in the small bowel (possible poor imaging)
■ Failure to remove radiopaque objects in X-ray field (possible poor imaging)

Urea clearance

The urea clearance test is a quantitative analysis of urine levels of urea, the main nitrogenous component in urine and the end product of protein metabolism. (See *How urea is formed*.)

After filtration by the glomeruli, roughly 40% of the urea is reabsorbed by the renal tubules. Because of this reabsorption, urea clearance was once considered a precise fraction (60%) of the glomerular filtration rate (GFR). However, because the reabsorption rate of urea varies with the amount of water reabsorbed, this test actually assesses overall renal function; the creatinine clearance test provides a more accurate evaluation of the GFR.

With this test, blood urea content and the total amount of urea excreted in the urine are proportional only when the rate of urine flow is 2 ml/minute or higher (maximal clearance). At lower flow rates, the test's accuracy decreases. The equation for determining urea clearance is:

Clearance = (urine concentration of urea × volume of urine collected) ÷ plasma concentration of urea

Purpose
■ To assess overall renal function

Cost
Inexpensive

Patient preparation
■ Explain to the patient that this test evaluates kidney function.
■ Instruct the patient to fast from midnight before the test and to abstain from exercise before and during the test.
■ Tell the patient the test requires two timed urine specimens and a blood sam-

ple. Explain who will perform the venipuncture and when.

■ Explain to the patient that he may experience discomfort from the needle puncture and the tourniquet.

■ Tell the patient that he'll need to empty his bladder completely so that the total amount of urine is collected from each hour's specimen.

■ Restrict medications that may affect test results. If they must be continued, note this on the laboratory request.

Reference values
Normally, urea clearance ranges from 64 to 99 ml/minute with maximal clearance. If the flow rate is less than 2 ml/minute, normal clearance is 41 to 68 ml/minute. (If the urine flow rate is less than 1 ml/minute, this test shouldn't be performed.)

Abnormal findings
Low urea clearance values may indicate decreased renal blood flow (caused by shock or renal artery obstruction), acute or chronic glomerulonephritis, advanced bilateral chronic pyelonephritis, acute tubular necrosis, or nephrosclerosis. Low clearance rates may also result from advanced bilateral renal lesions (as in polycystic kidney disease, renal tuberculosis, or cancer), bilateral ureteral obstruction, heart failure, or dehydration.

High urea clearance rates usually aren't diagnostically significant.

Interfering factors
■ Caffeine and milk (increase)
■ Small doses of epinephrine (increase)
■ Antidiuretic hormone and large doses of epinephrine (decrease)
■ Amphotericin B, corticosteroids, streptomycin, and thiazide diuretics (altered test results)

How urea is formed

Urea, the main nitrogenous component in urine, is the end product of protein metabolism. Amino acids absorbed by the intestinal villi pass from the portal vein into the liver. Because the liver stores only small amounts of amino acids – which are later returned to the blood for use in the synthesis of enzymes, hormones, or new protoplasm – the excess is converted into other substances, such as glucose, glycogen, and fat.

Before this conversion, the amino acids are deaminated – they lose their nitrogenous amino groups. These amino groups are then converted to ammonia. Because ammonia is toxic, especially to the brain, it must be removed as quickly as it's formed. Serious liver disease causes elevated blood ammonia levels and eventually leads to hepatic coma.

In the liver, ammonia combines with carbon dioxide to form urea, which is released into the blood and ultimately secreted in urine.

■ Failure to observe pretest restrictions or to empty the bladder completely (altered test results)

Uric acid, urine

A quantitative analysis of urine uric acid levels may supplement serum uric acid testing when seeking to identify disorders that alter production or excretion of uric acid (such as leukemia, gout, and renal dysfunction).

The most specific laboratory method for detecting uric acid is spectrophotometric absorption after treatment of the specimen with the enzyme uricase.

Purpose
■ To detect enzyme deficiencies and metabolic disturbances that affect uric acid production such as gout
■ To help measure the efficiency of renal clearance and to determine the risk of stone formation

Cost
Inexpensive

Patient preparation
■ Explain to the patient that this test measures the body's production and excretion of a waste product known as uric acid.
■ Tell the patient that the test requires urine collection over a 24-hour period, discarding the first specimen and retaining the last for proper collection technique.
■ Restrict medications that may affect test results. If they must be continued, note this on the laboratory request.

Reference values
Normal urine uric acid values vary with diet but generally are 250 to 750 mg/24 hours (SI, 1.48 to 4.43 mmol/d).

Abnormal findings
Elevated urine uric acid levels may result from chronic myeloid leukemia, polycythemia vera, multiple myeloma, early remission in pernicious anemia, lymphosarcoma and lymphatic leukemia during radiotherapy, or tubular reabsorption defects, such as Fanconi's syndrome and hepatolenticular degeneration (Wilson's disease).

Low urine uric acid levels occur with gout (when associated with normal uric acid production but inadequate excretion)

and with severe renal damage, such as that resulting from chronic glomerulonephritis, diabetic glomerulosclerosis, and collagen disorders.

Interfering factors
■ Diuretics, such as benzthiazide, ethacrynic acid, and furosemide, (decrease); allopurinol, phenylbutazone, probenecid, pyrazinamide, and salicylates (increase)
■ High purine diet (increase)
■ Low purine diet (decrease)

Urinalysis

A routine urinalysis tests for urinary and systemic disorders. This test evaluates physical characteristics (color, odor, turbidity, and opacity) of urine; determines specific gravity and pH; detects and measures protein, glucose, and ketone bodies; and examines sediment for blood cells, casts, and crystals.

Diagnostic laboratory methods include visual examination, reagent strip screening, refractometry for specific gravity, and microscopic inspection of centrifuged sediment.

Purpose
■ To screen the patient's urine for renal or urinary tract disease
■ To help detect metabolic or systemic disease unrelated to renal disorders
■ To monitor therapy with drugs that may adversely affect the kidneys
■ To detect the use of drugs or other substances

Cost
Inexpensive

Patient preparation

■ Explain to the patient that this test aids in the diagnosis of renal or urinary tract disease and helps evaluate overall body function.

■ Restrict medications that may affect test results. If they must be continued, note this on the laboratory request.

■ Tell the patient that a random urine specimen will be collected.

Normal findings

See *Normal findings in routine urinalysis,* page 396.

Abnormal findings

Nonpathologic variations in normal values may result from diet, nonpathologic conditions, specimen collection time, and other factors.

Urine pH, which is greatly affected by diet and medications, influences the appearance of urine and the composition of crystals. An alkaline pH (above 7.0) — characteristic of a vegetarian diet — causes turbidity and the formation of phosphate, carbonate, and amorphous crystals. An acid pH (below 7.0) — typical of a high-protein diet — produces turbidity and the formation of oxalate, cystine, leucine, tyrosine, amorphous urate, and uric acid crystals.

Protein, normally absent from the urine, may be present in a benign condition known as orthostatic (postural) proteinuria. Most common in patients ages 10 to 20, this condition is intermittent, appears after prolonged standing, and disappears after recumbency. Transient benign proteinuria can also occur with fever, exposure to cold, emotional stress, or strenuous exercise. Systemic diseases that may cause proteinuria include lymphoma, hepatitis, diabetes mellitus, toxemia, hypertension, lupus erythematosus, and febrile illnesses.

Sugars, usually absent from the urine, may appear under normal conditions. The most common sugar in urine is glucose. Transient nonpathologic glycosuria may result from emotional stress or pregnancy and may follow ingestion of a high-carbohydrate meal.

Centrifuged urine sediment contains cells, casts, crystals, bacteria, yeast, and parasites. Red blood cells (RBCs) commonly don't appear in urine without pathologic significance; however, strenuous exercise can cause hematuria.

The following abnormal findings generally suggest pathologic conditions:

■ *Color:* Color change can result from diet, drugs, and many diseases.

■ *Odor:* In diabetes mellitus, starvation, and dehydration, a fruity odor accompanies the formation of ketone bodies. In urinary tract infections, a fetid odor commonly is associated with *Escherichia coli.* Maple syrup urine disease and phenylketonuria also cause distinctive odors. Other abnormal odors include those similar to a brewery, sweaty feet, cabbage, fish, and sulfur.

■ *Turbidity:* Turbid urine may contain red or white cells, bacteria, fat, or chyle and may reflect renal infection.

■ *Specific gravity:* Low specific gravity (less than 1.005) is characteristic of diabetes insipidus, nephrogenic diabetes insipidus, acute tubular necrosis, and pyelonephritis. Fixed specific gravity, in which values remain 1.010 regardless of fluid intake, occurs in chronic glomerulonephritis with severe renal damage. High specific gravity (greater than 1.035) occurs in nephrotic syndrome, dehydration, acute glomerulonephritis, heart failure, liver failure, and shock.

■ *pH:* Alkaline urine pH may result from Fanconi's syndrome, urinary tract infection, and metabolic or respiratory alkalosis. Acid urine pH is associated with renal tubercu-

Normal findings in routine urinalysis

ELEMENT	FINDINGS
Macroscopic	
Color	Pale yellow to amber
Odor	Slightly aromatic
Appearance	Clear
Specific gravity	1.005 to 1.035
pH	4.5 to 8
Protein	None
Glucose	None
Ketone bodies	None
Bilirubin	None
Urobilinogen	Normal
Hemoglobin	None
Erythrocytes (red blood cells [RBCs])	None
Nitrite (bacteria)	None
Leukocytes (white blood cells [WBCs])	None
Microscopic	
RBCs	0 to 3/high-power field
WBCs	0 to 4/high-power field
Epithelial cells	0 to 5/high-power field
Casts	None, except 1 to 2 hyaline casts/low-power field
Crystals	Present
Bacteria	None
Yeast cells	None
Parasites	None

losis, pyrexia, phenylketonuria, alkaptonuria, and acidosis.

■ *Protein:* Proteinuria suggests renal failure or disease (including nephrosis, glomerulosclerosis, glomerulonephritis, nephrolithiasis, nephrotic syndrome, and polycystic kidney disease) or, possibly, multiple myeloma.

■ *Sugars:* Glycosuria usually indicates diabetes mellitus, but it may result from pheochromocytoma, Cushing's syndrome, impaired tubular reabsorption, advanced renal disease, or increased intracranial pressure. I.V. solutions containing glucose and total parenteral nutrition containing from 10% to 50% glucose can cause glucose to spill over the renal threshold, leading to glycosuria. Fructosuria, galactosuria, and pentosuria generally suggest rare hereditary metabolic disorders (except for lactosuria during pregnancy and lactation). However, an alimentary form of pentosuria and fructosuria may follow excessive ingestion of pentose or fructose. When the liver fails to metabolize these sugars, they spill into the urine because the renal tubules don't reabsorb them.

■ *Ketone bodies:* Ketonuria occurs in diabetes mellitus when cellular energy needs exceed available cellular glucose. In the absence of glucose, cells metabolize fat for energy. Ketone bodies — the end products of incomplete fat metabolism — accumulate in plasma and are excreted in the urine. Ketonuria may also occur with starvation states, low- or no-carbohydrate diets, and diarrhea or vomiting.

■ *Bilirubin:* Bilirubin in urine may occur with liver disease resulting from obstructive jaundice, hepatotoxic drugs or toxins, or from fibrosis of the biliary canaliculi (which may occur with cirrhosis).

■ *Urobilinogen:* Intestinal bacteria in the duodenum change bilirubin into urobilinogen. The liver reprocesses the remainder into bile. Increased urobilinogen in the urine may indicate liver damage, hemolytic disease, or severe infection. Decreased levels may occur with biliary obstruction, inflammatory disease, antimicrobial therapy, severe diarrhea, or renal insufficiency.

■ *Cells:* Hematuria indicates bleeding within the genitourinary tract and may result from infection, obstruction, inflammation, trauma, a tumor, glomerulonephritis, renal hypertension, lupus nephritis, renal tuberculosis, renal vein thrombosis, renal calculi, hydronephrosis, pyelonephritis, scurvy, malaria, parasitic infection of the bladder, subacute bacterial endocarditis, polyarteritis nodosa, or a hemorrhagic disorder. Strenuous exercise or exposure to toxic chemicals may also cause hematuria. An excess of white blood cells (WBCs) in urine usually implies urinary tract inflammation, especially cystitis or pyelonephritis. WBC and WBC casts in urine suggest renal infection or noninfective inflammatory disease. Numerous epithelial cells suggest renal tubular degeneration, such as heavy metal poisoning, eclampsia, and kidney transplant rejection.

■ *Casts (plugs of gelled proteinaceous material [high-molecular-weight mucoprotein]):* Casts form in the renal tubules and collecting ducts by agglutination of protein cells or cellular debris and are flushed loose by urine flow. Excessive numbers of casts indicate renal disease. Hyaline casts are associated with renal parenchymal disease, inflammation, trauma to the glomerular capillary membrane, and some physiologic states (such as after exercise); epithelial casts, with renal tubular damage, nephrosis, eclampsia, amyloidosis, and heavy metal poisoning; coarse and fine granular casts, with acute or chronic renal failure, pyelonephritis, and chronic lead intoxication; fatty and waxy casts, with nephrotic syndrome, chronic renal disease, and diabetes mellitus; RBC casts, with renal parenchymatous disease (especially glomerulonephritis), renal infarction, subacute bacterial endocarditis, vascular disorders, sickle cell anemia, scurvy, blood dyscrasias, malignant hypertension, collagen disease, and acute inflammation; and white blood cell casts, with acute pyelonephritis and glomerulonephritis, nephrotic syndrome, pyogenic infection, and lupus nephritis.

■ *Crystals:* Some crystals normally appear in urine, but numerous calcium oxalate crystals suggest hypercalcemia or ethylene glycol ingestion. Cystine crystals (cystinuria) reflect an inborn error of metabolism.

■ *Other components:* Bacteria, yeast cells, and parasites in urine sediment reflect genitourinary tract infection or contamination of external genitalia. Yeast cells, which may be mistaken for RBCs, are identifiable by their ovoid shape, lack of color, variable size and, frequently, signs of budding. The most common parasite in sediment is *Trichomonas vaginalis,* which causes vaginitis, urethritis, and prostatovesiculitis.

Interfering factors
■ Strenuous exercise before routine urinalysis (transient myoglobulinuria)
■ Insufficient urinary volume, less than 2 ml (possible limitation of the range of procedures)
■ Failure to send specimen to the laboratory immediately after the urine is collected (false-low urobilinogen)
■ Foods, such as beets, berries, and rhubarb (false change in color)
■ Certain drugs (possibly altered results)
■ Highly dilute urine such as in diabetes insipidus

Urine culture

Laboratory examination and culture of urine are used to evaluate urinary tract infections (UTIs), especially bladder infections. Urine in the kidneys and bladder is normally sterile, but a urine specimen may contain various organisms due to bacteria in the urethra and on external genitalia. Bacteriuria generally results from one prevalent bacteria type; the presence of more than two bacterial species in a specimen strongly suggests contamination during collection. A single negative culture doesn't always rule out infection.

Purpose
■ To diagnose a UTI
■ To monitor microorganism colonization after urinary catheter insertion

Cost
Inexpensive

Patient preparation
■ Explain to the patient that this test is used to detect UTI.
■ Inform the patient that the test requires a urine specimen and that no restriction of food or fluid is necessary. Tell him that the first voided specimen of the day is preferred because it will reflect a high colony count after an overnight incubation period.
■ Instruct the patient how to collect a clean voided midstream specimen; emphasize that external genitalia must be cleaned thoroughly.
■ If appropriate, explain catheterization or suprapubic aspiration to the patient, and inform him that he may experience some discomfort during specimen collection.

Reference values

A urine culture that contains 10,000 or fewer organisms per milliliter is considered negative.

Abnormal findings

Bacterial counts of 100,000/ml or more of a single microbe species indicates a probable UTI. Counts under 100,000/ml may be significant, depending on the patient's age, sex, history, and other individual factors. Counts under 10,000/ml usually suggest that the organisms are contaminants, except in symptomatic patients, those with urologic disorders, and those whose urine specimens were collected by suprapubic aspiration. A special test for acid-fast bacteria isolates *Mycobacterium tuberculosis,* thus indicating tuberculosis of the urinary tract. Isolation of more than two species of organisms or of vaginal or skin organisms usually suggests contamination and requires a repeat culture. Prolonged catheterization or urinary diversion may cause polymicrobial infection.

Interfering factors

■ Failure to use proper collection technique
■ Failure to preserve the specimen properly or to send it to the laboratory immediately after collection
■ Fluid- or drug-induced diuresis and antimicrobial therapy (possible decrease)

V

Vaginal smear

Although the Papanicolaou (Pap) test wasn't developed to detect vaginitis, a cytologist can usually identify cells associated with vaginitis while examining the stained cells for cancer. The most reliably detected cells are *Trichomonas vaginalis, Candida,* and herpes simplex type 2. If such cells are present, the Pap test indicates atypical cells with no evidence of malignancy.

The conventional way to detect vaginitis is the vaginal smear. Using a cotton-tipped applicator or wooden spatula, the examiner collects vaginal secretions and places them at opposite ends of a slide. After adding a drop of normal saline solution to one end of the slide and a drop of 10% to 20% potassium hydroxide (KOH) to the other end (wet-mount preparation), he immediately examines the slide. Trichomonads, white cells, epithelial cells, "clue" cells, and bacteria readily appear at the saline-treated end; *Candida,* at the KOH-treated end.

In the vaginal pool smear, secretions are aspirated through a pipette that's attached to a bulb for suction. Part of the secretion is smeared on a slide and fixed.

Scrapings for cytohormonal evaluation can also be taken from the vaginal pool. In this procedure, the lateral vaginal wall is gently scraped, and the scrapings are spread on a glass slide and fixed. Using the pyknotic index, the estrogenic effect is assessed by determining the percentage of superficial and intermediate squamous cells with a fatty pyknotic nucleus.

Purpose
■ To detect inflammatory tissue changes
■ To detect infection by microorganisms

Cost
Moderately expensive

Patient preparation
■ Explain to the patient that the test allows the study of vaginal cells.
■ The test shouldn't be scheduled during the patient's menstrual period; the best time is mid-cycle.
■ Describe the test for the patient. Tell her who will perform it, where it will take place, and its expected duration.
■ Tell the patient that the test requires that a specimen from the vagina and that she

may experience slight discomfort if a speculum is used.

■ Instruct the patient to avoid having intercourse for 24 hours, not to douche for 48 hours, and not to insert vaginal medications for 1 week before the test because doing so can wash away cellular deposits and change the vaginal pH.

Normal findings

No abnormalities are present.

Abnormal findings

A smear may detect organisms suggesting an infection. To confirm a suggestive or positive cytology report, the test may be repeated or followed by a biopsy.

Interfering factors

■ Douching within 48 hours or having intercourse within 24 hours before the test (washes away cellular deposits)
■ Excessive use of lubricating jelly on the speculum (false-negative)
■ Collection of the specimen during menstruation

Vanillylmandelic acid

Using spectrophotofluorometry, the vanillylmandelic acid (VMA) test determines urine levels of VMA, a phenolic acid. VMA is the catecholamine metabolite that's normally most prevalent in the urine and is the product of hepatic conversion of epinephrine and norepinephrine; urine VMA levels reflect endogenous production of these major catecholamines. As with the test for urine total catecholamines, this test helps to detect catecholamine-secreting tumors — especially pheochromocytoma — and helps evaluate the function of the adrenal medulla, the primary site of catecholamine production.

The VMA test ideally should be performed on a 24-hour urine specimen (not a random specimen) to overcome the effects of diurnal variations in catecholamine secretion. Other catecholamine metabolites — metanephrine, normetanephrine, and homovanillic acid (HVA) — may be measured at the same time. If evaluating hypertension, specimen collection may be of greatest value during the hypertensive episode.

Purpose

■ To help detect pheochromocytoma, neuroblastoma, or ganglioneuroma
■ To evaluate the function of the adrenal medulla

Cost

Moderately expensive

Patient preparation

■ Explain to the patient that this test evaluates hormonal secretion.
■ Instruct the patient to restrict foods and beverages containing phenolic acid — such as bananas, carbonated beverages, citrus fruits, chocolate, coffee, tea, and vanilla — for 3 days before the test.
■ Advise the patient to avoid stressful situations and excessive physical activity during the urine collection period.
■ Inform the patient that the test requires collection of urine over a 24-hour period, discarding the first specimen and retaining the last in a bottle containing a preservative, which is placed on ice or refrigerated.
■ Restrict medications that may affect test results. If they must be continued, note this on the laboratory request.

Reference values

Normally, VMA levels in adults are 1.4 to 6.5 mg/24 hours (SI, 7 to 33 µmol/d).

Although a pheochromocytoma is a cate-cholamine-producing tumor, causing hyper-secretion of epinephrine and norepinephrine by the adrenal medulla, not every patient with this disorder has elevated urine catecholamine levels. Moreover, hypertension, a prime clue in this condition, is sometimes absent. Thus, an analysis of one or more catecholamine metabolites is helpful in confirming the diagnosis.

Interpreting test results

When urine catecholamine levels remain normal in patients with hypertension, elevated urine vanillylmandelic acid (VMA) levels may signal a tumor. Alternatively, metanephrine may be high when VMA and catecholamines are essentially unchanged. VMA assay is also an alternative method when catecholamine analysis has been compromised by interfering food or drugs. Increased excretion of homo-vanillic acid (HVA) typically indicates malignant pheochromocytoma, although the incidence of malignancy is low.

Measurement of urine VMA is also useful for diagnosing two neurogenic tumors — neuroblastoma, a common soft-tissue tumor that's a leading cause of death in infants and young children, and ganglioneuroma, a well-defined tumor of the sympathetic nervous system that occurs in older children and young adults. Both tumors primarily produce dopamine and thus show the expected high readings of dopamine's metabolite, HVA, especially in their malignant forms. However, both tumors also show abnormal increases in urine VMA levels.

Abnormal findings

Elevated urine VMA levels may result from a catecholamine-secreting tumor. Further testing, such as the measurement of urine HVA levels to rule out pheochromocytoma, is necessary for precise diagnosis. (See *Diagnosing catecholamine-secreting tumors*.) If pheochromocytoma is confirmed, the patient may be tested for multiple endocrine neoplasia, an inherited condition commonly associated with pheochromocytoma. (Family members of a patient with confirmed pheochromocytoma should also be carefully evaluated for multiple endocrine neoplasia.)

Interfering factors

- Excessive exercise or emotional stress (increase)
- Failure to observe restrictions
- Failure to properly store the specimen during the collection period or to send the specimen to the laboratory immediately after the collection is completed
- Epinephrine, lithium carbonate, methocarbamol, norepinephrine (increase)
- Chlorpromazine, clonidine, guanethidine, monoamine oxidase inhibitors, reserpine (decrease)
- Levodopa and salicylates (increase or decrease)

Venereal Disease Research Laboratory test

The Venereal Disease Research Laboratory (VDRL) test is widely used to screen for primary and secondary syphilis. Usually, a serum sample is used in the VDRL test, but

The fluorescent treponemal antibody absorption (FTA-ABS) test—which uses a strain of the *Treponema pallidum* antigen itself as a reagent—is more sensitive than the Venereal Disease Research Laboratory (VDRL) test or the rapid plasma reagin (RPR) test in detecting all stages of untreated syphilis (as shown in the graph below). However, the test's complexity and the incidence of false-positive results make it an impractical screening tool. The VDRL and RPR tests are preferred for wide-scale screening and also when primary- or secondary-stage disease is suspected. With advanced syphilis, when the VDRL test may be negative for more than one-third of infected people, the FTA-ABS test is preferred for sensitivity.

The VDRL test can also be used to monitor response to treatment. Untreated syphilis produces titers that are low in the primary stage (less than 1:32), elevated in the secondary stage (greater than 1:32), and variable in the tertiary stage. Successful therapy markedly reduces titers, with two-thirds of patients reverting to a negative VDRL, especially during the first two stages of the disease. Third-stage therapy seldom produces a nonreactive VDRL, but maintenance of low-reactive values during the 6- to 12-month posttherapy period indicates success. A subsequent rise signals reinfection. By comparison, FTA-ABS test results usually remain positive following treatment.

A significant number of patients with infectious diseases show temporary false-positive VDRL test results. Chronic false-positive VDRL and FTA-ABS test readings are associated with the immune complex diseases.

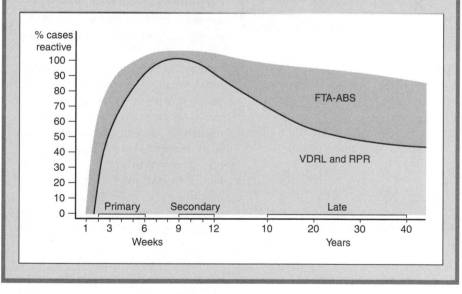

this test may also be performed on a cerebrospinal fluid (CSF) specimen obtained by lumbar puncture to test for tertiary syphilis. The VDRL test of CSF is less sensitive than the fluorescent treponemal antibody absorption test. (See *Serodiagnostic tests for untreated syphilis.*)

The rapid plasma reagin test can also be used to diagnose syphilis. (See *Rapid plasma reagin test,* page 404.)

The rapid plasma reagin test (RPR) is an acceptable substitute for the Venereal Disease Research Laboratory (VDRL) test in diagnosing syphilis. This rapid, macroscopic serologic test, available as a kit, uses a cardiolipin antigen to detect reagin, the antibody relatively specific for *Treponema pallidum* and the cause of syphilis.

In the RPR test, the patient's serum is mixed with cardiolipin on a plastic-coated card, rotated mechanically, and then examined with the unaided eye. If flocculation occurs, the test sample is diluted until no visible reaction occurs. The last dilution to show visible flocculation is the titer of the reagin antibody.

In the RPR test, like the VDRL test, normal serum shows no flocculation.

Purpose

■ To screen for primary and secondary syphilis
■ To confirm primary or secondary syphilis in the presence of syphilitic lesions
■ To monitor response to treatment

Cost

Moderately expensive

Patient preparation

■ Explain to the patient that this test detects syphilis.
■ Tell the patient that he doesn't need to restrict food, fluids, or medications, but that he should abstain from alcohol for 24 hours before the test.
■ Tell the patient that the test requires a blood sample. Explain who will perform the venipuncture and when.

■ Explain to the patient that he may experience discomfort from the needle puncture and the tourniquet.
■ If the test is nonreactive or borderline, but syphilis hasn't been ruled out, instruct the patient to return for follow-up testing. Explain that borderline test results don't necessarily mean that he's free from the disease.
■ If the test is reactive but the patient is experiencing no syphilitic symptoms, explain that many uninfected people experience false-positive reactions. Stress the need for further specific tests to rule out syphilis.

Normal findings

Normal serum shows no flocculation and is reported as a nonreactive test.

Abnormal findings

Definite flocculation is reported as a reactive test; slight flocculation is reported as a weakly reactive test. A reactive VDRL test occurs in about 50% of patients with primary syphilis and in nearly all patients with secondary syphilis. If syphilitic lesions exist, a reactive VDRL test is diagnostic. If no lesions are evident, a reactive VDRL test necessitates repeat testing. Biological false-positive reactions can be caused by conditions unrelated to syphilis — for example, hepatitis, infectious mononucleosis, leprosy, malaria, nonsyphilitic treponemal diseases (such as pinta and yaws), rheumatoid arthritis, and systemic lupus erythematosus.

A nonreactive test doesn't rule out syphilis because *Treponema pallidum* causes no detectable immunologic changes in the serum for 14 to 21 days after infection. Darkfield microscopy of exudate from suspicious lesions can provide early diagnosis by identifying the causative spirochetes.

A reactive VDRL test using a CSF specimen indicates neurosyphilis, which can follow the primary and secondary stages in patients who remain untreated.

Interfering factors
■ Ingestion of alcohol within 24 hours of the test (possible transient nonreactive results)
■ Immunosuppression (possible nonreactive results)

Vertebral radiography

Vertebral radiography visualizes all or part of the vertebral column. A commonly performed test, it's used to evaluate the vertebrae for deformities, fractures, dislocations, tumors, and other abnormalities. Bone films determine bone density, texture, erosion, and changes in bone relationships. X-rays of the cortex of the bone reveal any widening, narrowing, and signs of irregularity; joint X-rays, any fluid, spur formation, narrowing, and changes in the joint structure.

The type and extent of vertebral radiography depend on the patient's clinical condition. For example, a patient with lower back pain requires only a study of the lumbar and sacral segments.

ALERT! ▼ ▼ ▼ ▼ ▼ ▼ ▼ ▼ ▼
Vertebral radiography is contraindicated during the first trimester of pregnancy, unless the benefits outweigh the risk of fetal radiation exposure.

Purpose
■ To detect vertebral fractures, dislocations, subluxations, and deformities
■ To detect vertebral degeneration, infection, and congenital disorders
■ To detect disorders of the intervertebral disks

■ To determine the vertebral effects of arthritic and metabolic disorders

Cost
Expensive

Patient preparation
■ Explain to the patient that this test permits examination of the spine.
■ Describe the test for the patient. Tell him who will perform it, where it will take place, and its expected duration.
■ Advise the patient that he'll be placed in various positions for the X-ray films.
■ Tell the patient that although some positions may cause slight discomfort, his cooperation is needed to ensure accurate results.

Normal findings
Normal vertebrae show no curvatures, dislocations, fractures, subluxations, or other abnormalities. Specific positions and spacing of the vertebrae vary with the patient's age.

In the lateral view, adult vertebrae are aligned to form four alternately concave and convex curves. The cervical and lumbar curves are convex anteriorly; the thoracic and sacral curves are concave anteriorly. Although the structure of the coccyx varies, it usually points forward and downward.

AGE ISSUE ✻ ✻ ✻ ✻ ✻
Neonatal vertebrae form only one curve, which is concave anteriorly.

Abnormal findings
The vertebral radiograph readily shows dislocations, fractures, spondylolisthesis, subluxations, wedging, and such deformities as kyphosis, lordosis, and scoliosis.

To confirm other disorders, spinal structures and their spatial relationships on the radiograph must be examined, and the patient's history and clinical status must be considered. These disorders include congenital abnormalities, such as the absence of sacral or lumbar vertebrae, hemivertebrae, Klippel-Feil syndrome, and torticollis (wryneck); degenerative processes, such as hypertrophic spurs, narrowed disk spaces, and osteoarthritis; tuberculosis (Pott's disease); benign or malignant intraspinal tumors; ruptured disk and cervical disk syndrome; and systemic disorders, such as ankylosing spondylitis, Charcot's disease, osteoporosis, Paget's disease, and rheumatoid arthritis.

Depending on the radiographic results, a definitive diagnosis may also require additional tests, such as myelography or computed tomography scanning.

Interfering factors
■ Improper positioning of the patient or patient movement (possible poor imaging)

Vitamin A and carotene

The vitamin A and carotene test measures serum levels of vitamin A (retinol) and its precursor, carotene. A fat-soluble vitamin normally supplied by diet, vitamin A is important for reproduction, vision (especially night vision), and epithelial tissue and bone growth. Vitamin A is found mostly in fruits, vegetables, eggs, poultry, meat, and fish. Carotene is present in leafy green vegetables and in yellow fruits and vegetables.

In this serum test, the color reactions produced by vitamin A and related compounds with various reagents provide quantitative and qualitative information.

Purpose
■ To investigate suspected vitamin A deficiency or toxicity

■ To aid in the diagnosis of visual disturbances, especially night blindness and xerophthalmia
■ To aid in the diagnosis of skin diseases, such as ichthyosis or keratosis follicularis
■ To screen for malabsorption

Cost
Moderately expensive

Patient preparation
■ Explain to the patient that this test measures the vitamin A level in the blood.
■ Instruct the patient to fast overnight, but tell him that he doesn't need to restrict water intake.
■ Tell the patient that the test requires a blood sample. Explain who will perform the venipuncture and when.
■ Explain to the patient that he may experience discomfort from the needle puncture and the tourniquet.

Reference values
Normal serum levels for carotene are 10 to 85 µg/dl (SI, 0.19 to 1.58 µmol/L). Normal serum levels for vitamin A are 30 to 80 µg/dl (SI, 1.05 to 2.8 µmol/L).

Abnormal findings
Low serum levels of vitamin A (hypovitaminosis A) may indicate impaired fat absorption, as in celiac disease, cystic fibrosis of the pancreas, infectious hepatitis, or obstructive jaundice. Low levels are also associated with protein-calorie malnutrition (marasmic kwashiorkor). Similar decreases in vitamin A levels may also result from chronic nephritis.

Elevated vitamin A levels (hypervitaminosis A) usually indicate long-term excessive intake of vitamin A supplements or of foods high in vitamin A. Increased levels are also associated with hyperlipemia and the hypercholesterolemia of uncontrolled diabetes mellitus.

Decreased serum carotene levels may indicate impaired fat absorption or, rarely, insufficient dietary intake of carotene. Carotene levels may also be suppressed during pregnancy. Elevated carotene levels indicate grossly excessive dietary intake.

Interfering factors

■ Failure to observe overnight fast
■ Cholestyramine, mineral oil, and neomycin (possible decrease)
■ Glucocorticoids and hormonal contraceptives (possible increase)

Vitamin B$_{12}$

The vitamin B$_{12}$ radioisotope assay of competitive binding is a quantitative analysis of serum levels of vitamin B$_{12}$ (also called cyanocobalamin, antipernicious anemia factor, or extrinsic factor). This test is usually performed concurrently with the measurement of serum folic acid levels.

A water-soluble vitamin containing cobalt, vitamin B$_{12}$ is essential to hematopoiesis, deoxyribonucleic acid synthesis and growth, myelin synthesis, and central nervous system (CNS) integrity. This vitamin is found almost exclusively in animal products, such as meat, shellfish, milk, and eggs. (See *Cobalt: Critical trace element*.)

Purpose

■ To aid in the differential diagnosis of megaloblastic anemia, which may be due to a deficiency of vitamin B$_{12}$ or folic acid
■ To aid in the differential diagnosis of CNS disorders that are affecting peripheral and spinal myelinated nerves

Cobalt: Critical trace element

A trace element found mainly in the liver, cobalt is an essential component of vitamin B$_{12}$ and therefore is a critical factor in hematopoiesis. A balanced diet supplies sufficient cobalt to maintain hematopoiesis, primarily through foods containing vitamin B$_{12}$.

However, excessive ingestion of cobalt may have toxic effects. Toxicity has occurred, for example, in individuals who consumed large quantities of beer containing cobalt as a stabilizer, resulting in heart failure from cardiomyopathy. Quantitative analysis of cobalt alone is difficult because only a minute amount is found in the body, so cobalt is commonly measured by bioassay as part of vitamin B$_{12}$.

Normal cobalt concentration in human plasma is 60 to 80 pg/ml.

Cost
Inexpensive

Patient preparation

■ Explain to the patient that this test determines the amount of vitamin B$_{12}$ in the blood.
■ Instruct the patient to fast overnight before the test.
■ Tell the patient that the test requires a blood sample. Explain who will perform the venipuncture and when.
■ Explain to the patient that he may experience discomfort from the needle puncture and the tourniquet.
■ Restrict medications that may affect test results. If they must be continued, note this on the laboratory request.

Reference values

Normally, serum vitamin B_{12} values range from 200 to 900 pg/ml (SI, 148 to 664 pmol/L).

Abnormal findings

Decreased serum levels may indicate inadequate dietary intake, especially if the patient is a strict vegetarian. Low levels are also associated with malabsorption syndromes such as celiac disease; the isolated malabsorption of vitamin B_{12}; hypermetabolic states such as hyperthyroidism; pregnancy; and CNS damage, such as posterolateral sclerosis or funicular degeneration.

Elevated levels of serum vitamin B_{12} may result from excessive dietary intake; hepatic disease, such as cirrhosis or acute or chronic hepatitis; and myeloproliferative disorders such as myelocytic leukemia.

Interfering factors

- Failure to observe overnight fast
- Intake of substances that decrease vitamin B_{12} absorption
- Anticonvulsants, ethanol, metformin, and neomycin (possible decrease)
- Hormonal contraceptives (increase)

Vitamin C

Vitamin C chemical assay measures plasma levels of vitamin C (ascorbic acid), a water-soluble vitamin required for collagen synthesis and cartilage and bone maintenance. Vitamin C also promotes iron absorption, influences folic acid metabolism, and may be necessary for withstanding the stresses of injury and infection.

This vitamin is present in generous amounts in citrus fruits, berries, tomatoes, raw cabbage, green peppers, green, leafy vegetables, and fortified juices. Severe vitamin C deficiency, or scurvy, causes capillary fragility, joint abnormalities, and multisystemic symptoms.

Purpose

- To aid in the diagnosis of scurvy, scurvy-like conditions, and metabolic disorders, such as malnutrition and malabsorption syndromes

Cost

Expensive

Patient preparation

- Explain to the patient that this test detects the amount of vitamin C in the blood.
- Instruct the patient to fast overnight before the test.
- Tell the patient that the test requires a blood sample. Explain who will perform the venipuncture and when.
- Explain to the patient that he may experience discomfort from the needle puncture and the tourniquet.

Reference values

Normal plasma vitamin C levels range from 0.2 to 2 mg/dl (SI, 11 to 114 µmol/L).

Abnormal findings

Values less than 0.3 mg/dl (16.5 µmol/L) indicate significant deficiency. Vitamin C levels diminish during pregnancy to a low point immediately postpartum. Depressed levels occur with infection, fever, and anemia. Severe deficiencies result in scurvy.

High plasma levels can indicate increased ingestion of vitamin C. Excess vitamin C is converted to oxalate, which is excreted in the urine. Excessive concentration of oxalate can produce urinary calculi.

Interfering factors

- Failure to observe pretest dietary restrictions

Vitamin D₃

Vitamin D_3 (cholecalciferol), the major form of vitamin D, is endogenously produced in the skin by the sun's ultraviolet rays and occurs naturally in fish liver oils, egg yolks, liver, and butter. This test, a competitive protein-binding assay, determines serum levels of 25-hydroxycholecalciferol after chromatography has separated it from other vitamin D metabolites and contaminants. It's commonly combined with the measurement of serum calcium and alkaline phosphatase levels.

Purpose
- To evaluate skeletal disease, such as osteomalacia and rickets
- To aid in the diagnosis of hypercalcemia
- To detect vitamin D toxicity
- To monitor therapy with vitamin D_3

Cost
Expensive

Patient preparation
- Explain to the patient that this test measures vitamin D in the body.
- Tell the patient not to eat or drink for 8 to 12 hours before the test.
- Tell the patient that the test requires a blood sample. Explain who will perform the venipuncture and when.
- Explain to the patient that he may experience discomfort from the needle puncture and the tourniquet.
- Restrict medications that may affect test results, such as corticosteroids or anticonvulsants. If they must be continued, note this on the laboratory request.

Reference values
The range for serum 25-hydroxycholecalciferol values is from 10 to 60 ng/ml (SI, 25 to 150 nmol/L).

Abnormal findings
Low or undetectable levels may result from vitamin D deficiency, which can cause osteomalacia or rickets. Such deficiency may stem from poor diet, decreased exposure to the sun, or impaired absorption of vitamin D (secondary to celiac disease, cystic fibrosis, hepatobiliary disease, pancreatitis, or gastric or small-bowel resection). Low levels may also be related to various hepatic, parathyroid, and renal diseases that directly affect vitamin D metabolism.

Elevated levels (> 100 ng/ml [SI, > 250 nmol/L]) may indicate toxicity due to excessive self-medication or prolonged therapy. Elevated levels associated with hypercalcemia may be due to hypersensitivity to vitamin D, as in sarcoidosis.

Interfering factors
- Aluminum hydroxide, anticonvulsants, cholestyramine, colestipol, corticosteroids, isoniazid, and mineral oil (possible decrease)

Voiding cystourethrography

With voiding cystourethrography, a contrast medium is instilled by gentle syringe pressure or gravity into the bladder through a urethral catheter. Fluoroscopic films or overhead radiographs demonstrate bladder filling and then show excretion of the contrast medium as the patient voids.

ALERT! ▼ ▼ ▼ ▼ ▼ ▼ ▼ ▼ ▼

Voiding cystourethrography is contraindicated in patients with an acute or exacerbated urethral or bladder infection or an acute urethral injury. Hypersensitivity to the contrast medium may also contraindicate this test.

Purpose

■ To detect abnormalities of the bladder and urethra, such as vesicoureteral reflux, neurogenic bladder, prostatic hyperplasia, urethral strictures, or diverticula

Cost

Very expensive

Patient preparation

■ Explain to the patient that this test permits assessment of the bladder and urethra.

■ Describe the test for the patient. Inform him that a catheter will be inserted into his bladder and that a contrast medium will be instilled through the catheter.

■ Tell the patient he may experience a feeling of fullness and an urge to void when the contrast medium is instilled. Explain that X-rays will be taken of his bladder and urethra and that he'll be asked to assume various positions.

■ Tell the patient who will perform the test, where it will take place, and its expected duration.

■ Obtain informed consent, if necessary.

■ Check the patient's history for hypersensitivity to contrast media or iodine-containing foods such as shellfish.

■ Tell the patient that he may receive a sedative before the test.

■ Tell the patient that after the test, he should drink plenty of fluids to reduce burning on urination and to flush out any residual contrast medium.

Normal findings

Delineation of the bladder and urethra shows normal structure and function, with no regurgitation of contrast medium into the ureters.

Abnormal findings

Voiding cystourethrography may show cystocele, neurogenic bladder, prostate enlargement, ureterocele, urethral or vesical diverticula, urethral stricture, or vesicoureteral reflux. The severity and location of such abnormalities are then evaluated to determine whether surgical intervention is necessary.

Interfering factors

■ Embarrassment (inhibits patient from voiding on command)

■ Interrupted or less vigorous voiding, muscle spasm, or incomplete sphincter relaxation (due to urethral trauma during catheterization)

■ Presence of contrast media from recent tests, stool, or gas in the bowel (possible poor imaging)

WXYZ

White blood cell count

A white blood cell (WBC) count, also called a *leukocyte count*, is part of a complete blood cell count. It indicates the number of white cells in a microliter (µl, or cubic millimeter) of whole blood.

WBC counts can vary by as much as 2,000 cells/µl (SI, 2×10^9/L) on any given day, due to strenuous exercise, stress, or digestion. The WBC count may increase or decrease significantly with certain diseases, but is diagnostically useful only when the patient's white cell differential and clinical status are considered.

Purpose
- To determine infection or inflammation
- To determine the need for further tests, such as the WBC differential or bone marrow biopsy
- To monitor response to chemotherapy or radiation therapy

Cost
Inexpensive

Patient preparation
- Explain to the patient that the test is used to detect an infection or inflammation.
- Tell the patient that the test requires a blood sample. Explain who will perform the venipuncture and when.
- Explain to the patient that he may experience discomfort from the needle puncture and the tourniquet.
- Inform the patient that he should avoid strenuous exercise for 24 hours before the test. Also tell him that he should avoid eating a heavy meal before the test.
- If the patient is being treated for an infection, advise him that this test will be repeated to monitor his progress.
- Restrict medications that may affect test results. If they must be continued, note this on the laboratory request.

Reference values
The WBC count ranges from 4,000 to 10,000/µl (SI, 4 to 10×10^9/L).

Abnormal findings
An elevated WBC count (leukocytosis) often signals infection, such as an abscess,

meningitis, appendicitis, or tonsillitis. A high count may also result from leukemia or from tissue necrosis due to burns, a myocardial infarction, or gangrene.

A low WBC count (leukopenia) indicates bone marrow depression that may result from viral infections or from toxic reactions, such as those after treatment with an antineoplastic, ingestion of mercury or other heavy metals, or exposure to benzene or arsenicals. Leukopenia characteristically accompanies influenza, typhoid fever, measles, infectious hepatitis, mononucleosis, and rubella.

Interfering factors
■ Exercise, stress, or digestion
■ Most antineoplastics; anti-infectives, such as metronidazole and flucytosine; anticonvulsants such as phenytoin derivatives; thyroid hormone antagonists; and nonsteroidal anti-inflammatory drugs such as indomethacin (decrease)

White blood cell differential

The white blood cell (WBC) differential is used to evaluate the distribution and morphology of WBCs, providing more specific information about a patient's immune system than the WBC count alone.

WBCs are classified as one of five major types of leukocytes — neutrophils, eosinophils, basophils, lymphocytes, and monocytes. The differential count is the percentage of each type of WBC in the blood. The total number of each type of WBC is obtained by multiplying the percentage of each type by the total WBC count.

High levels of these leukocytes are associated with various allergic diseases and reactions to parasites. An eosinophil count is sometimes ordered as a follow-up test when an elevated or depressed eosinophil level is reported.

Purpose
■ To evaluate the body's capacity to resist and overcome infection
■ To detect and identify various types of leukemia (See *LAP stain.*)
■ To determine the stage and severity of an infection
■ To detect allergic reactions and parasitic infections and to assess their severity (eosinophil count)
■ To distinguish viral from bacterial infections

Cost
Moderately expensive

Patient preparation
■ Explain to the patient that this test is used to evaluate the immune system.
■ Restrict medications that may affect test results. If they must be continued, note this on the laboratory request.
■ Tell the patient that the test requires a blood sample. Explain who will perform the venipuncture and when.
■ Explain to the patient that he may experience discomfort from the needle puncture and the tourniquet.
■ Inform the patient that he doesn't need to restrict food and fluids but should refrain from strenuous exercise for 24 hours before the test.

Reference values
For normal values for the five types of WBCs classified in the differential for adults and children, see *Interpreting WBC differential values,* page 414.

LAP stain

Levels of leukocyte alkaline phosphatase (LAP), an enzyme found in neutrophils, may be altered by infection, stress, chronic inflammatory diseases, Hodgkin's disease, and hematologic disorders. Most of these conditions elevate LAP levels; only a few, notably chronic myelogenous leukemia (CML), depress them. Thus, this test is most commonly used to differentiate CML from other disorders that produce an elevated white blood cell count.

Procedure

To perform this test, a blood sample is obtained by venipuncture or fingerstick. The venous blood sample is collected in a 7-ml EDTA tube and transported immediately to the laboratory, where a blood smear is prepared. The peripheral blood sample is smeared on a 3″ (7.6 cm) glass slide and fixed in cold formalin-methanol. The blood smear is then stained to show the amount of LAP present in the cytoplasm of the neutrophils. One-hundred neutrophils are counted and assessed; each is as-signed a score of 0 to 4, according to the degree of LAP staining. Normally, values for LAP range from 40 to 100, depending on the laboratory's standards.

Implications of results

Depressed LAP values typically indicate CML; however, values may also be low in patients with paroxysmal nocturnal hemoglobinuria, aplastic anemia, and infectious mononucleosis. Elevated levels may indicate Hodgkin's disease, polycythemia vera, or a neutrophilic leukemoid reaction — a response to such conditions as infection, chronic inflammation, or pregnancy.

After a diagnosis of CML, the LAP stain may also be used to help detect the onset of the blastic phase of the disease, when LAP levels typically rise. However, LAP levels also increase toward normal in response to therapy; because of this, test results must be correlated with the patient's condition.

For an accurate diagnosis, differential test results must always be interpreted in relation to the total WBC count.

Abnormal findings

Abnormal differential patterns provide evidence for a wide range of disease states and other conditions. (See *Influence of disease on blood cell count,* pages 415 and 416.)

Interfering factors

■ Failure to completely fill the collection tube, to use the proper anticoagulant, or to adequately mix the sample and the anticoagulant

■ Desipramine and methysergide (increase or decrease eosinophil count)
■ Indomethacin and procainamide (decrease eosinophil count)
■ Anticonvulsants, capreomycin, cephalosporins, D-penicillamine, gold compounds, isoniazid, nalidixic acid, novobiocin, para-aminosalicylic acid, paromomycin, penicillins, phenothiazines, rifampin, streptomycin, sulfonamides, and tetracyclines (increase eosinophil count by provoking an allergic reaction)

Wound culture

Performed to confirm infection, a wound culture is a microscopic analysis of a specimen from a lesion. Wound cultures may be aerobic, for detection of organisms that usually appear in a superficial wound, or anaerobic, for organisms that need little or no oxygen and appear in areas of poor tissue perfusion, such as postoperative wounds, ulcers, and compound fractures. Indications for wound culture include fever as well as inflammation and drainage in damaged tissue.

Purpose
■ To identify an infectious microbe in a wound

Cost
Inexpensive

Patient preparation
■ Explain to the patient that this test is used to identify infectious microbes.
■ Describe the procedure to the patient. Inform him that drainage from the wound is withdrawn by a syringe or removed on sterile cotton swabs.
■ Tell him who will perform the procedure, where it will take place, and its expected duration.

Normal findings
Normally, no pathogenic organisms are present in a clean wound.

Abnormal findings
The most common aerobic pathogens for wound infection include *Staphylococcus aureus,* group A beta-hemolytic streptococci, *Proteus, Escherichia coli* and other Enterobacteriaceae, and some *Pseudomonas* species; the most common anaerobic

Influence of disease on blood cell count

CELL TYPE	CELL COUNT
Neutrophils 	*Increased by:* ■ Infections: chickenpox, endocarditis, herpes, gonorrhea, osteomyelitis, otitis media, Rocky Mountain spotted fever, salpingitis, septicemia, smallpox ■ Burns, carcinoma, ischemic necrosis due to myocardial infarction ■ Metabolic disorders: diabetic acidosis, eclampsia, thyrotoxicosis, uremia ■ Stress response due to acute hemorrhage, childbirth, emotional distress, excessive exercise, surgery, third trimester of pregnancy ■ Inflammatory disease: acute gout, myositis, rheumatic fever, rheumatoid arthritis, vasculitis *Decreased by:* ■ Bone marrow depression due to cytotoxic drugs or radiation ■ Infections: brucellosis, hepatitis, infectious mononucleosis, influenza, measles, mumps, rubella, tularemia, typhoid ■ Hypersplenism: hepatic disease and storage diseases ■ Collagen vascular disease, such as systemic lupus erythematosus ■ Deficiency of folic acid or vitamin B_{12}
Eosinophils	*Increased by:* ■ Allergic disorders: angioneurotic edema, asthma, food or drug sensitivity, hay fever, serum sickness ■ Parasitic infections: amebiasis, hookworm, roundworm, trichinosis ■ Skin diseases: dermatitis, eczema, herpes, pemphigus, psoriasis ■ Neoplastic diseases: chronic myelocytic leukemia, Hodgkin's disease, metastases and necrosis of solid tumors ■ Miscellaneous: adrenocortical hypofunction, collagen vascular disease, excessive exercise, pernicious anemia, polyarteritis nodosa, post-splenectomy, scarlet fever, sickle cell disease, ulcerative colitis *Decreased by:* ■ Stress response due to burns, mental distress, shock, surgery, trauma ■ Cushing's syndrome, infectious mononucleosis
Basophils	*Increased by:* ■ Some chronic hemolytic anemias, chronic hypersensitivity states, chronic myelocytic leukemia, Hodgkin's disease, myxedema, nephrosis, polycythemia vera, systemic mastocytosis, ulcerative colitis *Decreased by:* ■ Hyperthyroidism ■ Pregnancy, ovulation ■ Stress
Lymphocytes	*Increased by:* ■ Infections: brucellosis, cytomegalovirus, hepatitis, infectious mononucleosis, mumps, pertussis, rubella, syphilis, tuberculosis ■ Addison's disease, hypoadrenalism, immune diseases, lymphocytic leukemia, thyrotoxicosis, ulcerative colitis *Decreased by:* ■ Severe debilitating illness, such as heart failure, renal failure, advanced tuberculosis ■ Defective lymphatic circulation, high levels of adrenal corticosteroids, immunodeficiency due to immunosuppressants

(continued)

CELL TYPE	CELL COUNT
Monocytes 	*Increased by:* ■ Infections: hepatitis, malaria, Rocky Mountain spotted fever, subacute bacterial endocarditis, tuberculosis ■ Collagen vascular disease: polyarteritis nodosa, rheumatoid arthritis, systemic lupus erythematosus ■ Carcinomas ■ Monocytic leukemia ■ Lymphomas *Decreased by:* ■ Hairy cell leukemia ■ Human immunodeficiency virus infection ■ Rheumatoid arthritis ■ Prednisone therapy

pathogens include some *Clostridium, Peptococcus, Bacteroides,* and *Streptococcus* species.

Interfering factors

■ Failure to report recent or current antimicrobial therapy (possible false-negative)
■ Failure to use proper collection technique
■ Failure to use the proper transport medium, allowing the specimen to dry and the bacteria to deteriorate

PART THREE

Disease flowcharts to guide test selection

In today's fast-paced working environment, time is one of your most precious commodities. The faster you handle your patient load, the better. Proper use of medical flowcharts, also known as algorithms, can help you diagnose your patients quickly and accurately.

In this section, you'll review the flowcharts that are most commonly used in the clinical setting. Beginning with signs and symptoms or laboratory values, you'll be guided through the appropriate steps of test selection and interpretation that will lead you to a proper patient diagnosis.

Abbreviations used in Part Three

The following list shows abbreviations that are used throughout Part Three.

ACTH	Adrenocorticotropic hormone	NG	Nasogastric
ANA	Antinuclear antibody	PT	Prothrombin time
BP	Blood pressure	PTH	Parathyroid hormone
BUN	Blood urea nitrogen	PTT	Partial thromboplastin time
CRH	Corticotropin-releasing hormone	RAIU	Radioactive iodine uptake test
CT	Computed tomography	RBC	Red blood cell
ESR	Erythrocyte sedimentation rate	SIADH	Syndrome of inappropriate antidiuretic hormone secretion
FSH	Follicle-stimulating hormone		
GI	Gastrointestinal	T_3	Triiodothyronine
Hb A_2	Hemoglobin electrophoresis	T_4	Thyroxine
HCG	Human chorionic gonadotropin	TIBC	Total iron-binding capacity
HIV	Human immunodeficiency virus	TRH	Thyrotropin-releasing hormone
HPF	High-powered field	TS	Transferrin saturation
IVP	Intravenous pyelogram	TSH	Thyroid-stimulating hormone
LDH	Lactate dehydrogenase	UTI	Urinary tract infection
LH	Luteinizing hormone	VDRL	Venereal Disease Research Laboratory test
MCV	Mean corpuscular volume		
Mg	Magnesium	WBC	White blood cell
MMA	Methylmalonic acid		
MRI	Magnetic resonance imaging		

Adrenal insufficiency

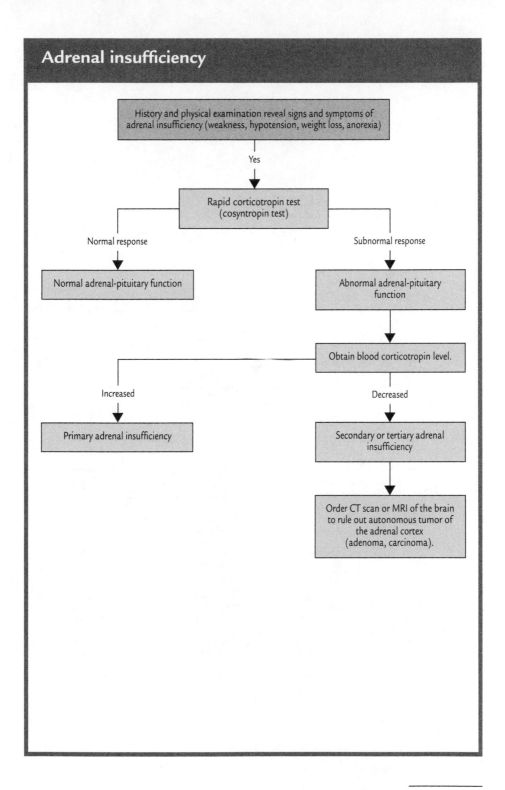

History and physical examination reveal signs and symptoms of
adrenal insufficiency (weakness, hypotension, weight loss, anorexia)

Yes

Rapid corticotropin test
(cosyntropin test)

Normal response

Normal adrenal-pituitary function

Subnormal response

Abnormal adrenal-pituitary
function

Obtain blood corticotropin level.

Increased

Primary adrenal insufficiency

Decreased

Secondary or tertiary adrenal
insufficiency

Order CT scan or MRI of the brain
to rule out autonomous tumor of
the adrenal cortex
(adenoma, carcinoma).

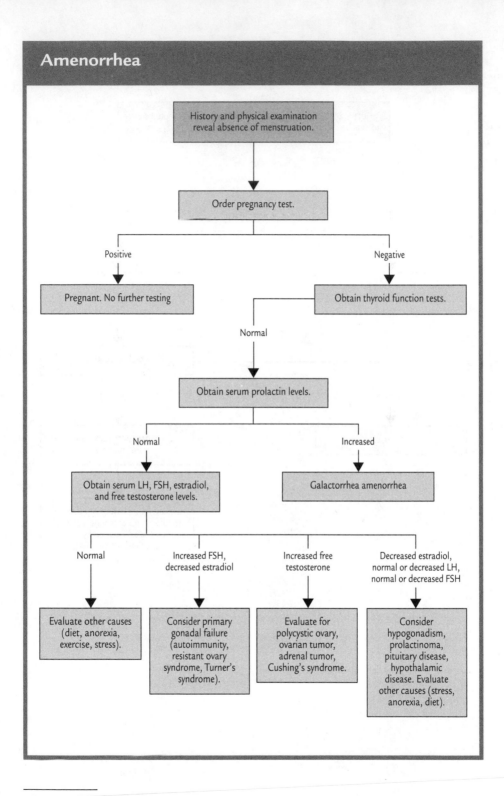

Amenorrhea

History and physical examination reveal absence of menstruation.

↓

Order pregnancy test.

Positive → Pregnant. No further testing

Negative → Obtain thyroid function tests.

Normal

↓

Obtain serum prolactin levels.

Normal → Obtain serum LH, FSH, estradiol, and free testosterone levels.

Increased → Galactorrhea amenorrhea

Normal → Evaluate other causes (diet, anorexia, exercise, stress).

Increased FSH, decreased estradiol → Consider primary gonadal failure (autoimmunity, resistant ovary syndrome, Turner's syndrome).

Increased free testosterone → Evaluate for polycystic ovary, ovarian tumor, adrenal tumor, Cushing's syndrome.

Decreased estradiol, normal or decreased LH, normal or decreased FSH → Consider hypogonadism, prolactinoma, pituitary disease, hypothalamic disease. Evaluate other causes (stress, anorexia, diet).

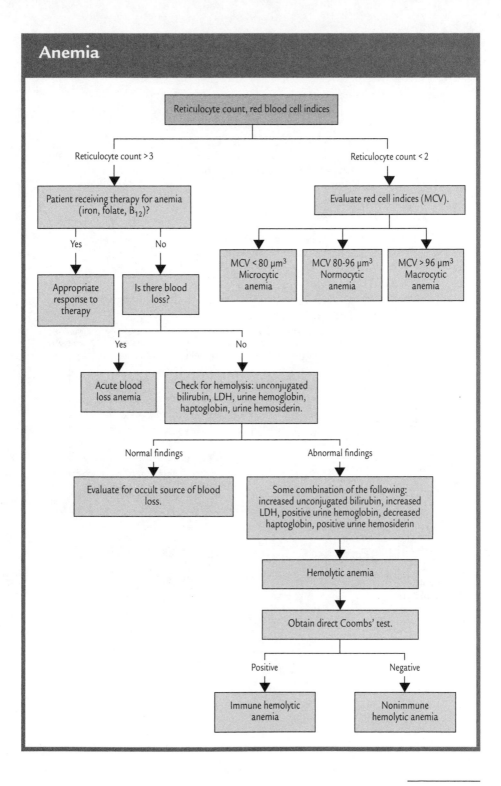

Anemia, macrocytic

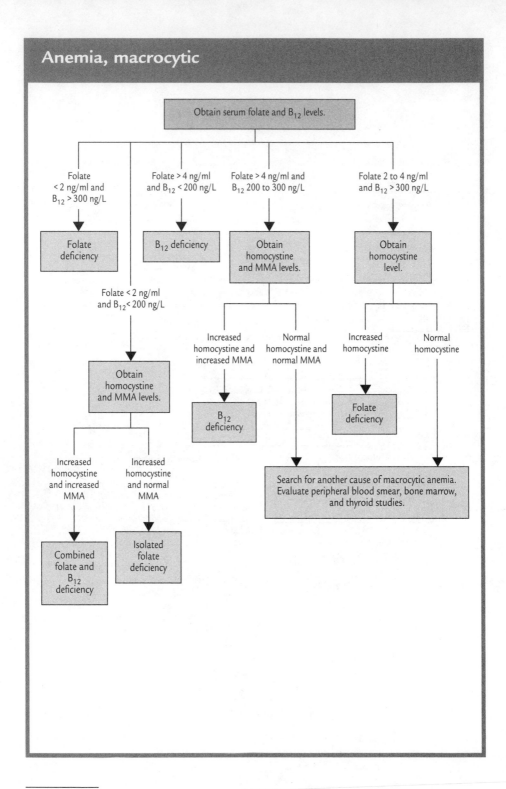

Anemia, microcytic

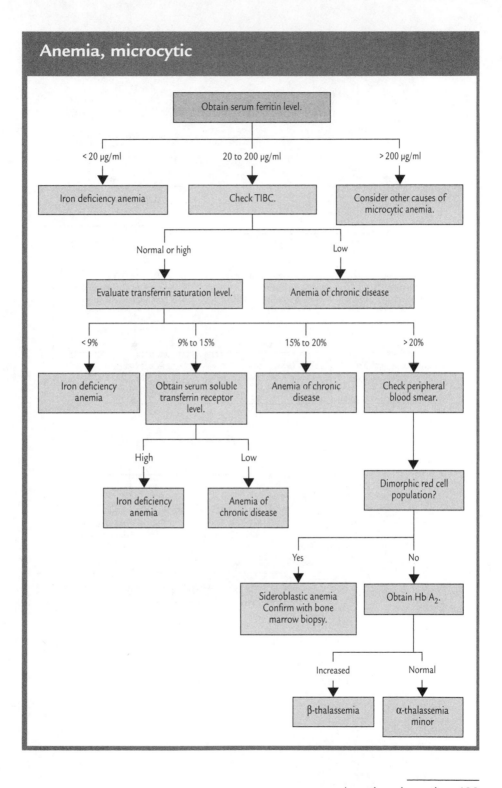

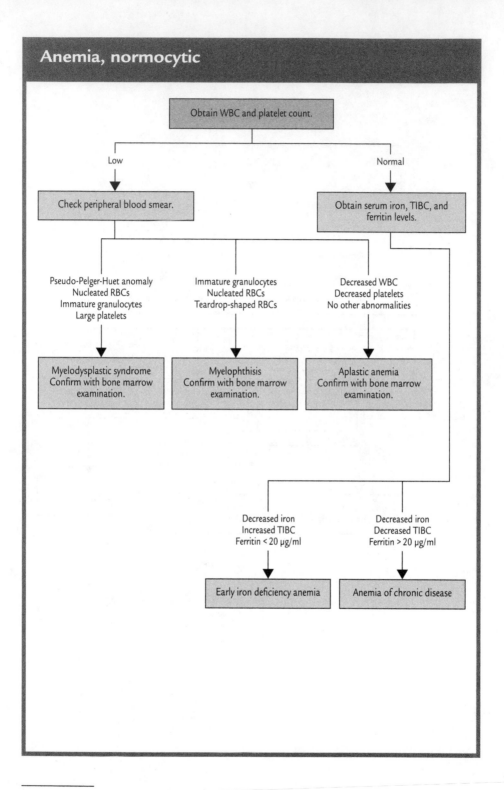

Cushing's syndrome

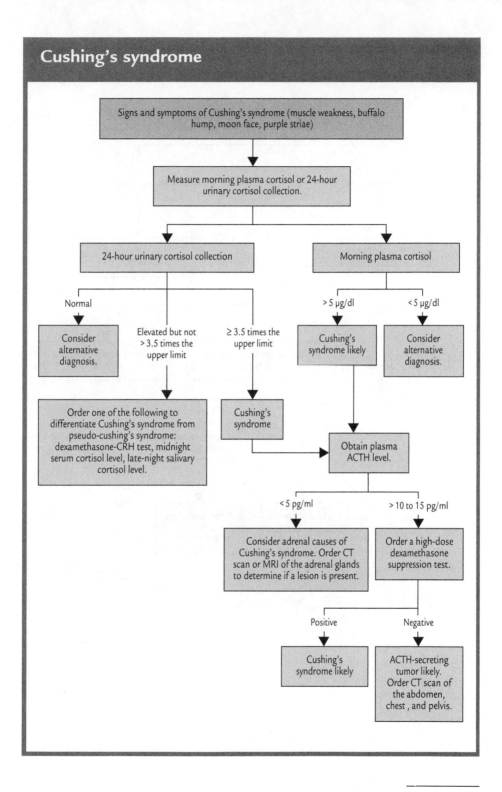

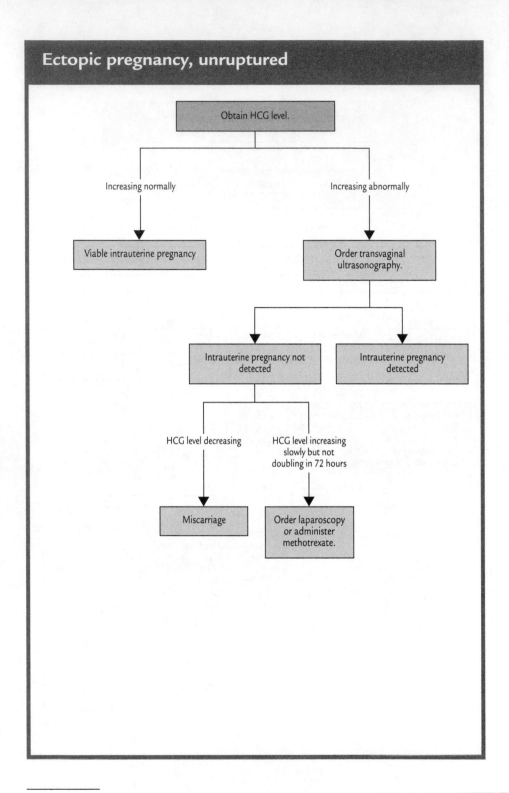

Hematuria

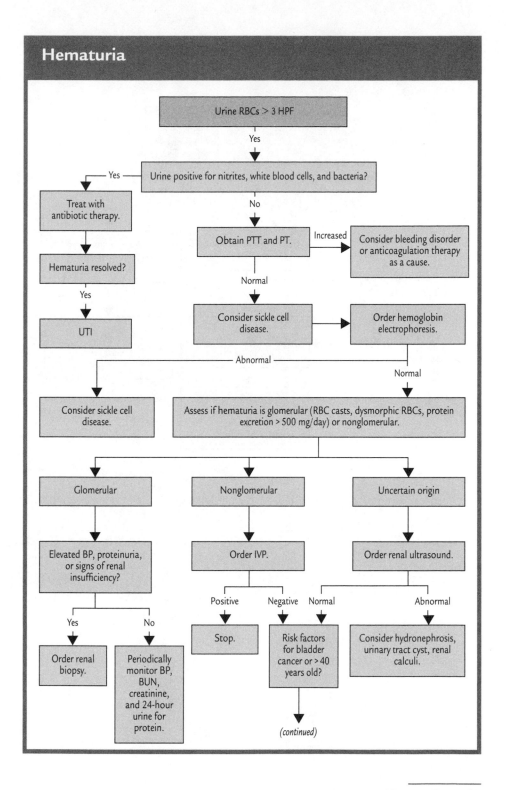

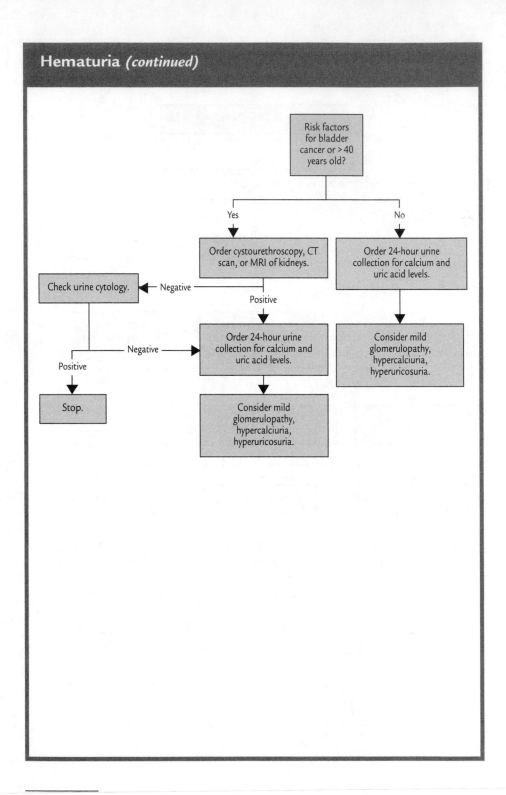

Hemochromatosis

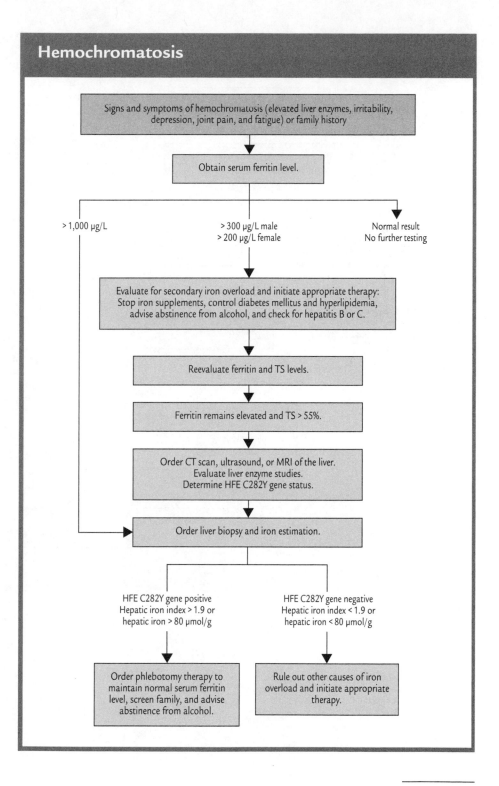

Signs and symptoms of hemochromatosis (elevated liver enzymes, irritability, depression, joint pain, and fatigue) or family history

Obtain serum ferritin level.

> 1,000 µg/L

> 300 µg/L male
> 200 µg/L female

Normal result
No further testing

Evaluate for secondary iron overload and initiate appropriate therapy: Stop iron supplements, control diabetes mellitus and hyperlipidemia, advise abstinence from alcohol, and check for hepatitis B or C.

Reevaluate ferritin and TS levels.

Ferritin remains elevated and TS > 55%.

Order CT scan, ultrasound, or MRI of the liver.
Evaluate liver enzyme studies.
Determine HFE C282Y gene status.

Order liver biopsy and iron estimation.

HFE C282Y gene positive
Hepatic iron index > 1.9 or
hepatic iron > 80 µmol/g

HFE C282Y gene negative
Hepatic iron index < 1.9 or
hepatic iron < 80 µmol/g

Order phlebotomy therapy to maintain normal serum ferritin level, screen family, and advise abstinence from alcohol.

Rule out other causes of iron overload and initiate appropriate therapy.

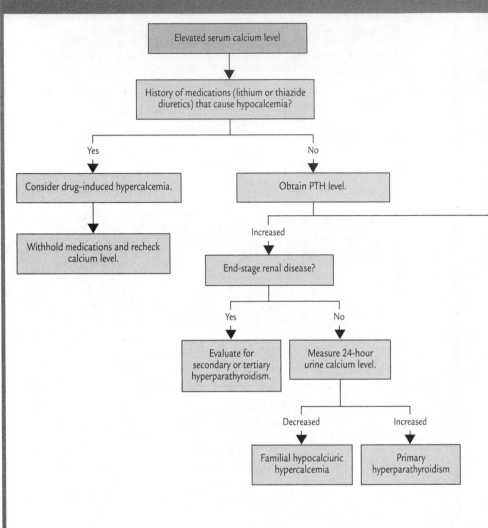

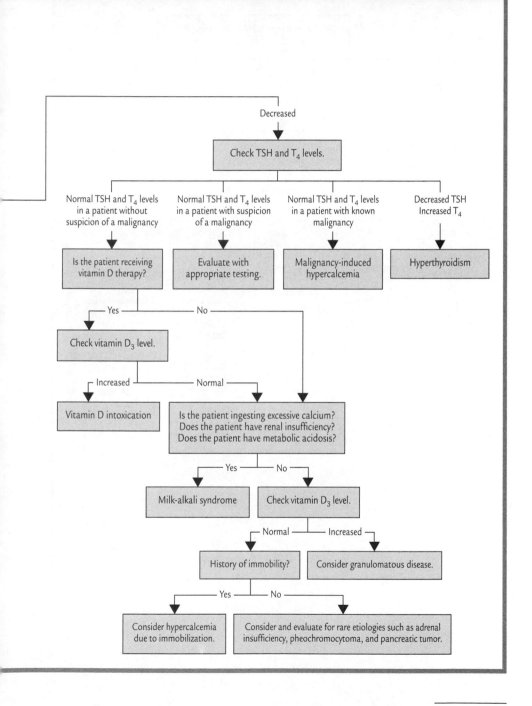

Hypernatremia

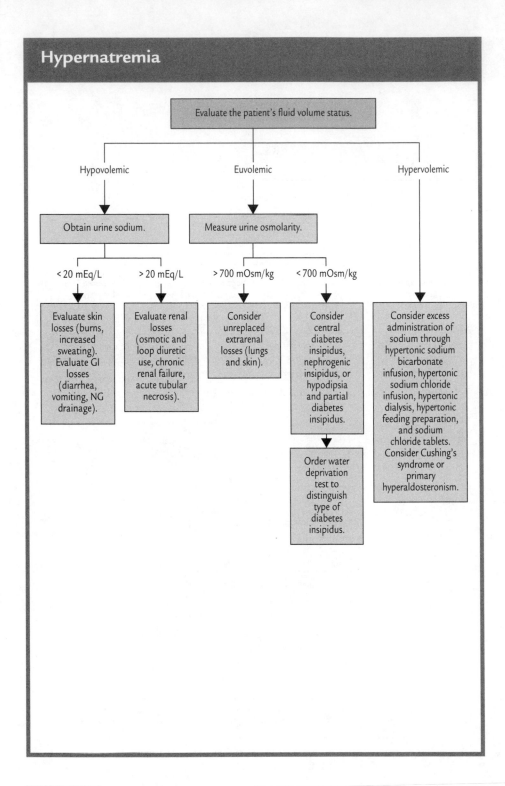

Evaluate the patient's fluid volume status.

Hypovolemic — Euvolemic — Hypervolemic

Obtain urine sodium.

Measure urine osmolarity.

< 20 mEq/L — > 20 mEq/L — > 700 mOsm/kg — < 700 mOsm/kg

Evaluate skin losses (burns, increased sweating). Evaluate GI losses (diarrhea, vomiting, NG drainage).

Evaluate renal losses (osmotic and loop diuretic use, chronic renal failure, acute tubular necrosis).

Consider unreplaced extrarenal losses (lungs and skin).

Consider central diabetes insipidus, nephrogenic insipidus, or hypodipsia and partial diabetes insipidus.

Order water deprivation test to distinguish type of diabetes insipidus.

Consider excess administration of sodium through hypertonic sodium bicarbonate infusion, hypertonic sodium chloride infusion, hypertonic dialysis, hypertonic feeding preparation, and sodium chloride tablets. Consider Cushing's syndrome or primary hyperaldosteronism.

Hyperthyroidism

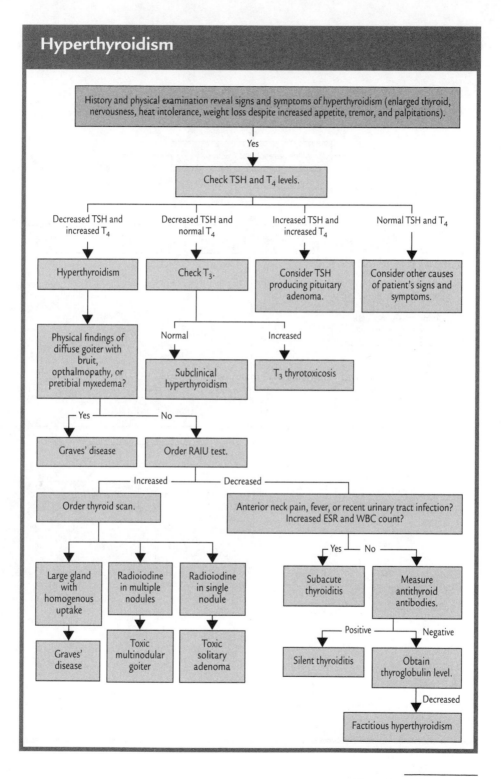

History and physical examination reveal signs and symptoms of hyperthyroidism (enlarged thyroid, nervousness, heat intolerance, weight loss despite increased appetite, tremor, and palpitations).

Yes

Check TSH and T_4 levels.

Decreased TSH and increased T_4 → Hyperthyroidism

Decreased TSH and normal T_4 → Check T_3.

Increased TSH and increased T_4 → Consider TSH producing pituitary adenoma.

Normal TSH and T_4 → Consider other causes of patient's signs and symptoms.

Hyperthyroidism → Physical findings of diffuse goiter with bruit, opthalmopathy, or pretibial myxedema?

Check T_3:
- Normal → Subclinical hyperthyroidism
- Increased → T_3 thyrotoxicosis

Physical findings of diffuse goiter with bruit, opthalmopathy, or pretibial myxedema?
- Yes → Graves' disease
- No → Order RAIU test.

Order RAIU test.
- Increased → Order thyroid scan.
- Decreased → Anterior neck pain, fever, or recent urinary tract infection? Increased ESR and WBC count?

Order thyroid scan.
- Large gland with homogenous uptake → Graves' disease
- Radioiodine in multiple nodules → Toxic multinodular goiter
- Radioiodine in single nodule → Toxic solitary adenoma

Anterior neck pain, fever, or recent urinary tract infection? Increased ESR and WBC count?
- Yes → Subacute thyroiditis
- No → Measure antithyroid antibodies.

Measure antithyroid antibodies.
- Positive → Silent thyroiditis
- Negative → Obtain thyroglobulin level.

Obtain thyroglobulin level.
- Decreased → Factitious hyperthyroidism

Hypocalcemia

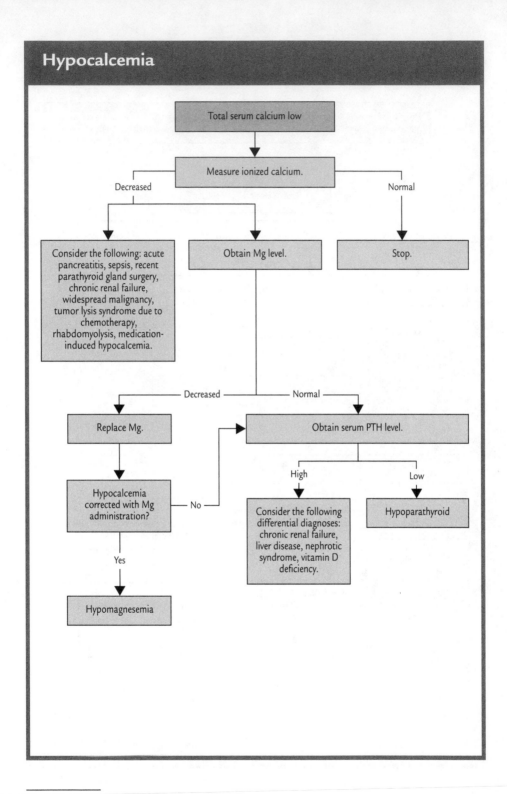

Hypoglycemia

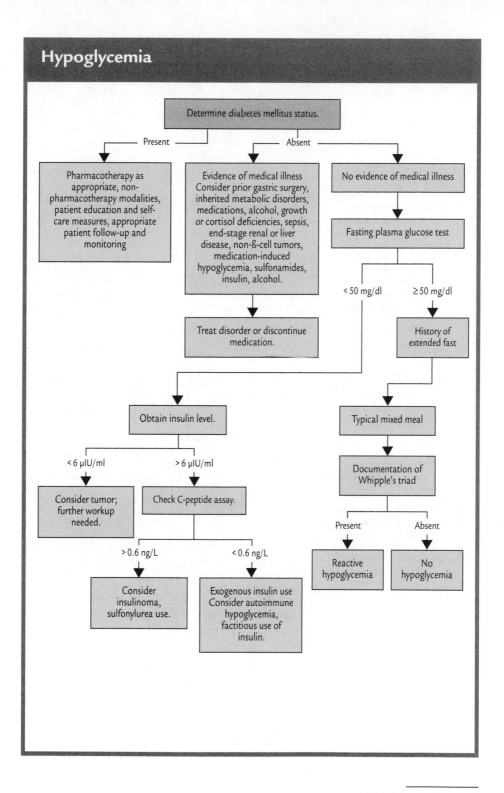

Hyponatremia

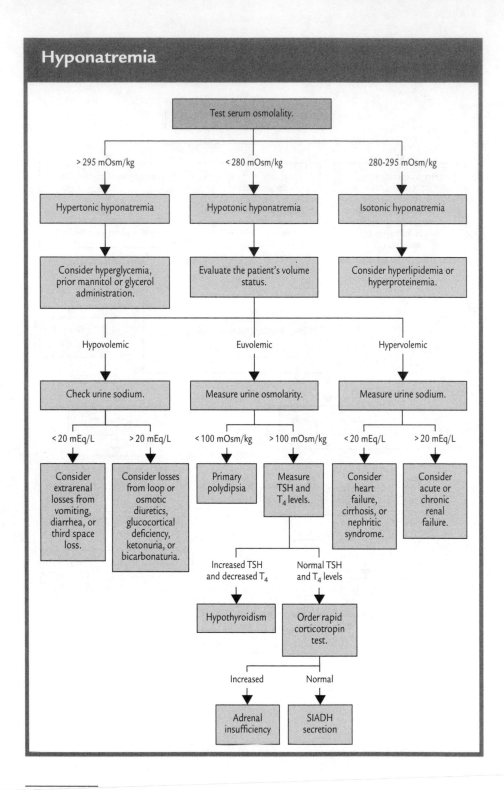

Hypothyroidism

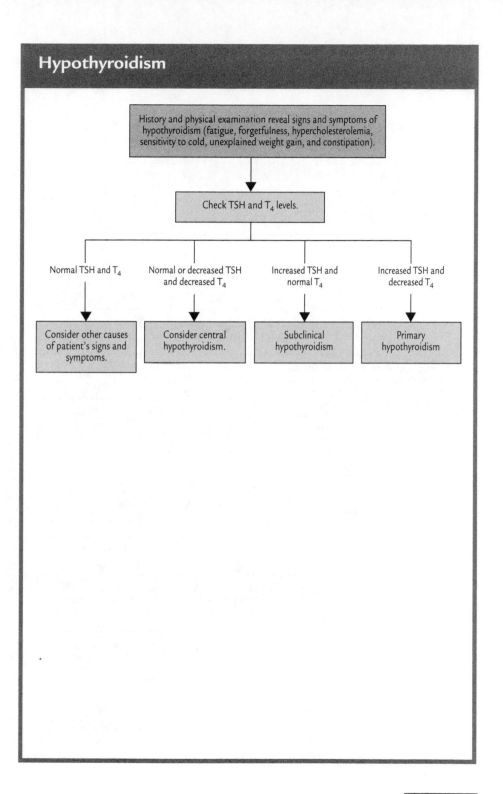

History and physical examination reveal signs and symptoms of hypothyroidism (fatigue, forgetfulness, hypercholesterolemia, sensitivity to cold, unexplained weight gain, and constipation).

Check TSH and T_4 levels.

Normal TSH and T_4

Normal or decreased TSH and decreased T_4

Increased TSH and normal T_4

Increased TSH and decreased T_4

Consider other causes of patient's signs and symptoms.

Consider central hypothyroidism.

Subclinical hypothyroidism

Primary hypothyroidism

Proteinuria

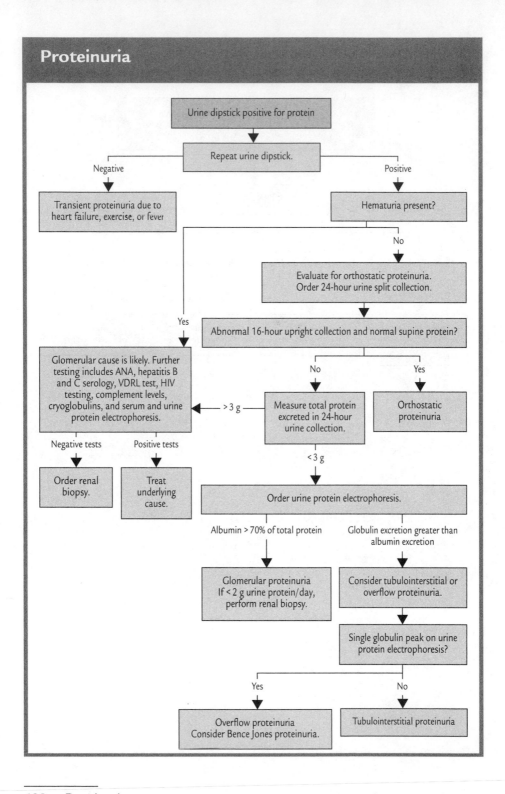

Urine dipstick positive for protein

↓

Repeat urine dipstick.

Negative → Transient proteinuria due to heart failure, exercise, or fever

Positive → Hematuria present?

No ↓

Evaluate for orthostatic proteinuria. Order 24-hour urine split collection.

↓

Abnormal 16-hour upright collection and normal supine protein?

No → Measure total protein excreted in 24-hour urine collection.

Yes → Orthostatic proteinuria

Yes →
Glomerular cause is likely. Further testing includes ANA, hepatitis B and C serology, VDRL test, HIV testing, complement levels, cryoglobulins, and serum and urine protein electrophoresis.

> 3 g → Glomerular cause is likely...

Negative tests → Order renal biopsy.

Positive tests → Treat underlying cause.

< 3 g ↓

Order urine protein electrophoresis.

Albumin > 70% of total protein → Glomerular proteinuria If < 2 g urine protein/day, perform renal biopsy.

Globulin excretion greater than albumin excretion → Consider tubulointerstitial or overflow proteinuria.

↓

Single globulin peak on urine protein electrophoresis?

Yes → Overflow proteinuria Consider Bence Jones proteinuria.

No → Tubulointerstitial proteinuria

ECG Interpretation

Normal ECG   441

Arrhythmias   444

12-lead ECGs   463

Normal ECG

How to read any ECG: An 8-step guide

An electrocardiogram (ECG) waveform has three basic elements: a P wave, a QRS com-plex, and a T wave. They're joined by five other useful diagnostic elements: the PR interval, the U wave, the ST segment, the J point, and the QT interval. The diagram below shows how these elements are related.

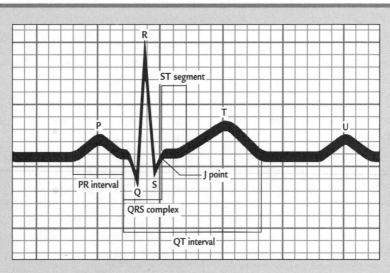

The following 8-step guide will enable you to read any electrocardiogram (ECG).

Step 1: Evaluate the P wave

Observe the P wave's size, shape, and location in the waveform. If the P wave consistently precedes the QRS complex, the sinoatrial (SA) node is initiating the electrical impulse, as it should be.

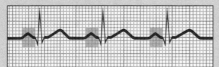

Step 2: Evaluate the atrial rhythm

The P wave should occur at regular intervals, with only small variations associated with respiration. Using a pair of calipers, you can easily measure the interval between P waves — the P-P interval. Compare the P-P intervals in several ECG cycles. Make sure that the calipers are set at the same point — at the beginning of the wave or on its peak. Instead of lifting the calipers, rotate one of the legs to the next P wave, to ensure accurate measurements. If the P-P interval is consistent, the atrial rhythm is regular.

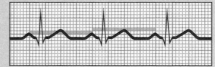

Step 3: Determine the atrial rate

To determine the atrial rate quickly, count the number of P waves in two 3-second segments. Multiply this number by 10. For a more accurate determination, count the number of small squares between two P waves, using either the

(continued)

(continued)

apex of the wave or the initial upstroke of the wave. Each small square equals 0.04 second; 1,500 squares equal 1 minute (0.04 × 1,500 = 60 seconds). So, divide 1,500 by the number of squares you counted between the P waves. This gives you the atrial rate — the number of contractions per minute.

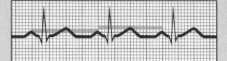

Step 6: Determine the ventricular rate

To determine the ventricular rate, use the same formula as in Step 3. In this case, however, count the number of small squares between two R waves to do the calculation. Also, check that the QRS complex is shaped appropriately for the lead you're monitoring.

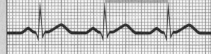

Step 4: Calculate duration of the PR interval

Count the number of small squares between the beginning of the P wave and the beginning of the QRS complex. Multiply the number of squares by 0.04 second. The normal interval is between 0.12 and 0.20 second, or between 3 and 5 small squares wide. A wider interval indicates delayed conduction of the impulse through the atrioventricular node to the ventricles. A short PR interval indicates the impulse originated in an area other than the SA node.

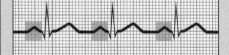

Step 7: Calculate the duration of the QRS complex

Count the number of squares between the beginning and the end of the QRS complex and multiply by 0.04 second. A normal QRS complex is less than 0.12 second, or less than 3 small squares wide. Some references specify 0.06 to 0.10 second as the normal duration for the QRS complex.

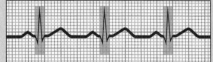

Step 8: Calculate the duration of the QT interval

Count the number of squares from the beginning of the QRS complex to the end of the T wave. Multiply this number by 0.04 second. The normal range is 0.36 to 0.44 second, or 9 to 11 small squares wide when the rate is 60 to 100. Otherwise, the QT interval will be different and must be calculated for rate.

Step 5: Evaluate the ventricular rhythm

Use the calipers to measure the R-R intervals. Remember to place the calipers on the same point of the QRS complex. If the R-R intervals remain consistent, the ventricular rhythm is regular.

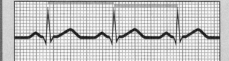

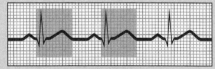

Normal sinus rhythm

When the heart functions normally, the sinoatrial (SA) node acts as the primary pacemaker, initiating the electrical impulses that set the rhythm for cardiac contractions. The SA node assumes this role because its automatic firing rate (automaticity) exceeds that of the heart's other pacemakers, allowing cells to depolarize spontaneously. Two factors account for increased automaticity. First, during the resting phase of the depolarization-repolarization cycle, SA node cells have the least negative charge. Second, depolarization actually begins during the resting phase.

Based on the location of the electrical disturbance, an arrhythmia can be classified as a sinus, atrial, junctional, or ventricular arrhythmia or as an atrioventricular (AV) block. Functional disturbances in the SA node produce sinus arrhythmias. Enhanced automaticity of atrial tissue or reentry of electrical impulses may produce atrial arrhythmias, the most common arrhythmias.

Junctional arrhythmias originate in the area around the AV node and the bundle of His. These arrhythmias usually result from a suppressed higher pacemaker or blocked impulses at the AV node.

Ventricular arrhythmias originate in ventricular tissue below the bifurcation of the bundle of His. These rhythms may result from reentry, enhanced automaticity, or after depolarization.

An AV block results from an abnormal interruption or delay of an atrial impulse conduction to the ventricles. It may be partial or total and may occur in the AV node, bundle of His, or Purkinje system.

Characteristics and interpretation

Regular rhythm ___ P wave ___ QRS complex

LEAD II

Atrial rhythm: regular
Ventricular rhythm: regular
Atrial rate: 60 to 100 beats/minute (80 beats/minute shown)
Ventricular rate: 60 to 100 beats/minute (80 beats/minute shown)
P wave: normally shaped (All P waves have a similar size and shape; a P wave precedes each QRS complex.)
PR interval: within normal limits (0.12 to 0.20 second) and constant (0.20-second duration shown)

QRS complex: within normal limits (0.06 to 0.10 second) (All QRS complexes have the same configuration. The duration shown here is 0.12 second.)
T wave: normally shaped; upright and rounded (Each QRS complex is followed by a T wave.)
QT interval: within normal limits (0.36 to 0.44 second) and constant (0.44-second duration shown)

Arrhythmias

Sinus arrhythmia

In sinus arrhythmia, the heart rate stays within normal limits, but the rhythm is irregular and corresponds to the respiratory cycle and variations in vagal tone. During inspiration, an increased volume of blood returns to the heart, reducing vagal tone and increasing sinus rate. During expiration, venous return decreases, vagal tone increases, and sinus rate slows.

Conditions unrelated to respiration may also produce sinus arrhythmia. These conditions include an inferior-wall myocardial infarction, digoxin toxicity, and increased intracranial pressure.

Sinus arrhythmia is easily recognized in elderly, pediatric, and sedated patients. The patient's pulse rate increases with inspiration and decreases with expiration. Usually, the patient is asymptomatic.

Intervention

Treatment usually isn't necessary, unless the patient is symptomatic or the sinus arrhythmia stems from an underlying cause. If the patient is symptomatic and his heart rate falls below 40 beats/minute, atropine may be administered.

Characteristics and interpretation

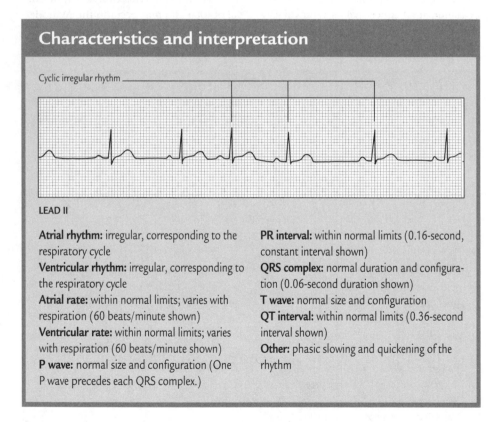

Cyclic irregular rhythm

LEAD II

Atrial rhythm: irregular, corresponding to the respiratory cycle

Ventricular rhythm: irregular, corresponding to the respiratory cycle

Atrial rate: within normal limits; varies with respiration (60 beats/minute shown)

Ventricular rate: within normal limits; varies with respiration (60 beats/minute shown)

P wave: normal size and configuration (One P wave precedes each QRS complex.)

PR interval: within normal limits (0.16-second, constant interval shown)

QRS complex: normal duration and configuration (0.06-second duration shown)

T wave: normal size and configuration

QT interval: within normal limits (0.36-second interval shown)

Other: phasic slowing and quickening of the rhythm

Sinus bradycardia

Characterized by a sinus rate of less than 60 beats/minute, sinus bradycardia usually occurs as the normal response to a reduced demand for blood flow. It's common among athletes, whose well-conditioned hearts can maintain stroke volume with reduced effort. Certain drugs — such as cardiac glycosides, calcium channel blockers, and beta-adrenergic blockers — may cause sinus bradycardia. It may occur after an inferior-wall myocardial infarction involving the right coronary artery, which provides the blood supply to the sinoatrial node. The rhythm may develop during sleep and in patients with increased intracranial pressure. It may also result from vagal stimulation during vomiting or defecation. Pathological sinus bradycardia may occur with sick sinus syndrome.

A patient with sinus bradycardia is asymptomatic if he's able to compensate for the drop in heart rate by increasing stroke volume. If not, he may have signs and symptoms of decreased cardiac output, such as hypotension, syncope, confusion, and blurred vision.

Intervention

If the patient is asymptomatic, treatment isn't necessary. If he has signs and symptoms, treatment aims to identify and correct the underlying cause. The heart rate may be increased with atropine. A temporary or permanent pacemaker may be inserted if the bradycardia persists. A transcutaneous pacemaker can also be applied and used.

Characteristics and interpretation

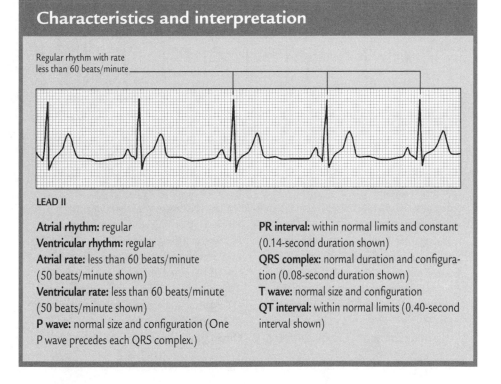

Regular rhythm with rate less than 60 beats/minute

LEAD II

Atrial rhythm: regular
Ventricular rhythm: regular
Atrial rate: less than 60 beats/minute (50 beats/minute shown)
Ventricular rate: less than 60 beats/minute (50 beats/minute shown)
P wave: normal size and configuration (One P wave precedes each QRS complex.)

PR interval: within normal limits and constant (0.14-second duration shown)
QRS complex: normal duration and configuration (0.08-second duration shown)
T wave: normal size and configuration
QT interval: within normal limits (0.40-second interval shown)

Sinus tachycardia

Sinus tachycardia is defined as a sinus rhythm ranging from 100 to 160 beats/minute. Sinus tachycardia is a normal response to cellular demands for increased oxygen delivery and blood flow. Conditions that cause such a demand include heart failure, shock, anemia, exercise, fever, hypoxia, pain, and stress. Drugs that stimulate the beta receptors in the heart also cause sinus tachycardia. They include isoproterenol (Isuprel), aminophylline (Phyllocontin), and inotropic agents such as dobutamine. Alcohol, caffeine, and nicotine may also produce sinus tachycardia.

An elevated heart rate increases myocardial oxygen demands. If the patient can't meet these demands (for example, because of coronary artery disease), ischemia and further myocardial damage may occur. If tachycardia exceeds 140 beats/minute for longer than 30 minutes, the electrocardiogram may show ST-segment and T-wave changes, indicating ischemia.

Intervention

Treatment focuses on finding the primary cause. If the cause is high catecholamine levels, a beta-adrenergic blocker or calcium channel blocker may slow the heart rate. After myocardial infarction, persistent sinus tachycardia may precede heart failure or cardiogenic shock.

Characteristics and interpretation

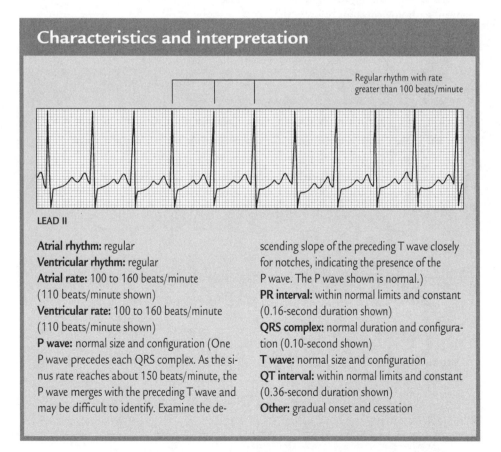

Regular rhythm with rate greater than 100 beats/minute

LEAD II

Atrial rhythm: regular
Ventricular rhythm: regular
Atrial rate: 100 to 160 beats/minute (110 beats/minute shown)
Ventricular rate: 100 to 160 beats/minute (110 beats/minute shown)
P wave: normal size and configuration (One P wave precedes each QRS complex. As the sinus rate reaches about 150 beats/minute, the P wave merges with the preceding T wave and may be difficult to identify. Examine the descending slope of the preceding T wave closely for notches, indicating the presence of the P wave. The P wave shown is normal.)
PR interval: within normal limits and constant (0.16-second duration shown)
QRS complex: normal duration and configuration (0.10-second shown)
T wave: normal size and configuration
QT interval: within normal limits and constant (0.36-second duration shown)
Other: gradual onset and cessation

Sinus arrest

Failure of the sinoatrial node to generate an impulse interrupts the sinus rhythm, producing "sinus pause" when one or two beats are dropped or "sinus arrest" when three or more beats are dropped. Such failure may result from an acute inferior-wall myocardial infarction, increased vagal tone, or use of certain drugs (cardiac glycosides, calcium channel blockers, and beta-adrenergic blockers). The arrhythmia may also be linked to sick sinus syndrome. The patient has an irregular pulse rate associat-ed with the sinus rhythm pauses. If the pauses are infrequent, the patient may be asymptomatic. If they occur frequently or last for several seconds, the patient may have signs of decreased cardiac output (CO).

Intervention

For a symptomatic patient, treatment focuses on maintaining CO and discovering the cause of the sinus arrest. If indicated, atropine may be given or a temporary or permanent pacemaker may be inserted.

Characteristics and interpretation

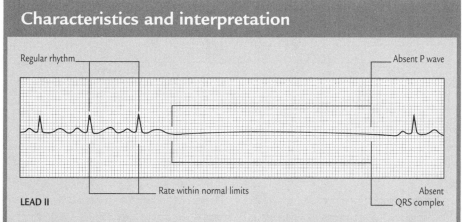

Regular rhythm — Absent P wave

Rate within normal limits

Absent QRS complex

LEAD II

Atrial rhythm: regular, except for the missing complexes

Ventricular rhythm: regular, except for the missing complexes

Atrial rate: within normal limits but varies because of the pauses (94 beats/minute shown)

Ventricular rate: within normal limits but varies because of pauses (94 beats/minute shown)

P wave: normal size and configuration (One P wave precedes each QRS complex but is absent during a pause.)

PR interval: within normal limits and constant when the P wave is present; not measurable when the P wave is absent (0.20-second duration shown on all complexes surrounding the arrest)

QRS complex: normal duration and configuration; absent during a pause (0.08-second duration shown)

T wave: normal size and configuration; absent during a pause

QT interval: within normal limits; not measurable during pause (0.40-second, constant interval shown)

Premature atrial contractions

Premature atrial contractions (PACs) usually result from an irritable focus in the atria that supersedes the sinoatrial node as the pacemaker for one or two beats. Although PACs commonly occur in normal hearts, they're also associated with coronary artery disease and valvular heart disease. In an inferior-wall myocardial infarction (MI), PACs may indicate a concomitant right atrial infarct. In an anterior-wall MI, PACs are an early sign of left-sided heart failure.

They also may warn of a more severe atrial arrhythmia, such as atrial flutter or fibrillation.

Possible causes include digoxin toxicity, hyperthyroidism, elevated catecholamine levels, acute respiratory failure, and chronic obstructive pulmonary disease.

Intervention

In most cases, no treatment is necessary or is directed at the underlying cause.

Characteristics and interpretation

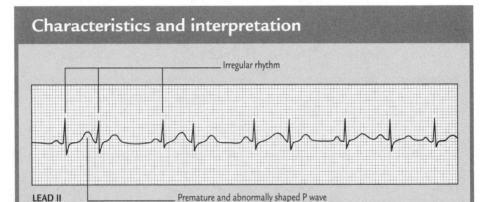

Irregular rhythm

LEAD II — Premature and abnormally shaped P wave

Atrial rhythm: irregular (Incomplete compensatory pause follows premature atrial contraction [PAC]. Underlying rhythm may be regular.)

Ventricular rhythm: irregular (Incomplete compensatory pause follows PAC. Underlying rhythm may be regular.)

Atrial rate: varies with underlying rhythm (90 beats/minute shown)

Ventricular rate: varies with underlying rhythm (90 beats/minute shown)

P wave: premature and abnormally shaped; possibly lost in previous T wave (Varying configurations indicate multiform PACs.)

PR interval: usually normal but may be shortened or slightly prolonged, depending on the origin of ectopic focus (0.16-second, constant interval shown)

QRS complex: usually normal duration and configuration (0.08-second, constant duration shown)

T wave: usually normal configuration; may be distorted if the P wave is hidden in the previous T wave

QT interval: usually normal (0.36-second, constant interval shown)

Other: may occur in bigeminy or couplets

Supraventricular tachycardia

In supraventricular tachycardia (SVT), the atrial rhythm is ectopic and the atrial rate is rapid, shortening diastole. This results in a loss of atrial kick, reduced systemic perfusion, a decrease in the atrial contraction's contribution to cardiac output, commonly referred to as *reduced coronary perfusion*, and potential ischemic myocardial changes.

Although SVT occurs in healthy patients, it's usually associated with high catcholamine levels, digoxin toxicity, myocardial infarction, cardiomyopathy, hyperthyroidism, hypertension, and valvular heart disease. Atrial tachycardia with block and multifocal atrial tachycardia are other types of SVT.

Intervention

If the patient is symptomatic, immediate cardioversion is necessary. If the patient's condition is stable, vagal stimulation, such as carotid sinus massage or Valsalva's maneuver, may be performed. If cardiac function is preserved, the treatment priority is a calcium channel blocker, beta-adrenergic blocker, digoxin, and cardioversion. If unsuccessful, consider procainamide (Pronestyl), amiodarone (Cordarone), or sotalol (Betapace) if each preceding treatment is ineffective in rhythm conversion. If these measures fail, cardioversion may be necessary.

Characteristics and interpretation

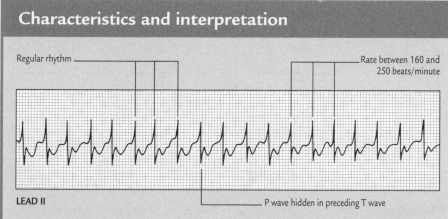

Regular rhythm

Rate between 160 and 250 beats/minute

LEAD II

P wave hidden in preceding T wave

Atrial rhythm: regular
Ventricular rhythm: regular
Atrial rate: three or more successive ectopic atrial beats at a rate of 160 to 250 beats/minute (210 beats/minute shown)
Ventricular rate: varies with atrioventricular conduction ratio (210 beats/minute shown)
P wave: 1:1 ratio with QRS complex, though generally indiscernible because of rapid rate; may be hidden in previous ST segment or T-wave
PR interval: may be unmeasurable if P wave can't be distinguished from preceding T wave (If P wave is present, PR interval is short when conduction through the AV node is 1:1. On this strip, the PR interval is indiscernible.)
QRS complex: usually normal unless aberrant intraventricular conduction is present (0.10-second duration shown)
T wave: may be normal or inverted if ischemia is present (inverted T waves shown)
QT interval: usually normal but may be shorter because of rapid rate (0.20-second interval shown)
Other: appearance of ST-segment and T-wave changes if tachyarrhythmia persists longer than 30 minutes or if coronary perfusion is greatly reduced

Atrial flutter

Characterized by an atrial rate of 300 beats/minute or more, atrial flutter results from multiple reentry circuits within the atrial tissue. Causes include conditions that enlarge atrial tissue and elevate atrial pressures. Atrial flutter is associated with myocardial infarction, increased catecholamine levels, hyperthyroidism, and digoxin toxicity. A ventricular rate of 300 beats/minute suggests the presence of an accessory pathway.

If the patient's pulse rate is normal, he probably has no symptoms. If his pulse rate is high, he probably has signs and symptoms of decreased cardiac output, such as hypotension and syncope.

Intervention

If the patient is unstable and symptomatic, immediate cardioversion is necessary. If the patient is stable, follow ACLS protocol for cardioversion and drug therapy, including calcium channel blockers, beta-adrenergic blockers, or antiarrhythmics. Anticoagulation therapy may also be necessary.

Characteristics and interpretation

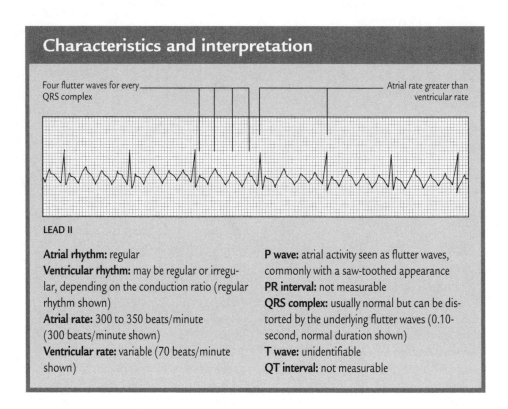

Four flutter waves for every QRS complex

Atrial rate greater than ventricular rate

LEAD II

Atrial rhythm: regular
Ventricular rhythm: may be regular or irregular, depending on the conduction ratio (regular rhythm shown)
Atrial rate: 300 to 350 beats/minute (300 beats/minute shown)
Ventricular rate: variable (70 beats/minute shown)

P wave: atrial activity seen as flutter waves, commonly with a saw-toothed appearance
PR interval: not measurable
QRS complex: usually normal but can be distorted by the underlying flutter waves (0.10-second, normal duration shown)
T wave: unidentifiable
QT interval: not measurable

Atrial fibrillation

Atrial fibrillation is defined as chaotic, asynchronous electrical activity in the atrial tissue. It results from multiple, multidirectional impulses (traveling in many reentry pathways) that cause the atria to quiver instead of contract regularly.

With this arrhythmia, blood may pool in the left atrium and form thrombi that can be ejected into the systemic circulation. An associated rapid ventricular rate can decrease cardiac output.

Possible causes include valvular disorders, hypertension, coronary artery disease, myocardial infarction, chronic lung disease, ischemia, thyroid disorders, and Wolff-Parkinson-White syndrome. Atrial fibrillation may also result from high adrenergic tone secondary to physical exertion, sepsis or alcohol withdrawal, or the use of such drugs as aminophylline (Phyllocontin) and cardiac glycosides.

Intervention

If the patient is symptomatic, synchronized cardioversion should be used immediately. Vagal stimulation may be used to slow the ventricular response, but it won't convert the arrhythmia. If the patient is stable, follow ACLS protocol for cardioversion and drug therapy, which may include calcium channel blockers, beta-adrenergic blockers, or antiarrhythmics. If atrial fibrillation lasts several days, anticoagulant therapy is recommended before pharmacologic or electrical conversion. If atrial fibrillation is of recent onset, ibutilide (Corvert) may be used to convert the rhythm.

Characteristics and interpretation

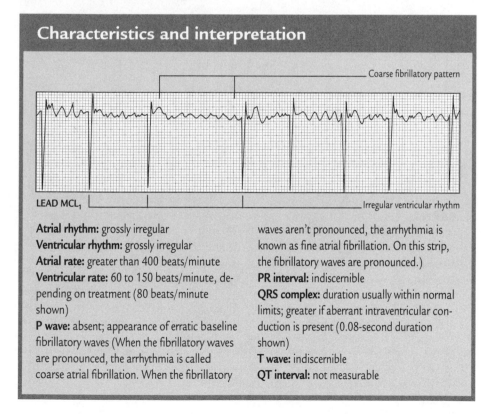

Coarse fibrillatory pattern

LEAD MCL₁

Irregular ventricular rhythm

Atrial rhythm: grossly irregular
Ventricular rhythm: grossly irregular
Atrial rate: greater than 400 beats/minute
Ventricular rate: 60 to 150 beats/minute, depending on treatment (80 beats/minute shown)
P wave: absent; appearance of erratic baseline fibrillatory waves (When the fibrillatory waves are pronounced, the arrhythmia is called coarse atrial fibrillation. When the fibrillatory waves aren't pronounced, the arrhythmia is known as fine atrial fibrillation. On this strip, the fibrillatory waves are pronounced.)
PR interval: indiscernible
QRS complex: duration usually within normal limits; greater if aberrant intraventricular conduction is present (0.08-second duration shown)
T wave: indiscernible
QT interval: not measurable

Junctional rhythm

Junctional rhythm occurs in the atrio-ventricular junctional tissue, producing retrograde depolarization of the atrial tissue and antegrade depolarization of the ventricular tissue. It results from conditions that depress sinoatrial node function, such as an inferior-wall myocardial infarction (MI), digoxin toxicity, and vagal stimulation. The arrhythmia may also stem from increased automaticity of the junctional tissue, which can be caused by digoxin toxicity or ischemia associated with an inferior-wall MI.

A junctional rhythm with a ventricular rate of 60 to 100 beats/minute is known as an accelerated junctional rhythm. If the ventricular rate exceeds 100 beats/minute, the arrhythmia is called junctional tachycardia.

Intervention

Treatment aims to identify and manage the arrhythmia's primary cause. If the patient is symptomatic, treatment may include atropine to increase the sinus or junctional rate. Pacemaker insertion may be necessary to maintain an effective heart rate if the patient doesn't respond to drugs.

Characteristics and interpretation

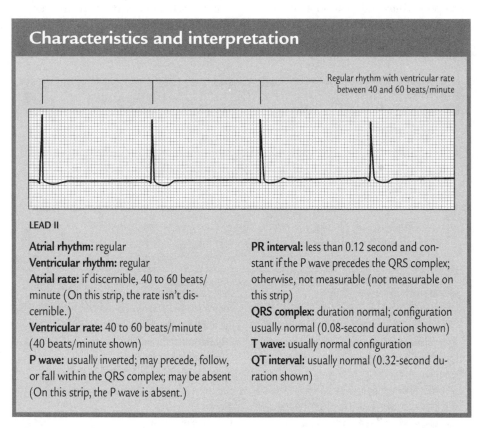

Regular rhythm with ventricular rate between 40 and 60 beats/minute

LEAD II

Atrial rhythm: regular
Ventricular rhythm: regular
Atrial rate: if discernible, 40 to 60 beats/minute (On this strip, the rate isn't discernible.)
Ventricular rate: 40 to 60 beats/minute (40 beats/minute shown)
P wave: usually inverted; may precede, follow, or fall within the QRS complex; may be absent (On this strip, the P wave is absent.)

PR interval: less than 0.12 second and constant if the P wave precedes the QRS complex; otherwise, not measurable (not measurable on this strip)
QRS complex: duration normal; configuration usually normal (0.08-second duration shown)
T wave: usually normal configuration
QT interval: usually normal (0.32-second duration shown)

Premature junctional contractions

In premature junctional contractions (PJCs), a junctional beat occurs before the next normal sinus beat. PJCs, which are ectopic beats, commonly result from increased automaticity in the bundle of His or the surrounding junctional tissue, which interrupts the underlying rhythm. The patient may complain of palpitations if PJCs are frequent.

PJCs most commonly result from digoxin toxicity. Other causes include ischemia associated with an inferior-wall myocardial infarction, excessive caffeine ingestion, and high levels of amphetamines in the body.

Intervention

In most cases, treatment is directed at the underlying cause.

Characteristics and interpretation

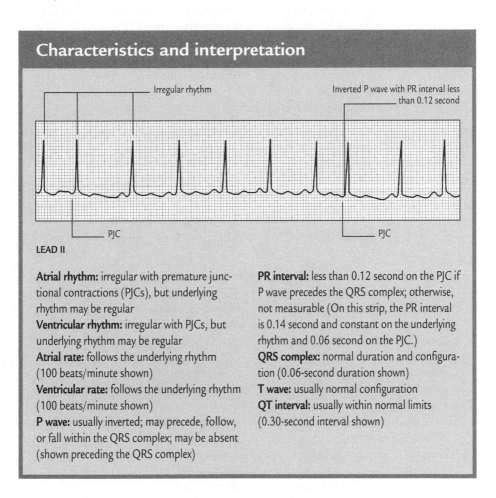

Irregular rhythm

Inverted P wave with PR interval less than 0.12 second

PJC

PJC

LEAD II

Atrial rhythm: irregular with premature junctional contractions (PJCs), but underlying rhythm may be regular
Ventricular rhythm: irregular with PJCs, but underlying rhythm may be regular
Atrial rate: follows the underlying rhythm (100 beats/minute shown)
Ventricular rate: follows the underlying rhythm (100 beats/minute shown)
P wave: usually inverted; may precede, follow, or fall within the QRS complex; may be absent (shown preceding the QRS complex)

PR interval: less than 0.12 second on the PJC if P wave precedes the QRS complex; otherwise, not measurable (On this strip, the PR interval is 0.14 second and constant on the underlying rhythm and 0.06 second on the PJC.)
QRS complex: normal duration and configuration (0.06-second duration shown)
T wave: usually normal configuration
QT interval: usually within normal limits (0.30-second interval shown)

Premature ventricular contractions

Among the most common arrhythmias, premature ventricular contractions (PVCs) occur in healthy and diseased hearts. These ectopic beats occur singly, in bigeminy, trigeminy, quadrigeminy, or clusters and may result from certain drugs, electrolyte imbalance, or stress.

When you detect PVCs, you must determine whether the pattern indicates danger. Paired PVCs can produce ventricular tachycardia because the second PVC usually meets refractory tissue. Three or more in a row is a run of ventricular tachycardia. Multiform PVCs look different from one another and may arise from different ventricular sites or be abnormally conducted.

In R-on-T phenomenon, the PVC occurs so early that it falls on the T wave of the preceding beat. Because the cells haven't fully depolarized, ventricular tachycardia or fibrillation can result.

Intervention

If the PVCs are thought to result from a serious cardiac problem, procainamide (Pronestyl), amiodarone (Cordarone), or lidocaine (Xylocaine) may be given to suppress ventricular irritability. When the PVCs are thought to result from a noncardiac problem, treatment aims at correcting the underlying cause — an acid-base or electrolyte imbalance, antiarrhythmic therapy, hypothermia, or high catecholamine levels.

Characteristics and interpretation

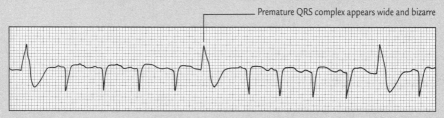

Premature QRS complex appears wide and bizarre

LEAD MCL₁

Atrial rhythm: irregular during premature ventricular contractions (PVCs); underlying rhythm may be regular
Ventricular rhythm: irregular during PVCs; underlying rhythm may be regular
Atrial rate: follows underlying rhythm (120 beats/minute shown)
Ventricular rate: follows underlying rhythm (120 beats/minute shown)
P wave: atrial activity independent of the PVCs (If retrograde atrial depolarization exists, a retrograde P wave will distort the ST segment of the PVC. On this strip, no P wave appears before the PVC, but one occurs with each QRS complex.)

PR interval: determined by underlying rhythm; not associated with the PVC (0.12-second, constant interval shown)
QRS complex: occurs earlier than expected; duration exceeds 0.12 second and complex has a bizarre configuration; may be normal in the underlying rhythm (On this strip, it's 0.08 second in the normal beats; it's bizarre and 0.12 second in the PVC.)
T wave: occurs in the direction opposite of the QRS complex; normal in the underlying complexes
QT interval: not usually measured in the PVC but may be within normal limits in the underlying rhythm (On this strip, the QT interval is 0.28 second in the underlying rhythm.)

Ventricular tachycardia

The life-threatening arrhythmia ventricular tachycardia develops when three or more premature ventricular contractions occur in a row and the rate exceeds 100 beats/minute. It may result from enhanced automaticity or reentry within the Purkinje system. The rapid ventricular rate reduces ventricular filling time; because atrial kick is lost, cardiac output drops. This puts the patient at risk for ventricular fibrillation.

Ventricular tachycardia usually results from acute myocardial infarction, coronary artery disease, valvular heart disease, heart failure, or cardiomyopathy. The arrhythmia can also stem from an electrolyte imbalance or from toxic levels of a drug, such as a cardiac glycoside, procainamide (Pron-

estyl), or quinidine. You may detect three variations of this arrhythmia: monomorphical V-tach, polymorphic V-tach, or torsades de pointe.

Intervention

This rhythm commonly degenerates into ventricular fibrillation and cardiovascular collapse, requiring immediate cardiopulmonary resuscitation and defibrillation. If the patient is symptomatic, prepare for immediate cardioversion, followed by antiarrhythmic therapy. Lidocaine (Xylocaine) or amiodarone (Cordarone) is usually administered immediately. If it proves ineffective, procainamide (Pronestyl) or sotalol (Betapace) is used, and magnesium sulfate if the patient is experiencing torsades de pointes.

Characteristics and interpretation

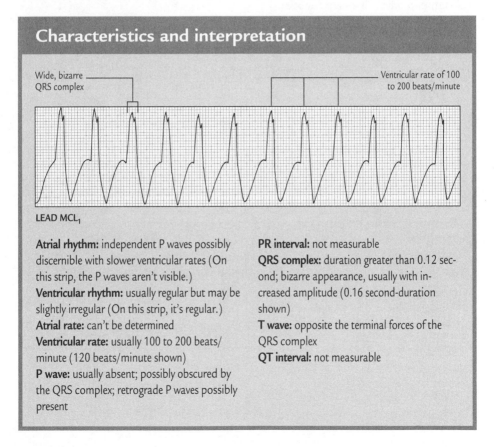

Wide, bizarre QRS complex

Ventricular rate of 100 to 200 beats/minute

LEAD MCL₁

Atrial rhythm: independent P waves possibly discernible with slower ventricular rates (On this strip, the P waves aren't visible.)
Ventricular rhythm: usually regular but may be slightly irregular (On this strip, it's regular.)
Atrial rate: can't be determined
Ventricular rate: usually 100 to 200 beats/minute (120 beats/minute shown)
P wave: usually absent; possibly obscured by the QRS complex; retrograde P waves possibly present

PR interval: not measurable
QRS complex: duration greater than 0.12 second; bizarre appearance, usually with increased amplitude (0.16 second-duration shown)
T wave: opposite the terminal forces of the QRS complex
QT interval: not measurable

Ventricular fibrillation

Defined as chaotic, asynchronous electrical activity within the ventricular tissue, ventricular fibrillation is a life-threatening arrhythmia that results in death if the rhythm isn't stopped immediately. Conditions leading to ventricular fibrillation include myocardial ischemia, hypokalemia, cocaine toxicity, hypoxia, hypothermia, severe acidosis, and severe alkalosis.

Patients with a myocardial infarction are at greatest risk for ventricular fibrillation during the initial 2 hours after the onset of chest pain. Those who experience ventricular fibrillation have a reduced risk of recurrence as healing progresses and scar tissue forms.

In ventricular fibrillation, a lack of cardiac output results in a loss of consciousness, pulselessness, and respiratory arrest. Initially, you may see coarse fibrillatory waves on the electrocardiogram strip. As the acidosis develops, the waves become fine and progress to asystole, unless defibrillation restores cardiac rhythm.

Intervention

Perform cardiopulmonary resuscitation until the patient can receive defibrillation. Administer epinephrine or vasopressin (Pitressin) if initial defibrillation series is unsuccessful. Other drugs that may be used include amiodarone (Cordarone), lidocaine (Xylocaine), and procainamide (Pronestyl). Magnesium sulfate may be used for torsades de pointes or refractory ventricular fibrillation.

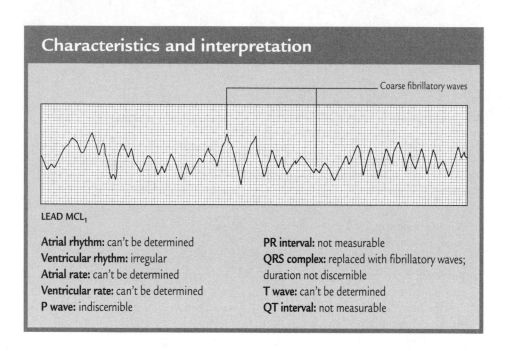

Characteristics and interpretation

Coarse fibrillatory waves

LEAD MCL₁

Atrial rhythm: can't be determined
Ventricular rhythm: irregular
Atrial rate: can't be determined
Ventricular rate: can't be determined
P wave: indiscernible

PR interval: not measurable
QRS complex: replaced with fibrillatory waves; duration not discernible
T wave: can't be determined
QT interval: not measurable

Idioventricular rhythm

A life-threatening arrhythmia, idioventricular rhythm acts as a safety mechanism when all potential pacemakers above the ventricles fail to discharge or when a block prevents supraventricular impulses from reaching the ventricles.

The slow ventricular rate and loss of atrial kick associated with this life-threatening arrhythmia markedly reduce cardiac output (CO), which in turn causes hypotension, confusion, vertigo, and syncope.

Intervention

Treatment aims to identify and manage the primary problem that triggered this safety mechanism.

Atropine or dopamine (Intropin) may be given to increase the atrial rate. A pacemaker may also be inserted to increase the heart rate and thereby improve CO.

Characteristics and interpretation

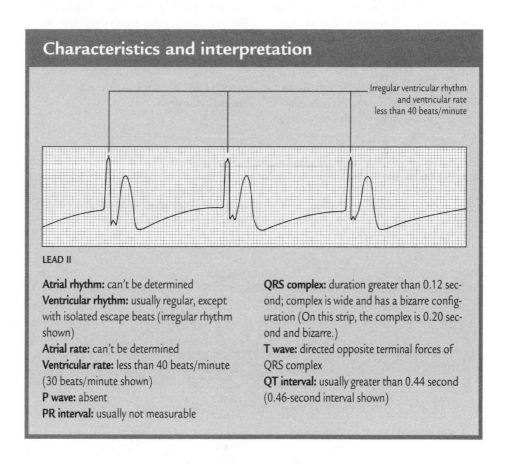

Irregular ventricular rhythm and ventricular rate less than 40 beats/minute

LEAD II

Atrial rhythm: can't be determined
Ventricular rhythm: usually regular, except with isolated escape beats (irregular rhythm shown)
Atrial rate: can't be determined
Ventricular rate: less than 40 beats/minute (30 beats/minute shown)
P wave: absent
PR interval: usually not measurable

QRS complex: duration greater than 0.12 second; complex is wide and has a bizarre configuration (On this strip, the complex is 0.20 second and bizarre.)
T wave: directed opposite terminal forces of QRS complex
QT interval: usually greater than 0.44 second (0.46-second interval shown)

Accelerated idioventricular rhythm

When the pacemaker cells above the ventricles fail to generate an impulse or when a block prevents supraventricular impulses from reaching the ventricles, idioventricular rhythms result. When the rate of an idioventricular rhythm ranges from 40 to 100 beats/minute, it's considered accelerated idioventricular rhythm, denoting a rate greater than the inherent pacemaker.

In this life-threatening arrhythmia, the cells of the His-Purkinje system operate as pacemaker cells. Causes for the loss of a supraventricular rate greater than the inherent pacemaker rate of 20 to 40 beats/minute include myocardial infarction, digoxin toxicity, or metabolic imbalances. Also, the arrhythmia commonly occurs during myocardial reperfusion after thrombolytic therapy.

The patient may be symptomatic, depending on his heart rate and ability to compensate for the loss of the atrial kick. If symptomatic, he may experience signs and symptoms of decreased cardiac output (CO), including hypotension, confusion, syncope, and blurred vision.

Intervention

An asymptomatic patient needs no treatment. For a symptomatic patient, treatment focuses on maintaining CO and identifying the cause of the arrhythmia. The patient may require a ventricular or atrioventricular pacemaker to enhance CO. Remember, this rhythm protects the heart from ventricular standstill and shouldn't be treated with lidocaine (Xylocaine) or other antiarrhythmics.

Characteristics and interpretation

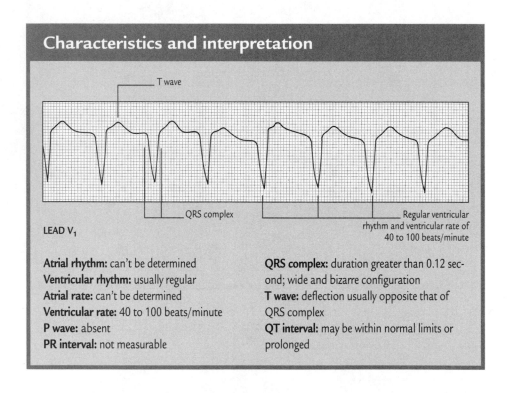

LEAD V₁

Regular ventricular rhythm and ventricular rate of 40 to 100 beats/minute

Atrial rhythm: can't be determined
Ventricular rhythm: usually regular
Atrial rate: can't be determined
Ventricular rate: 40 to 100 beats/minute
P wave: absent
PR interval: not measurable

QRS complex: duration greater than 0.12 second; wide and bizarre configuration
T wave: deflection usually opposite that of QRS complex
QT interval: may be within normal limits or prolonged

First-degree atrioventricular block

Defined as delayed conduction velocity through the atrioventricular (AV) node or His-Purkinje system, first-degree AV block is associated with an inferior-wall myocardial infarction and the effects of cardiac glycosides, amiodarone (Cordarone), or beta-adrenergic blocking agents. The arrhythmia is also associated with chronic degeneration of the conduction system.

Most patients with first-degree AV block are asymptomatic.

Intervention

Management of first-degree AV block includes identifying and treating the underlying cause as well as monitoring the patient for signs of progressive AV block.

Characteristics and interpretation

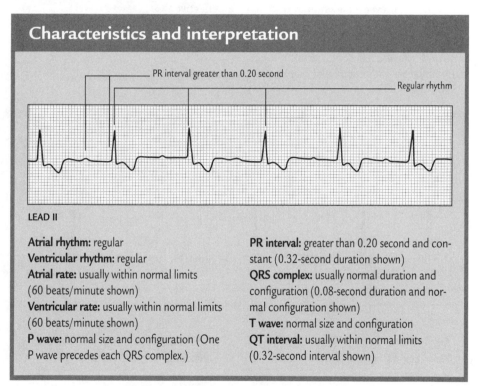

PR interval greater than 0.20 second

Regular rhythm

LEAD II

Atrial rhythm: regular
Ventricular rhythm: regular
Atrial rate: usually within normal limits (60 beats/minute shown)
Ventricular rate: usually within normal limits (60 beats/minute shown)
P wave: normal size and configuration (One P wave precedes each QRS complex.)

PR interval: greater than 0.20 second and constant (0.32-second duration shown)
QRS complex: usually normal duration and configuration (0.08-second duration and normal configuration shown)
T wave: normal size and configuration
QT interval: usually within normal limits (0.32-second interval shown)

Second-degree atrioventricular block, type I

In type I (Wenckebach or Mobitz I) second-degree atrioventricular (AV) block, diseased AV node tissues conduct impulses to the ventricles increasingly later, until one of the atrial impulses fails to be conducted or is blocked. Type I block most commonly occurs at the level of the AV node and is caused by an inferior-wall myocardial infarction, vagal stimulation, or digoxin toxicity.

The arrhythmia usually doesn't cause symptoms. However, a patient may have signs and symptoms of decreased cardiac output (CO), such as hypotension, confusion, and syncope. These effects occur especially if the patient's ventricular rate is slow.

Intervention

If the patient is asymptomatic, no intervention other than monitoring the electrocardiogram results frequently to see if a more serious form of AV block develops. Identifying the underlying cause may prevent further progression toward more life-threatening blocks.

If the patient is symptomatic, atropine may be needed to increase the rate and to stop the decremental conduction through the AV node. Occasionally, a temporary pacemaker may be necessary to maintain an effective CO.

Characteristics and interpretation

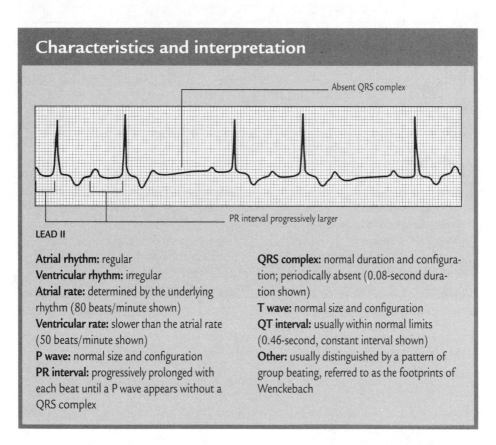

Absent QRS complex

PR interval progressively larger

LEAD II

Atrial rhythm: regular
Ventricular rhythm: irregular
Atrial rate: determined by the underlying rhythm (80 beats/minute shown)
Ventricular rate: slower than the atrial rate (50 beats/minute shown)
P wave: normal size and configuration
PR interval: progressively prolonged with each beat until a P wave appears without a QRS complex

QRS complex: normal duration and configuration; periodically absent (0.08-second duration shown)
T wave: normal size and configuration
QT interval: usually within normal limits (0.46-second, constant interval shown)
Other: usually distinguished by a pattern of group beating, referred to as the footprints of Wenckebach

Second-degree atrioventricular block, type II

A life-threatening arrhythmia produced by a conduction disturbance in the His-Purkinje system, a type II (Mobitz II) second-degree atrioventricular block causes an intermittent absence of conduction. In type II block, two or more atrial impulses are conducted to the ventricles with constant PR intervals, when, suddenly, the atrial impulse is blocked. This type of block occurs in an anterior-wall myocardial infarction (MI), severe coronary artery disease, and chronic degeneration of the conduction system.

Intervention

If the patient is hypotensive, treatment aims at increasing his heart rate to improve cardiac output. Because the conduction block occurs in the His-Purkinje system, drugs that act directly on the myocardium usually prove more effective than those that increase the atrial rate. As a result, dopamine (Intropin) instead of atropine may be administered to increase the ventricular rate.

If the patient has an anterior-wall MI, a temporary pacemaker may need to be inserted to prevent ventricular asystole. For long-term management, the patient usually needs a permanent pacemaker.

Characteristics and interpretation

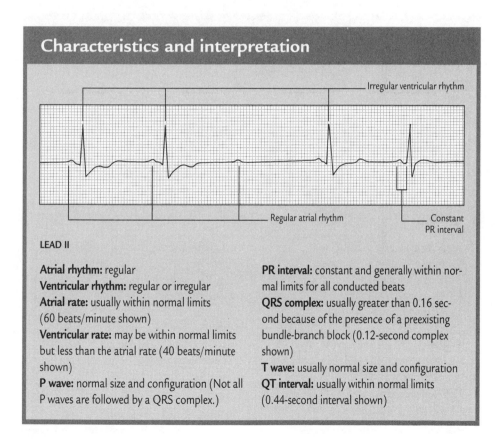

LEAD II

Atrial rhythm: regular
Ventricular rhythm: regular or irregular
Atrial rate: usually within normal limits (60 beats/minute shown)
Ventricular rate: may be within normal limits but less than the atrial rate (40 beats/minute shown)
P wave: normal size and configuration (Not all P waves are followed by a QRS complex.)

PR interval: constant and generally within normal limits for all conducted beats
QRS complex: usually greater than 0.16 second because of the presence of a preexisting bundle-branch block (0.12-second complex shown)
T wave: usually normal size and configuration
QT interval: usually within normal limits (0.44-second interval shown)

Third-degree atrioventricular block

Also called complete heart block, life-threatening third-degree atrioventricular (AV) block occurs when all supraventricular impulses are prevented from reaching the ventricles. If this type of block originates at the AV node, a junctional escape rhythm occurs; if it originates below the AV node, an idioventricular escape rhythm occurs.

Third-degree AV block involving the AV node may result from an inferior wall myocardial infarction (MI) or a toxic reaction to a drug, such as digoxin, a beta-adrenergic blocker, or a calcium channel blocker. Third-degree AV block below the AV node may result from an anterior-wall MI or chronic degeneration of the conduction system.

Intervention

If cardiac output is inadequate or if the patient's condition is deteriorating, atropine, dopamine (Intropin), or epinephrine may be administered to improve the ventricular rhythm. A temporary or permanent pacemaker may need to be inserted.

Characteristics and interpretation

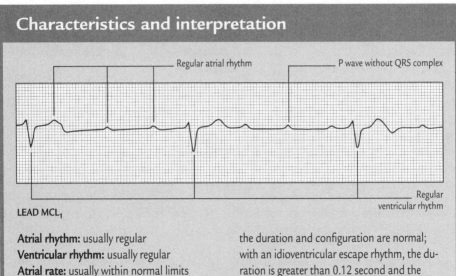

Regular atrial rhythm

P wave without QRS complex

Regular ventricular rhythm

LEAD MCL₁

Atrial rhythm: usually regular
Ventricular rhythm: usually regular
Atrial rate: usually within normal limits (90 beats/minute shown)
Ventricular rate: slow (30 beats/minute shown)
P wave: normal size and configuration
PR interval: not measurable because the atria and ventricles beat independently of each other
QRS complex: determined by the site of the escape rhythm (With a junctional escape rhythm, the duration and configuration are normal; with an idioventricular escape rhythm, the duration is greater than 0.12 second and the complex is distorted. In the complex shown, the duration is 0.16 second, the configuration is abnormal, and the complex is distorted.)
T wave: normal size and configuration
QT interval: may be within normal limits (0.56-second interval shown)

12-lead ECGs

Basic components and principles

Whereas rhythm strips are used to detect arrhythmias, the 12-lead, or standard, electrocardiogram (ECG) has a different purpose. The most common test for evaluating cardiac status, the 12-lead ECG helps identify various pathologic conditions — most commonly, acute myocardial infarction.

The 12-lead ECG provides 12 views of the heart's electrical activity. (See *12 views of the heart,* page 464.) The 12 leads include:

■ three bipolar limb leads (I, II, and III)
■ three unipolar augmented limb leads (aV$_R$, aV$_L$, and aV$_F$)
■ six unipolar precordial, or chest, leads (V$_1$, V$_2$, V$_3$, V$_4$, V$_5$, and V$_6$).

Leads

The six limb leads record electrical potential from the frontal plane, and the six precordial leads record electrical potential from the horizontal plane. Each waveform reflects the orientation of a lead to the wave of depolarization passing through the myocardium. Normally, this wave moves through the heart from right to left and from top to bottom.

BIPOLAR LEADS

Bipolar leads record the electrical potential difference between two points on the patient's body, where you place electrodes.

■ Lead I goes from the right arm (−) to the left arm (+).
■ Lead II goes from the right arm (−) to the left leg (+).
■ Lead III goes from the left arm (−) to the left leg (+).

Because of the orientation of these leads to the wave of depolarization, the QRS complexes typically appear upright. In lead II, these complexes are usually the tallest because this lead parallels the wave of depolarization.

UNIPOLAR LEADS

Each unipolar lead (the augmented limb leads and the precordial leads) has only one electrode, which represents the positive pole. The ECG computes the negative pole. Lead aV$_R$ typically records negative QRS complex deflections because the wave of depolarization moves away from it. In the aV$_F$ lead, QRS complexes are positive; in the aV$_L$ lead, they're biphasic.

Unipolar precordial leads V$_1$ and V$_2$ usually have a small R wave because the direction of ventricular activation is left to right initially. That's because conduction time is normally faster down the left bundle branch than it is down the right. However, the wave of depolarization moves toward the left ventricle and away from these leads, causing a low S wave.

In leads V$_3$ and V$_4$, the R and S waves may have the same amplitude, and you won't see a Q wave. In leads V$_5$ and V$_6$, the initial ventricular activation appears as a small Q wave; the following tall R wave represents the strong wave of depolarization moving toward the left ventricle. These leads record a small or absent S wave.

Determining electrical axis

As electrical impulses travel through the heart, they generate small electrical forces called instant-to-instant vectors. The mean of these vectors represents the direction and force of the wave of depolarization, also known as the heart's electrical axis.

In a healthy heart, the wave of depolarization (or the direction of the electrical axis) originates in the sinoatrial node and travels through the atria and the atrioventricular node and on to the ventricles. So the normal movement is downward and to the left — the direction of a normal electrical axis.

In an unhealthy heart, the wave of depolarization varies. That's because the direction of electrical activity swings away from areas of damage or necrosis.

A simple method for determining the direction of your patient's electrical axis is the quadrant method. Before you use this method, you need to understand the hexaxial reference system — a schematic view of the heart that uses the six limb leads.

12 views of the heart

The electrocardiogram's six limb leads view the heart from six different angles. This chart shows the direction of each lead relative to the wave of depolarization and lists the six views of the heart revealed by these leads.

PLANES OF THE HEART	LEADS	VIEW OF THE HEART
	Standard limb leads (bipolar)	
	I	Lateral wall
	II	Inferior wall
	III	Inferior wall
	Augmented limb leads (unipolar)	
	aV_R	Provides no specific view
	aV_L	Lateral wall
	aV_F	Inferior wall
	Precordial, or chest, leads (unipolar)	
	V_1	Anteroseptal wall
	V_2	Anteroseptal wall
	V_3	Anterior and anteroseptal wall
	V_4	Anterior wall
	V_5	Anterolateral wall
	V_6	Anterolateral wall

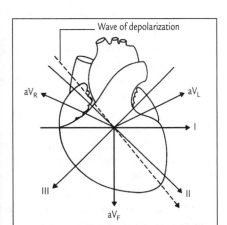

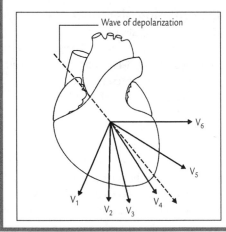

As you know, these leads include the three standard limb leads (I, II, and III), which are bipolar, and the three augmented limb leads (aV_R, aV_L, and aV_F), which are unipolar. Combined, these leads give a view of the wave of depolarization in the frontal plane, including the right, left, inferior, and superior portions of the heart.

Hexaxial reference system

The axes of the six limb leads also make up the hexaxial reference system, which divides the heart into six equal areas. To use the hexaxial reference system, picture in your mind the position of each lead: Lead I connects the right arm (negative pole) with the left arm (positive pole); lead II connects the right arm (negative pole) with the left leg (positive pole); and lead III connects the left arm (negative pole) with the left leg (positive pole). Each augmented limb lead has only one electrode, which represents the positive pole. As a result, lead aV_R goes from the heart toward the right arm (positive pole); aV_L goes from the heart toward the left arm (positive pole); and aV_F goes from the heart to the left leg (positive pole).

Next, take this mental picture one step further and draw an imaginary line to illustrate the axis of each lead. For example, for lead I, you would draw a horizontal line between the right and left arms; for lead II, between the right arm and left leg; and so on. All the lines should intersect near the center, somewhere over the heart. If you draw a circle to represent the heart, you would end up with a rough pie shape, with each wedge representing a portion of the heart monitored by each lead. (See *Understanding the hexaxial reference system.*)

This schematic representation of the heart allows you to plot your patient's electrical axis. If his axis falls in the right lower quadrant, between 0 degrees and + 90 de-

grees, it's considered normal. An axis between + 90 degrees and + 180 degrees indicates right axis deviation; one between 0 degrees and − 90 degrees, left axis deviation; and one between − 180 degrees and − 90 degrees, extreme axis deviation (sometimes called the northwest axis). Some experts, however, feel that the portion from 0 degrees to − 30 degrees has no clinical significance.

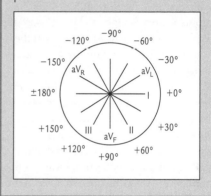

Quadrant method

A simple, rapid method for determining the heart's axis is the quadrant method, in which you observe the main deflection of the QRS complex in leads I and aV$_F$. The QRS complex serves as the traditional marker for determining the electrical axis because the ventricles produce the greatest amount of electrical force when they contract. Lead I indicates whether impulses are moving to the right or left; lead aV$_F$, whether they're moving up or down. (See *Using the quadrant method.*)

On the waveform for lead I, a positive main deflection of the QRS complex indicates that the electrical impulses are moving to the right, toward the positive pole of the lead, which is at the 0-degree position on the hexaxial reference system. Conversely, a negative deflection indicates that the impulses are moving to the left, toward the negative pole of the lead, which is at the + 180-degree position on the hexaxial reference system. On the waveform for lead aV$_F$, a positive deflection of the QRS complex indicates that the electrical impulses are traveling downward, toward the positive pole of the lead, which is at the + 90-degree position of the hexaxial reference system. A negative deflection indicates that impulses are traveling upward, toward the negative pole of the lead, which is at the + 90-degree position of the hexaxial reference system.

Plotting this information on the hexaxial reference system (with the horizontal axis representing lead I and the vertical axis representing lead aV$_F$) will reveal the patient's electrical axis. For example, if lead I shows a positive deflection of the QRS complex, darken the horizontal axis between the center of the hexaxial reference system and the 0-degree position. If lead aV$_F$ also shows a positive deflection of the QRS complex, darken the vertical axis be-

tween the center of reference system and the + 90-degree position. The quadrant between the two axes you have darkened indicates the patient's electrical axis. In this case, it's the left lower quadrant, which indicates a normal electrical axis.

Causes of axis deviation

Determining a patient's electrical axis can help confirm a diagnosis or narrow the range of clinical possibilities. Many factors influence the electrical axis, including the position of the heart within the chest, the size of the heart, the conduction pathways, and the force of electrical generation.

As you know, cardiac electrical activity swings away from areas of damage or necrosis. More specifically, electrical forces in the healthy portion of the heart take over for weak, or even absent, electrical forces in the damaged portion. For instance, after an inferior-wall myocardial infarction, portions of the inferior wall can no longer conduct electricity. As a result, the major electrical vectors shift to the left, resulting in a left axis deviation.

Typically, the damaged portion of the heart is the last area to be depolarized. For example, in a left anterior hemiblock, the left anterior fascicle of the left bundle branch can no longer conduct electricity. Therefore, the portion normally served by the left bundle branch is the last portion of the heart to be depolarized. This shifts electrical forces to the left; consequently, the ECG shows left axis deviation.

An opposite shift occurs with right bundle-branch block. In this condition, the wave of impulse travels quickly down the normal left side but much more slowly down the damaged right side. This shifts the electrical forces to the right, causing a right axis deviation.

An axis shift also takes place when the right or left ventricle is artificially paced. It

Using the quadrant method

This chart can help you quickly determine the direction of a patient's electrical axis, which is indicated by the gray arrow. First, observe the deflections of the QRS complexes in leads I and aV$_F$. Next, plot the deflections on the diagram. (Positive deflections are on the side that has positive degrees for that lead, and negative deflections are on the side that has negative degrees.) Then check the chart to determine if the patient's axis is normal or whether it has a left, right, or extreme deviation.

LEAD 1	LEAD aV$_F$	HEXAXIAL DIAGRAM	AXIS

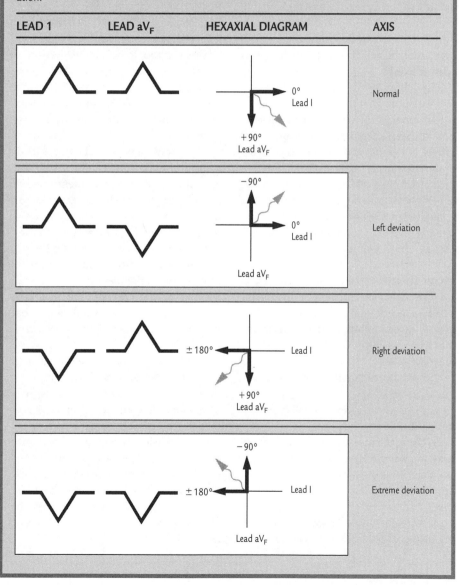

likewise takes place when the ventricles are depolarizing abnormally, such as occurs in ventricular tachycardia. Both of these conditions can cause a left axis deviation or, occasionally, an extreme axis deviation.

Axis deviation may also result from ventricular hypertrophy. For example, an enlarged right ventricle generates greater electrical forces than normal and would consequently shift the electrical axis to the right. Wolff-Parkinson-White syndrome may produce a right, left, or extreme axis deviation, depending on which part of the ventricle is activated early.

Sometimes axis deviation may be a normal variation, as in infants and children, who normally experience right axis deviation. It may also stem from noncardiac causes. For example, if the heart is shifted in the chest cavity because of a high diaphragm from pregnancy, expect to find a left axis deviation. Also, if a patient's heart is situated on the right side of the chest instead of the left (a condition called dextrocardia), expect to find right axis deviation.

How to interpret a 12-lead ECG

You can use various methods to interpret a 12-lead electrocardiogram (ECG). Here's a logical, easy-to-follow, seven-step method that will help ensure that you're interpreting it accurately.

1. Find the lead markers and note the leads.

2. Note whether there are full or half standardization marks.

3. Using the four-quadrant method, observe the waveforms for leads I and aV_F, and determine the heart's axis. This can provide an early clue to a possible problem.

4. Note the R-wave progression through the six precordial leads. Normally, in the precordial leads, the R wave (the first positive deflection of the QRS complex) appears progressively taller from lead V_1 to lead V_6. Conversely, the S wave (the negative deflection after an R wave) appears extremely deep in lead V_1 and becomes progressively smaller through lead V_6. (See *Normal findings*.)

5. Next, look at the T wave, which normally goes in the same direction as the QRS complex. If the main deflection of the QRS complex is positive, the T wave should be positive, too. If the main deflection of the QRS complex is negative, the T wave should be negative. The two exceptions to this are leads V_1 and V_2, in which a negative QRS complex with a positive T wave is normal.

If a T wave deflects in the opposite direction from the QRS complex, it's considered abnormal (except, as mentioned, in leads V_1 and V_2). Such a deflection is commonly referred to as an *inverted T wave* — a term that can be confusing when the QRS complex is negative and the T wave is actually positive. Keep in mind that in this case, inversion signifies that the T wave deflects in the direction opposite the QRS complex. It doesn't necessarily mean that the T wave is negative, as the word *inverted* suggests.

6. If you suspect a myocardial infarction (MI), start with lead I and continue through to lead V_6, observing the waveforms for changes in ECG characteristics that can indicate an acute MI, such as T-wave inversion, ST-segment elevation, and pathologic Q waves. Note the leads in which you see such changes and describe the changes. When first learning to interpret the 12-lead ECG, ignore lead aV_R, because it won't provide clues to left ventricular infarction or injury.

Normal findings

LEAD I

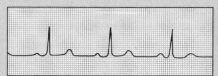

P wave: upright
Q wave: small or none
R wave: largest wave
S wave: none present, or smaller than R wave
T wave: upright
U wave: none present
ST segment: may vary from + 1 to − 0.5 mm

LEAD II

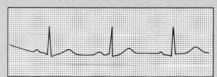

P wave: upright
Q wave: small or none
R wave: large (vertical heart)
S wave: none present, or smaller than R wave
T wave: upright
U wave: none present
ST segment: may vary from + 1 to − 0.5 mm

LEAD III

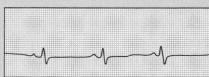

P wave: upright, biphasic, or inverted
Q wave: usually small or none (A Q wave must also be present in aV_F to be considered diagnostic.)
R wave: none present to large wave
S wave: none present to large wave, indicating a horizontal heart

T wave: upright, biphasic, or inverted
U wave: none present
ST segment: may vary from + 1 to − 0.5 mm

LEAD aV_R

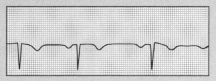

P wave: inverted
Q wave: none, small wave, or large wave present
R wave: none or small wave present
S wave: large wave (may be QS)
T wave: inverted
U wave: none present
ST segment: may vary from + 1 to − 0.5 mm

LEAD aV_L

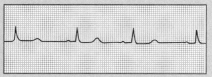

P wave: upright, biphasic, or inverted
Q wave: none, small wave, or large wave present (A Q wave must also be present in lead I or precordial leads to be considered diagnostic.)
R wave: none, small wave, or large wave present (A large wave indicates a horizontal heart.)
S wave: none present to large wave (A large wave indicates a vertical heart.)
T wave: upright, biphasic, or inverted
U wave: none present
ST segment: may vary from + 1 to − 0.5 mm

(continued)

Normal findings *(continued)*

LEAD aV_F

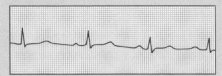

P wave: upright
Q wave: none, or small wave present
R wave: none, small wave, or large wave present (A large wave suggests a vertical heart.)
S wave: none to large wave present (A large wave suggests a horizontal heart.)
T wave: upright, biphasic, or inverted
U wave: none present
ST segment: may vary from + 1 to − 0.5 mm

LEAD V_1

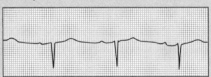

P wave: upright, biphasic, or inverted
Q wave: deep QS pattern may be present
R wave: none present or less than S wave
S wave: large (part of QS pattern)
T wave: usually inverted but may be upright and biphasic
U wave: none present
ST segment: may vary from 0 to + 1 mm

LEAD V_2

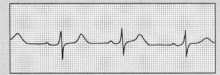

P wave: upright
Q wave: deep QS pattern may be present
R wave: none present or less than S wave (Wave may become progressively larger.)

S wave: large (part of QS pattern)
T wave: upright
U wave: upright, lower amplitude than T wave, if present
ST segment: may vary from 0 to + 1 mm

LEAD V_3

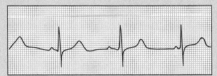

P wave: upright
Q wave: none or small wave present
R wave: less than, greater than, or equal to S wave (Wave may become progressively larger.)
S wave: large (greater than, less than, or equal to R wave)
T wave: upright
U wave: upright, lower amplitude than T wave, if present
ST segment: may vary from 0 to + 1 mm

LEAD V_4

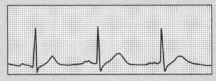

P wave: upright
Q wave: none or small wave present
R wave: progressively larger wave; R wave greater than S wave
S wave: progressively smaller (less than R wave)
T wave: upright
U wave: upright, lower amplitude than T wave, if present
ST segment: may vary from + 1 to − 0.5 mm

LEAD V₅

P wave: upright
Q wave: small
R wave: progressively larger but less than 26 mm
S wave: progressively smaller; less than the S wave in V₄
T wave: upright
U wave: none present

ST segment: may vary from +1 to −0.5 mm

LEAD V₆

P wave: upright
Q wave: small
R wave: largest wave but less than 26 mm
S wave: smallest; less than the S wave in V₅
T wave: upright
U wave: none present
ST segment: may vary from +1 to −0.5 mm

7. Determine the site and extent of myocardial damage. To do so, use *Locating myocardial damage,* page 472, and follow these steps:

■ Identify the leads recording pathologic Q waves. Look at the second column of the chart for those leads. Then look at the first column to find the corresponding myocardial wall, where infarction has occurred. Keep in mind that this chart serves as a guideline only. Actual areas of infarction may overlap or be larger or smaller than listed.

■ Identify the leads recording ST-segment elevation (or depression for reciprocal leads), and use the chart to locate the corresponding areas of myocardial injury.

■ Identify the leads recording T-wave inversion, and locate the corresponding areas of ischemia.

Acute myocardial infarction

An acute myocardial infarction (MI) can arise from any condition in which myocardial oxygen supply can't meet oxygen de-

mand. Starved of oxygen, the myocardium suffers progressive ischemia, leading to injury and, eventually, to infarction.

In most cases, an acute MI involves the left ventricle, although it can also involve the right ventricle or the atria, and is classified as either Q wave or non-Q wave.

In an acute transmural MI, the characteristic electrocardiogram (ECG) changes result from the three I's — ischemia, injury, and infarction.

■ Ischemia results from a temporary interruption of the myocardial blood supply. Its characteristic ECG change is T-wave inversion, a result of altered tissue repolarization. ST-segment depression may also occur.

ISCHEMIA

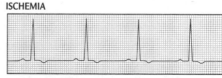

Ischemia produces T-wave inversion

Locating myocardial damage

WALL AFFECTED	LEADS	ECG CHANGES	ARTERY INVOLVED	RECIPROCAL CHANGES
Inferior (diaphragmatic)	II, III, aV_F	Q, ST, T	Right coronary artery (RCA)	I, aV_L and, possibly, V_4 through V_6
Posterolateral	I, aV_L, V_5, V_6	Q, ST, T	Circumflex or branch of left anterior descending (LAD) artery	V_1, V_2, or II, III, and aV_F
Anterior	V_1, V_2, V_3, V_4	Q, ST, T, loss of R-wave progression across precordial leads	Left coronary artery	II, III, aV_F
Posterior	V_1, V_2	None	RCA or circumflex, either of which supplies posterior descending artery	R greater than S in V_1 and V_2, ST-segment depression, T-wave elevation
Right ventricular	V_{4R}, V_{5R}, V_{6R}	Q, ST, T	RCA	None
Anterolateral	I, aV_L, V_4, V_5, V_6	Q, ST, T	LAD and diagonal branches, circumflex and obtuse marginal branches	II, III, aV_F
Anteroseptal	V_1, V_2, V_3	Q, ST, T, loss of R wave in V_1	LAD	None

■ Injury to myocardial cells results from a prolonged interruption of blood flow. Its characteristic ECG change, ST-segment elevation, reflects altered depolarization. Usually, an elevation greater than 0.1 mV is considered significant.

INJURY

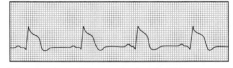

Injury produces ST-segment elevation

■ Infarction results from an absence of blood flow to myocardial tissue, leading to necrosis. The ECG shows pathologic Q waves, reflecting abnormal depolarization in damaged tissue or absent depolarization in scar tissue. The characteristic of a pathologic Q wave is a duration of 0.04 second or an amplitude measuring at least one-third the height of the entire QRS complex.

INFARCTION

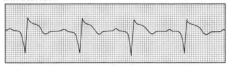

Infarction produces pathologic Q waves

Besides these three characteristic ECG changes, you may see reciprocal (or mirror image) changes. Reciprocal changes — most commonly, ST-segment depression or tall R waves — occur in the leads opposite those reflecting the area of ischemia, injury, or infarction.

Acute MI phases

To detect an acute MI, look for ST-segment elevation first, followed by T-wave inversion and pathologic Q waves.

Serial ECG recordings yield the best evidence of an MI. Normally, an acute MI progresses through the following phases.

HYPERACUTE PHASE

This phase begins a few hours after the onset of an acute MI. You'll see ST-segment elevation and upright (usually peaked) T waves.

FULLY EVOLVED PHASE

This phase starts several hours after MI onset. You'll see deep T-wave inversion and pathologic Q waves.

RESOLUTION PHASE

This appears within a few weeks of an acute MI. You'll see normal T waves.

STABILIZED CHRONIC PHASE

After the resolution phase, you'll see permanent pathologic Q waves revealing an old infarction.

Non-Q-wave MI

With an acute non–Q-wave MI, you'll see persistent ST-segment depression, T-wave inversion, or both. However, pathologic Q waves may not appear. To differentiate an acute non–Q-wave MI from myocardial ischemia, cardiac enzyme tests must be performed.

It's important to remember that for a true clinical diagnosis of an acute MI, a patient must have ECG changes and elevated cardiac enzyme levels. If the patient shows such signs as chest pain, left arm pain, diaphoresis, and nausea, proceed as if he has had an acute MI until this possibility has been ruled out.

Right-sided ECG, leads V_{1R} to V_{6R}

A right-sided electrocardiogram (ECG) provides information about the extent of damage to the right ventricle, especially during the first 12 hours of a myocardial infarction (MI). Right-sided ECG leads, placed over the right side of the chest in similar but reversed positions from the left precordial leads, are called unipolar right-sided chest leads.

Placing electrodes

Right-sided ECG leads are precordial leads designated by the letter V, a number representing the electrode position, and the letter R, indicating lead placement on the right side of the chest. Lead positions are:

- V_{1R}: fourth intercostal space, left sternal border
- V_{2R}: fourth intercostal space, right sternal border
- V_{3R}: midway between V_{2R} and V_{4R}, on a line joining these two locations
- V_{4R}: fifth intercostal space, right midclavicular line
- V_{5R}: fifth intercostal space, right anterior axillary line
- V_{6R}: fifth intercostal space, right midaxillary line.

Understanding polarity

The right-sided chest ECG leads measure the difference in electrical potential between a right-sided chest electrode and a central terminal. The chest electrode used in each of the right V leads is positive. The negative electrode is obtained by adding together leads I, II, and III, whose algebraic sum equals zero.

Viewing the heart

Chest leads, whether on the left or the right side of the chest, view the horizontal plane of the heart. The placement of left precordial leads gives a good picture of the electrical activity within the left ventricle. Because the right ventricle lies behind the left ventricle, the ability to evaluate right ventricular electrical activity when using only left precordial leads is limited. Right-sided ECG leads provide a better picture of the right ventricular wall. This may be especially useful when evaluating a patient for a right ventricular MI.

Leads V_{1R} and V_{2R} provide limited visualization of the right ventricle. Leads V_{3R} through V_{6R} are the most useful right ventricular leads. A decrease in the R wave with an increase in the S wave is normally seen from V_{1R} through V_{6R}, the reverse of the standard left precordial leads. V_{3R} to V_{6R} (particularly V_{4R}) are the most commonly used and the most helpful leads when looking for ECG changes indicating right ventricular ischemia and infarction.

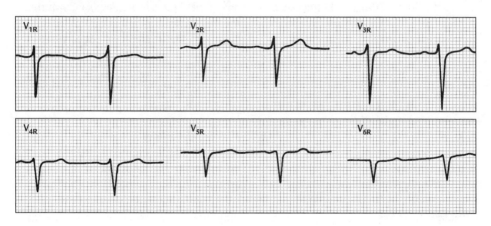

Left bundle-branch block

In left bundle-branch block, a conduction delay or block occurs in both the left posterior and the left anterior fascicles of the left bundle. This delay or block disrupts the normal left-to-right direction of depolarization. As a result, normal septal Q waves are absent. Because of the block, the wave of depolarization must move down the right bundle first and then spread from right to left.

This arrhythmia may indicate underlying heart disease such as coronary artery disease. It carries a more serious prognosis than right bundle-branch block because of its close correlation with organic heart disease, and it requires a large lesion to block the thick, broad left bundle branch.

Intervention

When left bundle-branch block occurs along with an anterior-wall myocardial infarction, it usually signals complete heart block, which requires insertion of a pacemaker.

Characteristics and interpretation

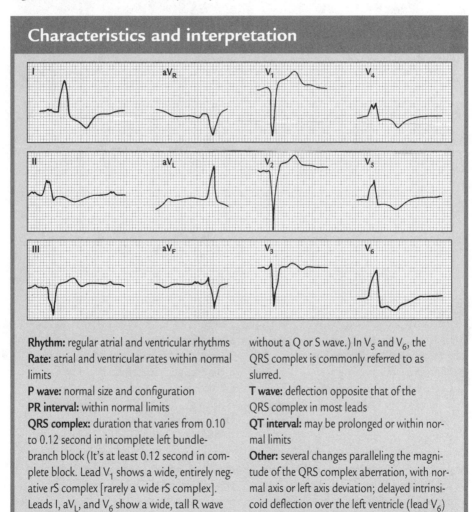

Rhythm: regular atrial and ventricular rhythms
Rate: atrial and ventricular rates within normal limits
P wave: normal size and configuration
PR interval: within normal limits
QRS complex: duration that varies from 0.10 to 0.12 second in incomplete left bundle-branch block (It's at least 0.12 second in complete block. Lead V_1 shows a wide, entirely negative rS complex [rarely a wide rS complex]. Leads I, aV_L, and V_6 show a wide, tall R wave without a Q or S wave.) In V_5 and V_6, the QRS complex is commonly referred to as slurred.
T wave: deflection opposite that of the QRS complex in most leads
QT interval: may be prolonged or within normal limits
Other: several changes paralleling the magnitude of the QRS complex aberration, with normal axis or left axis deviation; delayed intrinsicoid deflection over the left ventricle (lead V_6)

Right bundle-branch block

In the conduction delay or block associated with right bundle-branch block, the initial left-to-right direction of depolarization isn't affected. The left ventricle depolarizes on time, so the intrinsicoid deflection in leads V_5 and V_6 (the left precordial leads) takes place on time as well. However, the right ventricle depolarizes late, causing a late intrinsicoid deflection in leads V_1 and V_2 (the right precordial leads). This late de-polarization also causes the axis to deviate to the right.

Intervention

One potential complication of a myocardial infarction is a bundle-branch block. Some blocks require treatment with a temporary pacemaker. Others are monitored only to detect progression to a more complete block.

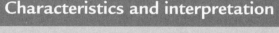

Characteristics and interpretation

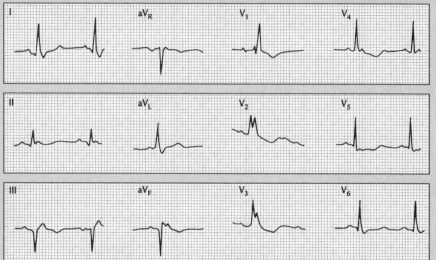

Rhythm: regular atrial and ventricular rhythms
Rate: atrial and ventricular rates within normal limits
P wave: normal size and configuration
PR interval: within normal limits
QRS complex: duration of at least 0.12 second in complete block and 0.10 to 0.12 second in incomplete block (In lead V_1, the QRS complex is wide and can appear in one of several patterns: an rSR' complex with a wide S and R' wave; an rS complex with a wide R wave; and a wide R wave with an M-shaped pattern. The complex is mainly positive, with the R wave oc-curring late. In leads I, aV_L, and V_6, a broad S wave can be seen.) In V_1 and V_2, the QRS complex is referred to as "rabbit-eared."
T wave: in most leads, deflection opposite that of the QRS-complex deflection
QT interval: may be prolonged or within normal limits
Other: in the precordial leads, occurrence of triphasic complexes because the right ventricle continues to depolarize after the left ventricle depolarizes, thereby producing a third phase of ventricular stimulation

Pericarditis

An inflammation of the pericardium, the fibroserous sac that envelops the heart, pericarditis can be acute or chronic. The acute form may be fibrinous or effusive, with a purulent serous or hemorrhagic exudate. Chronic constrictive pericarditis causes dense fibrous pericardial thickening. Regardless of the form, pericarditis can cause cardiac tamponade if fluid accumulates too quickly. It can also cause heart failure if constriction occurs.

In pericarditis, electrocardiogram changes occur in four stages. Stage 1 coincides with the onset of chest pain. Stage 2 begins within several days. Stage 3 starts several days after stage 2. Stage 4 occurs weeks later.

Intervention

Pericarditis is usually treated with aspirin or nonsteroidal anti-inflammatory drugs. A last resort is prednisone, quickly tapered over 3 days.

Characteristics and interpretation

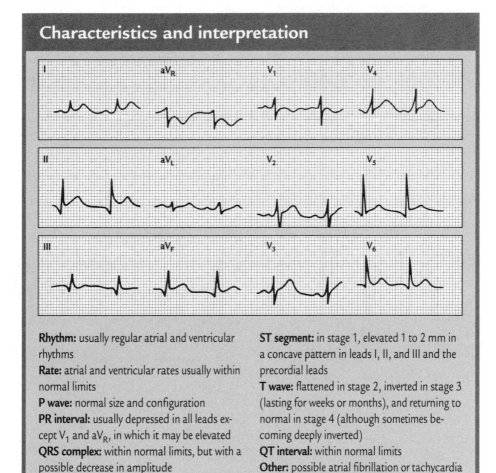

Rhythm: usually regular atrial and ventricular rhythms

Rate: atrial and ventricular rates usually within normal limits

P wave: normal size and configuration

PR interval: usually depressed in all leads except V_1 and aV_R, in which it may be elevated

QRS complex: within normal limits, but with a possible decrease in amplitude

ST segment: in stage 1, elevated 1 to 2 mm in a concave pattern in leads I, II, and III and the precordial leads

T wave: flattened in stage 2, inverted in stage 3 (lasting for weeks or months), and returning to normal in stage 4 (although sometimes becoming deeply inverted)

QT interval: within normal limits

Other: possible atrial fibrillation or tachycardia from sinoatrial node irritation

Digoxin: ECG effects

Digoxin increases the force of myocardial contraction, decreases conduction velocity through the atrioventricular (AV) node to slow the heart rate, and prolongs the effective refractory period of the AV node by direct and sympatholytic effects on the sino-atrial node. Excess amounts of this drug can slow conduction through the AV node and cause irritable ectopic foci in the ventricles.

Electrocardiogram (ECG) changes only indicate that the patient is receiving a form of digoxin. If an arrhythmia develops, these ECG changes can help identify the cause of the arrhythmia as digoxin toxicity.

Virtually any type of arrhythmia can be caused by an excess of digoxin. The most common ones include premature ventricular contractions (especially bigeminy), supraventricular tachycardias (with or without a block), second-degree heart block, and sinus arrest.

Intervention

Monitor the patient for noncardiac symptoms of digoxin toxicity. Withhold digoxin for 1 to 2 days before performing electrical cardioversion.

Characteristics and interpretation

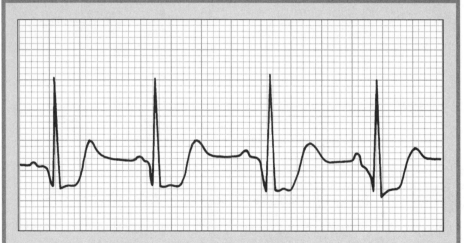

Rhythm: regular atrial and ventricular rhythms
Rate: atrial and ventricular rates are usually within normal limits, but bradycardia is possible
P wave: decreased voltage; may be notched
PR interval: within normal limits or prolonged
QRS complex: within normal limits
ST segment: gradual sloping, causing ST-segment depression in the direction opposite that of the QRS deflection

T wave: may be flattened and inverted in a direction opposite that of the QRS-complex deflection
Other: QT interval commonly shortened; ST-segment sloping and depression and QT-interval shortening from digoxin use but not necessarily signs of digoxin toxicity; ST-segment depression and T-wave inversion in leads with negatively deflected QRS complexes, possibly indicating a need to reduce the digoxin dose

Quinidine: ECG effects

An antiarrhythmic that decreases sodium transport through cardiac tissues, quinidine slows conduction through the atrioventricular (AV) node. It also prolongs the effective refractory period and decreases automaticity.

Although electrocardiogram (ECG) changes occur as a result of quinidine use, they aren't necessarily a sign of quinidine toxicity. At toxic levels, however, quinidine can cause sinoatrial and AV block and ventricular arrhythmias.

Intervention

Prolongation of the QT interval is a sign that the patient is predisposed to developing polymorphic ventricular tachycardia (torsade de pointes). Preventing ventricular tachyarrhythmias involves administering a cardiac glycoside for atrial tachyarrhythmias before quinidine.

Characteristics and interpretation

Rhythm: regular atrial and ventricular rhythms
Rate: atrial and ventricular rates within normal limits
P wave: may be widened and notched, especially in leads I and II
PR interval: within normal limits
QRS complex: widens slightly (Abnormal widening may be an early sign of developing quinidine toxicity.)

ST segment: commonly depressed
T wave: may be flattened or inverted
QT interval: may be prolonged (Abnormal lengthening of QT interval may be an early indication of quinidine toxicity.)
U wave: may be visible

Key diagnostic findings in major disorders

Abdominal aortic aneurysm

■ CT scan, MRI, or ultrasonography reveals the size, shape, and location of the aneurysm.

■ Anteroposterior and lateral X-rays of the abdomen may detect aortic calcification, which outlines the mass.

■ Aortography shows the condition of vessels proximal and distal to the aneurysm and the extent of the aneurysm. However, it may underestimate aneurysm diameter because it visualizes only the blood flow channel and not the surrounding clot.

Abnormal premenopausal bleeding

- Serum hormone levels reflect adrenal, pituitary, or thyroid dysfunction.
- Urine 17-KS reveal adrenal hyperplasia, hypopituitarism, or polycystic ovarian disease.
- Pelvic ultrasonography rules out uterine masses.
- Hysteroscopy allows visualization of the endometrium.
- Endometrial biopsy rules out malignancy and should be performed in all patients who experience abnormal premenopausal bleeding.
- Pelvic examination and Pap smear rule out local or malignant causes.

Abruptio placentae

- History includes mild to moderate vaginal bleeding (usually during second half of pregnancy).
- Amniocentesis reveals "port wine" fluid.
- Coagulation tests reveal a rise in fibrin split product levels.
- CBC reveals decreased Hb level and platelet counts.
- Pelvic ultrasonography reveals abnormal echo patterns.

Acceleration-deceleration cervical injuries

- Full cervical spine CT scans or X-rays indicate the absence of cervical fracture.
- If the X-rays are negative for obvious cervical fracture, examination emphasizes motor ability and sensation below the cervical spine to detect signs of nerve root compression.

Acquired immunodeficiency syndrome

- ELISA identifies the HIV-1 antibody.
- Western blot test may also reveal the HIV-1 antibody and should be performed after a positive ELISA to confirm the diagnosis (antibody may not be detected in late stages due to the body's inability to mount an antibody response).
- CD4+ T-lymphocyte assay reveals a lymphocyte count < 200 cells/μl in an HIV-infected individual.

Actinomycosis

- Culture of tissue or exudate identifies *Actinomyces israelii*.
- Gram staining of excised tissue or exudates reveals branching gram-positive rods.
- CXR reveals lesions in unusual locations such as the shaft of a rib.

Acute leukemia

- Bone marrow aspiration indicates a proliferation of immature WBCs.
- Bone marrow biopsy reveals cancerous cells.
- CBC indicates pancytopenia with circulating blasts.

Acute poststreptococcal glomerulonephritis

- History includes recent streptococcal infection.
- Serum electrolyte studies show elevated calcium, chloride, phosphate, potassium, and sodium levels.
- BUN and serum creatinine levels are elevated.
- Urinalysis reveals RBCs, WBCs, mixed cell casts, and protein.
- ASO test reveals elevated streptozyme titers, indicating a recent streptococcal infection (in 80% of patients).

- Anti-DNase B titers are elevated, indicating a recent streptococcal infection.
- Serum complement assay levels are low, indicating recent streptococcal infection.
- Throat culture may show group A beta-hemolytic streptococci.
- KUB X-rays show bilateral kidney enlargement.
- Renal biopsy reveals histologic changes indicating glomerulonephritis.

Acute pyelonephritis

- Urinalysis reveals sediment containing leukocytes (singly, in clumps, and in casts) and, possibly, a few RBCs; low specific gravity and osmolality, and a slightly alkaline urine pH.
- Urine culture reveals more than 100,000 organisms/ml of urine.
- KUB X-rays may reveal calculi, tumors, or cysts in the kidneys and the urinary tract.
- Excretory urography may show asymmetrical kidneys.

Acute renal failure

- History includes renal disease.
- BUN and serum creatinine levels are elevated.
- ABG analysis indicates a blood pH < 7.35 and HCO_3^- level < 22 mEq/L (SI, < 22 mmol/L).

Acute respiratory failure in chronic obstructive pulmonary disease

- ABG measurements show progressive deterioration when compared with normal values for patient; increased HCO_3^- level may indicate metabolic alkalosis or metabolic compensation for chronic respiratory acidosis.
- CXR reveals such pulmonary pathology as emphysema, atelectasis, lesions, pneumothorax, infiltrates, or effusions.
- Hb level and HCT are decreased.

- Serum electrolyte studies reveal hypokalemia.
- WBC count is elevated if bacterial infection is present.
- ECG indicates arrhythmias that suggest cor pulmonale and myocardial hypoxia.

Acute tubular necrosis

- Urinalysis reveals urinary sediment containing RBCs and casts, specific gravity of 1.010 or less, and osmolality < 400 mOsm/kg (SI, < 400 mmol/kg).
- Urine sodium level is between 40 and 60 mEq/L (SI, 40 to 60 mmol/d).
- BUN and serum creatinine levels are elevated.
- Serum electrolyte studies reveal hyperkalemia.
- ABG analysis indicates blood pH < 7.25 and HCO_3^- level < 22 mEq/L (SI, < 22 mmol/L).

Adenoid hyperplasia

- Nasopharyngoscopy or rhinoscopy reveals abnormal tissue mass.
- Lateral pharyngeal X-rays show oblation of the nasopharyngeal air column.

Adrenal hypofunction

- Plasma cortisol levels are decreased.
- Fasting blood glucose and serum sodium levels are decreased (in Addison's disease).
- Serum potassium and BUN levels are increased.
- CBC reveals increased HCT and elevated lymphocyte and eosinophil counts.
- X-rays reveal a small heart.
- Corticotropin level is increased.
- Rapid corticotropin test reveals low cortisol levels.
- Sweat test reveals elevated sodium level (> 46 mmol/L [SI, > 46 mEq/L]) and chloride level (> 43 mmol/L [SI, > 43 mEq/L]).

- Urine 17-hydroxycorticosteroid levels and urine 17-KS levels are decreased.

Adrenogenital syndrome

- Physical examination reveals pseudo-hermaphroditism in females or precocious puberty in patients of either sex.
- Urine 17-KS levels are elevated and can be suppressed by administering oral dexamethasone.
- Levels of urine hormone metabolites (particularly pregnanetriol) and plasma 17-hydroxyprogesterone are elevated.
- Urine 17-hydroxycorticosteroid levels are normal or decreased.
- Symptoms of adrenal hypofunction or adrenal crisis in the first week of life strongly suggest congenital adrenal hyperplasia; elevated serum calcium, chloride, and sodium levels (in the presence of excessive levels of urine 17-KS and pregnanetriol) and decreased urine aldosterone levels confirm it.

Age-related macular degeneration

- Indirect ophthalmoscopy reveals gross macular changes.
- I.V. fluorescein angiography reveals leaking vessels.
- Amsler's grid reveals visual field loss.

Albinism

- Family history suggests inheritance pattern.
- Inspection shows pale skin (in whites) and white-to-yellow hair.
- Microscopic examination of the skin and hair follicles reveals the amount of pigment present.
- Pigmentation testing of plucked hair roots by incubating them in tyrosine distinguishes tyrosinase-positive albinism from tyrosinase-negative albinism; tyrosinase-positive hair roots will develop color.

Alcoholism

- History includes chronic and excessive ingestion of alcohol.
- Liver function studies reveal increased levels of serum cholesterol, LD, ALT, AST, and CK in patients with liver damage.
- Serum amylase and lipase levels are elevated (in pancreatitis).

Allergic rhinitis

- Personal or family history includes allergies.
- Sputum and nasal smears reveal a large numbers of eosinophils.
- Skin test for specific allergen is positive, supported by tested response to environmental stimuli.

Alport's syndrome

- Family history includes recurrent hematuria, deafness, and renal failure (especially in men).
- Urinalysis indicates presence of RBCs.
- Renal biopsy reveals histologic changes characteristic of Alport's syndrome.
- Blood tests reveal Ig and complement components.
- Eye examination may reveal cataracts and, less commonly, keratoconus, microspherophakia, myopia, nystagmus, and retinitis pigmentosa.

Alzheimer's disease

- History includes progressive personality, mental status, and neurologic changes.
- PET scan reveals alteration in the metabolic activity of the cerebral cortex.
- Elevated Tau proteins with low levels of soluble amyloid beta-protein precursor in CSF correlate with Alzheimer's disease.
- EEG and CT scan may help diagnose later stages of illness.
- Autopsy reveals neurofibrillary tangles, neuritic plaques, and granulovascular degeneration.

Amebiasis

- Culture of stool, sputum, or aspirates from abscesses, ulcers, or tissue reveal *Entamoeba histolytica* (cysts and trophozoites).
- CT scan may reveal abscess.

Amputation, traumatic

- History and examination reveal trauma to an extremity.
- CBC reveals decreased Hb level and HCT, indicating hemorrhage.

Amyloidosis

- Histologic examination of tissue specimen (rectal mucosa, gingiva, skin, or nerve biopsy) or abdominal fat pad aspirate, using a polarizing or electron microscope and appropriate tissue staining, reveals amyloid deposits.
- Liver function studies are generally normal, except for slightly elevated serum alkaline phosphatase levels.
- ECG shows low voltage and conduction or rhythm abnormalities resembling those characteristic of myocardial infarction (with cardiac amyloidosis).
- Echocardiography (M-mode and two-dimensional) may detect myocardial infiltration.

Amyotrophic lateral sclerosis

- Upper and lower motor neuron degeneration occurs without sensory impairment.
- EMG may show abnormalities of electrical activity of involved muscles.
- Muscle biopsy may disclose atrophic fibers interspersed among normal fiber.
- Nerve conduction studies are usually normal.
- CSF analysis reveals increased protein content in one-third of patients.
- CT scan and EEG may help rule out other disorders.

Anal fissure

- Digital examination elicits pain and bleeding.
- Gentle traction on perianal skin allows for visualization of fistula.
- Anoscopy reveals longitudinal tear and confirms the diagnosis.
- Patient may complain of local itching, tenderness, or pain aggravated by bowel movements.

Anaphylaxis

- Patient's history, physical examination, and signs and symptoms establish the diagnosis. They may include a rapid onset of severe respiratory or cardiovascular symptoms after ingestion or injection of a drug, vaccine, diagnostic agent, food, or food additive or after an insect sting.

Ankylosing spondylitis

- Family history includes the disorder.
- X-rays reveal blurring of the bony margins of joints (in early stage), bilateral sacroiliac involvement, patchy sclerosis with superficial bony erosions, squaring of vertebral bodies, and "bamboo spine" (with complete ankylosis).
- Serum HLA-B27 is present in about 95% of patients with primary disease and 80% of patients with secondary disease.
- CBC reveals slightly elevated ESR and alkaline phosphatase and creatine phosphatase levels in active disease.
- Serum IgA levels may be elevated.

Anorectal abscess and fistula

Examination of rectum helps to distinguish type of abscess:

- Perianal abscess produces a red, tender, localized, oval swelling close to the anus, which may drain pus. Sitting or coughing increases pain.

- Ischiorectal abscess involves the entire perianal region on the affected side of the anus. Digital examination reveals a tender induration bulging into the anal canal, which may not produce drainage.
- Patient may report constipation, ribbon-formed stools, and pain with bowel movements.
- Submucous or high intramuscular abscess may produce a dull, aching pain in the rectum, tenderness and, occasionally, induration. Digital examination reveals a smooth swelling of the upper part of the anal canal or lower rectum.
- Pelvirectal abscess produces fever, malaise, and myalgia but no local anal or external rectal signs or pain. Digital examination reveals a tender mass high in the pelvis, perhaps extending into one of the ischiorectal fossae.
- Sigmoidoscopy, barium enema, and colonoscopy may be performed to rule out other conditions.

Anorectal stricture, stenosis, or contracture

- Visual inspection reveals narrowing of the anal canal.
- Digital examination reveals tenderness and tightness.

Anorexia nervosa

- History includes weight loss of 25% or greater with no organic basis, compulsive dieting and bulimic episodes or gorging and purging, and laxative or diuretic abuse.
- Emaciated appearance is accompanied by maintenance of physical vigor.
- CBC reveals decreased Hb level, platelet count, WBC count, and ESR.
- Bleeding time is prolonged (due to thrombocytopenia).
- Serum creatinine, BUN, uric acid, cholesterol, total protein, albumin, sodium, potassium, chloride, and calcium levels are decreased.
- Fasting blood glucose level is decreased.
- ECG reveals nonspecific ST interval, T-wave changes, prolonged PR interval, and ventricular arrhythmias.
- Additional diagnostic testing may be performed to rule out other disorders that may cause wasting.

Anthrax infection

- History includes exposure to wool, hides, or other animal products.
- Inspection reveals a large, pruritic, painless skin lesion.
- Tissue culture with Gram stain reveals large gram-positive rods.
- Drainage cultures reveal *Bacillus anthracis*.
- Indirect hemagglutination reveals a fourfold rise in titer.

Aortic insufficiency

- Cardiac catheterization shows reduced arterial diastolic pressure, aortic insufficiency, and valvular abnormalities.
- Echocardiography reveals left ventricular enlargement and changes in left ventricular function; it may show a dilated aortic root, a flail leaflet, thickening of the cusps, or valve prolapse.
- Doppler echocardiography readily detects mild degrees of aortic insufficiency that may be inaudible. It also shows a rapid, high-frequency, diastolic fluttering of the anterior mitral leaflet that results from aortic insufficiency.
- ECG may show left ventricular hypertrophy, ST-segment depression, and T-wave inversion.
- Radionuclide angiography helps to determine the degree of regurgitant blood flow and assess left ventricular function.

Aortic stenosis

■ Cardiac catheterization reveals the pressure gradient across the aortic valve (indicating the severity of obstruction), increased left ventricular end-diastolic pressures (indicating left ventricular dysfunction), and the number of cusps.

■ CXR shows valvular calcification, left ventricular enlargement, dilation of the ascending aorta, pulmonary venous congestion and, in later stages, left atrial, pulmonary artery, right atrial, and right ventricular enlargement.

■ Echocardiography demonstrates a thickened aortic valve and left ventricular wall and possible coexistent mitral valve stenosis.

■ Doppler echocardiography allows calculation of the aortic pressure gradient.

■ ECG reveals left ventricular hypertrophy and ST-segment and T-wave abnormalities. As hypertrophy progresses in severe aortic stenosis, left atrial enlargement is noted. Up to 10% of patients have atrioventricular and intraventricular conduction defects.

Aplastic or hypoplastic anemia

■ CBC reveals normochromic and normocytic RBCs with a total count of 1 million or less as well as decreased platelet, neutrophil, and WBC counts.

■ Serum iron is elevated. (Hemosiderin is present and tissue iron storage is visible microscopically.)

■ Bleeding time is prolonged.

■ Bone marrow biopsy yields a "dry tap" or shows severely hypocellular or aplastic marrow, with a varying amount of fat, fibrous tissue, or gelatinous replacement; absence of tagged iron and megakaryocytes; and depression of erythroid elements.

Appendicitis

■ History includes right upper quadrant abdominal pain that eventually localizes in lower right quadrant, plus patient complaints of nausea and vomiting, anorexia, and obstipation.

■ Temperature is elevated.

■ WBC count is elevated, with increased numbers of immature cells.

Arm and leg fractures

■ History includes trauma to extremity.

■ Physical examination reveals pain and difficulty moving parts distal to the injury.

■ Anteroposterior and lateral X-rays of extremity reveal fracture.

Arterial occlusive disease

■ Arteriography demonstrates the type (thrombus or embolus), location, and degree of obstruction and the collateral circulation.

■ Doppler ultrasonography and plethysmography show decreased blood flow distal to the occlusion.

■ Ophthalmodynamometry helps determine degree of obstruction in the internal carotid artery by comparing ophthalmic artery pressure to brachial artery pressure on the affected side. More than a 20% difference between pressures suggests insufficiency.

Asbestosis

■ History includes occupational, family, or neighborhood exposure to asbestos fibers.

■ CXR reveals fine, irregular, and linear diffuse infiltrates; extensive fibrosis results in "honeycomb" or "ground glass" appearance. X-rays also show pleural thickening and calcification, with bilateral oblation of costophrenic angles.

■ PFTs reveal decreased vital capacity, FVC, and total lung capacity; decreased or

normal FEV_1 in 1 second; a normal ratio of FEV_1 to FVC; and reduced diffusing capacity for CO_2.
- ABG analysis may reveal decreased Pao_2 and $Paco_2$.

Ascariasis
- Stools contain ova or roundworm.
- Vomitus contains roundworm.
- CXR reveals infiltrates, patchy areas of pneumonitis, and widening of hilar shadows.

Aspergillosis
- History includes ocular trauma or surgery.
- CXR reveals crescent-shaped radiolucency surrounding a circular mass.
- Culture of exudate identifies *Aspergillus*.

Asphyxia
- History includes change in mental status and alteration of respiratory pattern.
- ABG analysis reveals $Pao_2 < 60$ mm Hg (SI, < 8.02 kPa) and $Paco_2 > 50$ mm Hg (SI, > 6.64 kPa).
- CXR may reveal presence of foreign body, pulmonary edema, or atelectasis.
- Toxicology screening may reveal abnormal Hb level or ingestion of drugs or chemicals.
- PFTs may indicate respiratory muscle weakness.

Asthma
- PFTs may reveal:
  - forced expiratory flow $< 75\%$
  - FEV_1 of 83% or below
  - tidal volumes < 5 to 7 ml/kg of body weight
  - residual volume $> 35\%$ of total lung capacity.
- ABG analysis may demonstrate $Pao_2 < 75$ mm Hg (SI, < 10.03 kPa) and $Paco_2$

> 45 mm Hg (SI, > 5.3 kPa), indicating severe bronchial obstruction.
- CBC reveals eosinophil count $> 7\%$.
- CXR shows hyperinflation.

Asystole
ECG reveals a waveform that's almost a flat line. Characteristic findings include:
- Atrial rhythm is usually indiscernible; no ventricular rhythm is present.
- Atrial rate is usually indiscernible; no ventricular rate is present.
- P wave may be present.
- PR interval isn't measurable.
- QRS complex is absent, or occasional escape beats are present.
- T wave is absent.
- QT interval isn't measurable.

Ataxia-telangiectasia
- History and physical examination reveal the presence of ataxia, telangiectasia, and recurrent sinopulmonary infection.
- Serum analysis shows absent or deficient levels of IgA or IgE.
- Examination of thymic tissue reveals absence of Hassall's corpuscles.

Atelectasis
- Chest auscultation reveals decreased or absent breath sounds.
- CXR reveals characteristic horizontal lines in the lower lung zones (in widespread atelectasis) and dense shadows (with segmental or lobar collapse) with hyperinflation of neighboring lung.

Atopic dermatitis
- History includes clinical manifestations of allergy symptoms such as asthma, hay fever, or urticaria.
- CBC reveals elevated eosinophil count.
- Serum analysis shows elevated IgE levels.

- Tissue culture may be performed to rule out bacterial, viral, or fungal superinfections.

Atrial fibrillation

ECG findings include:
- Atrial and ventricular rhythms are grossly irregular.
- The atrial rate, almost indiscernible, usually exceeds 400 beats/minute. The ventricular rate usually varies from 100 to 150 beats/minute, but can be < 100 beats/minute.
- P wave is absent. Erratic baseline f (fibrillatory) waves appear instead. These chaotic f waves represent atrial tetanization from rapid atrial depolarizations. When f waves are pronounced, the arrhythmia is called *coarse atrial fibrillation*. When they aren't pronounced, the arrhythmia is called *fine atrial fibrillation*.
- PR interval is indiscernible.
- Duration and configuration of QRS complex are usually normal. If ventricular conduction is aberrant, the QRS complex may be wide and abnormally shaped.
- T wave is indiscernible.
- QT interval isn't measurable.
- Atrial fib-flutter, a rhythm that frequently varies between a fibrillatory line and flutter waves, may appear.

Atrial flutter

ECG findings include:
- Atrial rhythm is regular. Ventricular rhythm depends on the atrioventricular (AV) conduction pattern; it's often regular, although cycles may alternate. An irregular pattern may herald atrial fibrillation or indicate a block.
- Atrial rate is 250 to 400 beats/minute. Ventricular rate depends on the degree of AV block; usually, it's 60 to 100 beats/minute, but it may accelerate to 125 to 150 beats/minute.

- P wave is saw-toothed, referred to as flutter or F waves.
- PR interval isn't measurable.
- Usually, duration of QRS complex is within normal limits; however, the complex may be widened if F waves are buried within.
- T wave isn't identifiable.
- QT interval isn't measurable because T wave can't be identified.
- The patient may develop an atrial rhythm that frequently varies between a fibrillatory line and F waves. This is called *atrial fib-flutter*; the ventricular response is irregular.

Atrial septal defect

- Echocardiography measures right ventricular enlargement, may locate the defect, and shows volume overload in the right heart.
- ECG reveals incomplete or complete right bundle-branch block in nearly all cases.
- Cardiac catheterization reveals a left-to-right shunt, determines the extent of shunting and pulmonary vascular disease, detects the size and location of pulmonary venous drainage, and the atrioventricular valves' competence.

Atrial tachycardia

ECG findings include:
- Atrial and ventricular rhythms are regular.
- Atrial rate is characterized by three or more consecutive ectopic atrial beats occurring at a rate between 160 and 250 beats/minute; the rate rarely exceeds 250 beats/minute. The ventricular rate depends on the atrioventricular conduction ratio.
- Usually positive, the P wave may be aberrant, invisible, or hidden in the previous T wave. If visible, it precedes each QRS complex.

- PR interval may be unmeasurable if the P wave can't be distinguished from the preceding T wave.
- QRS complex duration and configuration are usually normal.
- T wave usually can't be distinguished.
- QT interval is usually within normal limits, but may be shorter because of the rapid rate.

Atrioventricular (AV) block, third-degree

ECG findings include:
- Atrial and ventricular rhythms are regular.
- Atrial rate, which is usually within normal limits, exceeds the ventricular rate. The slow ventricular rate ranges from 40 to 60 beats/minute, but this rate is determined by the block's location and the origin of the subsidiary impulse.
- P wave has normal size and configuration.
- PR interval isn't measurable because the atria and ventricles beat independently (AV dissociation).
- Configuration of the QRS complex depends on where the ventricular beat originates. A high AV junctional pacemaker produces a narrow QRS complex; a pacemaker in the bundle of His produces a wide QRS complex; a ventricular pacemaker produces a wide, bizarre QRS complex.
- T wave has normal size and configuration.
- QT interval may or may not be within normal limits.

Basal cell carcinoma

- Inspection reveals skin lesions.
- Tissue biopsy reveals basal cell carcinoma.

B-cell deficiency

- History includes recurrent infections.
- Family history includes infection as cause of death.
- IgM, IgA, and IgG levels are decreased (after age 6 months).
- Tissue biopsy may show B cells but no plasma cells (B cells mature to form plasma cells as part of a normal immune response) in acquired hypogammaglobulinemia.

Bell's palsy

- Inspection reveals facial paresthesia with an inability to raise the eyebrow, close the eyelid, smile, show the teeth, or puff the cheek.
- EEG distinguishes temporary conduction defect from pathologic interruption of nerve fibers (after 10 days).

Benign prostatic hyperplasia

- History includes problems with urination.
- Rectal examination reveals enlarged prostate gland.
- Prostate biopsy reveals histologic changes characteristic of benign prostatic hyperplasia.
- Excretory urography may indicate urinary tract obstruction, hydronephrosis, calculi, or tumors and filling and emptying defects in the bladder.
- Elevated BUN and creatinine levels suggest impaired renal function.
- Urinalysis and urine culture show hematuria, pyuria and, when the bacterial count exceeds 100,000/ml, infection.
- Cystourethroscopy indicates prostate enlargement (usually performed immediately before surgery to help determine the best operative procedure).

Berylliosis

■ History includes occupational, family, or neighborhood exposure to beryllium dust, fumes, or mists.

■ In acute berylliosis, CXR reveals acute miliary process or patchy acinous filling and diffuse infiltrates with prominent peribronchial markings.

■ In chronic berylliosis, CXR reveals reticulonodular infiltrates, hilar adenopathy, and large coalescent infiltrates in both lungs.

■ PFTs reveal decreased lung capacity.

Bladder cancer

■ Cystoscopy with biopsy reveals the presence of malignant cells and may reveal that the bladder is fixed to the pelvic wall or prostate.

■ Arylsulfatase A levels are elevated.

■ Retrograde cystography evaluates bladder structure and integrity and confirms the diagnosis.

■ Excretory urography reveals an early-stage or infiltrating tumor, ureteral obstruction, or a rigid deformity of the bladder wall. This test may also delineate functional problems in the upper urinary tract and help assess the degree of hydronephrosis.

■ Urinalysis indicates presence of blood and malignant cytology.

■ Ultrasonography may detect metastases in tissue beyond the bladder and can distinguish a bladder cyst from a bladder tumor.

■ Pelvic arteriography reveals tumor invasion of the bladder wall.

■ CT scan reveals the thickness of the involved bladder wall and detects enlarged retroperitoneal lymph nodes.

Blastomycosis

■ Culture of skin lesions, pus, sputum, or pulmonary secretions reveals *Blastomyces dermatitidis*.

Blepharitis

■ History includes irritated eyes and rubbing of the eyes.

■ Tissue culture of ulcerated lid margin reveals *Staphylococcus aureus* (with ulcerative blepharitis).

■ Inspection detects presence of nits (with pediculosis).

Blood transfusion reaction

■ Crossmatching reveals conflicting blood types.

■ Urinalysis reveals hemoglobinuria.

■ Antibody screening reveals anti-A or anti-B antibodies in the blood.

■ Serum haptoglobin level falls below pretransfusion level after 24 hours.

■ Blood cultures may indicate bacterial contamination.

Blunt and penetrating abdominal injuries

■ History includes trauma to abdomen or chest area.

■ CXR or abdominal X-ray indicates presence of free air.

■ Peritoneal lavage reveals blood, urine, bile, stool, or pus.

■ Serum amylase level > 239 U/L (SI, > 4.07 µkat/L) indicates pancreatic injury.

■ Hb level and HCT show a serial decrease.

■ Excretory urography and retrograde cystography indicate renal and urinary tract damage.

■ CT scan indicates abdominal organ rupture.

■ Exploratory laparotomy reveals specific injuries when other clinical evidence is incomplete.

Blunt chest injuries

- History includes trauma to chest area.
- With hemothorax, percussion reveals dullness.
- With tension pneumothorax, percussion reveals tympany.
- CXR may indicate rib and sternal injuries, pneumothorax, flail chest, pulmonary contusion, lacerated or ruptured aorta, diaphragmatic rupture, lung compression, or hemothorax.
- CT scan reveals aortic laceration or rupture, or diaphragmatic rupture.
- CK-MB level shows mild elevation.

Bone tumor, primary malignant

- Physical examination detects palpable mass over bony area.
- Biopsy reveals malignant cells.
- Bone X-ray and radioisotope bone scan reveal tumor location and size.
- CT scan reveals tumor location and size.
- MRI reveals tumor.
- Serum alkaline phosphatase level is elevated (in patients with sarcomas).

Botulism

- Offending toxin is detected in the patient's serum, stool, gastric content, or the suspected food.
- EMG shows diminished muscle action potential after a single supramaximal nerve stimulus.

Brain abscess

- History includes congenital heart disease or infection, especially of the middle ear, mastoid, nasal sinuses, heart, or lungs.
- CT scan or MRI reveals site of abscess.
- Arteriography highlights the abscess with a halo.
- Culture of drainage reveals causative organism, such as *Staphylococcus aureus*, *Streptococcus viridans*, or *Streptococcus hemolyticus*.

Breast cancer

- Breast examination is abnormal.
- Mammography, ultrasonography, or thermography indicates presence of mass.
- Surgical biopsy reveals malignant cells.
- CEA levels are > 20 ng/ml (SI, > 20 µg/L).
- Serum or urine of woman who isn't pregnant contains hCG.

Bronchiectasis

- History includes recurrent bronchial infections, pneumonia, and hemoptysis.
- CXR show pleural thickening, areas of atelectasis, and scattered cystic changes.

Bronchitis, chronic

- CXRs may show hyperinflation and increased bronchovascular markings.
- PFTs demonstrate increased residual volume, decreased vital capacity and forced expiratory flow, and normal static compliance and diffusing capacity.
- ABG analysis reveals decreased Pao_2 and normal or increased $Paco_2$.
- Sputum culture reveals the presence of microorganisms and neutrophils.
- ECG may detect atrial arrhythmias; peaked P waves in leads II, III, and aV_F; and, occasionally, right ventricular hypertrophy.
- Bronchography reveals location and extent of disease.

Brucellosis

- History includes contact with animals.
- Agglutinin titers within 3 weeks of illness are elevated.
- Multiple blood cultures, bone marrow culture, and biopsy of infected tissue indicate presence of *Brucella* bacteria.

Buerger's disease

- History includes intermittent claudication of the palm of the hand and the instep.
- Doppler ultrasonography reveals diminished circulation in the peripheral vessels.
- Plethysmography reveals decreased circulation in the peripheral vessels.

Burns

- History includes exposure to heat, electricity, or chemicals.
- Examination reveals depth of skin and tissue damage and area affected.
- Urinalysis may reveal myoglobinuria and hemoglobinuria.
- ABG analysis reveals reduced respiratory function.
- Fiber-optic bronchoscopy may reveal epithelial damage to the trachea and bronchi.
- Serum protein studies show increased albumin levels.
- BUN level is increased due to increased protein catabolism.
- Fibrin split products are increased.
- Serum magnesium levels are suppressed.
- Osmotic fragility is high (increased tendency to hemolysis).
- Changes are noted in serum electrolyte levels, including elevated potassium and decreased sodium levels.
- WBC count reveals leukocytosis.

Calcium imbalance

- In hypocalcemia:
  - serum calcium level is < 4.5 mEq/L (SI, < 1.08 mmol/L).
- In hypercalcemia:
  - serum calcium level is > 5.5 mEq/L (SI, > 2.25 mmol/L)
  - urinalysis reveals increased calcium precipitation.

Note: Because approximately one-half of serum calcium is bound to albumin, changes in serum protein must be considered when interpreting serum calcium levels.

Cancer of the vulva

- Pap test reveals abnormal cells.
- Tissue biopsy reveals malignant cells.
- Vulva staining (with toluidine blue dye) indicates diseased tissues.

Candidiasis

- Culture of skin, vaginal scrapings, pus, sputum, blood, or tissue reveals *Candida albicans*.

Cardiac tamponade

- CXR reveals slightly widened mediastinum and cardiomegaly.
- Echocardiography reveals pericardial effusion with signs of right ventricular and atrial compression.
- Pulmonary artery monitoring reveals increased right atrial pressure, right ventricular diastolic pressure, and central venous pressure.

Cardiogenic shock

- Auscultation detects gallop rhythm, faint heart sounds, and a holosystolic murmur (with ruptured ventricular septum or papillary muscles).
- Pulmonary artery pressure monitoring reveals:
  - increased pulmonary artery pressure
  - increased PAWP
  - increased systemic vascular resistance
  - increased peripheral vascular resistance
  - decreased cardiac output.
- Invasive arterial pressure monitoring reveals hypotension.
- CK levels are increased.

- ABG analysis may show metabolic acidosis and hypoxia.
- ECG shows acute myocardial infarction, ischemia, or ventricular aneurysm.

Carpal tunnel syndrome
- Physical examination reveals decreased sensation to light touch or pinpricks in the affected fingers.
- Tinel's sign is positive.
- Wrist-flexion test reveals positive Phalen's sign.
- Compression test provokes pain and paresthesia along the distribution of the median nerve.
- EMG detects a median nerve motor conduction delay of more than 5 milliseconds.

Cataract
- Eye examination reveals the white area behind the pupil (unnoticeable until the cataract is advanced).
- Ophthalmoscopy or slit-lamp examination reveals a dark area in the normally homogeneous red reflex.

Celiac disease
- Tissue biopsy of the small bowel reveals a mosaic pattern of alternating flat and bumpy areas on the bowel surface (due to an almost total absence of villi) and an irregular, blunt, and disorganized network of blood vessels (usually prominent in the jejunum).
- Stool samples (after 72-hour collection) reveal excess fat.
- HLA test reveals presence of HLA-B8 antigen.
- D-xylose absorption test reveals depressed blood and urine d-xylose levels.
- Upper GI series followed by a small-bowel series demonstrates protracted barium passage: Barium shows up in a segmented, coarse, scattered, and clumped pattern; the jejunum shows generalized dilation.
- Glucose tolerance test indicates poor glucose absorption.
- Low serum carotene levels, indicating malabsorption.
- CBC indicates decreased Hb level and HCT as well as decreased WBC and platelet counts.
- Decreased serum albumin, sodium, potassium, cholesterol, and phospholipid levels.
- PT may be shortened.

Cerebral aneurysm
- History includes headache and change in mental status (usually with rupture or leakage).
- Angiography shows location and size of unruptured aneurysm.
- CT scan reveals location of clot, hydrocephalus, areas of infarction, and extent of blood spillage within the cisterns around the brain.

Cerebral contusion
- History includes head trauma.
- CT scan reveals ischemic tissue and hematoma.
- Skull X-ray indicates fracture is absent.

Cerebral palsy
Infant displays:
- difficulty sucking or keeping food in his mouth
- infrequent voluntary movement
- arm or leg tremors with movement
- crossing legs when lifted from behind rather than pulling them up or "bicycling"
- legs difficult to separate to change diapers
- persistent use of one hand, or ability to use hands well but not legs.

Cervical cancer

- Pap test reveals abnormal cells.
- Cone biopsy of cervical tissue reveals malignant cells.
- Colposcopy determines the source of the abnormal cells seen on the Pap test.

Cesarean birth

These test findings indicate the need for cesarean birth:
- X-ray pelvimetry may reveal cephalopelvic disproportion and malpresentation.
- Ultrasonography may reveal pelvic masses that interfere with vaginal delivery and fetal position.
- Amniocentesis may reveal Rh isoimmunization, fetal distress, or fetal genetic abnormalities.
- Auscultation of fetal heart rate (fetoscope, Doppler unit, or electronic fetal monitor) may reveal acute fetal distress.

Chalazion

- Visual examination and palpation of the eyelid reveal a small bump or nodule.
- Tissue biopsy rules out meibomian gland cancer.

Chancroid

- History includes sexual contact with a partner with chancroid.
- Tissue culture of ulcer exudate, bubo aspirate, or blood reveals *Haemophilus ducreyi*.

Chlamydial infections

- History includes sexual contact with a partner with chlamydial infection.
- Culture of site indicates *Chlamydia trachomatis* (findings may reveal urethritis, cervicitis, salpingitis, endometritis, or proctitis).
- Culture of blood, pus, or CSF reveals *C. trachomatis* (findings may reveal epididymitis, prostatitis, or lymphogranuloma venereum).

Chloride imbalance

- In hypochloremia, serum chloride level is < 98 mEq/L (SI, < 98 mmol/L).
- In hyperchloremia, serum chloride level is > 108 mEq/L (SI, > 108 mmol/L).

Cholelithiasis and related disorders

- Ultrasonography of the gallbladder indicates presence of stones.
- Percutaneous transhepatic cholangiography reveals gallbladder disease.
- Endoscopic retrograde cholangiopancreatography visualizes the biliary tree.
- Hida scan of the gallbladder reveals obstruction of the cystic duct.
- Oral cholecystography shows stones in the gallbladder and biliary duct obstruction.
- Technetium-labeled iminodiacetic acid scan of the gallbladder indicates cystic duct obstruction and acute or chronic cholecystitis if the gallbladder can't be seen.
- Blood studies may reveal elevated serum alkaline phosphatase, LD, AST, and total bilirubin levels and icteric index.
- WBC count is slightly elevated during a cholecystitis attack.

Cholera

- Patient reports voluminous, gray-tinged diarrhea.
- Stool or vomitus culture reveals presence of *Vibrio cholerae*.
- Agglutination and other clear reactions to group- and type-specific antisera provide definitive diagnosis.
- Dark-field microscopic examination of fresh stool shows rapidly moving bacilli.
- Immunofluorescence allows for rapid diagnosis.

Choriocarcinoma

■ Radioimmunoassay of hCG levels, performed frequently, provides early and accurate diagnosis; levels that are extremely elevated for early pregnancy indicate gestational trophoblastic disease.

■ Histologic examination of possible hydatid vessels confirms the diagnosis.

■ Ultrasonography performed after the third month shows grapelike clusters rather than a fetus.

■ Amniography reveals the absence of a fetus (performed only when the diagnosis is in question).

■ Doppler ultrasonography demonstrates the absence of fetal heart tones.

■ Hb level, HCT, and RBC count are abnormal.

■ Fibrinogen levels are abnormal.

■ PT and PTT are abnormal.

■ WBC count and ESR are increased.

■ CXR, CT scan, and MRI may identify choriocarcinoma metastasis.

■ Lumbar puncture may detect early cerebral metastasis if hCG is in CSF.

Chronic fatigue and immune dysfunction syndrome

■ History includes persistent or relapsing debilitating fatigue or tendency to tire easily.

■ Average level of activity is < 50% of normal for 6 months or more.

■ Fatigue doesn't resolve with bed rest.

■ Diagnostic tests rule out other illnesses, such as Epstein-Barr virus, leukemia, and lymphoma.

Chronic glomerulonephritis

■ Urinalysis reveals proteinuria, hematuria, cylindruria, and RBC casts.

■ BUN level is elevated.

■ Serum creatinine level is elevated.

■ Kidney X-rays or ultrasonography reveals small kidneys.

■ Renal biopsy indicates presence of underlying disease.

Chronic granulomatous disease

■ History includes osteomyelitis, pneumonia, liver abscess, or chronic lymphadenopathy in a young child.

■ Nitroblue tetrazolium (NBT) test reveals impaired NBT reduction, indicating abnormal neutrophil metabolism.

■ Neutrophil function test measures the rate of intracellular killing by neutrophils; in chronic granulomatous disease, killing is delayed or absent.

Chronic lymphocytic leukemia

■ CBC reveals numerous abnormal lymphocytes.

■ WBC count is mildly but persistently elevated in early stages.

■ Granulocytopenia is present.

■ Bone marrow aspiration and biopsy reveal lymphocytic invasion.

Chronic mucocutaneous candidiasis

■ Inspection reveals large, circular lesions.

■ Culture of affected area indicates presence of *Candida*.

Chronic renal failure

■ History includes chronic progressive debilitation.

■ BUN level is elevated.

■ Serum creatinine level is elevated.

■ Serum potassium level may be elevated.

■ ABG analysis reveals blood pH < 7.35 and HCO_3^- level < 22 mEq/L (SI, < 22 mmol/L).

■ Urinalysis may show proteinuria, glycosuria, erythrocytes, leukocytes, and casts.

■ Kidney biopsy identifies underlying pathology.

Cirrhosis and fibrosis

■ Liver biopsy reveals destruction and fibrosis of hepatic tissue.

■ Abdominal X-rays show liver size and cysts or gas within the biliary tract or liver, liver calcification, and massive ascites.

■ CT and liver scans determine the liver size, identify liver masses, and reveal hepatic blood flow and obstruction.

■ Esophagogastroduodenoscopy reveals bleeding esophageal varices, stomach irritation or ulceration, or duodenal bleeding and irritation.

■ ALT, AST, total serum bilirubin, and indirect bilirubin levels are elevated.

■ Serum albumin and protein levels are decreased.

■ PT is prolonged.

■ HCT, Hb, and serum electrolyte levels are decreased.

Coal worker's pneumoconiosis

■ History includes exposure to coal dust.

■ In simple coal worker's pneumoconiosis (CWP), CXR reveals small opacities (< 1 cm in diameter) prominent in the upper lung fields.

■ In complicated CWP, CXR reveals one or more large opacities (1 to 5 cm in diameter), possibly exhibiting cavitation.

■ PFTs reveal decreased lung capacity.

Coarctation of the aorta

■ Physical examination reveals resting systolic hypertension, absent or diminished femoral pulses, and wide pulse pressure.

■ CXR reveals notching of the undersurfaces of the ribs due to collateral circulation.

■ Echocardiography reveals left ventricular muscle thickening, coexisting aortic valve abnormalities, and the coarctation site.

■ Aortography locates the site and extent of coarctation.

■ ECG may reveal left ventricular hypertrophy.

Coccidioidomycosis

■ Skin test indicates a positive reaction for coccidioidin.

■ Immunodiffusion of sputum and pus from lesions and tissue biopsy reveal presence of *Coccidioides immitis* spores.

■ Complement fixation reveals presence of IgG antibodies.

■ Serum Ig levels help establish diagnosis.

Colorado tick fever

■ History includes recent exposure to ticks.

■ Serum studies indicate presence of Colorado tick fever virus.

■ Patient may have leukopenia.

Colorectal cancer

■ Hemoccult test (guaiac) reveals blood in stools.

■ Proctoscopy or sigmoidoscopy reveals presence of mass.

■ Colonoscopy reveals lesion.

■ Tissue biopsy reveals malignant cells.

■ Barium X-ray reveals lesion.

■ CEA level is > 5 ng/ml (SI, > 5 µg/L).

Common variable immunodeficiency

■ Circulating B-cell count is normal.

■ Serum IgM, IgA, and IgG levels are decreased, suggesting diminished synthesis or secretion.

■ Antigenic stimulation reveals an inability to produce specific antibodies.

■ X-rays may reveal signs of chronic lung disease or sinusitis.

Complement deficiencies

- Total serum complement level is low.
- Specific assays may confirm deficiency of specific complement components.

Concussion

- History includes head trauma, with or without loss of consciousness.
- Patient demonstrates amnesia with regard to traumatic event.
- Patient reports headache.
- Neurologic examination results are normal for patient.
- Skull X-ray and CT scan may be negative.

Congenital hip dysplasia

- Ortolani's or Trendelenburg's sign is positive.
- Inspection reveals extra thigh fold on affected side, higher buttock fold on the affected side, restricted abduction of the affected hip.
- X-ray reveals the location of the femur head and a shallow acetabulum.

Conjunctivitis

- Inspection reveals inflammation of the conjunctiva.
- Stained smear of conjunctival scrapings reveal monocytes (viral conjunctivitis), polymorphonuclear cells (bacterial conjunctivitis), or eosinophils (allergic conjunctivitis).
- Conjunctival culture reveals causative organism.

Corneal abrasion

- History includes eye trauma or prolonged wearing of contact lenses.
- Fluorescein stain of the cornea turns the injured area green during flashlight examination.
- Slit-lamp examination discloses the depth of the abrasion.

Corneal ulcers

- History includes eye trauma or use of contact lenses.
- Flashlight examination reveals irregular corneal surface.
- Fluorescein dye, instilled in the conjunctival sac, stains the outline of the ulcer.

Coronary artery disease

- History includes angina and risk factors for coronary artery disease.
- ECG reveals ischemia and, possibly, arrhythmias during an anginal attack. ECG returns to normal when pain ceases.
- Coronary angiography reveals coronary artery stenosis or obstruction, collateral circulation, and the arteries' condition beyond the narrowing.
- Myocardial perfusion imaging with thallium-201 during treadmill exercise detects ischemic areas.

Cor pulmonale

- Pulmonary artery pressure measurements reveal increased right ventricular and pulmonary artery pressures as well as elevated right ventricular systolic, pulmonary artery systolic, and pulmonary artery diastolic pressures.
- CXR reveals large central pulmonary arteries and rightward enlargement of cardiac silhouette.
- Echocardiography reveals right ventricular enlargement.

Corrosive esophagitis and stricture

- History includes chemical ingestion.
- Oropharyngeal burns (indicated by white membranes and edema of the soft palate and uvula).
- Endoscopy (in the first 24 hours after ingestion) delineates the extent and location of the esophageal injury and assesses

depth of the burn; 1 week after ingestion, this test helps assess stricture development.

■ Barium swallow, performed 1 week after ingestion and every 3 weeks thereafter, as ordered, identifies segmental spasm or fistula.

Cri du chat syndrome

■ History includes cat cry, facial disproportions, microencephaly, small birth size, and poor physical and mental development.

■ Karyotype reveals deleted short arms of chromosome 5.

Crohn's disease

■ History includes frequent stools and abdominal cramping.

■ Barium enema reveals the string sign (segments of stricture separated by normal bowel).

■ Sigmoidoscopy and colonoscopy reveal patchy areas of inflammation.

■ Biopsy of bowel tissue reveals histologic changes indicative of Crohn's disease.

Cryptococcosis

■ Inspection may reveal signs of meningeal irritation.

■ Sputum, urine, prostatic secretion culture; bone marrow aspirate or biopsy; or pleural biopsy reveals *Cryptococcus neoformans*.

■ Blood culture reveals *C. neoformans* (with severe infection).

■ CXR reveals pulmonary lesion.

■ Cryptococcal antigen and positive cryptococcal culture occurs in 90% of tests.

Cushing's syndrome

■ Serum cortisol levels are consistently elevated.

■ 24-hour urine sample demonstrates elevated free cortisol levels.

■ Dexamethasone suppression test reveals a cortisol level of 5 g/dl (SI, 140 nmol/L) or greater (failure to suppress).

■ Urine 17-hydroxycorticosteroid levels are elevated.

■ Urine 17-KS levels are elevated.

■ Ultrasonography, CT scan, or angiography localize adrenal tumors.

■ CT scan of the head identifies pituitary tumors.

Cutaneous larva migrans

■ Patient displays characteristic migratory lesions.

■ History includes contact with warm, moist soil within the past several months.

Cystic fibrosis

■ Family history includes the disorder.

■ Pulmonary disease or pancreatic insufficiency (absence of trypsin) is present.

■ Sweat test reveals sodium and chloride concentrations of 50 to 60 mEq/L (SI, 50 to 60 mmol/L) or greater.

■ DNA testing may locate the Delta 508 deletion and help to confirm the diagnosis.

■ PFTs evaluate lung function.

■ Sputum culture allows the detection of concurrent infectious disease.

■ ABG analysis helps determine pulmonary status.

■ CXR helps diagnose respiratory obstruction and monitor its progress.

Cystinuria

■ Family history includes renal disease or renal calculi.

■ Chemical analysis of calculi shows cystine crystals, with a variable amount of calcium.

■ Clearance of cystine, lysine, arginine, and ornithine is elevated.

■ Urinalysis with amino acid chromatography indicates aminoaciduria, as evi-

denced by the presence of cystine, lysine, arginine, and ornithine.
- Urine pH is usually < 5.
- Microscopic examination of urine shows hexagonal, flat cystine crystals.
- Cyanide-nitroprusside test is positive.
- Excretory urography or KUB X-rays reveal size and location of calculi.

Cytomegalovirus infection
- Culture of urine, saliva, throat, or blood or biopsy specimens reveal virus.
- Indirect immunofluorescent test reveals IgM antibody.

Dacryocystitis
- History includes constant tearing.
- Culture of discharge from tear sac reveals *Staphylococcus aureus* and, occasionally, beta-hemolytic streptococci in acute dacryocystitis; culture reveals *Streptococcus pneumoniae* or *Candida albicans* in the chronic form.
- Dacryocystography locates the atresia.

Decompression sickness
- History includes rapid decompression.
- Physical examination reveals incapacitating joint and muscle pain and neurologic and respiratory disturbance.

Dermatitis
- Family history includes allergy and chronic inflammation.
- Patient demonstrates characteristic distribution of skin lesions.
- Serum IgE levels are elevated.

Dermatophytosis
- Inspection reveals skin lesions.
- Microscopic examination or culture of lesion scrapings reveals infective organism.
- Wood's light examination may reveal types of tinea capitis.

Diabetes insipidus
- History includes head trauma or neurologic surgery.
- Urinalysis reveals almost colorless urine of low osmolality (< 300 mOsmol/kg [SI, < 300 mmol/kg]) and low specific gravity (< 1.005).

Diabetes mellitus
- In nonpregnant adults, findings include:
  - symptoms of uncontrolled diabetes and a random blood glucose level ≥ 200 mg/dl (SI, ≥ 10.6 mmol/L)
  - fasting plasma glucose level ≥ 126 mg/dl (SI, ≥ 7 mmol/L) on at least two occasions
  - in a patient with normal fasting glucose, a blood glucose level > 200 mg/dl (SI, > 10.6 mmol/L) during the second hour of a glucose tolerance test and on at least one other occasion during the glucose tolerance test.
- Ophthalmologic examination may show diabetic retinopathy.
- Urinalysis reveals presence of acetone.

DiGeorge's syndrome
- History includes facial anomalies in infant.
- T-lymphocyte assay shows decreased or absent T cells.
- B-lymphocyte assay shows elevated B cells.
- CT scan or MRI shows thymus is absent.
- Serum calcium levels are < 8 mg/dl (SI, < 2 mmol/L).

Dilated cardiomyopathy
- CXR reveals cardiomegaly, usually affecting all heart chambers, and may also show pulmonary congestion, pleural or pericardial effusion, or pulmonary venous hypertension.
- ECG may reveal ST-segment and T-wave changes.

- Echocardiography reveals left ventricular thrombi, global hypokinesia, and degree of left ventricular dilation.

Diphtheria

- Inspection reveals characteristic thick, patchy grayish green membrane over the mucous membranes of the pharynx, larynx, tonsils, soft palate, and nose.
- Throat culture or culture of other suspect lesions reveals *Corynebacterium diphtheriae*.

Dislocated or fractured jaw

- History includes trauma to jaw or face.
- Maxillary or mandibular mobility is abnormal.
- X-ray of the jaw shows fracture.

Dislocations and subluxations

- Inspection confirms joint deformity.
- X-ray is negative for fracture but may reveal dislocation or subluxation.
- Arthroscopy reveals dislocation or subluxation.

Disseminated intravascular coagulation

- Patient displays abnormal bleeding in the absence of a known hematologic disorder.
- Platelet count is < 100,000/µl (SI, < 100 × 10^9/L).
- Fibrinogen is < 175 mg/dl (SI, < 1.75 g/L).
- PT is > 15 seconds.
- PTT is > 60 seconds.
- Fibrin split products reveal fibrin degradation products > 100 mg/ml.
- D-dimer test (a specific fibrinogen test for disseminated intravascular coagulation) is positive.

- Fibrin degradation products are increased, > 45 µg/ml (SI, > 45 mg/L).

Diverticular disease

- Upper GI series reveals barium-filled pouches in the esophagus and upper bowel.
- Barium enema reveals barium-filled pouches in the lower bowel; barium outlines diverticula filled with stool.

Down syndrome

- History includes hypotonia at birth.
- Karyotype reveals chromosome abnormality.
- Prenatal ultrasonography may suggest Down syndrome if a duodenal obstruction or an atrioventricular canal defect is present.
- Maternal serum AFP levels are reduced.
- Amniocentesis reveals the translocated chromosome.

Dysfunctional uterine bleeding

- History includes excessive vaginal bleeding.
- Organic, systemic, psychogenic, and endocrine causes of bleeding are ruled out.
- D&C and biopsy reveal endometrial hyperplasia.

Dysmenorrhea

- History includes abdominal pain related to menstruation.
- Pelvic examination may reveal the physical cause.
- Laparoscopy may reveal an underlying cause such as endometriosis or uterine leiomyoma.
- D&C may reveal an underlying cause such as cervical stenosis or pelvic inflammatory disease.

Dyspareunia

■ History includes discomfort during sexual intercourse.

■ Pelvic examination may reveal a physical disorder as underlying cause of discomfort.

Ectopic pregnancy

■ Serum pregnancy test shows presence of hCG.

■ Real-time ultrasonography (performed if serum pregnancy test is positive) reveals no intrauterine pregnancy.

■ Culdocentesis (performed if ultrasonography detects the absence of a gestational sac in the uterus) reveals free blood in the peritoneum.

■ Laparoscopy (performed if culdocentesis is positive) reveals pregnancy outside the uterus.

Electric shock

■ History includes electrical contact, voltage, and length of contact.

■ Physical examination reveals electrical burn.

■ ECG reveals ventricular fibrillation or other arrhythmias that progress to fibrillation or myocardial infarction.

■ Urine myoglobin test is positive.

Emphysema

■ Examination reveals barrel chest, pursed-lip breathing, and use of accessory muscles of respiration; palpation may reveal decreased tactile fremitus and decreased chest expansion; percussion may reveal hyperresonance; auscultation may reveal decreased breath sounds, crackles and wheezing on inspiration, prolonged expiratory phase with grunting respirations, and distant heart sounds.

■ In advanced disease, CXR may show a flattened diaphragm, reduced vascular markings at the lung periphery, overaeration of the lungs, a vertical heart, enlarged anteroposterior chest diameter, and large retrosternal air space.

■ PFTs indicate increased residual volume and total lung capacity, reduced diffusing capacity, and increased inspiratory flow.

■ ABG analysis usually shows reduced Pa_{O_2} and normal Pa_{CO_2} until late in the disease when Pa_{CO_2} increases.

■ ECG may reveal tall, symmetrical P waves in leads II, III, and aV_F; a vertical QRS axis; and signs of right ventricular hypertrophy late in the disease.

■ RBC count usually demonstrates an increased Hb level late in the disease, when the patient has persistent severe hypoxia.

Encephalitis

■ Lumbar puncture reveals elevated CSF pressure and clear CSF, with slightly elevated WBC and protein levels.

■ CSF or blood culture reveals virus.

■ Serologic studies (in herpes encephalitis) may show rising titers of complement-fixing antibodies.

■ EEG reveals abnormalities such as generalized slowing of waveforms.

Endocarditis

■ Auscultation reveals a loud, regurgitant murmur.

■ Blood cultures (three or more during a 24- to 48-hour period) reveal infecting organism.

■ WBC count is elevated.

■ ESR is elevated.

■ Serum creatinine level is elevated.

■ Echocardiography or transesophageal echocardiography reveals valvular damage and endocardial vegetation.

Endometriosis

■ Pelvic examination reveals multiple tender nodules on uterosacral ligaments or in

the rectovaginal septum, which enlarge and become more tender during menses.
- Palpation may uncover ovarian enlargement in patients with endometrial cysts on the ovaries or thickened, nodular adnexa (as in pelvic inflammatory disease).
- Barium enema rules out malignant or inflammatory bowel disease.

Enterobiasis

- Collecting a sample from the perianal area with a cellophane tape swab leads to identification of the *Enterobius* ova.
- History includes pruritus ani as well as recent contact with infected person or infected articles.

Enterocolitis

- Stool Gram stain reveals numerous gram-positive cocci and polymorphonuclear leukocytes with few gram-negative rods.
- Stool culture identifies *Staphylococcus aureus* as the causative organism.
- Blood studies reveal leukocytosis, moderately increased BUN level, and decreased serum albumin level.

Epicondylitis

- History includes traumatic injury or strain associated with athletic activity.
- Examination reveals pain with wrist extension and supination with lateral involvement or with flexion and pronation with epicondyle involvement.
- X-rays are normal at first, but later bony fragments, osteophyte sclerosis, or calcium deposits appear.
- Arthrography is normal with some minor irregularities on the tendon undersurface.
- Arthrocentesis identifies causative organism if joint infection is suspected.

Epidermolysis bullosa

- Skin biopsy of a freshly induced blister reveals type of epidermolysis bullosa.
- Fetoscopy and biopsy provide prenatal diagnosis of the severe scarring forms (at 20 weeks' gestation).

Epididymitis

- History includes unilateral, dull aching pain radiating to the spermatic cord, lower abdomen, and flank.
- Physical examination shows characteristic waddle, as an attempt to protect the groin and scrotum when walking.
- WBC count in urine is increased.
- Urine culture and sensitivity tests reveal causative organism.
- Elevated serum WBC count indicates infection.

Epiglottiditis

- Throat examination reveals a large, edematous, bright red epiglottis.
- Direct laryngoscopy reveals swollen, beefy-red epiglottis (not done if significant obstruction is suspected or immediate intubation isn't possible).
- Lateral neck X-rays show an enlarged epiglottis and distended hypopharynx.

Epilepsy

- CT scan provides brain density readings indicating abnormalities in internal structures.
- EEG may show paroxysmal abnormalities and helps classify the disorder.
- MRI helps identify the cause of the seizure by providing clear images of the brain in regions where bone normally hampers visualization.

Epistaxis

- History includes trauma to the nose, chemical irritation, sinus infection, or coagulopathy.

- Inspection with a bright light and nasal speculum locates the site of bleeding.

Erectile dysfunction

- Detailed sexual history reveals persistent or recurrent partial or complete failure to attain or maintain erection until completion of sexual activity or a persistent or recurrent lack of a subjective sense of sexual excitement and pleasure during sexual activity.
- Urologic screening rules out urogenital problems.
- Neurologic evaluation rules out neurologic dysfunction.
- Drug history rules out medication use as a causative factor.

Erysipeloid

- History includes occupational exposure to *Erysipelothrix insidiosa* and skin injury.
- Examination reveals purple erythema of the skin, persisting over several days.
- Full-thickness skin biopsy taken from the edge of the lesion results in isolation of *E. insidiosa*.

Erythroblastosis fetalis

- Maternal history reveals risk factors for incompatibility of fetal and maternal blood, such as erythroblastotic stillbirths, abortions, previously affected children, previous anti-Rh titers, and blood transfusions.
- Maternal blood typing indicates mother is Rh-negative (titers determine changes in the degree of maternal immunization).
- Amniocentesis reveals an increase in bilirubin levels (indicating possible hemolysis) and elevations in anti-Rh titers.
- Radiologic studies may show edema and, in hydrops fetalis, the halo sign (edematous, elevated, subcutaneous fat layers) and the Buddha position (fetus's legs are crossed).

- Direct Coombs' test of umbilical cord blood confirms maternal-neonatal Rh incompatibility.
- An umbilical cord Hb count < 10 g/dl (SI, < 100 g/L) signals severe disease.
- Stained RBC examination reveals many nucleated peripheral RBCs.

Esophageal cancer

- X-rays of the esophagus, with barium swallow and motility studies, reveal structural and filling defects and reduced peristalsis.
- CXR or esophagography reveals pneumonitis.
- Esophagoscopy, punch-and-brush biopsies, and exfoliative cytologic tests confirm esophageal tumors.
- Bronchoscopy may reveal tumor growth in the tracheobronchial tree.
- Endoscopic ultrasonography (combined with endoscopy and ultrasonography) identifies depth of tumor penetration.
- Mediastinoscopy reveals lesion and extent of disease.
- Esophageal biopsy reveals malignant cells.

Esophageal diverticula

- Barium swallow reveals characteristic out-pouching in esophagus.
- Esophagoscopy rules out other lesions as cause.

Exophthalmos

- Physical examination reveals forward displacement of the eyeballs.
- Exophthalmometer readings reveal the degree of anterior projection and asymmetry between the eyes to be > 12 mm.
- X-rays show orbital fracture or bony erosion by an orbital tumor.
- CT scan identifies lesions in optic nerve, orbit, or ocular muscle within the orbit.

Extraocular motor nerve palsies

- Neuro-ophthalmologic examination reveals third nerve palsy (ptosis, exotropia, pupil dilation, and unresponsiveness to light, inability to move and accommodate), fourth nerve palsy (diplopia and inability to rotate eye downward and upward), or sixth nerve palsy (one eye turning, with the other eye unable to abduct beyond midline).
- Skull X-rays rule out intracranial tumor.
- CT scan and MRI rule out tumor.
- Cerebral angiography rules out vascular abnormalities.
- Blood studies rule out diabetes.
- Culture and sensitivity tests reveal infective organism (for sixth nerve palsy resulting from infection).

Extrapulmonary tuberculosis

- Acid-fast smear reveals *Mycobacterium tuberculosis*.
- Tuberculin skin test is positive.
- CXR reveals primary pulmonary nodular infiltrates and cavitations (often, however, CXR is negative in extrapulmonary tuberculosis).
- Fluid specimen culture (urine, synovial fluid) reveals *M. tuberculosis*.

Fallopian tube cancer

- History includes unexplained postmenopausal bleeding.
- Pap test reveals abnormal cells.
- Ultrasonography defines tumor mass.
- Barium enema rules out intestinal obstruction.
- Laparotomy and biopsy reveal malignant cells.

Fanconi's syndrome

- 24-hour urine testing reveals excessive excretion of glucose, phosphate, amino acids, HCO_3^-, and potassium.
- Phosphorus and nitrogen levels are elevated (with increased renal dysfunction).
- Serum alkaline phosphatase levels are elevated (with rickets).
- Serum potassium level is decreased.
- Serum HCO_3^- level is < 22 mEq/L (SI, < 22 mmol/L).

Fatty liver

- Examination reveals large, tender liver.
- Liver function studies reveal low albumin, elevated globulin, elevated total bilirubin, low aminotransferase and, commonly, elevated cholesterol levels.
- PT is prolonged.
- Liver biopsy reveals excessive fat.

Femoral and popliteal aneurysms

- Palpation reveals a pulsating mass above or below the inguinal ligament (in femoral aneurysm) or in the popliteal space (in popliteal aneurysm).
- Arteriography or ultrasonography reveals location and size of aneurysm.

Folic acid deficiency anemia

- Serum folate level is decreased.
- Reticulocyte count is decreased.
- Schilling test is positive.
- Serum blood studies show macrocytosis, increased mean corpuscular volume, and abnormal platelets.

Folliculitis, furunculosis, and carbunculosis

- Examination reveals pustule, painful nodule, or abscess on areas with hair growth.

- Wound culture identifies *Staphylococcus aureus*.
- CBC may reveal leukocytosis.
- In carbunculosis, history includes preexistent furunculosis.

Galactorrhea

- History includes milk secretion more than 21 days after weaning.
- Breast palpation results in expression of secretions.
- Microscopic examination reveals fat droplets in fluid.
- Prolactin levels are > 200 ng/ml (SI, > 200 µg/L).
- CT scan rules out pituitary tumor.
- Mammography rules out tumor.

Galactosemia

- Deficiency of the enzyme galactose-1-phosphate uridyl transferase in RBCs indicates classic galactosemia; decreased galactokinase level in RBCs indicates galactokinase deficiency.
- Serum and urine galactose levels are increased.
- Ophthalmoscopy reveals punctate lesions in the fetal lens nucleus.
- Liver biopsy reveals acinar formation.
- Liver enzyme levels (AST and ALT) are elevated.
- Urinalysis reveals presence of albumin.
- Amniocentesis provides prenatal diagnosis (recommended for heterozygous and homozygous parents).

Gallbladder and bile duct carcinoma

- Liver function test may show elevated urobilirubin levels and may show elevated levels of bile and bilirubin.
- Serum bilirubin levels are elevated (5 to 390 mg/dl [SI, > 90 µmol/L]).
- Patient may be jaundiced.
- PT is prolonged.

- Serum alkaline phosphatase levels are consistently elevated.
- Liver-spleen scan identifies abnormality.
- Cholecystography shows stones or calcifications.
- MRI may show areas of tumor growth.
- Cholangiography outlines common bile duct obstruction.
- Ultrasonography of the gallbladder shows a mass.
- Endoscopic retrograde cholangiopancreatography identifies tumor site.
- Biopsy reveals malignant cells.

Gas gangrene

- History includes recent surgery or a deep puncture wound with rapid onset of pain and crepitation around the wound.
- Anaerobic cultures of wound drainage reveal *Clostridium perfringens*.
- Gram stain of wound drainage reveals large, gram-positive, rod-shaped bacteria.
- X-rays reveal gas in tissues.
- Blood studies reveal leukocytosis and, later, hemolysis.

Gastric carcinoma

- Barium X-rays with fluoroscopy reveal tumor or filling defect in the outline of the stomach, loss of flexibility and distensibility, and abnormal gastric mucosa with or without ulceration.
- Gastroscopy with fiber-optic endoscope visualizes mucosal lesions and allows gastroscopic biopsy (biopsy reveals malignant cells).
- Photography with fiber-optic endoscope provides a permanent record of gastric lesions that may help determine disease progression and effect of treatment.
- CT scans, CXR, liver and bone scans, and liver biopsy may rule out specific organ metastasis.

Gastritis

- History includes gastric discomfort or bleeding.
- Gastroscopy demonstrates inflammation of mucosa and confirms diagnosis.
- Stools or vomitus may contain occult blood.
- Hb level and HCT are decreased if bleeding has occurred.

Gastroenteritis

- History includes acute onset of diarrhea accompanied by abdominal pain and discomfort.
- Stool or blood culture reveals causative bacteria, parasites, or amoebae.
- Barium enema reveals inflammation.

Gastroesophageal reflux

- Barium swallow with fluoroscopy may be normal except in patients with advanced disease; in children, barium esophagography under fluoroscope reveals reflux.
- Esophageal acidity test reveals pH of 1.5 to 2.0.
- Acid perfusion test elicits pain or burning.
- Gastroesophageal reflux scanning detects radioactivity in the esophagus.
- Endoscopy and biopsy identify pathologic mucosal changes.

Gaucher's disease

- Bone marrow aspiration reveals Gaucher's cells.
- Direct assay of glucocerebrosidase activity, which can be performed on venous blood, shows absent or deficient activity.
- Liver biopsy reveals increased glucosylceramide accumulation.
- Serum acid phosphatase levels are increased.
- Platelet count and serum iron level are decreased.

Genital herpes

- History includes oral, vaginal, or anal sexual contact with an infected person or other direct contact with lesions.
- Examination reveals vesicles on the genitalia, mouth, or anus.
- Tissue culture and histologic biopsy of vesicular fluid reveals herpes simplex virus type 2.

Genital warts

- Dark-field examination of scrapings from wart cells shows marked vascularization of epidermal cells, which helps to differentiate genital warts from condylomata lata.
- Applying 5% acetic acid (white vinegar) to the warts turns them white, indicating papillomas.

Giardiasis

- History includes such risk factors as recent travel to an endemic area, participation in sexual activity involving oral-anal contact, ingestion of suspect water, or institutionalization.
- Stool specimen shows cysts.
- Duodenal aspirate or biopsy shows trophozoites.
- Small-bowel biopsy shows parasitic infection.

Glaucoma

- History includes gradual loss of peripheral vision.
- Tonometry (using an applanation, Schiøtz, or pneumatic tonometer) reveals increased intraocular pressure.
- Gonioscopy determines the angle of the anterior chamber of the eye, differentiating between chronic open-angle glaucoma and acute angle-closure glaucoma.
- Ophthalmoscopy reveals cupping and atrophy of the optic disk.

- Slit-lamp examination visualizes anterior structures of the eye, demonstrating effects of glaucoma.
- Perimetry or visual field tests evaluate the extent of visual field loss of open-angle deterioration.
- Fundus photography reveals changes in the optic disk.

Glycogen storage diseases

- Type Ia:
  - Liver biopsy reveals normal glycogen synthetase and phosphorylase enzyme activities but reduced or absent glucose-6-phosphatase activity.
  - Liver biopsy reveals normal glycogen structure, but elevated amounts.
  - Serum glucose levels are low.
  - Plasma studies reveal high levels of free fatty acids, triglycerides, cholesterol, and uric acid.
  - Injection of glucagon or epinephrine increases pyruvic and lactic acid levels but doesn't increase blood glucose levels.
  - Glucose tolerance test curve reveals depletional hypoglycemia and reduced insulin output.
- Type II (Pompe's):
  - Muscle biopsy reveals increased concentration of glycogen with normal structure and decreased alpha-1, 4-glucosidase level.
  - ECG (in infants) shows large QRS complexes in all leads, inverted T waves, and a shortened PR interval.
  - EMG (in adults) demonstrates muscle fiber irritability and myotonic discharges.
  - Amniocentesis reveals a deficiency in alpha-1,4-glucosidase level.
  - Placenta or umbilical cord examination shows an alpha-1,4-glucosidase deficiency.

- Liver biopsy shows deficient debranching activity and increased glycogen concentration.
- Type III (Cori's):
  - Laboratory tests (in children only) may reveal elevated AST or ALT levels and an increase in erythrocyte glycogen.
- Type IV (Andersen's):
  - Liver biopsy demonstrates deficient branching enzyme activity and that the glycogen molecule has longer outer branches.
- Type V (McArdle's):
  - Serum studies indicate no increase in venous levels of lactate in sample drawn from extremity after ischemic exercise.
  - Muscle biopsy reveals a lack of phosphorylase activity and an increased glycogen content.
- Type VI (Hers'):
  - Liver biopsy shows decreased phosphorylase beta activity and increased glycogen concentration.
- Type VII:
  - Serum studies indicate no increase in venous levels of lactate in sample drawn from extremity after ischemic exercise.
  - Blood studies reveal low erythrocyte phosphofructokinase activity and reduced half-life of RBCs.
  - Muscle biopsy shows deficient phosphofructokinase with a marked rise in glycogen concentration with normal structure.
- Type VIII:
  - Liver biopsy shows deficient phosphorylase beta activity and increased liver glycogen levels.
  - Blood studies show deficient phosphorylase beta kinase in leukocytes.

Goiter, simple

- History includes residence in an area known for nutritionally related risk factors (such as iodine-depleted soil or malnutrition) or ingestion of goitrogenic medications or foods.
- Serum TSH or T_3 concentration is high or normal.
- T_4 concentrations are low to normal.
- Uptake of ^{131}I is normal or increased.
- Protein-bound iodine is low to normal.
- Urinary excretion of iodine is low.

Gonorrhea

- History includes sexual contact with a partner with gonorrhea.
- Culture from site of infection (urethra, cervix, rectum, pharynx) reveals *Neisseria gonorrhoeae*.
- Culture of joint fluid and skin lesions reveals gram-negative diplococci (gonococcal arthritis).
- Culture of conjunctival scrapings confirms gonococcal conjunctivitis.
- Complement fixation and immunofluorescent assays of serum reveal antibody titers four times the normal rate.

Goodpasture's syndrome

- Immunofluorescence of alveolar basement membrane shows linear deposition of Ig as well as complement 3 and fibrinogen.
- Immunofluorescence of glomerular basement membrane (GBM) shows linear deposition of Ig combined with detection of circulating anti-GBM antibody.
- Lung biopsy shows interstitial and intra-alveolar hemorrhage with hemosiderin-laden macrophages.
- CXR reveals pulmonary infiltrates in a diffuse, nodular pattern.
- Renal biopsy reveals focal necrotic lesions and cellular crescents.

- Serum creatinine and BUN levels typically increase two to three times normal.
- Urinalysis may reveal RBCs and cellular casts, granular casts, and proteinuria.

Gout

- Microscopic analysis of synovial fluid obtained by needle aspiration reveals needlelike intracellular crystals of sodium urate; presence of monosodium urate monohydrate crystals confirms diagnosis.
- Serum uric acid levels are normal, but may be increased; the higher the level, the more likely a gout attack.
- Urine uric acid levels are increased (in approximately 20% of patients).
- X-rays reveal damage to the articular cartilage and subchondral bone (in chronic gout).

Granulocytopenia

- Patient demonstrates marked neutropenia.
- WBC count is markedly decreased.
- CBC reveals few observable granulocytes.
- Bone marrow aspiration reveals a scarcity of granulocytic precursor cells beyond the most immature forms.

Guillain-Barré syndrome

- History includes minor febrile illness 1 to 4 weeks before current symptoms.
- Examination reveals progressive muscle weakness.
- CSF analysis reveals normal WBC count, rising protein levels (peaks in 4 to 6 weeks), and increasing pressure.
- EMG reveals repeated firing of the same motor unit instead of widespread sectional stimulation.
- Electrophysiologic studies may reveal marked slowing of nerve conduction velocities.

Haemophilus influenzae infection

■ Blood culture reveals *H. influenzae* infection.

■ CBC reveals polymorphonuclear leukocytosis and, in young children with severe infection, leukopenia.

Hearing loss

■ Audiometry identifies and quantifies hearing loss.

■ The Weber, the Rinne, and Schwabach tests differentiate between conductive and sensorineural hearing loss.

■ Auditory brain stem response and behavioral tests may help to identify neonatal or infant hearing loss.

■ CT scan evaluates vestibular and auditory pathways.

■ Pure tone audiometry identifies the presence and degree of hearing loss.

■ MRI detects acoustic tumors and lesions.

Heart failure

■ Auscultation reveals dyspnea or crackles.

■ CXR reveals increased pulmonary vascular markings, interstitial edema, or pleural effusion and cardiomegaly.

■ Pulmonary artery monitoring reveals elevated pulmonary artery and capillary wedge pressures and elevated left ventricular end-diastolic pressure in left-sided heart failure, and elevated right atrial pressure or central venous pressure in right-sided heart failure.

Hemochromatosis

■ Serum or plasma iron concentration is elevated.

■ Transferrin levels are increased to 70% to 100% saturation.

■ 24-hour urine collection shows excretion of iron after administration of deferoxamine, an iron-chelating agent.

■ Liver biopsy may also confirm diagnosis.

Hemophilia

■ History suggests disorder runs in family.

■ History includes prolonged bleeding after surgery or trauma or of episodes of spontaneous bleeding into muscles or joints.

■ Hemophilia A:
  – Factor VIII assay is 0% to 55% of normal.
  – PTT is prolonged.
  – Platelet count and function, bleeding time, and PT are normal.

■ Hemophilia B:
  – Factor IX assay is deficient.
  – PTT is prolonged.

■ Hemophilia C:
  – Assay testing reveals deficient factor XI but normal factors VIII and IX levels (rules out hemophilias A and B).
  – PTT is prolonged.

■ CT scan rules out intracranial bleeding.

■ Arthroscopy rules out joint bleeding.

■ Endoscopy rules out GI bleeding.

Hemorrhoids

■ History includes intermittent rectal bleeding after defecation.

■ Examination reveals hemorrhoids protruding from rectum.

■ Proctoscopy reveals internal hemorrhoids.

■ Anoscopy and flexible sigmoidoscopy identify internal hemorrhoids and rule out polyps or fistulae.

Hemothorax

■ History includes recent trauma to chest area.

■ Chest percussion reveals dullness.

■ Chest auscultation reveals decreased to absent breath sounds on the affected side.

■ Thoracentesis reveals blood or serosanguineous fluid.

- CXR reveals pleural fluid with or without mediastinal shift.
- ABG studies show respiratory failure.
- Hb levels may be decreased depending on the degree of blood loss.

Hepatic encephalopathy

- History includes liver disease, with symptoms beginning with slight personality changes progressing to mental confusion and coma.
- Serum ammonia levels are > 33 µmol/L (SI, > 33 µmol/L).
- EEG shows slowing waves as the disease progresses.

Hepatitis, viral

- Hepatitis profile identifies serum antigens and antibodies (serum markers) specific to the causative virus, establishing the type of hepatitis (types A, B, C, D, and E).
- PT is prolonged (more than 3 seconds longer than normal indicates liver damage).
- AST and ALT levels are elevated.
- Serum alkaline phosphatase levels are elevated.
- Serum and urine bilirubin levels are elevated (with jaundice).
- Serum albumin is decreased and serum globulin is increased.
- Liver biopsy and liver scan show patchy necrosis.

Hereditary hemorrhagic telangiectasia

- History includes an established family pattern of bleeding disorders.
- Examination reveals localized aggregations of dilated capillaries on the skin of the face, ears, scalp, hands, arms, and feet, and under the nails; characteristic telangiectases are raised or flat, nonpulsatile, violet in color, blanche under pressure, and bleed easily.

- Bone marrow aspiration shows depleted iron stores, which confirms secondary iron deficiency anemia.
- Platelet count may be abnormal.

Herniated disk

- History includes unilateral low back pain radiating to the buttocks, legs, and feet, often associated with a previous traumatic injury or back strain.
- X-rays show degenerative changes and rule out other abnormalities.
- MRI also rules out spinal compression.
- Lasègue's test causes resistance and pain as well as loss of ankle or knee-jerk reflex.
- Myelography pinpoints the level of herniation and reveals spinal canal compression by herniated disk material.
- CT scan identifies soft tissue and bone abnormalities.
- EMG confirms nerve involvement.
- Neuromuscular tests identify motor and sensory loss and leg muscle weakness.

Herpangina

- Examination reveals vesicular lesions on the mucous membranes of the soft palate, tonsillar pillars, and throat.
- Cultures of mouth washings or stool reveal the coxsackieviruses.
- Antibody titers are elevated.

Herpes simplex

- Examination reveals edema with small vesicles on an erythematous base that rupture, leaving a painful ulcer followed by yellow crusting.
- Isolation of virus from local lesions and biopsy reveal *Herpesvirus hominis*.

Herpes zoster

- Examination reveals small red, nodular skin lesions that spread unilaterally around the thorax or vertically over the arms or

legs and vesicles filled with clear fluid or pus.
- Examination of vesicular fluid and infected tissue reveals eosinophilic intranuclear inclusions and varicella virus.
- Lumbar puncture shows increased CSF pressure; CSF analysis shows increased protein levels and, possibly, pleocytosis (with central nervous system involvement).

Hiatal hernia
- CXR reveals air shadow behind the heart (with large hernia).
- Barium swallow with fluoroscopy reveals outpouching at lower end of the esophagus and identifies diaphragmatic abnormalities.
- Serum Hb level and HCT may be decreased (with paraesophageal hernia).
- Endoscopy and biopsy rule out varices and other small gastroesophageal lesions.
- Esophageal motility studies reveal esophageal motor or lower esophageal pressure abnormalities.
- pH studies reveal reflux of gastric contents.
- Acid perfusion test reveals heartburn resulting from esophageal reflux.

Hirschsprung's disease
- Rectal biopsy reveals absence of ganglion cells.
- Barium enema studies reveal a narrowed segment of distal colon with a sawtooth appearance and a funnel-shaped segment above it; barium is retained longer than the usual 12 to 24 hours.
- Rectal manometry detects failure of the internal anal sphincter to relax and contract.
- Upright films of the abdomen show marked colonic distention.

Histoplasmosis
- History includes an immunocompromised condition or exposure to contaminated soil in an endemic area.
- Tissue biopsy and sputum culture reveal *Histoplasma capsulatum* (in acute primary and chronic pulmonary histoplasmosis).
- Histoplasmosis skin test is positive.
- Complement fixation test results and agglutination titers are increased.

Hodgkin's disease
- Lymph node biopsy reveals Reed-Sternberg's abnormal histiocyte proliferation and nodular fibrosis and necrosis.
- CT scan shows lymph node abnormality.
- Lymphangiography shows lymph node abnormality.
- Bone marrow, liver, mediastinal, and spleen biopsies; abdominal CT scan; and lung and bone scans identify organ involvement.
- Blood studies show normochromic anemia (in 50% of patients) and elevated, normal, or reduced WBC count and differential showing any combination of neutrophilia, lymphocytopenia, monocytosis, and eosinophilia.
- Serum alkaline phosphatase levels are increased.

Hookworm disease
- Stool specimen reveals hookworm ova.
- Blood studies show decreased Hb level (in severe cases) and markedly increased WBC count with eosinophil count elevation.

Huntington's disease
- History includes family inheritance pattern along with progressive chorea and dementia, with usual onset between ages 35 and 40.
- PET scan identifies disease.

- DNA analysis identifies marker for gene linked to the disease.
- Evoked potential studies reveal bilateral abnormal P100 latencies.
- Pneumoencephalography reveals the characteristic butterfly dilation of the brain's lateral ventricles.
- CT scan reveals brain atrophy.

Hydatidiform mole

- History includes vaginal bleeding, ranging from brownish red spotting to bright red hemorrhage.
- Examination reveals an abnormally enlarged uterus; pelvic examination reveals grapelike vesicles.
- Histologic identification of hydatid vesicles after passage helps confirm diagnosis.
- Ultrasonography shows grapelike structures rather than a fetus; use of a Doppler ultrasonic flowmeter demonstrates the absence of fetal heart tones.
- Amniography reveals the absence of a fetus.
- WBC count and ESR are increased.
- Hb level, HCT, RBC count, PT, PTT, fibrinogen levels, and hepatic and renal function studies are abnormal.
- Serum hCG levels are elevated 100 days or more after the last menstrual period.
- Serum human placental lactogen levels are subnormal.

Hydrocephalus

- Examination reveals an abnormally large head size for age.
- Skull X-rays reveal thinning of the skull with separation of sutures and widening of the fontanels.
- Ventriculography reveals enlargement of the brain's ventricles.
- Angiography, CT scan, or MRI of the brain reveals areas of altered density and rules out intracranial lesions.

Hydronephrosis

- KUB X-rays reveal bilateral kidney enlargement.
- Renal ultrasonography reveals large, echo-free, central mass that compromises the renal cortex.
- Excretory urography reveals abnormal kidneys.
- Urine studies reveal the inability to concentrate urine, a decreased GFR and, possibly, pyuria (if infection is present).

Hyperaldosteronism

- Serum potassium levels are persistently low (in the absence of edema, diuretic use, GI loss, or abnormal sodium intake).
- Low plasma renin level after volume depletion by diuretic administration and upright posture and a high plasma aldosterone level after volume expansion by salt loading confirms primary hyperaldosteronism in a hypertensive patient without edema.
- Serum HCO_3^- level is elevated with ensuing alkalosis resulting from the loss of hydrogen and potassium in the distal tubules.
- Serum and urine aldosterone levels are increased.
- Plasma volume levels are increased.
- Adrenal angiography or CT scan reveals adrenal tumor.
- Suppression testing reveals decreased plasma aldosterone and urine metabolites (secondary hyperaldosteronism) or normal plasma aldosterone and urine metabolites (primary hyperaldosteronism).
- ECG reveals ST-segment depression and the presence of U waves, indicating hypokalemia.
- CXR shows left ventricular hypertrophy from chronic hypertension.
- CT scan, ultrasonography, or MRI identifies tumor location.

Hyperbilirubinemia

■ Patient is jaundiced.

■ Serum bilirubin levels are > 10 mg/dl (SI, > 180 μmol/L).

Hyperemesis gravidarum

■ History includes uncontrolled nausea and vomiting that persists beyond the first trimester of pregnancy.

■ Examination reveals substantial weight loss.

■ Serum sodium, chloride, potassium, and protein levels are decreased.

■ BUN level is elevated.

■ Urinalysis reveals ketonuria and proteinuria.

Hyperlipoproteinemia

■ Type I (Fredrickson's hyperlipoproteinemia, fat-induced hyperlipemia, idiopathic familial):

– Chylomicrons (very-low-density lipoproteins [VLDL], low-density lipoproteins [LDL], high-density lipoproteins [HDL]) are present in plasma 14 hours or more after last meal.

– Serum chylomicron and triglyceride levels show high elevation; serum cholesterol levels are slightly elevated.

– Serum lipoprotein lipase levels are decreased.

– Leukocytosis is present.

■ Type II (familial hyperbetalipoproteinemia, essential familial hypercholesterolemia):

– Plasma concentrations of LDL are increased.

– Serum LDL and cholesterol levels are elevated.

– Increased LDL levels are detected by amniocentesis.

■ Type III (familial broad-beta disease, xanthoma tuberosum):

– Serum beta-lipoprotein levels are abnormal.

– Cholesterol and triglyceride levels are elevated.

– Glucose levels are slightly elevated.

■ Type IV (endogenous hypertriglyceridemia, hyperbetalipoproteinemia):

– Plasma VLDL levels are elevated.

– Plasma triglyceride levels are moderately increased.

– Serum cholesterol levels are normal or slightly elevated.

– Glucose tolerance is mildly abnormal.

– History includes early coronary artery disease.

■ Type V (mixed hypertriglyceridemia, mixed hyperlipidemia):

– Chylomicrons are present in plasma.

– Plasma VLDL levels are elevated.

– Serum cholesterol and triglyceride levels are elevated.

Hyperparathyroidism

■ Serum parathyroid hormone levels are increased.

■ Serum calcium levels are increased.

■ Urine cyclic adenosine monophosphate test reveals failure to respond to parathyroid hormone.

■ X-rays show diffuse demineralization of bones, bone cysts, outer cortical bone absorption, and subperiosteal erosion of the radial aspect of the middle fingers.

■ X-ray spectrophotometry demonstrates increased bone turnover.

■ Radioimmunoassay shows increased concentration of parathyroid hormone with accompanying hypercalcemia.

■ Serum phosphorus levels are increased.

■ Serum and urine chloride, uric acid, creatinine, and alkaline phosphatase levels are increased; basal acid secretion is present.

■ Serum immunoreactive gastrin levels are increased.

Hyperpituitarism

- Growth hormone (GH) immunoassay shows increased plasma GH levels.
- Glucose suppression test shows failure to suppress GH level to below accepted norm of 5 ng/ml (SI, 5 µg/L).
- Skull X-rays, CT scan, arteriography, and pneumoencephalography reveal the presence and extent of a pituitary lesion.
- Bone X-rays reveal a thickening of the cranium (especially of frontal, occipital, and parietal bones) and of the long bones as well as osteoarthritis in the spine.

Hypersplenism

- I.V. infusion of chromium-labeled RBCs or platelets reveals high spleen-liver ratio of radioactivity, indicating splenic destruction or sequestration.
- CBC shows decreased Hb levels, WBC count, and platelet count, and elevated reticulocyte count.
- Examination reveals splenomegaly.

Hypertension

- Serial blood pressure measurements on a sphygmomanometer are more than 140/90 mm Hg.
- Urinalysis reveals presence of protein, RBCs, WBCs, or glucose.
- Excretory urography may reveal renal atrophy.
- BUN and serum creatinine levels are normal or elevated, suggesting renal disease.

Hyperthyroidism

- Radioimmunoassay shows increased serum T_4 and T_3 levels.
- Thyroid scan reveals increased uptake of ^{131}I.
- Thyroid-releasing hormone (TRH) stimulation test reveals failure of the TSH level to rise within 30 minutes after administration of TRI I.

- Autoantibody tests reveal presence of thyroid-stimulating Ig.

Hypervitaminoses A and D

- History includes accidental or misguided use of supplemental vitamin preparations.
- Serum vitamin A level is > 90 µg/dl (SI, > 2.8 µmol/L) in hypervitaminosis A.
- Serum vitamin D level is > 100 ng/ml (SI, > 250 nmol/L) in hypervitaminosis D.
- Serum carotene level is > 250 µg/dl (SI, > 4.74 µmol/L) in hypercarotenemia.
- X-rays show calcification of tendons, ligaments, and subperiosteal tissues in hypervitaminosis D.

Hypoglycemia

- Blood glucose studies reveal abnormally low levels (< 45 mg/dl [SI, < 2.6 mmol/L]).
- C-peptide assay identifies fasting hypoglycemia.

Hypogonadism

- Serum and urine gonadotropin levels are increased in primary, or hypergonadotropic; hypogonadism and decreased in secondary, or hypogonadotropic, hypogonadism.
- Chromosomal analysis identifies the cause.
- Testicular biopsy and semen analysis reveal impaired spermatogenesis and low testosterone levels.
- X-rays and bone scans show delayed closure of epiphyses and immature bone age.

Hypoparathyroidism

- Radioimmunoassay shows decreased serum parathyroid hormone levels.
- Urine and serum calcium levels are decreased.
- Serum phosphorus levels are increased.
- Urine creatinine levels are decreased.

- X-rays show increased bone density and malformation.
- Cyclic adenosine monophosphate test demonstrates a 10- to 20-fold increase.
- ECG shows increased QT and ST intervals due to hypercalcemia.

Hypopituitarism

- Radioimmunoassay shows decreased plasma levels of some or all pituitary hormones.
- Serum T_4 levels are decreased (with thyroid dysfunction).
- Arginine test reveals failure of hGH levels to rise after arginine infusion (with pituitary dysfunction).
- Insulin tolerance test reveals failure of stimulation or a blunted response of hGH levels (with hypothalamic-pituitary-adrenal axis dysfunction).
- Urine 17-KS levels are decreased (with hypoadrenalism).
- Levels of serum pituitary hormones (FSH, LH, and TSH) are decreased.
- CT scan, pneumoencephalography, or cerebral angiography confirms the presence of tumors inside or outside the sella turcica.

Hypothermic injuries

- History includes severe and prolonged exposure to cold.
- Core body temperature is < 95° F (35° C).
- Physical examination shows burning, tingling, numbness, swelling, pain, and mottled blue-gray skin in exposed areas.

Hypothyroidism in adults

- Radioimmunoassay shows low serum levels of thyroid hormones.
- Serum TSH level may be increased (due to thyroid insufficiency) or decreased (due to hypothalamic or pituitary insufficiency).

- Radioactive iodine uptake test reveals below normal percentages of iodine uptake.
- Radionuclide thyroid imaging reveals "cold spots."
- Thyroid ultrasonography identifies cysts or tumors.
- Serum antithyroid antibodies are elevated (in autoimmune thyroiditis).

Hypothyroidism in children

- Elevated serum TSH levels are associated with low T_3 and T_4 levels.
- Thyroid scan (^{131}I uptake test) shows decreased uptake levels and confirms the absence of thyroid tissue in athyroid children.
- Gonadotropin levels are increased and compatible with sexual precocity in older children.
- Hip, knee, and thigh X-rays reveal absence of the femoral or tibial epiphyseal line and delayed skeletal development that's markedly inappropriate for the child's chronological age.

Hypovolemic shock

- History includes recent loss of blood volume.
- Blood pressure auscultation reveals mean arterial pressure under 60 mm Hg in adults and a narrowing pulse pressure.
- Blood studies show low Hb level and HCT, low RBC count, and low platelet levels.
- Serum potassium, sodium, LD, creatinine, and BUN levels are elevated.
- Urine specific gravity is > 1.020.
- Urine osmolality is elevated.
- Urine creatinine levels are decreased.
- ABG measurements show decreased pH, decreased Pao_2, and increased $Paco_2$ levels.

Idiopathic hypertrophic subaortic stenosis

■ Echocardiography shows increased thickness of the intraventricular septum and abnormal motion of the anterior mitral leaflet during systole, occluding left ventricular outflow in obstructive disease.
■ Cardiac catheterization reveals elevated left ventricular end-diastolic pressure and, possibly, mitral insufficiency.
■ ECG usually demonstrates left ventricular hypertrophy, T wave inversion, left anterior hemiblock, Q waves in precordial and inferior leads, ventricular arrhythmias and, possibly, atrial fibrillation.
■ Phonocardiography confirms an early systolic murmur.

Idiopathic thrombocytopenic purpura

■ Platelet count is markedly decreased.
■ Bleeding time is prolonged.
■ Bone marrow studies show an abundance of megakaryocytes (platelet precursors) and a shortened circulating platelet survival time.

IgA deficiency

■ Serum IgA levels are < 15% of total Ig or < 60 mg/dl (SI, < 0.60 g/L).
■ IgA is usually absent from secretions.

Impetigo

■ Inspection reveals characteristic lesions.
■ Microscopic visualization, Gram stain, or culture of exudate identifies *Staphylococcus aureus* as causative organism.
■ WBC count may be elevated.

Inactive colon

■ History includes dry, hard, infrequent stools.
■ Digital rectal examination reveals stools in the lower portion of the rectum and a palpable colon.

■ Proctoscopy reveals unusually small colon lumen, prominent veins, and an abnormal amount of mucus.
■ Upper GI series and barium enema rule out tumor.
■ Fecal occult blood test is negative.

Inclusion conjunctivitis

■ History includes sexual contact with a partner infected with *Chlamydia trachomatis*.
■ Examination reveals swollen, reddened lower eyelids, excessive tearing, and a moderately purulent discharge.
■ Conjunctival scraping reveals cytoplasmic inclusion bodies in conjunctival epithelial cells and many polymorphonuclear leukocytes; culture for bacteria is negative.

Infantile autism

■ History includes symptom development before age 30 months.
■ Denver Developmental Screening Test shows delayed development, especially of social and language skills.
■ IQ testing indicates retardation.
■ Evaluation reveals impairment in social interaction skills, verbal and nonverbal communication, and imaginative activity and a markedly restricted range of activities and interests.

Infectious mononucleosis

■ WBC count is elevated during 2nd and 3rd week of illness, with lymphocytes and monocytes making up 50% to 70% of WBCs (10% of lymphocytes are abnormal).
■ Heterophil agglutination tests indicate the presence of heterophil antibodies; testing at 3- to 4-week intervals reveals a rise to four times normal levels.
■ Indirect immunofluorescence shows antibodies to Epstein-Barr virus and cellular antigens.
■ Liver function studies are abnormal.

Infectious myringitis

■ Otoscopic examination shows small, reddened, inflamed blebs in the ear canal, on the tympanic membrane, and in the middle ear (with bacterial invasion).
■ Culture of exudate identifies infective organism.

Infertility, female

■ History includes inability to achieve pregnancy after having regular intercourse, without contraception, for at least 1 year.
■ Progesterone blood levels reveal a luteal phase deficiency.
■ FSH levels are decreased.
■ Hysterosalpingography reveals tubal obstruction or uterine abnormalities.
■ Endoscopy shows tubal obstruction or uterine abnormalities.
■ Laparoscopy visualizes abdominal and pelvic areas and may reveal peritubular adhesions or ureterotubal obstruction.
■ Postcoital (Sims-Huhner) test shows inadequate motile sperm cells in cervical fluid after intercourse.
■ Immunologic or antibody testing detects spermicidal antibodies in the sera of the female.

Infertility, male

■ History includes abnormal sexual development, delayed puberty, or infertility in previous relationships.
■ Medical history also includes prolonged fever, mumps, impaired nutritional status, previous surgery, or trauma to genitalia.
■ Semen analysis reveals subnormal sperm counts, decreased sperm motility, abnormal morphology, or absence of viable spermatozoa.
■ Urine 17-KS levels are decreased.
■ Serum testosterone levels are decreased.

Influenza

■ Nose and throat culture identifies the causative virus.
■ Cold agglutinin titers are elevated.
■ Serum antibody titers are increased.
■ WBC count is decreased and lymphocytes are increased (uncomplicated cases).

Inguinal hernia

■ History includes sharp or "catching" pain when lifting or straining, with excessive coughing, or following a recent pregnancy.
■ Examination reveals a swelling or lump in the inguinal area.
■ Palpation of the inguinal area, while the patient is performing Valsalva's maneuver, reveals pressure against the fingertip (indirect hernia) or pressure against the side of the finger (direct hernia).
■ Abdominal X-ray rules out obstruction.
■ WBC count may be elevated.

Insect bites and stings

■ Tick:
 – History reveals exposure in woods and fields and complaints of itching.
 – After several days, tick paralysis (acute flaccid paralysis, starting as paresthesia and pain in legs and resulting in respiratory failure from bulbar paralysis) occurs.
■ Bee, wasp, or yellow jacket:
 – History reveals painful sting.
 – Examination reveals protruding stinger (bees), edema, urticaria, or pruritus.
 – Systemic reaction (anaphylaxis), indicating hypersensitivity, usually appears within 20 minutes and may include weakness, chest tightness, dizziness, nausea, vomiting, abdominal cramps, and throat constriction.
■ Brown recluse (violin) spider:

– History reveals exposure to dark areas (outdoor privy, barn, woodshed) in south-central United States with reaction within 2 to 8 hours of the bite.
– Examination reveals localized vasoconstriction with ischemic necrosis at bite site and small, reddened puncture wound forming a bleb and becoming ischemic, proceeding to a dark, hard center in 3 to 4 days and an ulcer within 2 to 3 weeks.
– Pain is minimal initially, but increases over time.
– Commonly, fever, chills, malaise, weakness, nausea, vomiting, edema, seizures, joint pains, petechiae, cyanosis, and phlebitis develop.
– Rarely, thrombocytopenia and hemolytic anemia develop and lead to death within 24 to 48 hours (usually in a child or patient with previous history of cardiac disease).
■ Scorpion:
– In nonlethal types, history reveals symptoms lasting from 24 to 78 hours and including local swelling and tenderness, sharp burning sensation, skin discoloration, paresthesia, lymphangitis with regional gland swelling, and anaphylaxis (rare).
– In lethal types, history reveals symptoms including immediate sharp pain, hyperesthesia, drowsiness, itching (nose, throat, mouth), impaired speech, and generalized muscle spasms (including jaw muscle spasms, laryngospasm, incontinence, seizures, nausea, and vomiting).
■ Black widow spider:
– History reveals exposure to dark areas (outdoor privy, barn, woodshed) in southern United States between April and November and report of pinprick sensation followed by dull, numbing pain.

– Examination reveals edema and tiny red bite marks, rigidity of stomach muscles, and severe abdominal pain (10 to 40 minutes after bite).
– Muscle spasms develop in extremities.
– Ascending paralysis occurs, causing difficulty in swallowing and labored, grunting respirations.
– Other symptoms include extreme restlessness, vertigo, sweating, chills, pallor, seizures (especially in children), hyperactive reflexes, hypertension, tachycardia, thready pulse, circulatory collapse, nausea, vomiting, headache, ptosis, eyelid edema, urticaria, pruritus, and fever.

Intestinal obstruction

■ History includes progressive, colicky abdominal pain and distention.
■ Abdominal X-ray reveals the presence and location of intestinal gas or fluid.
■ In X-ray, small-bowel obstruction appears as a typical "stepladder" pattern of alternating gas and fluid levels.
■ In X-ray, large-bowel obstruction reveals a distended, air-filled colon or a closed loop of sigmoid with extreme distention.
■ Serum sodium, chloride, and potassium levels may decrease because of vomiting.
■ WBC count may be normal or slightly elevated if necrosis, peritonitis, or strangulation occurs.
■ Serum amylase level may increase.
■ Sigmoidoscopy, colonoscopy, or barium enema may help identify the cause of obstruction.

Intussusception

■ Barium enema reveals characteristic coiled spring sign and delineates the extent of intussusception.
■ Upright abdominal X-rays may show a soft-tissue mass and signs of complete or partial obstruction, with dilated loops of bowel.

- Elevated WBC count may indicate obstruction, strangulation, or bowel infarction.

Iodine deficiency

- Serum T_4 levels are low, with high ^{131}I uptake.
- 24-hour urine collection reveals low iodine levels.
- Serum TSH levels are high.
- Radioiodine uptake test traces ^{131}I in the thyroid 24 hours after administration.

Iron deficiency anemia

- Bone marrow studies reveal depleted or absent iron stores and normoblastic hyperplasia.
- Hb level is decreased.
- HCT is decreased.
- Serum iron levels are low, with high iron binding capacity.
- Serum ferritin levels are low.
- RBC count is low, with microcytic and hypochromic cells.
- GI studies rule out or confirm the bleeding.

Irritable bowel syndrome

- History includes diarrhea alternating with constipation and bowel upset related to diet or psychological stress.
- Sigmoidoscopy may reveal spastic contraction.
- Barium enema may reveal colonic spasm and tubular appearance of descending colon.
- Colonoscopy, rectal examination, or rectal biopsy may rule out other disorders.
- Fecal tests for occult blood, parasites, and pathogenic bacteria are negative.

Junctional tachycardia

ECG findings include:

- Atrial and ventricular rhythms are usually regular. The atrial rhythm may be difficult to determine if the P wave is absent or hidden in the QRS complex or preceding T wave.
- Atrial and ventricular rates exceed 100 beats/minute (usually between 100 and 200 beats/minute). The atrial rate may be difficult to determine if the P wave is absent or hidden in the QRS complex, or precedes the T wave.
- P wave is usually inverted. It may occur before or after the QRS complex, be hidden in the QRS complex, or be absent.
- If the P wave precedes the QRS complex, the PR interval is shortened (< 0.12 second). Otherwise, the PR interval can't be measured.
- Duration of QRS complex is within normal limits. The configuration is usually normal.
- T-wave configuration is usually normal, but may be abnormal if the P wave is hidden in the T wave. Fast rate may make the T wave indiscernible.
- QT interval is usually within normal limits.

Juvenile angiofibroma

- Nasopharyngeal mirror or nasal speculum reveals a blue mass in the nose or nasopharynx.
- Nasal X-rays reveal a bowing of the posterior wall of the maxillary sinus.
- Angiography reveals the size and location of the tumor and also shows the source of vascularization.

Keratitis

- History includes recent infection of the upper respiratory tract accompanied by cold sores.

■ Slit-lamp examination reveals one or more small branchlike (dendritic) lesions (caused by herpes simplex virus).
■ Touching the cornea with cotton reveals reduced corneal sensation.

Kidney cancer
■ Renal ultrasonography and CT scan identify renal tumor.
■ Excretory urography, nephrotomography, and KUB X-ray identify renal tumor.
■ Liver function studies show increased alkaline phosphatase, bilirubin, and transaminase levels.
■ PT is prolonged.
■ Blood studies show anemia, polycythemia, hypercalcemia, and increased ESR.
■ Urinalysis reveals hematuria.
■ Antegrade urography and cytologic studies reveal malignancy.
■ Renal biopsy reveals malignant cells.
■ Radionuclide renal imaging reveals malignant tumor.

Klinefelter syndrome
■ Karyotype obtained by culturing lymphocytes from the patient's peripheral blood shows chromosome abnormality.
■ Testosterone level is depressed after puberty.
■ Urine 17-KS levels are decreased.
■ FSH levels are increased.

Kyphosis
■ History includes severe pain.
■ Examination reveals curvature of the thoracic spine and bone destruction.
■ X-rays reveal vertebral wedging, Schmorl's nodes, irregular plates and, possibly, mild scoliosis of 10 to 20 degrees.

Labyrinthitis
■ History includes nausea and vomiting, hearing loss, and severe vertigo from any movement of the head.
■ Examination reveals spontaneous nystagmus with jerking movements of the eyes toward the unaffected ear.
■ Culture of drainage identifies infective organism.
■ Audiometry reveals sensorineural hearing loss.
■ CT scan rules out brain lesion.

Laryngeal cancer
■ History includes hoarseness that lasts longer than 2 weeks.
■ Laryngoscopy reveals lesion.
■ Laryngeal tomography, CT scan, or laryngography defines the borders of a lesion.
■ Laryngeal biopsy reveals malignant cells.
■ CXR identifies metastasis.

Laryngitis
■ History includes hoarseness, ranging from mild to complete loss of voice.
■ Indirect laryngoscopy reveals red, inflamed and, occasionally, hemorrhagic vocal cords, with rounded rather than sharp edges, and exudate; bilateral swelling may be present, which restricts movement but doesn't cause paralysis.

Lassa fever
■ History includes recent travel to an endemic area.
■ Throat washings, pleural fluid, or blood cultures reveal Lassa virus.
■ Antibody titer reveals Lassa Ig.

Legg-Calvé-Perthes disease
■ Examination reveals restricted abduction and rotation of the hip.

■ Hip X-rays (taken every 3 to 4 months) reveal flattening of the femoral head or deformity, new bone formation, and eventually regeneration of the joint.
■ Bone scan reveals involvement of anterolateral portion of the femoral head.
■ Aspiration and culture of synovial fluid rule out joint sepsis.

Legionnaires' disease
■ Cultures of respiratory tract secretions and tissue culture identify *Legionella pneumophila*.
■ Direct immunofluorescence testing reveals *L. pneumophila*.
■ Indirect fluorescent serum antibody testing shows convalescent serum with a fourfold or greater rise in antibody titer for *L. pneumophila*.
■ CXR reveals patchy, localized infiltration, which progresses to multilobar consolidation, pleural effusions and, in fulminant disease, opacification of the entire lung.
■ Blood studies show leukocytosis, increased ESR, and increases in alkaline phosphatase, ALT, and AST levels.
■ ABG measurements show decreased Pao_2 and, initially, decreased $Paco_2$.
■ Bronchial washings, blood and pleural fluid cultures, and transtracheal aspirate studies rule out pulmonary infections.

Leishmaniasis
■ Scrapings from edges of lesion identify species of *Leishmania*.
■ *Leishmania* skin test is positive.

Leprosy
■ Examination reveals skin lesions and muscular and neurologic deficits.
■ Biopsy of skin lesions, peripheral nerves, or smear of skin or ulcerated mucous membranes allows identification of *Mycobacterium leprae*.

Lichen planus
■ Examination reveals generalized eruptions of flat, glistening purple papules marked with white lines or spots appearing linearly or coalescing into plaques.
■ Skin biopsy reveals lichen planus.

Listeriosis
■ Cultures of blood, CSF, cervical or vaginal lesion drainage, or lochia from a mother with an infected fetus reveal *Listeria monocytogenes*.
■ CBC reveals monocytosis.

Liver abscess
■ Liver scan reveals filling defects at the area of the abscess longer than $3/4''$ (1.9 cm).
■ Hepatic ultrasonography reveals defects caused by abscess.
■ CT scan reveals a low-density, homogenous area with well-defined borders.
■ CXR reveals the diaphragm on the affected side to be raised and fixed.
■ Blood tests show elevated levels of AST, ALT, alkaline phosphatase, and bilirubin.
■ Serum albumin is decreased.
■ WBC count is elevated.
■ Blood cultures and percutaneous liver aspiration identify causative organism.
■ Stool cultures and serologic and hemagglutination tests isolate *Entamoeba histolytica* (in amoebic abscesses).

Liver cancer
■ Needle biopsy or open biopsy reveals malignant cells.
■ AFP levels are elevated in 70% of patients with hepatocellular carcinoma.
■ Liver scan shows filling defects.
■ Liver function tests are abnormal.
■ CXR rule out metastasis to lungs.
■ Arteriography may define large tumors.
■ Serum electrolyte measurements show increased levels of sodium.

- Serum glucose and cholesterol levels are decreased.

Lower urinary tract infection

- Microscopic urinalysis reveals RBC and WBC counts > 10 per high-power field.
- Clean-catch urinalysis reveals bacterial count of more than 100,000/ml.
- Voiding cystoureterography or excretory urography shows congenital anomalies predisposing the patient to urinary tract infections.

Lung abscess

- Auscultation of the chest may reveal crackles and decreased breath sounds.
- CXR shows a localized infiltrate with one or more clear spaces, usually containing air or fluid.
- Percutaneous aspiration of an abscess or bronchoscopy may be used to obtain cultures to identify the causative organism.
- Blood and sputum cultures and Gram stain identify causative organism.
- WBC count is elevated.

Lung cancer

- CXR reveals lesion or mass.
- Sputum cytology reveals malignant cells.
- Bronchoscopy reveals site of mass.
- Biopsy reveals malignant cells.
- Tissue biopsy reveals evidence of metastasis.

Lupus erythematosus

- Examination reveals classic butterfly rash occurring over the nose and cheeks.
- ANA, anti-DNA, and lupus erythematosus cell tests are positive.
- Urine studies may show RBCs, WBCs, urine casts, sediment, and protein loss.
- CXR reveals pleurisy or lupus pneumonitis.

- Blood studies may show decreased serum complement 3 and complement 4 levels, indicating active disease; ESR is usually elevated; leukopenia, mild thrombocytopenia, and anemia also may be evident.
- ECG may show a conduction defect (with cardiac involvement or pericarditis).
- Renal biopsy identifies progression and extent of renal involvement.

Lyme disease

- History includes recent travel to endemic areas or exposure to ticks.
- Examination reveals the classic skin lesion called *erythema chronicum migrans*, beginning as a red macule or papule at the tick bite site growing in size to as large as 2″ (5 cm), described as hot and pruritic, with bright red outer rims and white centers.
- Mild anemia and elevated ESR, leukocyte count, serum IgM level, and AST level support the diagnosis.
- Antibody titers, ELISA, or blood culture may reveal *Borrelia burgdorferi*; lumbar puncture with CSF analysis allows for identification of antibodies to *B. burgdorferi* (if Lyme disease involves the central nervous system).

Lymphocytopenia

- Lymphocyte count is markedly decreased.
- Bone marrow aspiration and lymph node biopsies identify the cause.

Magnesium imbalance

- Hypomagnesemia:
  – Serum magnesium levels are < 1.5 mEq/L (SI, < 15 mg/L).
  – Serum potassium and calcium levels are decreased.
  – ECG shows tachyarrhythmias, slightly prolonged PR interval, prolonged QT interval, slightly prolonged QRS complex, ST-segment depression, prominent U waves, and broad flattened T waves.

- Hypermagnesemia:
  - Serum magnesium levels are > 2.5 mEq/L (SI, > 25 mg/L).
  - Serum potassium and calcium levels are elevated.
  - ECG shows prolonged PR interval, prolonged QRS complex, and elevated T wave.

Malaria

- History includes travel to an endemic area, recent blood transfusion, or I.V. drug use.
- Blood smears reveal parasites in RBCs.
- Indirect immunofluorescent serum antibody tests reveal malaria (2 weeks after onset).
- CBC shows decreased Hb level and a normal or decreased WBC count.
- Urinalysis reveals protein and WBCs in urine sediment.
- Serum blood studies show a reduced platelet count, prolonged PT, prolonged PTT, and decreased plasma fibrinogen levels (in falciparum malaria).

Malignant brain tumor

- Skull X-ray, brain scan, CT scan, or MRI reveals lesion.
- Biopsy of lesion reveals malignant cells.
- Lumbar puncture shows increased protein levels and decreased glucose levels in CSF; increased CSF pressure, indicating increased intracranial pressure; and, occasionally, tumor cells in CSF.

Malignant lymphoma

- Examination reveals enlarged lymph nodes.
- Biopsy of lymph nodes, tonsils, bone marrow, liver, bowel, or skin reveals malignant cells.
- CXR; lymphangiography; liver, bone, and spleen scans; CT scan of the abdomen; and excretory urography show disease progression.
- Serum uric acid level is normal or elevated.
- Serum calcium level may be elevated, indicating bone lesions.

Malignant melanoma

- Examination reveals skin lesion or nevus with recent changes in appearance.
- Excisional biopsy and full-depth punch biopsy reveal malignant cells.
- Urine test reveals melanin.

Mallory-Weiss syndrome

- History includes recent bout of forceful vomiting followed by vomiting blood or passing blood rectally (after a few hours to several days).
- Endoscopy identifies esophageal tear.
- Angiography reveals bleeding site.
- Serum HCT is decreased. (Measurements help to quantify blood loss.)

Marfan syndrome

- History includes disease in close relatives.
- Examination reveals skeletal deformities and ectopia lentis.
- X-rays reveal skeletal abnormalities.
- Echocardiography detects aortic root dilation.

Mastitis and breast engorgement

- History includes breast discomfort or other symptoms of inflammation in a lactating woman.
- Examination reveals redness, swelling, warmth, hardness, tenderness, cracks or fissures of the nipple, and enlarged lymph nodes.
- Cultures of expressed milk identify infective organism (generalized mastitis).

■ Cultures of breast skin identify infective organism (localized mastitis).

Mastoiditis

■ X-rays of the mastoid area reveal hazy mastoid air cells, and the bony walls between the cells appear decalcified.
■ Otoscopy reveals a dull, thickened, and edematous tympanic membrane, if the membrane isn't concealed by obstruction.
■ Culture and sensitivity tests identify causative organism.
■ Audiometry shows a conductive hearing loss.

Medullary cystic disease

■ Family history includes medullary cystic disease.
■ Arteriography and excretory urography reveal small kidneys.
■ Kidney biopsy shows structural abnormalities.
■ Blood studies show profound anemia.
■ Serum alkaline phosphatase level is elevated (in young patients).

Medullary sponge kidney

■ Excretory urography reveals a characteristic flowerlike appearance of the pyramidal cavities when they fill with contrast material.
■ Urinalysis is normal, but may show increased WBC count and casts (with infection) or an increased RBC count (with hematuria).

Ménière's disease

■ History includes vertigo, tinnitus, and hearing loss or distortion.
■ Audiometric studies indicate a sensorineural hearing loss and loss of discrimination and recruitment.
■ MRI rules out brain lesions or tumors.

■ Auditory brain stem response test rules out cochlear or retrocochlear lesion as the cause of hearing loss.

Meningitis

■ Lumbar puncture reveals cloudy CSF, elevated CSF pressure, high protein level, and depressed glucose concentration.
■ CSF culture and sensitivity tests reveal gram-positive or gram-negative organisms.
■ CXR shows pneumonitis or lung abscess, tubercular lesions, or granulomas (secondary to fungal infection).
■ Sinus and skull X-rays may help identify cranial osteomyelitis, paranasal sinusitis, or skull fracture.
■ WBC count shows leukocytosis.
■ CT scan rules out cerebral hematoma, hemorrhage, or tumor.
■ Brudzinski's and Kernig's signs are positive.

Meningococcal infection

■ Blood, CSF, or lesion culture reveals *Neisseria meningitidis*.
■ Platelet and clotting levels are decreased (with skin or adrenal hemorrhages).

Menopause

■ History includes menstrual cycle irregularities.
■ Pap test results show changes indicating the influence of estrogen deficiency on vaginal mucosa.
■ Radioimmunoassay blood studies show decreased estrogen levels and plasma estradiol level of 0 to 30 pg/ml (SI, 9 to 92 pmol/L).
■ Pelvic examination, endometrial biopsy, and D&C rule out suspected organic disease.
■ Serum FSH level is 30 to 100 mIU/ml (SI, 30 to 100 IU/L).
■ Plasma LH level is 20 to 100 mIU/ml (SI, 20 to 100 IU/ml).

Metabolic acidosis

- ABG analysis reveals:
  - pH < 7.35 (in severe acidosis, pH may fall to 7.10)
  - $Paco_2$ normal or < 34 mm Hg (SI, < 5.3 kPa)
  - HCO_3^- level may be < 22 mEq/L (SI, < 22 mmol/L).
- Anion gap is > 14 mEq/L (SI, > 14 mmol/L).
- Serum potassium levels are usually elevated.
- Blood glucose and serum ketone body levels are elevated (in diabetes mellitus).
- Plasma lactic acid levels are elevated (in lactic acidosis).

Metabolic alkalosis

- ABG analysis reveals:
  - pH > 7.45
  - $Paco_2$ may be > 45 mm Hg (SI, > 5.3 kPa) (indicating respiratory compensation)
  - HCO_3^- level > 29 mEq/L (SI, > 29 mmol/L).
- Serum electrolyte levels usually show decreased potassium, calcium, and chloride levels.
- ECG shows a low T wave merging with a P wave and atrial or sinus tachycardia.

Mitral insufficiency

- Cardiac catheterization may indicate signs of mitral insufficiency, including increased left ventricular end-diastolic volume and pressure, increased PAWP and atrial pressure, and decreased cardiac output.
- CXR may demonstrate left atrial and ventricular enlargement, pulmonary venous congestion, and calcification of the mitral leaflets.
- Echocardiography may reveal abnormal motion of the valve leaflets, left atrial enlargement, and a hyperdynamic left ventricle.
- ECG may show left atrial and ventricular hypertrophy, sinus tachycardia, or atrial fibrillation.

Mitral stenosis

- Cardiac catheterization shows a diastolic pressure gradient across the mitral valve and elevated left atrial and pulmonary artery pressures as well as an elevated PAWP. Catheterization may also reveal elevated right ventricular pressure, decreased cardiac output, and abnormal contraction of the left ventricle. Note that this test may not be indicated in patients who have isolated mitral stenosis with mild symptoms.
- CXR shows left atrial and left ventricular enlargement (in severe mitral stenosis), straightening of the left border of the cardiac silhouette, enlarged pulmonary arteries, dilation of the pulmonary veins of the upper lobes of the lungs, and mitral valve calcification.
- Echocardiography may disclose thickened mitral valve leaflets and left atrial enlargement.
- ECG can reveal atrial fibrillation, right ventricular hypertrophy, left atrial enlargement (in sinus rhythm), and right axis deviation.

Motion sickness

- History includes nausea, vomiting, dizziness, headache, fatigue, diaphoresis, or difficulty breathing related to a sensation of motion.
- If problem is persistent and affects the person's lifestyle, audiometry and vestibular tests may rule out vertigo.

Multiple endocrine neoplasia

- Family history reveals inheritance pattern, confirmed by genetic testing.
- Evaluation of signs and symptoms suggests multiple endocrine neoplasia.
- Diagnostic tests reveal hyperplasia, adenoma, or carcinoma in two or more endocrine glands, confirmed by biopsy.

Multiple myeloma

- CBC shows moderate to severe anemia; differential may show 40% to 50% lymphocytes but seldom more than 3% plasma cells.
- Rouleaux formation is seen on differential smear results.
- Analysis of urine proteins reveals Bence Jones protein, proteinuria, and hypercalciuria.
- Serum calcium levels are elevated.
- Serum electrophoresis shows an elevated globulin spike, which is electrophoretically and immunologically abnormal.
- Excretion tests show phenolsulfonphthalein level > 25% in 15 minutes, > 80% in 2 hours.
- Bone marrow aspiration detects myelomatous cells.
- KUB X-rays reveal bilateral renal enlargement.
- X-rays reveal multiple, sharply circumscribed osteolytic lesions, especially on the skull, pelvis, and spine.

Multiple sclerosis

- History includes multiple neurologic attacks with characteristic remissions and exacerbations.
- EEG results are abnormal.
- CSF analysis reveals elevated gamma globulin fraction of IgG (with normal serum gamma globulin levels).
- MRI reveals multifocal white matter lesions resulting from demyelination.

- Evoked potential studies show slowed conduction of nerve impulses (in 80% of patients).
- CT scan may show lesions within the brain's white matter.

Mumps

- History includes inadequate immunization and exposure to person infected with mumps.
- Examination reveals swelling and tenderness of the parotid glands and one or more of the other salivary glands.
- Antibody titer increases fourfold 3 weeks after acute phase of illness.
- Serum amylase level may be elevated.

Muscular dystrophy

- History includes progressive muscle weakness and evidence of genetic transmission.
- Muscle biopsy reveals fat and connective tissue deposits, degeneration and necrosis of muscle fibers and, in Duchenne's and Becker's dystrophies, a deficiency of the muscle protein dystrophin.
- EMG shows short, weak bursts of electrical activity in affected muscles.
- Genetic testing identifies the gene defect (in some patients).
- Urine creatinine, serum CK, LD, ALT, and AST levels are elevated.

Myasthenia gravis

- History includes progressive muscle weakness and muscle fatigability that improves with rest.
- Tensilon test is positive, showing improved muscle function after an I.V. injection of edrophonium or neostigmine.
- Serum acetylcholine receptor antibodies test is positive in symptomatic adults.
- EMG reveals motor unit potentials that are initially normal but progressively di-

minish in amplitude with continuing contractions.
- CXR or CT scan may show a thymoma.

Mycosis fungoides
- History includes multiple, varied, and progressively severe skin lesions.
- Biopsy of lesions reveals lymphoma cells.
- Fingerstick smear reveals Sézary cells (abnormal circulating lymphocytes), found in the erythrodermic variants of mycosis fungoides (Sézary syndrome).

Myelitis and acute transverse myelitis
- WBC count is normal or slightly elevated.
- CSF analysis may show normal or increased lymphocyte and protein levels and allows for isolation of the causative agent.
- Throat washings may reveal the causative virus (in poliomyelitis).
- CT scan or MRI may rule out spinal tumor.
- Examination may reveal focal neck and back pain with development of paresthesia and sensory loss.

Myocardial infarction
- History includes substernal chest pain, with radiation.
- Serial 12-lead ECG may be normal or inconclusive during the first hours after a myocardial infarction (MI); may reveal serial ST-segment depression (in subendocardial MI) and ST-segment elevation and Q waves (in transmural MI).
- Cardiac enzyme tests reveal elevated CK levels, with CK-MB isoenzyme > 5% of total CK over a 72-hour period.
- Cardiac protein tests reveal elevated troponin T and I levels. Elevations of troponin I are specific for myocardial injury.

- Echocardiography shows ventricular wall dyskinesia (with a transmural MI).
- Radioisotope scans using I.V. technetium 99m pertechnetate show "hot spots," indicating damaged muscle.
- Myocardial perfusion imaging with thallium-210 reveals a "cold spot" in most patients during the first few hours after a transmural MI.

Myocarditis
- History includes recent febrile upper respiratory tract infection, viral pharyngitis, or tonsillitis.
- Cardiac examination reveals supraventricular and ventricular arrhythmias, S_3 and S_4 gallops, a faint S_1, possibly a murmur of mitral insufficiency, and a pericardial friction rub (in patients with pericarditis).
- Endomyocardial biopsy reveals histologic changes consistent with myocarditis.
- Cardiac enzyme levels, including CK, CK-MB, serum AST, and LD, are elevated.
- WBC count and ESR are elevated.
- Antibody titers such as ASO are elevated.
- ECG shows diffuse ST-segment and T-wave abnormalities, conduction defects, and other ventricular and supraventricular arrhythmias.
- Cultures of stool, throat, pharyngeal washings, or other body fluids identify the causative bacteria or virus.

Nasal papillomas
- Examination reveals inverted papillomas as large, bulky, highly vascular, and edematous; color varies from dark red to gray; consistency, from firm to friable.
- Examination may also reveal exophytic papillomas that are raised, firm, and rubbery; color varies from pink to gray; papillomas are securely attached by a broad or

pedunculated base to the mucous membrane.
- Biopsy reveals histologic findings characteristic of papillomas.

Nasal polyps
- X-rays of sinuses and nasal passages reveal soft tissue shadows over the affected areas.
- Examination with a nasal speculum reveals nasal obstruction and a dry, red surface with clear or gray growths; large growths may resemble tumors.

Near drowning
- History includes recent water submersion.
- Auscultation of the lungs reveals rhonchi and crackles.
- ABG analysis reveals:
    - pH < 7.35
    - PaO_2 < 75 mm Hg (SI, < 10.03 kPa)
    - HCO_3^- level < 22 mEq/L (SI, < 22 mmol/L).
- ECG may show supraventricular tachycardia, premature ventricular contractions, and nonspecific ST-segment and T-wave abnormalities.

Necrotizing enterocolitis
- Anteroposterior and lateral abdominal X-rays reveal nonspecific intestinal dilation and, in later stages, gas or air in the intestinal wall.
- Platelet count is decreased.
- Serum sodium levels are < 135 mEq/L (SI, < 135 mmol/L).
- Serum bilirubin levels (indirect, direct, and total) may be elevated.
- Blood and stool cultures are positive for *Escherichia coli*, *Clostridia*, *Salmonella*, *Pseudomonas*, or *Klebsiella*.
- Hb level is decreased.
- PT and PTT are prolonged.

- Fibrin degradation products are increased.
- Guaiac test detects occult blood in stool.

Nephrotic syndrome
- Urinalysis shows marked proteinuria and reveals increased number of hyaline, granular, and waxy, fatty casts and oval fat bodies.
- Renal biopsy provides histologic identification of the lesion.
- T_3 resin uptake percentage is high with a low or normal free T_4 level.
- Serum protein electrophoresis reveals decreased albumin and gamma globulin levels and markedly increased alpha$_2$ and beta globulin levels.
- Serum triglyceride, phospholipid, and cholesterol levels are elevated.

Neurofibromatosis
- Examination reveals café-au-lait spots and multiple pedunculated nodules (neurofibromas) of varying sizes on the nerve trunks of the extremities and on the nerves of the head, neck, and body.
- X-rays and CT scan reveal widening internal auditory meatus and intervertebral foramen.
- Myelography reveals spinal cord tumors.
- Lumbar puncture with CSF analysis reveals elevated protein concentration.

Neurogenic arthropathy
- History includes painless joint deformity.
- X-rays reveal soft-tissue swelling or effusion (early stage), articular fracture, subluxation, erosion of articular cartilage, periosteal new bone formation, and excessive growth of marginal new bodies or resorption.

- Vertebral examination reveals narrowing of vertebral disk spaces, deterioration of vertebrae, and osteophyte formation.
- Synovial biopsy reveals bony fragments and bits of calcified cartilage.

Neurogenic bladder

- History includes neurologic disease or spinal cord injury.
- CSF analysis shows increased protein level indicating cord tumor; increased gamma globulin level may indicate multiple sclerosis.
- X-rays of the skull and vertebral column show fracture, dislocation, congenital anomalies, or metastasis.
- Myelography shows spinal cord compression.
- EMG confirms presence of peripheral neuropathy.
- Cystometry reveals abnormal micturition and vesical function.
- External sphincter EMG reveals detrusor-external sphincter dyssynergia.
- Voiding cystourethrography reveals neurogenic bladder.
- Whitaker test reveals bladder abnormality.

Nezelof syndrome

- History includes failure to thrive, poor eating habits, weight loss, and recurrent infections in children.
- Family history may reveal genetic transmission.
- T-lymphocyte assay reveals defective T cells that are moderately to markedly decreased in number.

Nocardiosis

- History reveals progressive pneumonia despite antibiotic therapy.
- Culture of sputum or discharge identifies *Nocardia*.

- Biopsy of lung or other tissue identifies *Nocardia*.
- CXR shows fluffy or interstitial infiltrates, nodules, or abscesses.

Nonspecific genitourinary infections

- History includes sexual contact with a partner with a nonspecific genitourinary infection.
- Cultures of prostatic, cervical, or urethral secretions reveal excessive polymorphonuclear leukocytes but few, if any, specific organisms.

Nonviral hepatitis

- History includes exposure to hepatotoxic chemicals or drugs.
- Serum ALT levels are > 56 U/L (SI, > 0.96 µkat/L).
- Serum AST levels are > 40 U/L (SI, > 0.68 µkat/L).
- Serum total and direct bilirubin levels are elevated (with cholestasis).
- Serum alkaline phosphatase levels are elevated.
- Differential WBC count reveals elevated eosinophils.

Nystagmus

- Inspection reveals involuntary eye movement.
- Positional testing causes nystagmus to occur.
- Electronystagmography reveals nystagmus.
- Vestibular acuity tests may rule out a vestibular lesion as the cause.
- X-rays may rule out structural defects.

Obesity

- Observation and comparison of height and weight to a standardized table reveals weight exceeding ideal body weight by

20% or more. In morbid obesity, body weight > 200% of standard range.

■ Measurement of the thickness of subcutaneous fat folds with calipers reveals excess body fat.

Optic atrophy

■ Slit-lamp examination reveals a pupil that reacts sluggishly to direct light stimulation.

■ Ophthalmoscopy shows pallor of the nerve head from loss of microvascular circulation in the disk and deposit of fibrous or glial tissue.

■ Visual field testing reveals a scotoma and, possibly, major visual field impairment.

Orbital cellulitis

■ Examination reveals eyelid edema and purulent discharge.

■ Culture of eye discharge identifies *Streptococcus, Staphylococcus,* or *Pneumococcus* as the causative organism.

Ornithosis

■ History includes recent exposure to birds.

■ *Chlamydia psittaci* is recovered from mice, eggs, or tissue culture inoculated with the patient's blood or sputum.

■ Comparison of acute and convalescent sera shows a fourfold rise in antibody titers during convalescent phase.

■ CXR reveals patchy lobar infiltrate.

Osgood-Schlatter disease

■ Examination reveals pain during internal rotation of the tibia while extending the knee from 90 degrees flexion, which subsides immediately with external rotation of the tibia.

■ X-rays may reveal epiphyseal separation and soft tissue swelling (up to 6 months after onset) and eventual bone fragmentation.

Osteoarthritis

■ History includes deep, aching joint pain, particularly after exercise or weight bearing, usually relieved by rest; and morning stiffness that lasts < 30 minutes.

■ Examination may reveal nodes in the distal and proximal joints that become red, swollen, and tender.

■ X-rays reveal narrowing of the joint space or margin, cystlike bony deposits in joint space and margins, sclerosis of the subchondral space, joint deformity due to degeneration or articular damage, bony growths at weight-bearing areas, and fusion of joints.

Osteogenesis imperfecta

■ Examination reveals blue sclera and deafness.

■ X-rays reveal multiple old fractures and skeletal deformities.

■ Skull X-ray shows wide sutures with small, irregularly shaped islands of bone (wormian bones).

Osteomyelitis

■ History includes sudden pain in the affected bone accompanied by tenderness, heat, swelling, and restricted movement.

■ Blood cultures identify *Staphylococcus aureus, Streptococcus pyogenes, Pneumococcus, Pseudomonas aeruginosa, Escherichia coli,* or *Proteus vulgaris* as the causative organism.

■ Bone scan shows infection site in early stages of illness.

■ X-ray reveals abnormal areas of calcification (may not be evident until 2 to 3 weeks).

■ ESR is elevated (> 20 mm/hour [SI, > 20 mm/h]).

■ WBC count reveals leukocytosis.

Osteoporosis

■ X-rays may reveal typical degeneration in the lower thoracic and lumbar vertebrae; vertebral bodies may appear flattened and more dense than normal.

■ Photon absorptiometry reveals deterioration of bone mass.

■ Bone biopsy reveals thin, porous, but otherwise normal-looking bone.

■ Bone densitometry reveals decreased bone density.

Otitis externa

■ Examination reveals pain on palpation of the tragus or auricle.

■ Otoscopy reveals a swollen external ear canal (sometimes to the point of complete closure), periauricular lymphadenopathy (tender nodes in front of the tragus, behind the ear, or in the upper neck) and, occasionally, regional cellulitis.

■ In fungal otitis externa, examination reveals thick, red epithelium after removal of growth.

■ Microscopic examination or culture and sensitivity tests identify *Aspergillus niger* or *Candida albicans* as the causative organism for fungal otitis externa; *Pseudomonas, Proteus vulgaris, Streptococcus,* or *Staphylococcus aureus* as the causative organism for bacterial otitis externa.

■ In chronic otitis externa, examination of the ear canal reveals a thick red epithelium.

Otitis media

■ In acute suppurative otitis media:
– Otoscopy reveals obscured or distorted bony landmarks of the tympanic membrane.
– Pneumatoscopy may show decreased tympanic membrane mobility.
– Examination shows that pulling on the auricle doesn't exacerbate the pain.

■ In acute secretory otitis media:
– Otoscopy demonstrates tympanic membrane retraction, causing the bony landmarks to appear more prominent, with clear or amber fluid detected behind the tympanic membrane, possibly with a meniscus and bubbles.
– If hemorrhage into the middle ear has occurred, the tympanic membrane appears blue-black.

■ In chronic otitis media:
– History discloses recurrent or unresolved otitis media; otoscopy shows thickening and, sometimes, scarring and decreased mobility of the tympanic membrane.
– Pneumatoscopy reveals decreased or absent tympanic membrane movement.

■ History of recent air travel or scuba diving suggests barotitis media.

Otosclerosis

■ Rinne test reveals bone conduction lasting longer than air conduction (normally, the reverse is true); as otosclerosis progresses, bone conduction deteriorates.

■ Audiometric testing reveals hearing loss ranging from 60 dB in early stages to total loss as the disease advances.

■ Weber's test reveals sound lateralizing to the more affected ear.

Ovarian cancer

■ Examination reveals abdominal mass.

■ CT scan shows the abdominal tumor.

■ Pelvic ultrasonography reveals mass.

■ Exploratory laparotomy with biopsy reveals malignant cells.

■ Transvaginal ultrasonography shows ovarian enlargement and growth.

■ Transvaginal Doppler color flow imaging reveals ovarian growth.

■ CEA levels are > 20 ng/ml (SI, > 20 µg/L).

- Serum hCG levels are elevated in a non-pregnant woman.
- Barium enema reveals obstruction and size of tumor.

Ovarian cysts
- Pelvic ultrasonography reveals ovarian mass.
- Laparoscopy reveals a bubble on the surface of the ovary, which may be clear, serous, or mucus-filled.
- hCG titers are highly elevated (with theca-lutein cysts).
- Progesterone levels are elevated.

Paget's disease
- X-rays reveal increased bone expansion and density (before overt symptoms appear).
- Bone scan reveals radioisotope concentrates in areas of active lesions (early pagetic lesions).
- Bone biopsy reveals characteristic mosaic pattern.
- Serum alkaline phosphatase level is highly elevated.
- Urine hydroxyproline levels are increased.

Pancreatic cancer
- Ultrasonography, CT scan, or MRI reveals mass size and locations.
- Laparotomy and biopsy reveal malignant cells.
- Barium swallow shows neoplasm or changes in the duodenum or stomach indicating carcinoma of the head of the pancreas.
- Endoscopic retrograde cholangiopancreatography shows mass and abnormalities of the pancreatic ducts.
- Cholangiography shows obstructed bile ducts caused by carcinoma of the pancreas.
- Secretin test reveals an abnormal volume of secretions, HCO_3^-, or enzymes.

- Serum alkaline phosphatase and serum bilirubin levels are markedly elevated with biliary obstruction.
- Plasma insulin immunoassay reveals measurable serum insulin (with islet cell tumors).
- Stool guaiac testing shows presence of occult blood, suggesting ulceration in GI tract or ampulla of Vater.

Parainfluenza
- History includes symptoms of respiratory illness.
- Serum antibody titers differentiate parainfluenza from other respiratory illnesses.
- Blood culture reveals virus (rarely done).

Parkinson's disease
- History and examination reveal muscle rigidity, akinesia, and pill-roll tremors increasing during stress or anxiety.
- Urinalysis reveals decreased dopamine levels.
- Evoked potential studies reveal bilateral abnormal P100 latencies.

Pediculosis
- In pediculosis capitis, examination reveals oval, grayish nits that can't be shaken loose.
- In pediculosis corporis, examination reveals characteristic skin lesions and nits found on clothing.
- In pediculosis pubis, examination reveals nits attached to pubic hairs, which feel coarse and grainy to the touch.

Pelvic inflammatory disease
- History includes recent sexual intercourse, intrauterine device insertion, childbirth, or abortion.

- Cultures and Gram stain of secretions from the endocervix or cul-de-sac identify *Neisseria gonorrhoeae* or *Chlamydia trachomatis* as the infective organism.
- Ultrasonography reveals an adnexal or uterine mass.
- Laparoscopy reveals infection or abscess.

Penetrating chest wounds

- Examination reveals chest wound and a sucking sound during breathing.
- Hb level and HCT are markedly decreased, indicating severe blood loss.
- CXR reveals pneumothorax and possible lung laceration.

Penile cancer

- Tissue biopsy reveals malignant cells.
- Examination reveals small circumscribed lesion, pimple, or sore on the penis, which may be accompanied by pain, hemorrhage, dysuria, purulent discharge, and urinary meatal obstruction (in late stages).

Peptic ulcers

- History includes heartburn, midepigastric pain, or gastric bleeding.
- Endoscopy reveals ulcer.
- Upper GI X-rays show abnormalities in the mucosa.
- Gastric secretory studies show hyperchlorhydria.
- Biopsy rules out malignancy.
- Stool guaiac testing reveals presence of occult blood.

Perforated eardrum

- History includes trauma to the ear accompanied by severe earache and bleeding from the ear.
- Direct visual inspection of the tympanic membrane with an otoscope confirms perforation; flaccid, thin areas indicate previous perforation.
- Audiometric testing reveals hearing loss.

Pericarditis

- Chest auscultation reveals pericardial friction rub.
- Pericardial fluid culture identifies infecting organism (in bacterial or fungal pericarditis).
- ECG reveals ST-segment elevation in the standard limb leads and most precordial leads without the significant changes in QRS morphology that occur with myocardial infarction.
- ECG may also reveal atrial ectopic rhythms and diminished QRS voltage (with pericardial effusion).
- Echocardiography reveals an echofree space between the ventricular wall and the pericardium (with pericardial effusion).

Peritonitis

- Examination reveals severe abdominal pain with direct or rebound tenderness.
- Abdominal X-rays reveal edematous and gaseous distention of the small and large bowel, or air in the abdominal cavity (with perforation of a visceral organ).
- Paracentesis reveals bacteria in fluid, exudate, pus, blood, or urine.
- CXR may show elevation of the diaphragm.
- Elevated WBC count indicates leukocytosis.

Pernicious anemia

- Hb level is markedly decreased.
- RBC count is decreased.
- Mean corpuscular volume is increased.
- Serum vitamin B_{12} assay reveals levels < 190 pg/ml (SI, < 162 pmol/L).
- Schilling test reveals < 3% excretion of radioactive B_{12} in urine in 24 hours.

- Bone marrow aspiration reveals erythroid hyperplasia with increased numbers of megaloblasts but few normally developing RBCs.
- Gastric analysis reveals absence of free hydrochloric acid after histamine or pentagastrin injection.

Pharyngitis

- Examination reveals generalized redness and inflammation of the posterior wall of the pharynx and red, edematous mucous membranes studded with white or yellow follicles.
- Exudate is usually confined to the lymphoid areas of the throat, sparing the tonsillar pillars.
- Throat culture identifies the infective organism, most commonly *Streptococcus.*

Phenylketonuria

- Family history indicates presence of autosomal recessive gene.
- Guthrie screening test reveals elevated serum phenylalanine levels.
- Drops of 10% ferric chloride solution added to a wet diaper turns a deep, bluish-green color, indicating phenylpyruvic acid in the urine.
- Low serum tyrosine level in neonates age 1 week or less.
- Urine testing reveals presence of phenylpyruvic acid.

Pheochromocytoma

- History includes acute episodes of hypertension, headache, sweating, and tachycardia, particularly in a patient with hyperglycemia, glycosuria, and hypermetabolism.
- 24-hour urine test reveals increased excretion of total free catecholamine and its metabolites, vanillylmandelic acid, and metanephrine.

- Total plasma catecholamines may show levels 10 to 50 times higher than normal.
- Angiography reveals an adrenal medullary tumor.
- Excretory urography with nephrotomography, adrenal venography, or CT scan helps localize a tumor.

Phosphate imbalance

- Hypophosphatemia: Serum phosphate level is < 2.7 mg/dl (SI, < 0.87 mmol/L) in adults and < 4.5 mg/dl (SI, < 1.45 mmol/L) in children.
- Hyperphosphatemia: Serum phosphate level is > 4.5 mg/dl (SI, > 1.45 mmol/L) in adults and > 6.7 mg/dl (SI, > 1.78 mmol/L) in children.

Photosensitivity reactions

- History includes recent exposure to light or certain chemicals.
- Examination reveals erythema, edema, desquamation, and hyperpigmentation (characteristic skin eruptions).
- Photopatch test for ultraviolet A and B may identify the causative light wavelength.

Pilonidal disease

- Examination reveals a series of openings along the midline of the intergluteal fold with thin, brown, foul-smelling drainage or a protruding tuft of hair; pressure on the sinus tract produces purulent drainage.
- Culture of discharge from the infected sinus reveals staphylococci or skin bacteria (usually not bowel bacteria).

Pituitary tumors

- Skull X-rays with tomography reveal enlargement of the sella turcica or erosion of its floor and enlargement of the paranasal sinuses and mandible, thickened cranial bones, and separated teeth (if growth hormone predominates).

- Carotid angiography reveals displacement of the anterior cerebral and internal carotid arteries (with enlarging tumor mass).
- Intracranial CT scan may confirm the existence of the adenoma and accurately depict its size.
- Orbital radiography shows superior orbital fissure enlargement.
- MRI of the brain differentiates healthy, benign, and malignant tissues and blood vessels.
- Tangent screen examination reveals bitemporal hemianopia.
- Urine free cortisol levels are > 108 µg/24 hours (SI, > 276 mmol/24 h).
- HGH levels are > 5 ng/ml (SI, > 5 µg/L) in men, > 10 ng/ml (SI, > 10 µg/L) in women.
- Urine 17-hydroxycorticosteroid levels are > 10 mg/24 hours (SI, > 27.6 µmol/24 h as cortisol) in men, > 6 mg/24 hours (SI, > 16.5 µmol/24 h as cortisol) in women, and > 5 mg/24 hours (SI, > 13.8 µmol/24 h as cortisol) in children.

Pityriasis rosea

- Examination reveals slightly raised oval lesion, approximately 2 to 6 cm in diameter, changing to yellow-tan or erythematous patches with scaly edges approximately 0.5 to 1 cm in diameter on the trunk and extremities.

Placenta previa

- History includes painless bleeding during third trimester of pregnancy.
- Pelvic ultrasonography reveals abnormal echo patterns.
- Pelvic examination (performed only immediately before delivery) reveals only cervix and minimal descent of fetal presenting part.

Plague

- History includes exposure to rodents (bubonic plague).
- Culture of skin lesion reveals *Yersinia pestis.*
- WBC count is elevated; WBC differential reveals increased polymorphonuclear leukocytes.
- CXR reveals fulminating pneumonia (with pneumonic plague).

Platelet function disorders

- History includes excessive bleeding or bruising.
- Bleeding time is prolonged.
- PT and PTT are normal.
- Platelet count is normal.
- Platelet function tests measure platelet release reaction and aggregation to identify defective mechanism.

Pleural effusion and empyema

- CXR reveals radiopaque fluid in dependent regions.
- Lung auscultation reveals decreased breath sounds.
- Percussion detects dullness over the effused area, which doesn't change with respiration.
- Pleural fluid analysis reveals:
  – transudative effusions with decreased specific gravity
  – empyema with acute inflammatory WBCs and microorganisms
  – empyema or rheumatoid arthritis with extremely decreased pleural fluid glucose levels.

Pleurisy

- Auscultation of the chest reveals characteristic pleural friction rub — a coarse, creaky sound heard during late inspiration and early expiration, directly over the area of pleural inflammation.

- Palpation may reveal coarse vibration.

Pneumocystis carinii pneumonia

- History includes an immunocompromising condition (such as HIV infection, leukemia, and lymphoma) or procedure (such as organ transplantation).
- Histologic studies of sputum specimen confirm presence of *P. carinii*.
- CXR shows slowly progressing, fluffy infiltrates and occasional nodular lesions or a spontaneous pneumothorax.
- Gallium scan of the chest shows increased uptake over the lungs even if the CXR appears relatively normal.

Pneumonia

- Percussion reveals dullness; auscultation discloses crackles, wheezing, or rhonchi over the affected lung area as well as decreased breath sounds and decreased vocal fremitus.
- CXR discloses infiltrates, confirming the diagnosis.
- Gram stain and culture of sputum show acute inflammatory cells.
- WBC count indicates leukocytosis in bacterial pneumonia and a normal or low count in viral or mycoplasmal pneumonia.
- Blood cultures reflect bacteremia and help determine the causative organism.

Pneumothorax

- History includes sudden, sharp pain and shortness of breath.
- CXR reveals air in the pleural space and, possibly, mediastinal shift.
- Examination reveals overexpansion and rigidity of the affected chest side; in tension pneumothorax, examination may reveal neck vein distention.
- Palpation of chest reveals crackling beneath the skin and decreased vocal fremitus.

- Chest auscultation reveals decreased or absent breath sounds on the affected side.
- ABG measurements reveal pH < 7.35, $Pao_2 < 80$ mm Hg (SI, < 10.6 kPa), and $Paco_2 > 45$ mm Hg (SI, > 5.3 kPa).

Poisoning

- History includes ingestion, inhalation, injection of, or skin contact with a poisonous substance.
- Toxicologic studies (including drug screens) reveal poison in the mouth, vomitus, urine, stool, or blood or on the victim's hands or clothing.
- CXR (with inhalation poisoning) reveals pulmonary infiltrates or edema or aspiration pneumonia (with petroleum distillate inhalation).

Poliomyelitis

- Throat culture or stool examination reveals poliovirus.
- Convalescent serum antibody titers rise fourfold from acute titers.
- CSF pressure and protein levels may be slightly increased.
- WBC count may be elevated initially, mostly due to polymorphonuclear leukocytes, which constitute 50% to 90% of the total count; thereafter, the number of cells is diminished with mononuclear leukocytes accounting for most of them.

Polycystic kidney disease

- Family history includes polycystic kidney disease.
- Physical examination reveals large bilateral, irregular masses in the flanks.
- Excretory or retrograde urography reveals enlarged kidneys, with elongation of pelvis, flattening of the calyces, and indentations caused by cysts.
- Excretory urography of the neonate shows poor excretion of contrast agent.

- Ultrasonography, CT scan, and radioisotope scans of the kidney show kidney enlargement and presence of cysts. CT scan also demonstrates multiple areas of cystic damage.

Polycythemia, secondary

- RBC mass is increased.
- Hb level, HCT, mean corpuscular volume, and mean corpuscular Hb level are increased.
- Urine erythropoietin and blood histamine levels are elevated.
- Arterial oxygen saturation may be decreased.
- Bone marrow biopsies reveal hyperplasia confined to the erythroid series.

Polycythemia, spurious

- Hb level, HCT, and RBC count are elevated.
- RBC mass is normal.
- WBC count is normal.

Polycythemia vera

- Laboratory studies confirm polycythemia vera by showing increased RBC mass and normal arterial oxygen saturation in association with splenomegaly or two of the following:
    - elevated platelet count
    - elevated WBC count
    - elevated leukocyte alkaline phosphatase level
    - elevated serum B_{12} elevation or unbound B_{12}-binding capacity.
- Bone marrow biopsy reveals panmyelosis.
- Serum and urine uric acid levels are increased.

Polymyositis and dermatomyositis

- Muscle biopsy reveals necrosis, degeneration, regeneration, and interstitial chronic lymphocytic infiltration.
- Muscle enzyme levels (CK, aldolase, AST) are elevated and not attributable to hemolysis of RBCs or hepatic or other diseases.
- Urine creatine level is markedly increased.
- EMG reveals polyphasic short-duration potentials, fibrillation, and bizarre high-frequency repetitive changes.
- ANA test is positive.

Porphyrias

- Screening tests reveal porphyrins or their precursors (such as aminolevulinic acid and porphobilinogen) in urine, stool, blood, or skin biopsy.
- Urinary lead level is > 400 mg/24-hour collection.

Potassium imbalance

- Hypokalemia:
    - Serum potassium levels are < 3.5 mEq/L (SI, < 3.5 mmol/L).
    - ECG shows flattened T waves, elevated U waves, and depressed ST segment.
- Hyperkalemia:
    - Serum potassium levels are > 5 mEq/L (SI, > 5 mmol/L).
    - ECG shows tall, tented T waves; widened QRS complex; prolonged PR interval; flattened or absent P waves; and depressed ST segment.

Precocious puberty in females

- X-rays of hands, wrists, knees, and hips reveal advanced bone age and possible premature epiphyseal closure.
- Androstenedione level is > 3 ng/ml.

- Radioimmunoassays for estrogen levels and FSH levels are abnormally high for age.
- Vaginal smear for estrogen secretion reveals abnormally high levels.
- Urinary test for gonadotropic activity and excretion of 17-KS show abnormally high levels.

Precocious puberty in males

- Detailed patient history reveals recent growth pattern, behavior changes, family history of precocious puberty, or hormonal ingestion.
- In true precocious puberty:
  - Serum levels of LH, FSH, and corticotropin are elevated.
  - Plasma tests for testosterone demonstrate elevated levels (equal to those of an adult male).
  - Evaluation of ejaculate indicates true precocity by revealing presence of live spermatozoa.
  - Skull and hand X-rays reveal advanced bone age.
- In pseudoprecocious puberty:
  - Chromosome analysis may demonstrate an abnormal pattern of autosomes and sex chromosomes.
  - Steroid excretion levels, such as testosterone and 24-hour 17-KS levels, are elevated.

Pregnancy

- Serum hCG level is elevated.
- Urine hCG level is elevated.
- Pelvic examination reveals changes to uterus consistent with pregnancy.
- Ultrasonography reveals presence of fetus in the uterus.

Pregnancy-induced hypertension

- Mild preeclampsia:
  - Systolic blood pressure is 140 mm Hg or shows a rise of 30 mm Hg or more above the patient's normal systolic pressure (measured on two occasions, 6 hours apart).
  - Diastolic blood pressure is 90 mm Hg or shows a rise of 15 mm Hg or more above the patient's normal diastolic pressure (measured on two occasions, 6 hours apart).
  - Proteinuria (urine protein level is > 500 mg/24 hours).
- Severe preeclampsia:
  - Blood pressure measurements are 160/110 mm Hg or higher (measured on two occasions, 6 hours apart) on bed rest.
  - Proteinuria is increased (urine protein level ≥ 5 g/24 hours).
  - Patient has oliguria (urine output ≤ 400 ml/24 hours).
  - Deep tendon reflexes are hyperactive.
- Eclampsia:
  - History and examination reveal signs of severe preeclampsia and seizure activity.
  - Ophthalmoscopic examination may reveal vascular spasm, papilledema, retinal edema or detachment, and arteriovenous nicking or hemorrhage.

Premature labor

- Physical examination reveals rhythmic uterine contractions, cervical dilation and effacement, possible rupture of membranes, expulsion of cervical mucus plug, and bloody discharge occurring before expected date of delivery.
- Vaginal examination reveals progressive cervical effacement and dilation.
- Pelvic ultrasonography identifies fetus' position in the mother's pelvis.

Premature rupture of the membranes

■ History includes passage of amniotic fluid before the expected date of delivery.
■ Examination reveals amniotic fluid in the vagina.
■ Nitrazine paper test of fluid from posterior fornix turns deep blue.
■ Fluid from posterior fornix smeared on slide and allowed to dry takes on a fernlike pattern.

Premenstrual syndrome

■ History includes menstruation-related symptoms, including mild to severe personality changes, nervousness, irritability, fatigue, lethargy, depression, breast tenderness or bloating, joint pain, headache, diarrhea, and exacerbations of skin, respiratory, or neurologic problems recorded for 2 to 3 months.
■ Serum estrogen and progesterone levels are normal (ruling out hormonal imbalance).

Pressure ulcers

■ History includes immobility, malnutrition, or skin irritation.
■ Inspection reveals skin breakdown.
■ Wound culture and sensitivity identify the infecting organisms.

Proctitis

■ In acute proctitis, sigmoidoscopy reveals edematous, bright-red or pink rectal mucosa that's thick, shiny, friable, and possibly ulcerated.
■ In chronic proctitis, sigmoidoscopy reveals thickened mucosa, loss of vascular pattern, and stricture of the rectal lumen.
■ Biopsy reveals absence of malignant cells.

Progressive systemic sclerosis

■ History includes Raynaud's phenomenon.
■ ANA test is positive, revealing low titer and speckled pattern.
■ Hand X-rays reveal terminal phalangeal tuft resorption, subcutaneous calcification, and joint space narrowing and erosion.
■ CXR shows bilateral basilar pulmonary fibrosis.
■ RF is positive in approximately one third of patients.
■ ESR is elevated.
■ Urinalysis reveals proteinuria, microscopic hematuria, and casts (with renal involvement).

Prostatic cancer

■ Digital rectal examination reveals small, hard nodule in prostate area.
■ Serum prostate-specific antigen levels are elevated.
■ Serum prostatic acid phosphatase is > 3.7 ng/ml (SI, > 3.7 µg/L).
■ Serum alkaline phosphatase level is elevated.
■ Biopsy reveals malignant cells.

Prostatitis

■ Examination reveals tender, indurated, swollen, and warm prostate.
■ Urine samples, taken at start of voiding, midstream, after a physician massages the prostate, and final specimen, reveal a significant increase in colony count of the prostatic specimens.

Protein-calorie malnutrition

■ History includes poor diet lacking in protein.
■ Examination reveals a small, gaunt, and emaciated appearance with no adipose tissue; dry and "baggy" skin; general weak-

ness; sparse hair and dull brown or reddish yellow eyes; and slow pulse rate and respirations.
■ Anthropometry reveals height and weight < 80% of standard for the patient's age and sex, and below standard arm circumference and triceps skinfolds.
■ Serum albumin and pre-albumin levels are markedly decreased.

Pruritus ani

■ History includes perianal itching, irritation, or superficial burning.
■ Rectal examination identifies no fissures or fistulas.
■ Biopsy rules out carcinoma.

Pseudomembranous enterocolitis

■ History includes sudden onset of copious, watery or bloody diarrhea; abdominal pain; and fever.
■ Rectal biopsy reveals characteristic histologic changes, such as plaquelike lesions on the colonic mucosal surface consisting of fibrinopurulent exudate and necrotic epithelial debris.
■ Stool cultures identify *Clostridium difficile*.

Pseudomonas infections

■ Culture of blood, spinal fluid, urine, exudate, or sputum identifies the *Pseudomonas* organism.
■ Gram stain reveals gram-negative bacillus.

Psoriasis

■ Examination reveals dry, cracked, encrusted lesions (erythematous plaques) accompanied by itching on the scalp, chest, elbows, knees, back, or buttocks.
■ Skin biopsy reveals psoriasis.
■ Serum uric acid level is elevated, without indications of gout.

Psoriatic arthritis

■ Examination reveals psoriatic lesions.
■ X-rays reveal erosion of terminal phalangeal tufts, "whittling" of the distal end of the terminal phalanges, "pencil-in-cup"' deformity of the distal interphalangeal joints, sacroiliitis, and atypical spondylitis with syndesmophyte formation, resulting in hyperostosis and vertebral ossification.
■ Rheumatoid screening test is nonreactive.
■ ESR is elevated.
■ Serum uric acid levels are increased.

Ptosis

■ Examination reveals drooping of the upper eyelid.
■ Measurement of palpebral fissure widths, range of lid movement, and relation of lid margin to upper border of the cornea reveal the severity of illness.

Puerperal infection

■ History includes fever within 48 hours after delivery or abortion.
■ Culture of lochia, blood, incisional exudate (from cesarean incision or episiotomy), uterine tissue, or material collected from the vaginal cuff reveals *Streptococcus,* coagulase-negative staphylococci, *Clostridium perfringens, Bacteroides fragilis,* or *Escherichia coli* as the causative organism.
■ Elevated WBC count shows leukocytosis and an increased sedimentation rate.
■ Pelvic examination reveals induration without purulent discharge (parametritis).
■ Culdoscopy shows adnexal induration and thickening.

Pulmonary edema

■ Examination reveals respiratory distress.
■ Chest auscultation reveals crackles in the lung fields.
■ ABG analysis usually shows decreased Pao_2 (hypoxia) and variable $Paco_2$. Pro-

found respiratory alkalosis and acidosis may occur; metabolic acidosis occurs when cardiac output is low.

■ CXR shows diffuse haziness of the lung fields and, often, cardiomegaly and pleural effusions.

■ Pulmonary artery catheterization reveals elevated pulmonary wedge pressures.

Pulmonary embolism and infarction

■ Lung scan reveals perfusion defects in areas beyond occluded vessels.

■ Pulmonary angiography reveals emboli.

■ CXR shows areas of atelectasis, elevated diaphragm and pleural effusion, prominent pulmonary artery and, occasionally, a wedge-shaped infiltrate suggesting pulmonary infarction.

■ ECG may show right axis deviation; right bundle-branch block; tall, peaked P waves; ST-segment depression; T-wave inversion; and supraventricular tachycardia.

■ Auscultation reveals right ventricular gallop, increased intensity of the pulmonic component of S_2, crackles, and pleural rub at the site of the embolism.

■ ABG analysis may show decreased Pao_2 and $Paco_2$ levels.

Pulmonary hypertension

■ Pulmonary artery catheterization reveals elevated pulmonary systolic pressure and PAWP.

■ Pulmonary angiography reveals filling defects in pulmonary vasculature.

■ PFTs may show decreased flow rates and increased residual volume (with underlying obstructive disease); total lung capacity may be decreased (with underlying restrictive disease).

■ ABG analysis reveals decreased Pao_2.

■ ECG shows right axis deviation and tall or peaked P waves in inferior leads (with right ventricular hypertrophy).

Pulmonic insufficiency

■ Cardiac catheterization shows pulmonic insufficiency, increased right ventricular pressure, and associated cardiac defects.

■ CXR shows enlargement of the right ventricle and pulmonary artery.

■ Echocardiography shows right ventricular or right atrial enlargement.

■ ECG may be normal in mild cases or show right ventricular or right atrial hypertrophy.

Pulmonic stenosis

■ Cardiac catheterization reveals increased right ventricular pressure, decreased pulmonary artery pressure, and an abnormal valve orifice.

■ CXR usually reveals a normal heart size and normal lung vascularity, although the pulmonary arteries may be evident. With severe obstruction and right-sided heart failure, CXR may reveal right atrial and ventricular enlargement.

■ Echocardiography reveals the abnormality in the pulmonic valve.

■ ECG results may be normal in mild cases, or they may indicate right axis deviation and right ventricular hypertrophy. High amplitude P waves in leads II, III, aV_F, and V_1 indicate right atrial enlargement.

Rabies

■ History reveals recent animal bite.

■ Throat and saliva culture identifies virus.

■ Serum fluorescent rabies antibody test is positive.

■ WBC count is elevated, with increased polymorphonuclear and large mononuclear cells.

■ Urine glucose, acetone, and protein levels are elevated.

Radiation exposure

■ History includes exposure to radiation and nausea and vomiting.
■ CBC reveals decreased Hb level and HCT and decreased WBC, platelet, and lymphocyte counts.
■ Bone marrow studies reveal blood dyscrasias.
■ X-rays may show bone necrosis.
■ Geiger counter measurement reveals the amount of radiation in an open wound.

Rape-trauma syndrome

■ History includes rape or attempted rape, accompanied by feelings of anxiety, grief, anger, fear, or revenge.
■ Examination shows signs of physical trauma.
■ X-rays reveal fractures.
■ Vaginal specimen is positive for semen.
■ Fingernail and pubic hair scrapings and semen analysis may help to identify alleged rapist.

Raynaud's disease

■ History and examination reveal changes in skin color induced by cold or stress, bilateral involvement, minimal cutaneous gangrene or absence of gangrene, and clinical symptoms of 2 years' duration or more.
■ Cold stimulation test demonstrates Raynaud's syndrome.
■ Arteriography reveals no underlying secondary disease.

Rectal polyps

■ Proctosigmoidoscopy or colonoscopy reveals type, size, and location of polyps.
■ Biopsy reveals histologic changes consistent with polyps.
■ Barium enema reveals polyps high in the colon.
■ Stool guaiac testing reveals presence of occult blood.

Rectal prolapse

■ In complete prolapse, visual examination reveals the full thickness of the bowel wall and, possibly, the sphincter muscle protruding and mucosa falling into bulky, concentric folds.
■ In partial prolapse, visual examination reveals only partially protruding mucosa and a smaller mass of radial mucosal folds.

Reiter's syndrome

■ History includes venereal or enteric infection.
■ HLA testing reveals presence of HLA-B27.
■ Analysis of urethral discharge and synovial fluid reveals numerous WBCs, mostly polymorphonuclear leukocytes.
■ Synovial fluid analysis reveals increased complement and protein; fluid is grossly purulent.
■ WBC count and ESR are elevated.

Relapsing fever

■ History includes recurrent fever for 5 to 15 days.
■ Blood smear shows spirochetes.
■ WBC count is elevated, with increase in lymphocytes (although WBC count may be within normal limits).
■ ESR is increased.

Renal calculi

■ KUB X-rays reveal renal calculi.
■ Excretory urography reveals size and location of calculi.
■ Kidney ultrasonography reveals obstructive changes.
■ Urine culture may reveal urinary tract infection.
■ Urinalysis may be normal or may show increased specific gravity, acid or alkaline pH (depending on the type of stone), hematuria, crystals, casts, and pyuria (with or without WBCs).

- 24-hour urine collection shows presence of calcium oxalate, phosphorus, or uric acid.

Renal infarction

- Urinalysis reveals proteinuria and microscopic hematuria.
- Urine enzyme levels, especially LD and alkaline phosphatase, are elevated.
- Serum ALT, AST, and LD levels are elevated.
- Excretory urography shows diminished or absent excretion of contrast dye (with vascular occlusion or urethral obstruction).
- Isotopic renal scan demonstrates absent or reduced blood flow to the kidneys.
- Renal arteriography reveals infarction.

Renal tubular acidosis

- Urine studies reveal pH > 6, low titratable acids and ammonia content, increased HCO_3^- and potassium levels, and low specific gravity (> 1.005).
- Blood pH is < 7.35.
- Serum HCO_3^- level is < 22 mEq/L (SI, < 22 mmol/L).
- Serum potassium and phosphorus levels are decreased.

Renal vein thrombosis

- Excretory urography reveals enlarged kidneys and diminished excretory function (in acute thrombosis); urography contrast medium seems to "smudge" necrotic renal tissue.
- In chronic thrombosis, excretory urography may show ureteral indentations that result from collateral venous channels.
- Renal venography reveals filling defects.
- Renal biopsy reveals characteristic histologic changes.
- Urinalysis reveals gross or microscopic hematuria, proteinuria (> 2 g/day in chronic disease), casts, and oliguria.

- Blood studies show leukocytosis, hypoalbuminemia, hyperlipemia, and thrombocytopenia.

Renovascular hypertension

- Isotopic renal blood flow scan and rapid-sequence excretory urography demonstrate abnormal renal blood flow and discrepancies in kidney size and shape.
- Renal arteriography reveals the arterial stenosis or obstruction.
- Samples from both the right and left renal veins allow for comparison of plasma renin levels with those in the inferior vena cava; renin level is increased in the affected kidney.

Respiratory acidosis

- ABG measurements reveal:
  - pH < 7.35
  - $Paco_2$ > 45 mm Hg (SI, > 5.3 kPa)
  - HCO_3^- level of 22 to 26 mEq/L (SI, 22 to 26 mmol/L) in the acute stage and > 26 mEq/L (SI, > 26 mmol/L) in the chronic stage.

Respiratory alkalosis

- ABG measurements reveal:
  - pH > 7.45
  - $Paco_2$ < 35 mm Hg (SI, < 4.7 kPa) in acute stage
  - HCO_3^- level normal in acute stage and < 22 mEq/L (SI, < 22 mmol/L) in chronic stage.

Respiratory distress syndrome, adult

- Initial ABG measurements reveal:
  - pH > 7.45
  - Pao_2 < 60 mm Hg (SI, < 8.02 kPa)
  - $Paco_2$ < 35 mm Hg (SI, < 4.7 kPa).
- ABG measurements following progression of illness reveal:
  - pH < 7.35

– decreased Pa_{O_2} (despite oxygen therapy)

– Pa_{CO_2} level > 45 mm Hg (SI,> 5.3 kPa)

– HCO_3^- level < 22 mEq/L (SI, < 22 mmol/L).

■ Serial CXRs initially show bilateral infiltrates; later X-rays reveal ground glass appearance and eventually "whiteouts" of both lungs.

Respiratory distress syndrome, child

■ CXR reveals fine reticulonodular pattern (may be normal for first 6 to 12 hours after birth).

■ ABG measurements reveal pH < 7.35 and Pa_{O_2} < 75 mm Hg (SI, < 10.03 kPa).

■ Chest auscultation reveals normal or diminished air entry and crackles (rare in early stages).

■ Amniocentesis reveals lecithin-sphingomyelin ratio of < 2 (used to assess risk of respiratory distress syndrome).

Respiratory syncytial virus infection

■ Cultures of nasal and pharyngeal secretions identify respiratory syncytial virus infection (not always reliable).

■ Serum antibody titers elevated (maternal antibodies may impair results before age 6 months).

■ CXR may reveal pneumonia.

■ Indirect immunofluorescence and ELISA tests are positive.

Restrictive cardiomyopathy

■ CXR reveals massive cardiomegaly, affecting all four chambers of the heart, pericardial effusion, and pulmonary congestion (advanced stage).

■ Echocardiography detects increased left ventricular muscle mass and differences in end-diastolic pressures between the ventricles.

■ Carotid palpation reveals blunt carotid upstroke with small volume.

■ Cardiac catheterization demonstrates increased left ventricular end-diastolic pressure.

■ ECG may show low-voltage complexes, hypertrophy, atrioventricular conduction defects, or arrhythmias.

Retinal detachment

■ Ophthalmoscopy reveals the usually transparent retina to be gray and opaque.

■ In severe detachment, ophthalmoscopy reveals folds in the retina and a ballooning out of the area.

■ Indirect ophthalmoscopy reveals retinal tears.

■ Ocular ultrasonography shows a dense sheetlike echo on a B-scan.

Retinitis pigmentosa

■ Family history indicates a possible predisposition to retinitis pigmentosa.

■ Electroretinography shows a retinal response time slower than normal or absent.

■ Visual field testing (using a tangent screen) detects ring scotomata.

■ Fluorescein angiography shows white dots (areas of dyspigmentation) in the epithelium.

■ Ophthalmoscopy may initially show normal fundi but later reveals characteristic black pigmentary disturbance.

Reye's syndrome

■ History includes recent viral disorder with varying degrees of encephalopathy and cerebral edema.

■ ALT level is > 56 U/L (SI, > 0.96 µkat/L).

■ AST level is > 40 U/L (SI, > 0.68 −2 to + 13 µkat/L.

- Liver biopsy reveals fatty droplets uniformly distributed throughout cells.
- PT and PTT are prolonged.
- CSF analysis reveals WBCs < 10/ml; in coma, CSF pressure is increased.
- Serum ammonia levels are elevated.
- Serum fatty acid and lactate levels are elevated.
- Serum glucose levels are normal or low.

Rheumatic fever and rheumatic heart disease

- History includes streptococcal infection.
- Examination reveals joint pain and swelling and one or more of these symptoms: carditis, polyarthritis, chorea, erythema marginatum, or subcutaneous nodules.
- C-reactive protein is positive.
- ASO titer is elevated (within 2 months of onset).
- Echocardiography and cardiac catheterization reveal valvular damage.
- Cardiac enzymes may be elevated (in severe carditis).

Rheumatoid arthritis, adult

- Serum RF titer is above 1:80.
- X-rays reveal bone demineralization and soft-tissue swelling (in early stages), loss of cartilage and narrowing of joint spaces, and cartilage and bone destruction, erosion, subluxations, and deformities.
- Synovial fluid analysis reveals increased volume and turbidity but decreased viscosity and complement 3 and complement 4 levels, and elevated WBC count.
- ESR is increased.
- CBC shows moderate decrease in RBC count, Hb level, and HCT and slight leukocytosis.

Rheumatoid arthritis, juvenile

- History includes persistent joint stiffness and pain in the morning or after periods of inactivity.
- ANA test may be positive in patients who have pauciarticular juvenile rheumatoid arthritis (JRA) with chronic iridocyclitis.
- RF is present in 15% of patients with JRA, as compared with 85% of patients with rheumatoid arthritis.
- Early changes seen on X-ray include soft-tissue swelling, effusion, and periostitis in affected joints.
- In later X-ray studies, osteoporosis and accelerated bone growth may appear, followed by subchondral erosions, joint space narrowing, bone destruction, and fusion.
- CBC usually shows decreased Hb levels, increased neutrophil count, increased platelet levels, and elevated ESR.
- Blood studies reveal elevated C-reactive protein, serum haptoglobin, Ig, and complement 3 levels.
- HLA testing reveals presence of HLA-B27, forecasting later development of ankylosing spondylitis.

Rocky Mountain spotted fever

- History includes tick bite or travel to a tick-infested area.
- Complement fixation test shows a fourfold rise in convalescent antibodies compared to acute titers.
- Blood culture identifies *Rickettsia rickettsii*.
- Decreased platelet count indicates thrombocytopenia during second week of illness.
- WBC count is elevated during second week of illness.

Rosacea

- Examination reveals vascular and acneiform lesions without the comedones characteristically associated with acne vulgaris; in severe cases, rhinophyma is seen.

Roseola infantum

- History includes high fever (103° to 105° F [39.4° to 40.6° C]) followed by rash 48 hours after fever subsides.
- Examination reveals maculopapular, nonpruritic rash that blanches on pressure.

Rubella

- History includes exposure to infected person.
- Examination reveals maculopapular rash, beginning on the face and spreading to the trunk and extremities.
- Examination also reveals lymphadenopathy.
- Cell cultures of throat, blood, urine, and CSF reveal rubella virus.
- Convalescent serum antibody titers rise fourfold from acute titers.

Rubeola

- History includes exposure to person infected with the measles virus (patient may be unaware of contact).
- Examination reveals the pathognomonic Koplik's spots.
- Cultures of blood, nasopharyngeal secretions, and urine identify measles virus (during the febrile period).
- Serum antibody titers appear within 3 days after onset of the rash and reach peak titers 2 to 4 weeks later.

Salmonellosis

- Culture of blood, stool, urine, bone marrow, pus, or vomitus identifies gram-negative bacilli of the genus *Salmonella*.

- Widal's test reveals a fourfold rise in titer.

Sarcoidosis

- Kveim skin test confirms discrete epithelioid cell granuloma.
- CXR reveals bilateral hilar and right paratracheal adenopathy with or without diffuse interstitial infiltrates; occasionally, large nodular lesions appear in lung parenchyma.
- Lymph node, skin, or lung biopsy reveals noncaseating granulomas with negative cultures for mycobacteria and fungi.
- PFTs show decreased total lung capacity and compliance and decreased diffusing capacity.
- Tuberculin skin test, fungal serologies, and sputum cultures for mycobacteria and fungi and biopsy cultures are negative.

Scabies

- Visual examination of the contents of the scabietic burrow may reveal itch mite.
- Mineral oil placed over the burrow, followed by superficial scraping and examination of expressed material, reveals ova or mite feces.
- Pediculicide administration to affected area clears skin.

Scarlet fever

- History includes recent streptococcal pharyngitis.
- Examination reveals strawberry tongue and fine erythematous rash that blanches on pressure.
- Pharyngeal culture identifies group A beta-hemolytic streptococci.
- CBC reveals granulocytosis and, possibly, a reduced RBC count.

Schistosomiasis

- History includes travel to endemic areas.

- Urine, stool, or lesion biopsy reveals ova.
- WBC count reveals eosinophilia.

Scoliosis

- Examination reveals unequal shoulder height, elbow levels, and heights of iliac crests and asymmetry of the paraspinal muscles.
- Scoliosometer (an apparatus for measuring curvature of the spinal column) reveals angle of trunk rotation to be abnormal.
- Anterior, posterior, and lateral spinal X-rays reveal degree of curvature and flexibility of the spine.

Septal perforation and deviation

- History and examination reveal whistle on inspiration, rhinitis, epistaxis, nasal crusting, and watery discharge.
- Inspection of the nasal mucosa with bright light and a nasal speculum reveals perforation or deviation.

Septic arthritis

- Synovial fluid Gram stain and culture or biopsy of synovial membrane reveals gram-positive cocci (*Staphylococcus aureus, Streptococcus pyogenes, Streptococcus pneumoniae,* or *Streptococcus viridans*), gram-negative cocci (*Neisseria gonorrhoeae* or *Haemophilus influenzae*), or gram-negative bacilli (*Escherichia coli, Salmonella,* or *Pseudomonas*) as the causative organism.
- Joint fluid analysis reveals gross pus or watery, cloudy fluid of decreased viscosity, with markedly elevated WBCs/ml, containing primarily neutrophils.
- Culture of skin exudate, sputum, urethral discharge, stool, urine, blood, or nasopharyngeal secretions is positive for causative organism.

- Skeletal X-rays show distention of joint capsules, followed by narrowing of joint space (indicating cartilage damage), and erosions of bone (joint destruction).
- WBC count may be elevated with many polymorphonuclear cells; ESR is increased.

Septic shock

- History includes infection accompanied by fever, confusion, nausea, vomiting, and hyperventilation.
- Blood cultures identify gram-negative bacteria (*Escherichia coli, Klebsiella, Enterobacter, Pseudomonas, Proteus,* or *Bacteroides*) or gram-positive bacteria (*Streptococcus pneumoniae, S. pyogenes,* or *Actinomyces*) as the causative organism.
- WBC count is elevated.
- Pulmonary artery catheterization reveals decreased central venous pressure, pulmonary artery pressures, wedge pressure, cardiac output (may be initially elevated), and systemic vascular resistance.
- ABG measurements reveal decreased $Paco_2$, low or normal HCO_3^- level, and pH > 7.45 (in early stages); as shock progresses, decreasing $Paco_2$, Pao_2, HCO_3^- level, and pH indicate the development of metabolic acidosis with hypoxemia.
- Serum BUN and creatinine levels increase; creatinine clearance decreases.
- Urine osmolality is < 400 mOsm/kg serum water (SI, < 400 mmol/kg serum water); ratio of urine osmolality to plasma osmolality is < 1.5.
- ECG reveals ST-segment depression, inverted T waves, and arrhythmias.

Severe combined immunodeficiency disease

- History includes overwhelming infections during the first year of life.
- T-cell count and function are severely diminished.

■ Lymph node biopsy reveals absence of lymphocytes.

Shigellosis

■ Microscopic examination of a fresh stool may reveal mucus, RBCs, and polymorphonuclear leukocytes.
■ Stool culture identifies *Shigella*.
■ Hemagglutinating antibodies may be present, indicating severe infection.

Sickle cell anemia

■ Family history includes homozygous inheritance.
■ Stained blood smear reveals sickle cells.
■ Hb electrophoresis reveals HbS.
■ CBC may reveal decreased RBC count and elevated WBC and platelet counts.
■ ESR is decreased.
■ Serum iron levels are increased.

Sideroblastic anemias

■ Bone marrow aspirate reveals ringed sideroblasts.
■ Microscopic examination reveals RBCs that are hypochromic or normochromic and slightly macrocytic; red cell precursors may be megaloblastic, with anisocytosis and poikilocytosis.
■ Hb levels are decreased.
■ Serum iron and transferrin levels are increased.

Silicosis

■ History includes occupational exposure to silica dust.
■ Examination reveals decreased chest expansion, diminished intensity of breath sounds, areas of hyporesonance and hyperresonance, fine to medium crackles, and tachypnea (with chronic silicosis).
■ CXR reveals the following:
– small, discrete, nodular lesions distributed throughout both lung fields but typically concentrated in the upper lung zones
– enlarged hilar lung nodes that exhibit "eggshell" calcification (in simple silicosis)
– one or more conglomerate masses of dense tissue (in complicated silicosis).
■ PFTs reveal:
– reduced FVC (in complicated silicosis)
– reduced FEV_1 (in obstructed disease)
– reduced maximal voluntary ventilation (in restrictive and obstructive disease)
– reduced diffusing capacity for carbon monoxide when fibrosis destroys alveolar walls and oblates pulmonary capillaries, or when fibrosis thickens the alveolar capillary membrane.
■ ABG measurements reveal:
– significantly decreased Pao_2 (in the late stages of chronic or complicated disease)
– decreased or normal $Paco_2$ in early stages; may increase as restrictive pattern develops.

Sinus bradycardia

■ ECG reveals:
– regular atrial and ventricular rhythm
– atrial and ventricular rates < 60 beats/minute
– P wave of normal size and configuration with a P wave preceding each QRS complex
– PR interval within normal limits and constant
– QRS complex of normal duration and configuration
– T wave of normal size and configuration
– QT interval within normal limits, but possibly prolonged.

Sinusitis

■ Nasal examination reveals inflammation and pus.

■ Sinus X-rays reveal cloudiness in the affected sinus, air-fluid levels, or thickened mucosal lining.

■ Transillumination allows inspection of the sinus cavities by passing a light through them; in sinusitis, purulent drainage prevents passage of light.

Sinus tachycardia

■ ECG reveals:
  – regular atrial and ventricular rhythms
  – atrial and ventricular rates > 100 beats/minute (usually between 100 and 160 beats/minute)
  – P wave of normal size and configuration with a P wave preceding each QRS complex
  – PR interval within normal limits and constant
  – QRS complex of normal duration and configuration
  – T wave of normal size and configuration
  – QT interval within normal limits, but commonly shortened.

Sjögren's syndrome

■ History and examination reveal two of the following three conditions: xerophthalmia, xerostomia (with salivary gland biopsy showing lymphocytic infiltration), and associated autoimmune or lymphoproliferative disorder.

■ ESR is elevated.

■ Hypergammaglobulinemia is present.

■ RF test is positive (75% to 90% of patients).

■ ANA test is positive (50% to 80% of patients).

■ Schirmer's tearing test is positive for tearing deficiency.

■ Lower lip biopsy shows salivary gland infiltration by lymphocytes.

Skull fractures

■ History includes recent head trauma.

■ Skull X-ray shows fracture (minor vault fractures may not be visible).

■ Neurologic examination evaluates cerebral function.

■ Cerebral angiography reveals vascular disruption from internal pressure and injury.

■ CT scan, echoencephalography, air encephalography, MRI, and radioactive scanning reveal cranial nerve injury or intracranial hemorrhage from ruptured blood vessels. These tests also help to localize subdural or intracerebral hematomas.

Snakebites, poisonous

■ Examination reveals fang marks.

■ Bleeding time and PTT are prolonged.

■ Hb level and HCT are decreased.

■ Platelet count is sharply decreased.

■ Urinalysis may reveal hematuria.

■ CXR may show pulmonary edema or emboli.

■ ECG may reveal tachycardia and ectopic beats.

Sodium imbalance

■ Hyponatremia:
  – Serum sodium level is < 135 mEq/L (SI, < 135 mmol/L).
  – Urine sodium level is > 100 mEq/24 hours (SI, > 100 mmol/d).
  – Serum osmolality is low.

■ Hypernatremia:
  – Serum sodium level is > 145 mEq/L (SI, > 145 mmol/L).
  – Urine sodium level is < 40 mEq/24 hours (SI, < 40 mmol/d).
  – Serum osmolality is high.

Spinal cord defects

- Examination reveals a protruding sac on the spine.
- Transillumination of sac reveals meningocele.
- Spinal X-ray shows bone defect (in spina bifida occulta).
- CT scan reveals hydrocephalus (in 90% of patients).

Spinal injuries without cord damage

- History includes trauma, metastatic disease, infection, or endocrine disorder.
- Physical examination reveals the location and level of injury.
- Spinal X-rays reveal fracture.
- Myelography reveals spinal mass.
- Lumbar puncture reveals increased CSF pressure, indicating spinal trauma or lesion.

Spinal neoplasms

- Lumbar puncture reveals clear yellow CSF with increased protein levels.
- X-rays show distortions of intervertebral foramina, changes in vertebrae or collapsed areas in the vertebral body, and localized enlargement of the spinal canal indicating an adjacent block.
- Myelography identifies the level of the lesion.
- CT scan and MRI show cord compression and tumor location.
- Radioisotope bone scan reveals evidence of metastatic invasion of the vertebrae by showing increased osteoblastic activity.
- Biopsy reveals malignant cells.

Sporotrichosis

- Examination reveals small, painless, movable subcutaneous nodules with discoloration and ulceration.

- Cultures of either sputum, pus, or bone drainage identify *Sporothrix schenckii*.

Sprains and strains

- History includes recent injury or chronic overuse of extremity.
- Examination reveals pain (local with a sprain, sharp and transient with a strain), swelling, and ecchymoses (rapid onset with a sprain; may take several days with a strain).
- X-ray of the extremity doesn't indicate fracture.

Squamous cell carcinoma

- Examination reveals ulcerated nodule with indurated base.
- Biopsy reveals squamous cell carcinoma.

Staphylococcal scalded skin syndrome

- Examination reveals three-stage progression of erythema, exfoliation, and desquamation.
- Skin lesions are positive for Group 2 *Staphylococcus aureus*.

Stomatitis and other oral infections

- Examination reveals inflammation of the oral mucosa or surrounding area.
- Smear of ulcer exudate reveals fusiform bacillus or spirochete as the causative organism (in Vincent's angina).

Strabismus

- Visual acuity test reveals the degree of visual defect.
- Hirschberg's method detects malalignment.
- Retinoscopy identifies refractive error.
- Maddox rods test identifies specific muscle involvement.

- Convergence test shows distance at which convergence is sustained.
- Duction test reveals limitation of eye movement.
- Cover-uncover test demonstrates eye deviation and the rate of recovery to original alignment.
- Alternate-cover test shows intermittent or latent deviation.

Stroke
- Patient reports sudden onset of motor or sensory impairment.
- CT scan detects structural abnormalities, edema, and lesions, such as nonhemorrhagic infarction and aneurysms.
- Cerebral angiography reveals disruption or displacement of the cerebral circulation by occlusion or hemorrhage.
- Ultrasonography of carotid and cerebral arteries may reveal occlusion.
- Digital abstraction angiography evaluates the patency of the cerebral vessels and identifies their position in the head and neck. It also detects and evaluates lesions and vascular abnormalities.
- PET scan provides data on cerebral metabolism and cerebral blood flow changes, especially in ischemic stroke.
- Single-photon emission tomography identifies cerebral blood flow and helps diagnose cerebral infarction.
- EEG may detect reduced electrical activity in an area of cortical infarction.
- Transcranial Doppler studies examine the size of intracranial vessels and the direction of blood flow.
- MRI allows evaluation of the lesion's location and size.

Strongyloidiasis
- History includes travel to endemic area.
- Stool specimen contains *Strongyloides stercoralis* larvae.

- Sputum specimen contains eosinophils and larvae.
- Hb level is decreased.
- WBC count with differential shows eosinophils at 450 to 700/µl (SI, 4.5 to 7 × 10^9/L).

Stye
- Visual examination reveals abscess of the lid glands.
- Abscess culture reveals a staphylococcal organism.

Sudden infant death syndrome
- Autopsy reveals:
  - small or normal adrenal glands
  - petechiae over the visceral surface of the pleura, within the thymus, and in the epicardium
  - well-preserved lymphoid structures
  - pathologic changes suggesting chronic hypoxemia
  - edematous, congestive lungs fully expanded in the pleural cavities
  - liquid blood in the heart (not clotted)
  - curd from the stomach inside the trachea.

Syndrome of inappropriate antidiuretic hormone
- History includes recent weight gain despite anorexia, nausea, and vomiting.
- Serum osmolality is < 280 mOsm/kg of water.
- Serum sodium level is < 123 mEq/L (SI, < 123 mmol/L).
- Urine sodium level is > 20 mEq/L without diuretics (SI, > 20 mmol/L).

Syphilis
- History includes sexual contact with partner with syphilis.
- Culture of lesion identifies *Treponema pallidum*.

- The fluorescent treponemal antibody-absorption test identifies antigens of *T. pallidum* in tissue, ocular fluid, CSF, tracheobronchial secretions, and exudates from lesions.
- Venereal Disease Research Laboratory (VDRL) slide test and rapid plasma reagin test are positive, detecting nonspecific antibodies.
- In neurosyphilis:
  - CSF analysis reveals elevated total protein level.
  - VDRL slide test is reactive.
  - Cell count > 5 mononuclear cells/ml.

Taeniasis

- History includes travel to endemic areas; exposure to eating undercooked, infected beef, pork, or fish; or in dwarf tapeworm, exposure to an infected person.
- Laboratory observation reveals tapeworm ova or body segments in stool.
- Beef tapeworm reveals:
  - crawling sensation in perianal area
  - intestinal obstruction and appendicitis.
- Pork tapeworm reveals:
  - seizures, headaches, personality changes (often overlooked in adults).
- In fish tapeworm:
  - anemia (Hb as low as 6 to 8 g/dl; SI, 60 to 80 g/L).
- Dwarf tapeworm reveals:
  - no symptoms (mild infestation)
  - anorexia, diarrhea, restlessness, dizziness, and apathy (severe infestation).

Tay-Sachs disease

- Family history includes Eastern European Jewish ancestry or history of the disease. Diagnostic screening may detect carriers of autosomal recessive gene.
- Serum analysis shows deficiency of hexosaminidase A.

- Ophthalmic examination reveals optic nerve atrophy and a distinctive cherry-red spot on the retina.

Tendinitis and bursitis

- History includes unusual strain or injury 2 to 3 days before onset of pain or heat-aggravated joint pain.
- Examination reveals localized pain and inflammation at joint.
- X-rays (in late stages) reveal bony fragments, osteophyte sclerosis, or calcium deposits.
- Arthrography is usually normal, with occasional small irregularities on the undersurface of the tendon.

Testicular cancer

- Physical examination reveals testicular mass.
- Transillumination confirms tumor.
- Biopsy reveals malignant cells.
- Excretory urography reveals ureteral deviation (indicates node involvement).
- Testosterone levels are > 1,200 ng/dl (SI, > 41.6 nmol/L) or < 300 ng/dl (SI, < 10.4 nmol/L).
- Urine testing indicates presence of hCG.
- Serum AFP and beta-hCG levels are increased.

Testicular torsion

- Physical examination reveals tense, tender swelling in the scrotum or inguinal canal and hyperemia of the overlying skin.
- Doppler ultrasonography reveals testicular torsion.

Tetanus

- History includes trauma and absence of tetanus immunization.
- Meningitis, rabies, phenothiazine or strychnine toxicity, or other conditions that mimic tetanus are ruled out.

- Cultures are positive for an anaerobic spore forming rod clostridium tetani.

Tetralogy of Fallot

- Echocardiography reveals septal overriding of the aorta, the ventricular septal defect (VSD), and pulmonic stenosis, and detects hypertrophy of walls of the right ventricle.
- Cardiac catheterization shows pulmonic stenosis, the VSD, and the overriding aorta and rules out other cyanotic heart defects.
- Auscultation reveals a loud systolic heart murmur, which may diminish or obscure the pulmonic component of S_2.
- Palpation may reveal a cardiac thrill at the left sternal border and an obvious right ventricular impulse.
- ECG shows right ventricular hypertrophy, right axis deviation and, possibly, right atrial hypertrophy.
- CXR reveals decreased pulmonary vascular marking (depending on the severity of pulmonary obstruction) and a boot-shaped cardiac silhouette.

Thalassemia

- Thalassemia major reveals:
  - lowered RBC count and Hb level
  - elevated reticulocyte level
  - elevated bilirubin and urinary and fecal urobilinogen levels
  - low serum folate level
  - X-rays of the skull and long bones showing a thinning and widening of the marrow space
  - Hb electrophoresis revealing a significant rise in HbF and a slight increase in HbA_2
  - peripheral blood smear revealing extremely thin and fragile RBCs, pale nucleated RBCs, and marked anisocytosis.
- Thalassemia intermedia reveals:
  - hypochromic and microcytic RBCs.

- Thalassemia minor reveals:
  - hypochromic and microcytic RBCs
  - Hb electrophoresis revealing a significant increase in HbA_2 and a moderate rise in HbF.

Thoracic aortic aneurysm

- CXR reveals widening of the aorta.
- CT scan or MRI reveals location and size of aneurysm.
- Aortography reveals the lumen of the aneurysm, its size and location and, in dissecting aneurysm, the false lumen.

Throat abscesses

- History includes staphylococcal or streptococcal infection.
- Examination reveals swelling of the soft palate on the abscessed side of the throat, with displacement of the uvula to the opposite side; red, edematous mucous membranes; and tonsil displacement toward the midline.
- Retropharyngeal abscess is indicated by:
  - history of nasopharyngitis or pharyngitis
  - soft, red bulging of the posterior pharyngeal wall
  - X-rays that reveal the larynx pushed forward and a widened space between the posterior pharyngeal wall and vertebrae
  - pharyngeal culture that identifies infective organism.
- Throat culture reveals streptococcal or staphylococcal infection.

Thrombocytopenia

- Platelet count is markedly decreased.
- Bleeding time is prolonged.
- PT and PTT are normal.
- Bone marrow studies reveal an increased number of megakaryocytes (platelet precursors) and shortened platelet survival.

Thrombophlebitis

- Homans' sign is positive.
- Doppler ultrasonography reveals reduced blood flow to a specific area and obstruction to venous flow.
- Plethysmography reveals decreased circulation distal to affected area.
- Phlebography reveals filling defects and diverted blood flow.

Thyroid cancer

- History includes exposure to radiation therapy or a family history of thyroid cancer.
- Examination reveals an enlarged, palpable node in the thyroid gland, neck, lymph nodes of the neck, or vocal cords.
- Thyroid scan reveals a "cold," nonfunctioning nodule.
- Biopsy reveals a well-encapsulated, solitary nodule of uniform but abnormal structure.
- Serum calcitonin assay reveals an elevated fasting calcitonin and an abnormal response to calcium stimulation (with medullary cancer).

Thyroiditis

- Autoimmune thyroiditis reveals:
  - positive precipitin test
  - high titers of thyroglobulin
  - microsomal antibodies present in serum.
- Subacute granulomatous thyroiditis reveals:
  - elevated ESR
  - increased thyroid hormone levels
  - decreased thyroidal radioiodine uptake.

Tic disorders

- History identifies stressors that may be related to symptoms.
- Examination reveals recurrent, involuntary movements involving the facial muscles, coughing, sniffling, or jerking head movements.
- Psychogenic tics are ruled out.

Tinea versicolor

- Wood's light examination reveals lesions.
- Microscopic examination of skin scrapings shows hyphae and clusters of yeast.

Tonsillitis

- Examination reveals generalized inflammation of the pharyngeal wall and swollen tonsils that project from between the pillars of the fauces and exude white or yellow follicles, with inflamed uvula.
- Purulent drainage appears when pressure is applied to the tonsillar pillars.
- Throat culture identifies infective organism, commonly beta-hemolytic streptococci.

Torticollis

- History includes painless neck deformity.
- Examination reveals enlargement of the sternocleidomastoid muscle.
- Cervical spine X-rays are negative for bone or joint disease but may reveal an associated disorder such as tuberculosis, scar tissue formation, or arthritis (in acquired torticollis).

Toxic epidermal necrolysis

- Examination reveals scalded skin with no history of burn.
- Nikolsky's sign (skin sloughs off with slight friction) appears in erythematous areas.
- Culture and Gram stain identify infective organism.
- WBC count reveals leukocytosis.

Toxic shock syndrome

■ Culture of vaginal discharge or lesions identifies *Staphylococcus aureus*.
■ CK level is elevated.
■ BUN level is elevated.
■ Serum creatinine level is elevated.
■ AST level is > 56 U/L (SI, > 0.95 −2 to +3 μkat/L) and ALT level is > 40 U/L (SI, > 0.68 μkat/L).
■ Platelet count is markedly decreased.

Toxocariasis

■ History includes pica, eosinophilia, or recent exposure to a dog.
■ Massive leukocytosis develops.
■ Hypereosinophilia develops.
■ Antibodies to *Toxocara canis* are present in serum.
■ Liver biopsy contains *T. canis* larvae.

Toxoplasmosis

■ History includes exposure to a cat or ingestion of uncooked meat.
■ Blood, body fluid, or tissue tests positive for *Toxoplasma gondii* antibodies.
■ *T. gondii* is identified in mice after their inoculation with specimens of patient's body fluids, blood, and tissue.

Tracheoesophageal fistula and esophageal atresia

■ Examination reveals respiratory distress and drooling in a neonate.
■ Catheter (#10 or #12 French) meets obstruction when passed through the nose at 4″ to 5″ (10 to 12.5 cm) distal from the nostrils.
■ CXR demonstrates the position of the catheter and can show a dilated, air-filled upper esophageal pouch, pneumonia in the right upper lobe, or bilateral pneumonitis.
■ Abdominal X-ray reveals gas in the bowel in a distal fistula (but none in a proximal fistula or atresia without fistula).
■ Cinefluorography defines the upper pouch by allowing visualization on a fluoroscopic screen and differentiates between overflow aspiration from a blind end (atresia) and aspiration due to passage of liquids through a tracheoesophageal fistula.

Trachoma

■ Examination reveals follicular conjunctivitis with corneal infiltration and upper lid or conjunctival scarring, with symptoms persisting for 3 weeks.
■ Microscopic examination of a Giemsa-stained conjunctival scraping reveals cytoplasmic inclusion bodies, some polymorphonuclear reaction, plasma cells, Leber's cells (large macrophages containing phagocytosed debris), and follicle cells.

Transposition of the great arteries

■ Echocardiography reveals the reversed position of the aorta and the pulmonary artery and records echoes from both semilunar valves simultaneously, due to the aortic valve displacement.
■ Cardiac catheterization reveals decreased oxygen saturation in left ventricular blood and aortic blood; increased right atrial, right ventricular, and pulmonary artery oxygen saturation; and right ventricular systolic pressure equal to systemic pressure.
■ Dye injection during catheterization reveals the transposed vessels and the presence of any other cardiac defects.
■ CXR shows right atrial and ventricular enlargement causing the heart to appear oblong (within days to weeks) and increased vascular markings, except when pulmonic stenosis exists.

■ ECG reveals right axis deviation and right ventricular hypertrophy (may be normal in a neonate).
■ ABG measurements reveal hypoxia and secondary metabolic acidosis.

Trichinosis

■ History includes ingestion of raw or improperly cooked pork or pork products.
■ Stools contain mature worms and larvae during the invasion stage.
■ Skeletal muscle biopsy reveals encysted larvae 10 days after ingestion.
■ Antibody titers are elevated during acute and convalescent stage.
■ During acute stages, serum liver enzymes (AST, LD, and CK) are elevated.
■ Eosinophil count is elevated.

Trichomoniasis

■ History includes sexual contact with person with trichomoniasis.
■ Examination reveals vaginal erythema; edema; frank excoriation; a frothy, malodorous, greenish yellow vaginal discharge; and, rarely, a thin, gray pseudomembrane over the vagina.
■ Cervical examination shows punctate cervical hemorrhages, giving the cervix a strawberry appearance.
■ Microscopic examination of vaginal or seminal discharge identifies *Trichomonas vaginalis*.
■ Culture of clear urine specimens may also reveal *T. vaginalis*.

Trichuriasis

■ History includes ingestion of food contaminated with nematoid ova.
■ Stool specimen contains whipworm ova.

Tricuspid insufficiency

■ Cardiac catheterization shows markedly decreased cardiac output; mean right atrial

and right ventricular end-diastolic pressures may be elevated.
■ CXR reveals right atrial and ventricular enlargement.
■ Echocardiography shows right ventricular dilation and paradoxical septal motion. It may show prolapsing or flailing of the tricuspid valve leaflets. Doppler echocardiography provides estimates of pulmonary artery and right ventricular systolic pressure.
■ ECG reveals right atrial hypertrophy and right or left ventricular hypertrophy. ECG also may reveal atrial fibrillation or incomplete right bundle-branch block.

Tricuspid stenosis

■ Cardiac catheterization shows increased right atrial pressure and decreased cardiac output; it may also show an increased pressure gradient across the tricuspid valve.
■ CXR reveals right atrial and superior vena cava enlargement.
■ Echocardiography reveals a thick tricuspid valve with reduced mobility and right atrial enlargement.
■ ECG shows right atrial hypertrophy and right ventricular hypertrophy. Atrial fibrillation may be present. Tall, peaked P waves are seen in lead II and prominent, upright P waves are seen in lead V_1, indicating right atrial enlargement.

Trigeminal neuralgia

■ History includes pain in the superior mandibular or maxillary area, without sensory or motor impairment.
■ Examination reveals splinting on the affected side of the face while talking.
■ Skull X-rays, tomography, and CT scans rule out sinus or tooth infections and tumors.

Tuberculosis

- Stains and cultures of sputum, CSF, urine, and abscess drainage reveal heat-sensitive, nonmotile, aerobic, acid-fast bacilli.
- CXR shows nodular lesions, patchy infiltrates, cavity formation, scar tissue, and calcium deposits.
- Auscultation reveals crepitant crackles, bronchial breath sounds, wheezes, and whispered pectoriloquy.
- Chest percussion reveals a dullness over the affected area.
- Tuberculin skin test reveals that the patient has been infected with tuberculosis.

Tularemia

- History includes exposure to animals or ticks.
- Lymph nodes, sputum, or gastric washings identify *Francisella tularensis*.
- Agglutination test reveals a rise in antibody titers.
- Skin test (with a diluted specimen of *F. tularensis*) has a positive reaction (90% of patients).

Typhus, epidemic

- Weil-Felix reaction reveals a fourfold rise in agglutination titer 8 to 12 days after infection.
- Complement fixation for group-specific typhus antigens is positive 8 to 12 days after infection.

Ulcerative colitis

- History includes recurrent bloody diarrhea and GI disturbances.
- Sigmoidoscopy shows increased mucosal friability, decreased mucosal detail, and thick inflammatory exudate.
- Biopsy reveals histologic changes characteristic of ulcerative colitis.
- Colonoscopy identifies the extent of the disease.

- Barium enema identifies the extent of the disease and detects complications.
- ESR increases, correlating with severity of attack.
- Serum potassium and magnesium levels are decreased.
- CBC shows decreased Hb level and leukocytosis.
- Serum albumin level is decreased.
- PT is prolonged.

Undescended testes

- Examination of scrotum reveals unpalpable testes, either unilateral or bilateral.
- Buccal smear identifies genetic sex by showing a male sex chromatin pattern.
- Serum gonadotropin levels confirm the presence of testes.

Urticaria and angioedema

- History includes exposure to medications, food, and environmental influences.
- Skin testing reveals specific allergens.
- Serum complement 4 and complement 1 esterase inhibitor levels are decreased (confirming hereditary angioedema).
- CBC, urinalysis, ESR, and CXR rule out inflammatory infections.

Uterine cancer

- Endometrial, cervical, and endocervical biopsies reveal malignant cells.
- Schiller's test shows cancerous tissues resisting stain.
- Cervical biopsies and endocervical curettage identify degree of cervical involvement.
- Barium enema reveals bladder or rectal involvement.

Uterine leiomyomas

- History includes abnormal endometrial bleeding.
- Pelvic palpation reveals round or irregular mass.

- Ultrasonography shows a dense mass.
- Hysterosalpingography reveals asymmetric uterus.
- Laparoscopy reveals lumps on the uterus.
- CBC reveals decreased RBC count, Hb level, and HCT.

Uveitis

- Slit-lamp examination reveals a "flare and cell" pattern, which looks like light passing through smoke, and an increased number of cells over the inflamed area.
- Examination with a special lens, slit-lamp, and ophthalmoscope identifies active inflammatory fundus lesions involving the retina and choroid.
- Serologic tests indicate toxoplasmosis (in posterior uveitis).

Vaginal cancer

- Pap test reveals abnormal cells.
- Vaginal examination, aided by Lugol's solution, reveals lesion.
- Lesion biopsy reveals malignant cells.
- Gallium scan shows abnormal gallium activity.

Vaginismus

- History and examination rule out physical disorders causing muscle constriction.
- Pelvic examination reveals involuntary constriction of the musculature surrounding the outer portion of the vagina.
- Detailed sexual history reveals involuntary spastic contraction of the lower vaginal muscles, possibly coexisting with dyspareunia, preventing intercourse.

Varicella

- History includes exposure to person infected with chickenpox, although the patient may be unaware of contact.
- Examination reveals crops of small, erythematous macules on the trunk or scalp progressing to papules and then clear vesicles on a erythematous base; vesicles become cloudy and break, and then form a scab.
- Vesicular fluid tests positive for herpesvirus varicella-zoster.

Variola

- History includes exposure to infected person.
- Aspirate from vesicles and pustules reveals variola virus.
- Complement fixation detects antibodies to variola virus.
- Microscopic examination of smears from lesions shows variola virus.

Vascular retinopathies

- Central retinal artery occlusion:
  - Ophthalmoscopy (direct or indirect) shows emptying of retinal arterioles.
  - Slit-lamp examination reveals, within 2 hours of occlusion, clumps or segmentation in the artery. Later examination shows a milky white retina around the optic disk (resulting from swelling and necrosis of ganglion cells caused by reduced blood supply). Other findings include a cherry-red spot in the macula (which subsides after several weeks).
  - Ophthalmodynamometry measures approximate relative pressures in the central retinal arteries and indirectly assesses internal carotid artery blockage.
  - Ultrasonography reveals blood vessel conditions in the neck.
  - Digital subtraction angiography identifies carotid occlusion.
  - MRI helps identify the reason for obstruction by revealing carotid or other obstruction.
  - Contrast-enhanced CT scan discloses the diseased carotid artery.
- Central retinal vein occlusion:

– Ophthalmoscopy (direct or indirect) reveals retinal hemorrhage, retinal vein engorgement, white patches among hemorrhages, and edema around the optic disk.
– Ultrasonography confirms or rules out occluded blood vessels.

■ Diabetic retinopathy:
– Slit-lamp examination shows thickening of retinal capillary walls.
– Indirect ophthalmoscopy demonstrates retinal changes, such as microaneurysms (earliest change), retinal hemorrhages and edema, venous dilation and beading, exudates, vitreous hemorrhage, proliferation of fibrin into vitreous from retinal holes, growth of new blood vessels, and microinfarctions of nerve fiber layer.
– Fluorescein angiography shows leakage of fluorescein from dilated vessels and differentiates between microaneurysms and true hemorrhages.

■ Hypertensive retinopathy:
– History reveals hypertension and decreased vision.
– Ophthalmoscopy (direct or indirect) performed in early disease discloses hard and shiny deposits, tiny hemorrhages, narrowed arterioles, nicking of the veins where arteries cross them (referred to as arteriovenous nicking), and elevated arterial blood pressure. The same test in later disease shows cotton wool patches, exudates, retinal edema, papilledema caused by ischemia and capillary insufficiency, hemorrhages, and microaneurysms.

Vasculitis

■ Polyarteritis nodosa:
– History includes hypertension, abdominal pain, myalgia, headache, joint pain, and weakness.
– ESR is elevated.

– Leukocytosis, anemia, and thrombocytosis are present.
– C_3 complement is depressed.
– RF titer is > 1:80.
– Circulating immune complexes are present.
– Tissue biopsy shows necrotizing vasculitis.

■ Allergic angiitis and granulomatosis:
– History includes asthma.
– Eosinophilia is present.
– Tissue biopsy may show granulomatous inflammation with eosinophilic infiltration.

■ Polyangiitis overlap syndrome:
– History includes allergy.
– Eosinophilia is present.
– Tissue biopsy that may show granulomatous inflammation with eosinophilic infiltration.

■ Wegener's granulomatosis:
– Leukocytosis is present.
– Tissue biopsy reveals necrotizing vasculitis with granulomatous inflammation.
– ESR and IgA and IgG levels are elevated.
– RF titer is low.
– Circulating immune complexes are present.

■ Temporal arteritis:
– Hb level is decreased.
– ESR is elevated.
– Tissue biopsy shows panarteritis with infiltration of mononuclear cells, giant cells within vessel wall, fragmentation of internal elastic lamina, and proliferation of intima.

■ Takayasu's arteritis:
– Hb level is decreased.
– Leukocytosis is present.
– Lupus erythematosus cell preparation is positive and ESR is elevated.
– Arteriography shows calcification and obstruction of affected vessels.

– Tissue biopsy shows inflammation of adventitia and intima of vessels and thickening of vessel walls.

■ Hypersensitivity vasculitis:
– History includes exposure to an antigen, such as a microorganism or a drug.
– Tissue biopsy may show leukocytoclastic angiitis (usually in postcapillary venules), with infiltration of polymorphonuclear leukocytes, fibrinoid necrosis, and extravasation of erythrocytes.

■ Mucocutaneous lymph node syndrome:
– History and examination reveal fever, nonsuppurative cervical adenitis, edema, congested conjunctivae, desquamation of fingertips, and erythema of oral cavity, lips, and palms.
– Tissue biopsy may show intimal proliferation and infiltration of vessel walls with mononuclear cells.

Velopharyngeal insufficiency

■ Examination reveals unintelligible speech.
■ Fiber-optic nasopharyngoscopy permits monitoring of velopharyngeal patency during speech and may identify the insufficiency.
■ Ultrasonography shows air-tissue overlap reflecting the degree of velopharyngeal sphincter incompetence; an opening of > 20 mm^2 results in unintelligible speech.

Ventricular aneurysm

■ History includes persistent arrhythmias, onset of heart failure, or systemic embolization in a patient with left ventricular failure and a history of myocardial infarction.
■ CXR reveals an abnormal bulge distorting the heart's contour (with large aneurysm).
■ Left ventriculography reveals left ventricular enlargement, with an area of akinesia or dyskinesia and diminished cardiac function.
■ Echocardiography reveals abnormal motion in the left ventricular wall.

Ventricular fibrillation

■ ECG findings include:
– Atrial rhythm isn't measurable.
– Ventricular rhythm has no pattern or regularity.
– Atrial and ventricular rates aren't measurable.
– P wave and PR interval aren't measurable.
– Duration of the QRS complex isn't measurable; configuration is wide and irregular.
– T wave isn't measurable.

Ventricular septal defect

■ Echocardiography or MRI reveals a large defect and its location in the septum, estimates the size of a left-to-right shunt, suggests pulmonary hypertension, and identifies associated lesions and complications.
■ Cardiac catheterization determines the size and exact location of the defect, calculates the degree of shunting, determines the extent of pulmonary hypertension, and detects associated defects.
■ CXR is normal with small defects; in large defects, it shows cardiomegaly, left atrial and ventricular enlargement, and prominent pulmonary vascular markings.
■ ECG is normal with small defects; in large defects, it shows left and right ventricular hypertrophy.

Ventricular tachycardia

■ ECG findings include:
– Atrial rhythm isn't measurable. Ventricular rhythm is usually regular, but may be slightly irregular.

– Atrial rate can't be measured. Ventricular rate is usually rapid (140 to 220 beats/minute).

– P wave is usually absent. It may be obscured by and is dissociated from the QRS complex. Retrograde and upright P waves may be present.

– PR interval isn't measurable.

– QRS complex has a duration > 0.12 second, has a bizarre appearance, and usually has increased amplitude.

– T wave occurs in the opposite direction of the QRS complex.

– QT interval isn't measurable.

Vesicoureteral reflux

■ History includes symptoms of urinary tract infection.

■ Examination reveals hematuria or strong-smelling urine (in infants).

■ Palpation may reveal a hard, thickened bladder (if posterior urethral valves are causing an obstruction in male infants).

■ Cystoscopy reveals reflux.

■ Urinalysis reveals bacterial count > 100,000/ml; specific gravity < 1.010, and increased pH.

■ Excretory urography may show dilated lower ureter, ureter visible for its entire length, hydronephrosis, calyceal distortion, and renal scarring.

■ Voiding cystourethrography identifies and determines the degree of reflux, shows when reflux occurs, and may also pinpoint the cause.

■ Bladder catheterization identifies the amount of residual urine.

Vitamin A deficiency

■ History includes inadequate dietary intake of foods high in vitamin A.

■ Ocular examination reveals xerophthalmia, Bitot's spots, perforation, and scarring.

■ Serum levels of vitamin A are < 20 µg/dl (SI, < 0.70 µmol/L).

■ Carotene levels are < 40 µg/dl (SI, < 0.76 µmol/L).

Vitamin B deficiencies

■ History includes inadequate dietary intake of foods high in vitamin B.

■ Serum vitamin B_2 is < 2 µg/dl.

■ 24-hour urine test reveals:

– thiamine deficiency

– riboflavin deficiency

– niacin deficiency

– pyridoxine deficiency.

Vitamin C deficiency

■ History includes inadequate intake of ascorbic acid.

■ Serum ascorbic acid levels are < 0.2 mg/dl (SI, < 11.5 µmol/L).

Vitamin D deficiency

■ History includes inadequate dietary intake of preformed vitamin D.

■ Serum vitamin D_3 levels are low or undetectable.

■ Serum calcium levels are < 7.5 mg/dl (SI, < 1.88 mmol/L).

■ Alkaline phosphatase levels are < 4 Bodansky units/dl.

■ X-rays reveal characteristic bone deformities and abnormalities such as Looser's zones.

Vitamin E deficiency

■ History includes diet high in polyunsaturated fatty acids fortified with iron but not vitamin E.

■ Serum vitamin E levels are < 5 µg/ml (SI, < 12 µmol/L).

■ Serum CK levels are increased.

■ Platelet levels are increased.

Vitamin K deficiency

- PT is 25% longer than the normal range of 10 to 20 seconds (in the absence of anticoagulant therapy or hepatic disease).
- Capillary fragility test is positive.

Vitiligo

- Examination reveals stark white skin patches.
- Wood's light examination in a darkened room detects vitiliginous patches; depigmented skin reflects the light, while pigmented skin absorbs it.

Vocal cord nodules and polyps

- History includes persistent hoarseness.
- Indirect laryngoscopy initially shows small red nodes; later, white solid nodes appear on one or both cords.
- Indirect laryngoscopy shows unilateral or, occasionally, bilateral, sessile or pedunculated polyps of varying size anywhere on the vocal cords.

Vocal cord paralysis

- History and examination reveal hoarseness or airway obstruction.
- Indirect laryngoscopy reveals one or both cords fixed in an adducted or partially abducted position.

Volvulus

- History includes sudden onset of severe abdominal pain.
- Examination reveals palpable abdominal mass.
- Abdominal X-rays reveal obstruction and abnormal air-fluid levels in the sigmoid and cecum (in midgut volvulus, abdominal X-rays may be normal).
- Barium enema findings include:
  – In cecal volvulus, barium fills the colon distal to the section of cecum.
  – In sigmoid volvulus in children, barium may twist to a point; in adults, barium may take on an "ace of spades" configuration.
- In midgut volvulus, upper GI series reveals obstruction and possibly a twisted contour in a narrow area near the duodenojejunal junction where barium won't pass.
- WBC count is elevated, indicating strangulation or bowel infarction.

Von Willebrand's disease

- History reveals family inheritance pattern.
- Bleeding time is prolonged.
- PTT is prolonged.
- Factor VIII-related antigens are decreased and factor VIII activity level is low.
- Clot retraction and platelet aggregation are normal.

Vulvovaginitis

- Examination reveals vaginal discharge and inflammation of the vulva.
- Culture of vaginal exudate identifies presence of *Trichomonas vaginalis, Candida albicans, Gardnerella vaginitis, Neisseria gonorrhoeae,* or *Phthirus pubis.*

Warts

- Visual examination reveals evidence of irregular growth on skin.
- Sigmoidoscopy may rule out internal involvement in recurrent anal warts.

Whooping cough

- Examination reveals forceful coughing that ends in a characteristic whoop.
- Nasopharyngeal swabs and sputum cultures identify *Bordetella pertussis* (in the early stages of illness).
- WBC count is markedly elevated, with 60% to 90% lymphocytes.

Wilms' tumor

- Examination reveals palpable abdominal mass in early childhood.
- Gallium scan reveals abnormal activity.
- Percutaneous renal biopsy reveals malignant cells.
- Excretory urography doesn't indicate neoplasm or extrarenal mass.

Wilson's disease

- Slit-lamp ophthalmic examination reveals Kayser-Fleischer rings (in advanced disease).
- Liver biopsy reveals excessive copper deposits and tissue changes indicative of chronic active hepatitis, fatty liver, or cirrhosis.
- Serum ceruloplasmin is < 22.9 mg/dl (SI, < 0.22 g/L).
- Urine copper is > 100 µg/24 hours (SI, > 1.6 µmol/24 h); may be as high as 1,000 µg/24 hours (SI, > 16 µmol/24 h).

Wiskott-Aldrich syndrome

- History includes thrombocytopenia, bleeding disorders at birth, and recurrent infections.
- Platelet count is markedly decreased.
- IgE levels are normal or elevated, IgG and IgA levels are normal, and IgM levels are decreased.
- Isohemagglutinin levels are low or absent.
- Sputum and throat cultures commonly identify *Streptococcus pneumoniae,* meningococci, or *Haemophilus influenzae* as the causative organisms.

Wounds, open trauma

- History includes injury.
- Examination reveals open wound.
- X-rays show bone damage, extent of injury to the area and surrounding tissue, and retention of injuring object.

- EMG reveals isolated, irregular motor unit potentials with increased amplitude and duration indicating peripheral nerve injury.
- Nerve conduction studies reveal abnormal nerve conduction time indicating peripheral nerve injury.
- CBC reveals decreased Hb and HCT levels and increased WBC count.

X-linked infantile hypogammaglobulinemia

- Serum IgM, IgA, and IgG are decreased or absent (in patient at least age 9 months).
- Antigenic stimulation testing confirms an inability to produce specific antibodies, although cellular immunity remains intact.

Yellow fever

- Blood culture reveals presence of arbovirus.
- Urine albumin levels are increased (in 90% of patients).
- Antibody titer is elevated.

Zinc deficiency

- History includes excessive intake of foods containing iron, calcium, vitamin D, and the fiber and phytates in cereals.
- Serum zinc levels are < 121 µg/dl (SI, < 18.4 µmol/L).

Appendices
Selected references
Index

Therapeutic drug monitoring guidelines

DRUG	LABORATORY TEST MONITORED	THERAPEUTIC RANGES OF TEST

aminoglycoside antibiotics (amikacin, gentamicin, tobramycin)	Amikacin peak
	   trough
	Gentamicin/tobramycin
	   peak
	   trough
	Creatinine
		20 to 25 mcg/ml (SI, 43 to 60 µmol/L)
		5 to 10 mcg/ml (SI, 6.8 to 17 µmol/L)
		
		4 to 8 mcg/ml (SI, 4 to 16.7 µmol/L)
		1 to 2 mcg/ml (SI, 2.1 to 4.2 µmol/L)
		0.6 to 1.3 mg/dl (SI, 53 to 115 µmol/L)

amphotericin B	Creatinine BUN Electrolytes (especially potassium and magnesium) Liver function tests Complete blood count (CBC) with differential and platelets	0.6 to 1.3 mg/dl (SI, 53 to 115 µmol/L) 8 to 20 mg/dl (SI, 2.9 to 7.5 mmol/L) Potassium: 3.5 to 5 mEq/L (SI, 3.5 to 5 mmol/L) Magnesium: 1.5 to 2.5 mEq/L (SI, 16 to 26 mg/L) Sodium: 135 to 145 mEq/L (SI, 135 to 145 mmol/L) Chloride: 100 to 108 mEq/L (SI, 100 to 108 mmol/L) * *****
antibiotics	White blood cell (WBC) count with differential Cultures and sensitivities	*****
biguanides (metformin)	Creatinine Fasting glucose Glycosylated hemoglobin CBC	0.6 to 1.3 mg/dl (SI, 53 to 115 µmol/L) 70 to 110 mg/dl (SI, 4.1 to 5.9 mmol/L) 5.5% to 8.5% of total hemoglobin (SI, 0.055 to 0.085) *****
clozapine	WBC count with differential	*****

Note: *** For those areas marked with five asterisks, these values can be used:**

Hemoglobin: Women: 12 to16 g/dl (SI, 120 to 160 g/L)
     Men: 14 to 18 g/dl (SI, 140 to 180 g/L)
Hematocrit: Women: 37% to 48% (SI, 0.37 to 0.48)
     Men: 42% to 52% (SI, 0.42 to 0.52)
RBCs: 4 to 5.5 x 10⁶/mm³ (SI, 4.0 to 5.5 × 10¹²/L)
WBCs: 5 to 10 x 10³/mm³ (SI, 5 to 10 × 10³/mm³)

Differential: Neutrophils: 45% to 74% (SI, 0.45 to 0.74)
     Bands: 0% to 8% (SI, 0 to 0.08)
     Lymphocytes: 16% to 45% (SI, 0.16 to 0.45)
     Monocytes: 4% to 10% (SI, 0.04 to 0.10)
     Eosinophils: 0% to 7% (SI, 0 to 0.07)
     Basophils: 0% to 2% (SI, 0 to 0.02)

MONITORING GUIDELINES

Wait until the administration of the third dose to check drug levels. Obtain blood for peak level 30 minutes after I.V. infusion or 60 minutes after I.M. administration. For trough levels, draw blood just before next dose. Dosage may need to be adjusted accordingly. Recheck after three doses. Monitor creatinine and blood urea nitrogen (BUN) levels and urine output for signs of decreasing renal function.

Monitor creatinine, BUN, and electrolyte levels at least weekly during therapy. Also, regularly monitor blood counts and liver function test results during therapy.

Specimen cultures and sensitivities will determine the cause of the infection and the best treatment. Monitor WBC count with differential weekly during therapy.

Check renal function and hematologic parameters before initiating therapy and at least annually thereafter. If the patient has impaired renal function, don't use metformin because it may cause lactic acidosis. Monitor response to therapy by periodically evaluating fasting glucose and glycosylated hemoglobin levels. A patient's home monitoring of glucose levels helps monitor compliance and response.

Obtain WBC count with differential before initiating therapy, weekly during therapy, and 4 weeks after discontinuing the drug.

* For those areas marked with one asterisk, these values can be used:

ALT: 7 to 56 U/L (SI, 0.17 to 0.68 µkat/L)
AST: 5 to 40 U/L (SI, 0.17 to 1.00 −2 to +3 µkat/L)
LDH: 60 to 220 U/L (SI, 1.9 to 3.6 µkat/L)
GGT: < 40 U/L (SI, < 0.51 µkat/L)
Total bilirubin: 0.2 to 1 mg/dl (SI, 3 to 22 µmol/L)

DRUG	LABORATORY TEST MONITORED	THERAPEUTIC RANGES OF TEST
digoxin	Digoxin	0.8 to 2 ng/ml (SI, 1.0 to 2.6 nmol/L)
	Electrolytes (especially potassium, magnesium, and calcium)	Potassium: 3.5 to 5 mEq/L (SI, 3.5 to 5 mmol/L)
		Magnesium: 1.3 to 2.1 mEq/L (SI, 0.65 to 1.05 mmol/L)
		Sodium: 135 to 145 mEq/L (SI, 135 to 145 mmol/L)
		Chloride: 100 to 108 mEq/L (SI, 100 to 108 mmol/L)
		Calcium: 8.6 to 10 mg/dl (SI, 2.15 to 50 mmol/L)
	Creatinine	0.6 to 1.3 mg/dl (SI, 53 to 115 µmol/L)
diuretics	Electrolytes	Potassium: 3.5 to 5 mEq/L (SI, 3.5 to 5 mmol/L)
		Magnesium: 1.3 to 2.1 mEq/L (SI, 0.65 to 1.05 mmol/L)
		Sodium: 135 to 145 mEq/L (SI, 135 to 145 mmol/L)
		Chloride: 100 to 108 mEq/L (SI, 100 to 108 mmol/L)
		Calcium: 8.6 to 10 mg/dl (SI, 2.15 to 50 mmol/L)
	Creatinine	0.6 to 1.3 mg/dl (SI, 53 to 115 µmol/L)
	BUN	8 to 20 mg/dl (SI, 2.9 to 7.5 mmol/L)
	Uric acid	2 to 7 mg/dl (SI, 0.12 to 0.37 mmol/L)
	Fasting glucose	70 to 110 mg/dl (SI, 4.1 to 5.9 mmol/L)
erythropoietin	Hematocrit	Women: 36% to 48% (SI, 0.36 to 0.48)
		Men: 42% to 52% (SI, 0.42 to 0.52)
ethosuximide	Ethosuximide	40 to 100 mcg/ml (SI, 283 to 708 µmol/L)
gemfibrozil	Lipids	Total cholesterol: < 200 mg/dl (SI, < 5.2 mmol/L)
		LDL: < 130 mg/dl (SI, < 3.37 mmol/L)
		HDL: Women: 40 to 85 mg/dl (SI, 1.03 to 2.2 mmol/L)
		Men: 37 to 70 mg/dl (SI, 0.96 to 1.8 mmol/L)
		Triglycerides: 10 to 190 mg/dl (SI, 0.11 to 2.21 mmol/L)
heparin	Partial thromboplastin time (PTT)	1.5 to 2 times control

Note: *** For those areas marked with five asterisks, these values can be used:**

Hemoglobin: Women: 12 to16 g/dl (SI, 120 to 160 g/L)
      Men: 14 to 18 g/dl (SI, 140 to 180 g/L)
Hematocrit: Women: 37% to 48% (SI, 0.37 to 0.48)
      Men: 42% to 52% (SI, 0.42 to 0.52)
RBCs: 4 to 5.5 x 10^6/mm^3 (SI, 4.0 to 5.5 × 10^{12}/L)
WBCs: 5 to 10 x 10^3/mm^3 (SI, 5 to 10 × 10^3/mm^3)

Differential: Neutrophils: 45% to 74% (SI, 0.45 to 0.74)
      Bands: 0% to 8% (SI, 0 to 0.08)
      Lymphocytes: 16% to 45% (SI, 0.16 to 0.45)
      Monocytes: 4% to 10% (SI, 0.04 to 0.10)
      Eosinophils: 0% to 7% (SI, 0 to 0.07)
      Basophils: 0% to 2% (SI, 0 to 0.02)

Check digoxin levels at least 12 hours, but preferably 24 hours, after the last dose is administered. To monitor maintenance therapy, check drug levels at least 1 to 2 weeks after therapy is initiated or changed. Make any adjustments in therapy based on the entire clinical picture, not solely on drug levels. Also, check electrolyte levels and renal function periodically during therapy.

To monitor fluid and electrolyte balance, perform baseline and periodic determinations of electrolyte, calcium, BUN, uric acid, and glucose levels.

After therapy is initiated or changed, monitor the hematocrit twice weekly for 2 to 6 weeks until stabilized in the target range and a maintenance dose determined. Monitor hematocrit regularly thereafter.

Check drug level 8 to 10 days after therapy is initiated or changed.

Therapy is usually withdrawn after 3 months if response is inadequate. Patient must be fasting to measure triglyceride levels.

When drug is given by continuous I.V. infusion, check PTT every 4 hours in the early stages of therapy. When drug is given by deep S.C. injection, check PTT 4 to 6 hours after injection.

* For those areas marked with one asterisk, these values can be used:
ALT: 7 to 56 U/L (SI, 0.17 to 0.68 μkat/L)
AST: 5 to 40 U/L (SI, 0.17 to 1.00 −2 to +3 μkat/L)
LDH: 60 to 220 U/L (SI, 1.9 to 3.6 μkat/L)
GGT: < 40 U/L (SI, < 0.51 μkat/L)
Total bilirubin: 0.2 to 1 mg/dl (SI, 3 to 22 μmol/L)

DRUG	LABORATORY TEST MONITORED	THERAPEUTIC RANGES OF TEST
HMG-CoA reductase inhibitors (fluvastatin, lovastatin, pravastatin, simvastatin)	Lipids	Total cholesterol: < 200 mg/dl (SI, < 5.2 mmol/L) LDL: < 130 mg/dl (SI, < 3.37 mmol/L) HDL: Women: 40 to 85 mg/dl (SI, 1.03 to 2.2 mmol/L) Men: 37 to 70 mg/dl (SI, 0.96 to 1.8 mmol/L) Triglycerides: 10 to 190 mg/dl (SI, 0.11 to 2.21 mmol/L)
	Liver function tests	*
insulin	Fasting glucose	70 to 110 mg/dl (SI, 4.1 to 5.9 mmol/L)
	Glycosylated hemoglobin	5.5% to 8.5% of total hemoglobin (SI, 0.055 to 0.085)
lithium	Lithium	0.5 to 1.4 mEq/L (SI, 0.5 to 1.4 mmol/L)
	Creatinine	0.6 to 1.3 mg/dl (SI, 53 to 115 µmol/L)
	CBC	*****
	Electrolytes (especially potassium and sodium)	Potassium: 3.5 to 5 mEq/L (SI, 3.5 to 5 mmol/L) Magnesium: 1.3 to 2.1 mEq/L (SI, 0.65 to 1.05 mmol/L) Sodium: 135 to 145 mEq/L (SI, 135 to 145 mmol/L) Chloride: 100 to 108 mEq/L (SI, 100 to 108 mmol/L)
	Fasting glucose	70 to 110 mg/dl (SI, 4.1 to 5.9 mmol/L)
	Thyroid function tests	TSH: 0.2 to 5.4 microU/ml (SI, 0.2 to 5.4 mU/L) T_3: 80 to 200 ng/dl (SI, 1.2 to 3 nmol/L) T_4: 5.4 to 11.5 mcg/dl (SI, 60 to 165 nmol/L)
methotrexate	Methotrexate	Normal elimination: < 10 micromol 24 hours postdose (SI, < 10 micromol 24 h postdose) < 1 micromol 48 hours postdose (SI, < 1 micromol 48 h postdose) < 0.2 micromol 72 hours postdose (SI, < 0.2 micromol 72 h postdose)
	CBC with differential	*****
	Platelet count	150 to 450 $\times$ 10^3/mm^3
	Liver function tests	*
	Creatinine	0.6 to 1.3 mg/dl (SI, 53 to 115 µmol/L)

Note: *** For those areas marked with five asterisks, these values can be used:**

Hemoglobin: Women: 12 to16 g/dl (SI, 120 to 160 g/L)
          Men: 14 to 18 g/dl (SI, 140 to 180 g/L)
Hematocrit: Women: 37% to 48% (SI, 0.37 to 0.48)
          Men: 42% to 52% (SI, 0.42 to 0.52)
RBCs: 4 to 5.5 x 10^6/mm^3 (SI, 4.0 to 5.5 $\times$ 10^{12}/L)
WBCs: 5 to 10 x 10^3/mm^3 (SI, 5 to 10 $\times$ 10^3/mm^3)

Differential: Neutrophils: 45% to 74% (SI, 0.45 to 0.74)
          Bands: 0% to 8% (SI, 0 to 0.08)
          Lymphocytes: 16% to 45% (SI, 0.16 to 0.45)
          Monocytes: 4% to 10% (SI, 0.04 to 0.10)
          Eosinophils: 0% to 7% (SI, 0 to 0.07)
          Basophils: 0% to 2% (SI, 0 to 0.02)

MONITORING GUIDELINES

Perform liver function tests at baseline, 6 to 12 weeks after therapy is initiated or changed, and periodically thereafter. If adequate response isn't achieved within 6 weeks, consider changing the therapy.

Monitor response to therapy by evaluating glucose and glycosylated hemoglobin levels. Glycosylated hemoglobin level is a good measure of long-term control. A patient's home monitoring of glucose levels helps measure compliance and response.

Checking lithium levels is crucial to the safe use of the drug. Obtain lithium levels immediately before next dose. Monitor levels twice weekly until stable. Once at steady state, levels should be checked weekly; when the patient is on the appropriate maintenance dose, levels should be checked every 2 to 3 months. Monitor creatinine, electrolyte, and fasting glucose levels; CBC; and thyroid function test results before therapy is initiated and periodically during therapy.

Monitor methotrexate levels according to dosing protocol. Monitor CBC with differential, platelet count, and liver and renal function test results more frequently when therapy is initiated or changed and when methotrexate levels may be elevated, such as when the patient is dehydrated.

* For those areas marked with one asterisk, these values can be used:

ALT: 7 to 56 U/L (SI, 0.17 to 0.68 µkat/L)
AST: 5 to 40 U/L (SI, 0.17 to 1.00 −2 to +3 µkat/L)
LDH: 60 to 220 U/L (SI, 1.9 to 3.6 µkat/L)
GGT: < 40 U/L (SI, < 0.51 µkat/L)
Total bilirubin: 0.2 to 1 mg/dl (SI, 3 to 22 µmol/L)

DRUG	LABORATORY TEST MONITORED	THERAPEUTIC RANGES OF TEST
phenytoin	Phenytoin CBC	10 to 20 mcg/ml (SI, 40 to 79 µmol/L) *****
potassium chloride	Potassium	3.5 to 5 mEq/L (SI, 3.5 to 5 mmol/L)
procainamide	Procainamide N-acetylprocainamide CBC	4 to 8 mcg/ml (SI, 17 to 42 µmol/L) (procainamide) 5 to 30 mcg/ml (combined procainamide and NAPA) *****
quinidine	Quinidine CBC Liver function tests Creatinine Electrolytes (especially potassium)	2 to 6 mcg/ml (SI, 6 to 15 µmol/L) ***** * 0.6 to 1.3 mg/dl (SI, 53 to 115 µmol/L) Potassium: 3.5 to 5 mEq/L (SI, 3.5 to 5 mmol/L) Magnesium: 1.3 to 2.1 mEq/L (SI, 0.65 to 1.05 mmol/L) Sodium: 135 to 145 mEq/L (SI, 135 to 145 mmol/L) Chloride: 98 to 106 mEq/L (SI, 100 to 108 mmol/L)
sulfonylureas	Fasting glucose Glycosylated hemoglobin	70 to 110 mg/dl (SI, 4.1 to 5.9 mmol/L) 5.5% to 8.5% of total hemoglobin (SI, 0.055 to 0.085)
theophylline	Theophylline	10 to 20 mcg/ml (SI, 44 to 111 µmol/L)
thyroid hormone	Thyroid function tests	TSH: 0.2 to 5.4 microU/ml (SI, 4.1 to 5.9 mmol/L) T_3: 80 to 200 ng/dl (SI, 1.2 to 4 nmol/L) T_4: 5.4 to 11.5 mcg/dl (SI, 60 to165 nmol/L)
vancomycin	Vancomycin Creatinine	20 to 35 mcg/ml (SI, 14 to 28 µmol/L) (peak) 5 to 10 mcg/ml (SI, 3 to 7 µmol/L) (trough) 0.6 to 1.3 mg/dl (SI, 53 to 115 µmol/L)
warfarin	International Normalized Ratio (INR)	For an acute MI, atrial fibrillation, treatment of pulmonary embolism, prevention of systemic embolism, tissue heart valves, valvular heart disease, or prophylaxis or treatment of venous thrombosis: 2 to 3 (SI, 2 to 3) For mechanical prosthetic valves or recurrent systemic embolism: 2.5 to 3.5 (SI, 2.5 to 3.5)

Note: *** For those areas marked with five asterisks, these values can be used:**

Hemoglobin: Women: 12 to16 g/dl (SI, 120 to 160 g/L)
Men: 14 to 18 g/dl (SI, 140 to 180 g/L)
Hematocrit: Women: 37% to 48% (SI, 0.37 to 0.48)
Men: 42% to 52% (SI, 0.42 to 0.52)
RBCs: 4 to 5.5 x 10^6/mm^3 (SI, 4.0 to 5.5 × 10^{12}/L)
WBCs: 5 to 10 x 10^3/mm^3 (SI, 5 to 10 × 10^3/mm^3)

Differential: Neutrophils: 45% to 74% (SI, 0.45 to 0.74)
Bands: 0% to 8% (SI, 0 to 0.08)
Lymphocytes: 16% to 45% (SI, 0.16 to 0.45)
Monocytes: 4% to 10% (SI, 0.04 to 0.10)
Eosinophils: 0% to 7% (SI, 0 to 0.07)
Basophils: 0% to 2% (SI, 0 to 0.02)

MONITORING GUIDELINES

Monitor phenytoin levels immediately before next dose and 2 to 4 weeks after therapy is initiated or changed. Obtain a CBC at baseline and monthly early in therapy. Watch for toxic effects at therapeutic levels. Adjust the measured level for hypoalbuminemia or renal impairment, which can increase free drug levels.

Check level weekly after oral replacement therapy is initiated until stable and every 3 to 6 months thereafter.

Measure procainamide levels 6 to 12 hours after a continuous infusion is started or immediately before the next oral dose. Combined (procainamide and NAPA) levels can be used as an index of toxicity when renal impairment exists. Obtain CBC periodically during longer-term therapy.

Obtain levels immediately before next oral dose and 30 to 35 hours after therapy is initiated or changed. Periodically obtain blood counts, liver and kidney function test results, and electrolyte levels.

Monitor response to therapy by periodically evaluating fasting glucose and glycosylated hemoglobin levels. Patient should monitor glucose levels at home to help measure compliance and response.

Obtain theophylline levels immediately before next dose of sustained-release oral product and at least 2 days after therapy is initiated or changed.

Monitor thyroid function test results every 2 to 3 weeks until appropriate maintenance dose is determined.

Vancomycin levels may be checked with the third dose administered, at the earliest. Draw peak levels 15 minutes after the I.V. infusion is completed. Draw trough levels immediately before the next dose is administered. Renal function can be used to adjust dosing and intervals.

Check INR daily, beginning 3 days after therapy is initiated. Continue checking it until therapeutic goal is achieved, and monitor it periodically thereafter. Also, check levels 7 days after any change in warfarin dose or concomitant, potentially interacting therapy.

* For those areas marked with one asterisk, these values can be used:

ALT: 7 to 56 U/L (SI, 0.17 to 0.68 µkat/L)
AST: 5 to 40 U/L (SI, 0.17 to 1.00 −2 to +3 µkat/L)
LDH: 60 to 220 U/L (SI, 1.9 to 3.6 µkat/L)
GGT: < 40 U/L (SI, < 0.51 µkat/L)
Total bilirubin: 0.2 to 1 mg/dl (SI, 3 to 22 µmol/L)

Drug interference with test results

Drugs can interfere with the results of blood or urine tests in two ways. A drug in a blood or urine specimen may interact with the chemicals used in the laboratory test, causing a false result. Alternatively, a drug may cause a physiologic change in the patient, resulting in an actual increased or decreased blood or urine level of the substance being tested. This chart identifies drugs that can cause these two types of interference in some common blood and urine tests.

TEST AND DRUGS CAUSING CHEMICAL INTERFERENCE	DRUGS CAUSING PHYSIOLOGIC INTERFERENCE	
	Increase test values	Decrease test values
Alkaline phosphatase ■ Albumin ■ Fluorides	■ Anticonvulsants ■ Hepatotoxic drugs ■ Ticlopidine	■ Clofibrate ■ Estrogens ■ Vitamin D ■ Zinc salts
Ammonia, blood	■ Acetazolamide ■ Ammonium chloride ■ Asparaginase ■ Barbiturates ■ Diuretics, loop and thiazide ■ Ethanol	■ Kanamycin, oral ■ Lactulose ■ Neomycin, oral ■ Potassium salts ■ Tetracyclines
Amylase, serum ■ Chloride salts ■ Fluorides	■ Asparaginase ■ Cholinergic agents ■ Contraceptives, hormonal ■ Contrast media with iodine ■ Drugs inducing acute pancreatitis: azathioprine, corticosteroids, loop and thiazide diuretics ■ Methyldopa ■ Narcotics	■ Somatostatin
Aspartate aminotransferase ■ Erythromycin ■ Methyldopa	■ Cholinergic agents ■ Hepatotoxic drugs ■ Opium alkaloids	■ Interferon ■ Naltrexone

TEST AND DRUGS CAUSING CHEMICAL INTERFERENCE	DRUGS CAUSING PHYSIOLOGIC INTERFERENCE	
	Increase test values	Decrease test values
Bilirubin, serum		
■ Ascorbic acid	■ Hemolytic agents	■ Barbiturates
■ Dextran	■ Hepatotoxic drugs	■ Sulfonamides
■ Epinephrine	■ Methyldopa	
■ Levodopa	■ Rifampin	
■ Pindolol		
■ Propanolol		
■ Theophylline		
Blood urea nitrogen		
■ Chloral hydrate	■ Anabolic steroids	■ Tetracyclines
■ Chloramphenicol	■ Nephrotoxic drugs	
■ Streptomycin	■ Pentamidine	
Calcium, serum		
■ Aspirin	■ Anabolic steroids	■ Acetazolamide
■ Heparin	■ Calcium salts	■ Anticonvulsants
■ Hydralazine	■ Diuretics, loop and thiazide	■ Calcitonin
■ Sulfisoxazole	■ Lithium	■ Cisplatin
	■ Thyroid hormones	■ Contraceptives, hormonal
	■ Vitamin D	■ Corticosteroids
		■ Laxatives
		■ Magnesium salts
		■ Plicamycin
Chloride, serum		
	■ Acetazolamide	■ Corticosteroids
	■ Androgens	■ Diuretics, loop and thiazide
	■ Diuretics	■ Laxatives
	■ Estrogens	
	■ Nonsteroidal anti-inflammatory drugs (NSAIDs)	
Cholesterol, serum		
■ Androgens	■ Alcohol	■ Androgens
■ Aspirin	■ Beta-adrenergic blockers	■ Captopril
■ Corticosteroids	■ Contraceptives, hormonal	■ Chlorpropamide
■ Nitrates	■ Corticosteroids	■ Cholestyramine
■ Phenothiazines	■ Cyclosporine	■ Clofibrate
■ Vitamin D	■ Diuretics, thiazide	■ Colestipol
	■ Phenothiazines	■ Haloperidol
	■ Sulfonamides	■ Neomycin, oral
	■ Ticlopidine	
Creatine kinase		
	■ Aminocaproic acid	■ Not applicable
	■ Amphotericin B	
	■ Chlorthalidone	
	■ Ethanol (long-term use)	
	■ Gemfibrozil	

TEST AND DRUGS CAUSING CHEMICAL INTERFERENCE	DRUGS CAUSING PHYSIOLOGIC INTERFERENCE	
	Increase test values	Decrease test values

Creatinine, serum
- Cefoxitin
- Cephalothin
- Flucytosine

- Cimetidine
- Flucyxtosine
- Nephrotoxic drugs

- Not applicable

Glucose, serum
- Acetaminophen
- Ascorbic acid (urine)
- Cephalosporins (urine)

- Antidepressants, tricyclic
- Beta-adrenergic blockers
- Corticosteroids
- Cyclosporine
- Dextrothyroxine
- Diazoxide
- Diuretics, loop and thiazide
- Epinephrine
- Estrogens
- Isoniazid
- Lithium
- Phenothiazines
- Phenytoin
- Salicylates
- Somatostatin

- Acetaminophen
- Anabolic steroids
- Clofibrate
- Disopyramide
- Ethanol
- Gemfibrozil
- Monoamine oxidase inhibitors
- Pentamidine

Magnesium, serum

- Lithium
- Magnesium salts

- Albuterol
- Aminoglycosides
- Amphotericin B
- Calcium salts
- Cardiac glycosides
- Cisplatin
- Diuretics, loop and thiazide
- Ethanol

Phosphates, serum

- Vitamin D (excessive amounts)

- Antacids, phosphate-binding
- Lithium
- Mannitol

Potassium, serum

- Aminocaproic acid
- Angiotensin-converting enzyme (ACE) inhibitors
- Antineoplastics
- Cyclosporine
- Diuretics, potassium-sparing
- Isoniazid
- Lithium
- Mannitol
- Succinylcholine

- Aminoglycosides
- Ammonium chloride
- Amphotericin B
- Corticosteroids
- Diuretics, potassium-wasting
- Glucose
- Insulin
- Laxatives
- Penicillins, extended-spectrum
- Salicylates

TEST AND DRUGS CAUSING CHEMICAL INTERFERENCE	DRUGS CAUSING PHYSIOLOGIC INTERFERENCE	
	Increase test values	Decrease test values

Protein, serum

	Increase test values	Decrease test values
	■ Anabolic steroids ■ Corticosteroids ■ Phenazopyridine	■ Contraceptives, hormonal ■ Estrogens ■ Hepatotoxic drugs

Protein, urine

	Increase test values	Decrease test values
■ Aminoglycosides ■ Cephalosporins ■ Contrast media ■ Magnesium sulfate ■ Miconazole ■ Nafcillin ■ Phenazopyridine ■ Sulfonamides ■ Tolbutamide ■ Tolmetin	■ ACE inhibitors ■ Cephalosporins ■ Contrast media with iodine ■ Corticosteroids ■ Nafcillin ■ Nephrotoxic drugs ■ Sulfonamides	■ Not applicable

Prothrombin time

	Increase test values	Decrease test values
	■ Anticoagulants ■ Asparaginase ■ Aspirin ■ Azathioprine ■ Certain cephalosporins ■ Chloramphenicol ■ Cholestyramine ■ Colestipol ■ Cyclophosphamide ■ Hepatotoxic drugs ■ Propylthiouracil ■ Quinidine ■ Quinine ■ Sulfonamides	■ Anabolic steroids ■ Contraceptives, hormonal ■ Estrogens ■ Vitamin K

Sodium, serum

	Increase test values	Decrease test values
	■ Carbamazepine ■ Clonidine ■ Diazoxide ■ Estrogens ■ Guanabenz ■ Guanadrel ■ Guanethidine ■ Methyldopa ■ NSAIDs ■ Steroids	■ Ammonium chloride ■ Carbamazepine ■ Desmopressin ■ Diuretics ■ Lithium ■ Lypressin ■ Vasopressin ■ Vincristine

TEST AND DRUGS CAUSING CHEMICAL INTERFERENCE	DRUGS CAUSING PHYSIOLOGIC INTERFERENCE	
	Increase test values	Decrease test values

Uric acid, serum

■ Ascorbic acid	■ Acetazolamide	■ Acetohexamide
■ Caffeine	■ Cisplatin	■ Allopurinol
■ Hydralazine	■ Cyclosporine	■ Clofibrate
■ Isoniazid	■ Diazoxide	■ Contrast media with iodine
■ Levodopa	■ Diuretics	■ Diflunisal
■ Theophylline	■ Epinephrine	■ Glucose infusions
	■ Ethambutol	■ Guaifenesin
	■ Ethanol	■ Phenothiazines
	■ Levodopa	■ Phenylbutazone
	■ Niacin	■ Salicylates (small doses)
	■ Phenytoin	■ Uricosuric agents
	■ Propranolol	
	■ Spironolactone	

Laboratory value changes in elderly patients

Standard normal laboratory values reflect the physiology of adults ages 20 to 40. However, normal values for older patients usually differ because of age-related physiologic changes.

Certain test results, however, remain unaffected by age. These include partial thromboplastin time, prothrombin time, serum acid phosphatase, serum carbon dioxide, serum chloride, aspartate aminotransferase, and total serum protein. You can use this chart to interpret other changeable test values in your elderly patients.

TEST VALUES AGES 20 TO 40	AGE-RELATED CHANGES	CONSIDERATIONS
Serum		
Albumin 3.5 to 5 g/dl (SI, 35 to 50 g/L)	Under age 65: Higher in males Over age 65: Equal levels that then decrease at same rate	Increased dietary protein intake needed in older patients if liver function is normal; edema: a sign of low albumin level
Alkaline phosphatase 30 to 85 IU/L (SI, 42 to 128 U/L)	Increases 8 to 10 IU/L	May reflect liver function decline or vitamin D malabsorption and bone demineralization
Beta globulin 0.7 to 1.1 g/dl (SI, 7 to 11 g/L)	Increases slightly	Increases in response to decrease in albumin if liver function is normal; increased dietary protein intake needed
Blood urea nitrogen Men: 10 to 25 mg/dl (SI, 3.6 to 9.3 mmol/L) Women: 8 to 20 mg/dl (SI, 2.9 to 7.5 mmol/L)	Increases, possibly to 69 mg/dl (SI, 25.8 mmol/L)	Slight increase acceptable in absence of stressors, such as infection or surgery
Cholesterol Men: < 205 mg/dl (SI, < 5.30 mmol/L) Women: < 190 mg/dl (SI, < 4.90 mmol/L)	Men: Increases to age 50, then decreases Women: Lower than men until age 50, increases to age 70, then decreases	Rise in cholesterol level (and increased cardiovascular risk) in women as a result of postmenopausal estrogen decline; dietary changes, weight loss, and exercise needed

TEST VALUES AGES 20 TO 40	AGE-RELATED CHANGES	CONSIDERATIONS
Serum (continued)		
Creatine kinase 55 to 170 U/L (SI, 0.94 to 2.89 µkat/L)	Increases slightly	May reflect decreasing muscle mass and liver function
Creatinine 0.6 to 1.3 mg/dl (SI, 53 to 115 µmol/L)	Increases, possibly to 1.9 mg/dl in men (SI, 168 µmol/L)	Important factor to prevent toxicity when giving drugs excreted in urine
Creatinine clearance Men: 94 to 140 ml/min/1.73 m^2 (SI, 0.91 to 1.35 mL/s/m^2) Women: 72 to 110 mL/min/1.73 m^2 (SI, 0.69 to 1.06 mL/s/m^2)	Men: Decreases; formula: ([140 − age) × kg body weight]/(72 × serum creatinine) Women: 85% of men's rate	Reflects reduced glomerular filtration rate; important factor to prevent toxicity when giving drugs excreted in urine
Hematocrit Men: 45% to 52% (SI, 0.45 to 0.52) Women: 37% to 48% (SI, 0.37 to 0.48)	May decrease slightly (unproven)	Reflects decreased bone marrow and hematopoiesis, increased risk of infection (because of fewer and weaker lymphocytes and immune system changes that diminish antigen-antibody response)
Hemoglobin Men: 14 to 18 g/dl (SI, 140 to 180 g/L) Women: 12 to 16 g/dl (SI, 120 to 160 g/L)	Men: Decreases by 1 to 2 g/dl Women: Unknown	Reflects decreased bone marrow, hematopoiesis, and (for men) androgen levels
High-density lipoprotein Men: 37 to 70 mg/dl (SI, 0.96 to 1.8 mmol/L) Women: 40 to 85 mg/dl (SI, 1.03 to 2.2 mmol/L)	Levels higher in women than in men but equalize with age	Compliance with dietary restrictions required for accurate interpretation of test results
Lactate dehydrogenase 71 to 207 U/L (SI, 1.2 to 3.52 µkat/L)	Increases slightly	May reflect declining muscle mass and liver function
Leukocyte count 4,000 to 10,000/µl (SI, 4 to 10 × 10^9/L)	Decreases to 3,100 to 9,000/µl (SI, 3.1 to 9 × 10^9/L)	Decrease proportionate to lymphocyte count
Lymphocyte count 25% to 40% (SI, 0.25 to 0.40)	Decreases	Decrease proportionate to leukocyte count
Platelet count 140,000 to 400,000/µl (SI, 140 to 400 × 10^9/L)	Change in characteristics: decreased granular constituents, increased platelet-release factors	May reflect diminished bone marrow and increased fibrinogen levels

TEST VALUES AGES 20 TO 40	AGE-RELATED CHANGES	CONSIDERATIONS
Serum *(continued)*		
Potassium 3.5 to 5.5 mEq/L (SI, 3.5 to 5.5 mmol/L)	Increases slightly	Requires avoidance of salt substitutes composed of potassium, vigilance in reading food labels, and knowledge of hyperkalemia's signs and symptoms
Thyroid-stimulating hormone 0 to 15 µlU/ml (SI, 15 mU/L)	Increases slightly	Suggests primary hypothyroidism or endemic goiter at much higher levels
Thyroxine 5 to 13.5 µg/dl (SI, 60 to 165 mmol/L)	Decreases 25%	Reflects declining thyroid function
Triglycerides Men: 44 to 180 mg/dl (SI, 0.44 to 2.01 mmol/L) Women: 10 to 190 mg/dl (SI, 0.11 to 2.21 mmol/L)	Increases slightly	Suggests abnormalities at any other levels, requiring additional tests such as serum cholesterol
Triiodothyronine 80 to 220 ng/dl (SI, 1.2 to 3 nmol/L)	Decreases 25%	Reflects declining thyroid function
Urine		
Glucose 0 to 15 mg/dl (SI, 0 to 8 mmol/L)	Decreases slightly	May reflect renal disease or urinary tract infection (UTI); unreliable check for older diabetics because glucosuria may not occur until plasma glucose level exceeds 300 mg/dl
Protein 50 to 80 mg/24 hours (SI, 50 to 80 mg/d)	Increases slightly	May reflect renal disease or UTI
Specific gravity 1.032 (SI, 1.032)	Decreases to 1.024 (SI, 1.024) by age 80	Reflects 30% to 50% decrease in number of nephrons available to concentrate urine

Quick-reference guide to laboratory test results

A

Acetylcholine receptor antibodies, serum
Negative
Acid mucopolysaccharides, urine
Adults: < 13.3 µg glucuronic acid/mg/creatinine/
24 hours
Acid phosphatase, serum
0 to 3.7 U/L (SI, 0 to 3.7 U/L)
Adrenocorticotropic hormone, plasma
< 120 pg/ml (SI, < 26.4 pmol/L)
Alanine aminotransferase
8 to 50 IU/L (SI, 0.14 to 0.85 µkat/L)
Aldosterone, serum
Supine individuals: 3 to 16 ng/dl (SI, 80 to 440 pmol/L)
Upright individuals: 7 to 30 ng/dl (SI, 190 to
832 pmol/L)
Aldosterone, urine
3 to 19 µg/24 hours (SI, 8 to 51 nmol/d)
Alkaline phosphatase, peritoneal fluid
Males > 18 years: 90 to 239 U/L (SI, 90 to 239 U/L)
Females < 45 years: 76 to 196 U/L (SI, 76 to 196 U/L);
>45 years: 87 to 250 U/L (87 to 250 U/L)
Alkaline phosphatase, serum
30 to 85 IU/ml (SI, 42 to 128 U/L)
Alpha-fetoprotein, serum
Males and nonpregnant females: < 15 ng/ml (SI,
< 15 mg/L)
Ammonia, peritoneal fluid
< 50 µg/dl (SI, < 29 µmol/L)
Amniotic fluid analysis
Lecithin-sphingomyelin ratio: > 2
Meconium: absent (except in breech presentation)
Phosphatidylglycerol: present
Amylase, peritoneal fluid
138 to 404 U/L (SI, 138 to 404 U/L)
Amylase, serum
Adults ≥ 18 years: 25 to 85 U/L (SI, 0.39 to
1.45 µkat/L)
Amylase, urine
1 to 17 U/hour (SI, 0.017 to 0.29 µkat/h)
Androstenedione (radioimmunoassay)
Males: 75 to 205 ng/dl (SI, 2.6 to 7.2 nmol/L)
Females: 85 to 275 ng/dl (SI, 3.0 to 9.6 nmol/L)

Angiotensin-converting enzyme
Adults ≥ 20 years: 8 to 52 U/L (SI, 0.14 to 0.88 µkat/L)
Anion gap
8 to 14 mEq/L (SI, 8 to 14 mmol/L)
Antibody screening, serum
Negative
Antidiuretic hormone, serum
1 to 5 pg/ml (SI, 1 to 5 mg/L)
Antiglobulin test, direct
Negative
Antimitochondrial antibodies, serum
Negative
Anti–smooth-muscle antibodies, serum
Negative
Antistreptolysin-O, serum
Preschoolers and adults: 85 Todd units/ml
School-age children: 170 Todd units/ml
Antithrombin III
80% to 120% of normal control values
Antithyroid antibodies, serum
Normal titer < 1:100
Arginine test
Human growth hormone levels
– *Males:* increase to > 10 ng/ml (SI, > 10 µg/L)
– *Females:* increase to > 15 ng/ml (SI, > 15 µg/L)
– *Children:* increase to > 48 ng/ml (SI, > 48 µg/L)
Arterial blood gases
pH: 7.35 to 7.45 (SI, 7.35 to 7.45)
PaO$_2$: 80 to 100 mm Hg (SI, 10.6 to 13.3 kPa)
PaCO$_2$: 35 to 45 mm Hg (SI, 4.7 to 5.3 kPa)
O$_2$ CT: 15% to 23% (SI, 0.15 to 0.23)
SaO$_2$: 94% to 100% (SI, 0.94 to 1.00)
HCO$_3$$^-$: 22 to 25 mEq/L (SI, 22 to 25 mmol/L)
Arylsufatase A, urine
Random: 16 to 42 µ/g creatinine
24-hour: 0.37 to 3.60 µ/day creatinine
1-hour test: 2 to 19 µ/1 hour (SI, 2 to 19 µ/h)
2-hour test: 4 to 37 µ/2 hours (SI, 4 to 37 µ/h)
24-hour test: 170 to 2,000 µ/24 hours (SI, 2.89 to
34.0 µkat/L)
Aspartate aminotransferase
Males: 8 to 46 U/L (SI, 0.14 to 0.78 µkat/L)
Females: 7 to 34 U/L (SI, 0.12 to 0.58 µkat/L)

Aspergillosis antibody, serum
Normal titer < 1:8
Atrial natriuretic factor, plasma
20 to 77 pg/ml

B

Bacterial meningitis antigen
Negative
Bence Jones protein, urine
Negative
Beta-hydroxybutyrate
< 0.4 mmol/L (SI, 0.4 mmol/L)
Bilirubin, amniotic fluid
Early: < 0.075 mg/dl (SI, < 1.3 Umol/L)
Term: < 0.025 mg/dl (SI, < 0.41 Umol/L)
Bilirubin, serum
Adults
– *Direct:* < 0.5 mg/dl (SI, < 6.8 μmol/L)
– *Indirect:* 1.1 mg/dl (SI, 19 μmol/L)
Neonates
– *Total:* 1 to 12 mg/dl (SI, 34 to 205 μmol/L)
Bilirubin, urine
Negative
Blastomycosis antibody, serum
Normal titer < 1:8
Bleeding time
Template: 3 to 6 minutes (SI, 3 to 6 m)
Ivy: 3 to 6 minutes (SI, 3 to 6 m)
Duke: 1 to 3 minutes (SI, 1 to 3 m)
Blood urea nitrogen
8 to 20 mg/dl (SI, 2.9 to 7.5 mmol/L)
B-lymphocyte count
270 to 640/μl

C

Calcitonin, plasma
Baseline
– *Males:* 40 pg/ml (SI, 40 ng/L)
– *Females:* 20 pg/ml (SI, 20 ng/L)
Calcium infusion
– *Males:* 190 pg/ml (SI, 190 ng/L)
– *Females:* 130 pg/ml (SI, 130 ng/L)
Pentagastrin infusion
– *Males:* 110 pg/ml (SI, 110 ng/L)
– *Females:* 30 pg/ml (SI, 30 ng/L)
Calcium, serum
Adults: 8.2 to 10.2 mg/dl (SI, 2.05 to 2.54 mmol/L)
Children: 8.6 to 11.2 mg/dl (SI, 2.15 to 2.79 mmol/L)
Ionized: 4.65 to 5.28 mg/dl (SI, 1.1 to 1.25 mmol/L)

Calcium, urine
100 to 300 mg/24 hours (SI, 2.50 to 7.50 mmol/d)
***Candida* antibodies, serum**
Negative
Capillary fragility

Petechiae per 5 cm:	*Score:*
11 to 20	2+
21 to 50	3 +
over 50	4 +

Carbon dioxide, total, blood
22 to 26 mEq/L (SI, 22 to 26 mmol/L)
Carcinoembryonic antigen, serum
< 5 ng/ml (SI, < 5 mg/L)
Catecholamines, plasma
Supine
– *Epinephrine:* undetectable to 110 pg/ml (SI, undetectable to 600 pmol/L)
– *Norepinephrine:* 70 to 750 pg/ml (SI, 413 to 4,432 pmol/L)
Standing
– *Epinephrine:* undetectable to 140 pg/ml (SI, undetectable to 764 pmol/L)
– *Norepinephrine:* 200 to 1,700 pg/ml (SI, 1182 to 10,047 pmol/L)
Catecholamines, urine
Epinephrine: 0 to 20 μg/24 hours (SI, 0 to 109 nmol/24 h)
Norepinephrine: 15 to 80 μg/24 hours (SI, 89 to 473 nmol/24 h)
Dopamine: 65 to 400 μg/24 hours (SI, 425 to 2,610 nmol/24 h)
Cerebrospinal fluid
Pressure: 50 to 180 mm H_2O
Appearance: clear, colorless
Gram stain: no organisms
Ceruloplasmin, serum
22.9 to 43.1 g/dl (SI, 0.22 to 0.43 g/L)
Chloride, cerebrospinal fluid
118 to 130 mEq/L (SI, 118 to 130 mmol/L)
Chloride, serum
100 to 108 mEq/L (SI, 100 to 108 mmol/L)
Chloride, urine
Adults: 110 to 250 nmol/24 hours (SI, 110 to 250 mmol/d)
Children: 15 to 40 nmol/24 hours (SI, 15 to 40 mmol/d)
Infants: 2 to 10 mmol/24 hours (SI, 2 to 10 mmol/d)
Cholinesterase (pseudocholinesterase)
204 to 532 IU/dl (SI, 2.04 to 5.32 kU/L)
Coccidioidomycosis antibody, serum
Normal titer < 1:2
Cold agglutinins, serum
Normal titer < 1:64

Complement, serum
Total
– 40 to 90 U/ml (SI, 0.4 to 0.9 g/L)
C3
– *Males:* 80 to 180 mg/dl (SI, 0.8 to 1.8 g/L)
– *Females:* 76 to 120 mg/dl (SI, 0.76 to 1.2 g/L)
C4
– *Males:* 15 to 60 mg/dl (SI, 0.15 to 0.6 g/L)
– *Females:* 15 to 52 mg/dl (SI, 0.15 to 0.52 g/L)
Copper, urine
3 to 35 µg/24 hours (SI, 0.05 to 0.55 µmol/d)
Cortisol, free, urine
< 50 µg/24 hours (SI, < 138 mmol/d)
Cortisol, plasma
Morning: 9 to 35 µg/dl (SI, 250 to 690 nmol/L)
Afternoon: 3 to 12 µg/dl (SI, 80 to 330 nmol/L)
C-reactive protein, serum
< 0.8 mg/dl (SI, < 8 mg/L)
Creatine kinase
Total
– *Males:* 55 to 170 U/L (SI, 0.94 to 2.89 µkat/L)
– *Females:* 30 to 135 U/L (SI, 0.51 to 2.3 µkat/L)
Creatinine clearance
Males: 94 to 140 ml/min/1.73 m² (SI, 0.91 to
1.35 ml/s/m²)
Females: 72 to 110 ml/min/1.73 m² (SI, 0.69 to
1.06 ml/s/m²)
Creatinine, serum
Males: 0.8 to 1.2 mg/dl (SI, 62 to 115 µmol/L)
Females: 0.6 to 0.9 mg/dl (SI, 53 to 97 µmol/L)
Creatinine, urine
Males: 14 to 26 mg/kg body weight/24 hours (SI,
124 to 230 µmol/kg body weight/d)
Females: 11 to 20 mg/kg body weight/24 hours (SI,
97 to 177 µmol/kg body weight/d)
Cryoglobulins, serum
Negative
Cyclic adenosine monophosphate, urine
0.3 to 3.6 mg/day (SI, 100 to 723 µmol/d)
or
0.29 to 2.1 mg/g creatinine (SI, 100 to 723 µmol/mol
creatinine)
Cytomegalovirus antibodies, serum
Negative

D

D-xylose absorption
Blood
– *Adults:* 25 to 40 mg/dl in 2 hours
– *Children:* > 30 mg/dl in 1 hour

Urine
– *Adults:* > 3.5 g excreted in 5 hours (age 65 of older,
> 5 g in 24 hours)
– *Children:* 16% to 33% excreted in 5 hours

E

Epstein-Barr virus antibodies
Negative
Erythrocyte sedimentation rate
Males: 0 to 10 mm/hour (SI, 0 to 10 mm/h)
Females: 0 to 20 mm/hour (SI, 0 to 20 mm/h)
Esophageal acidity
pH > 5.0
Estrogens, serum
Females
– *Menstruating:* 26 to 149 pg/ml (SI, 90 to 550 pmol/
L)
– *Postmenopausal:* 0 to 34 pg/ml (SI, 0 to 125 pmol/L)
Males
– 12 to 34 pg/ml (SI, 40 to 125 pmol/L)
Children
– *< 6 years:* 3 to 10 pg/ml (SI, 10 to 36 pmol/L)
Euglobulin lysis time
2 to 4 hours (SI, 2 to 4 h)

F

Factor assay, one-stage
50% to 150% of normal activity (SI, 0.50 to 1.50)
Febrile agglutination, serum
Salmonella antibody: < 1:80
Brucellosis antibody: < 1:80
Tularemia antibody: < 1:40
Rickettsial antibody: < 1:40
Ferritin, serum
Males
– 20 to 300 ng/ml (SI, 20 to 300 µg/L)
Females
– 20 to 120 ng/ml (SI, 20 to 120 µg/L)
Infants
– *1 month:* 200 to 600 ng/ml (SI, 200 to 600 µg/L)
– *2 to 5 months:* 50 to 200 ng/ml (SI, 50 to 200 µg/L)
– *6 months to 15 years:* 7 to 140 ng/ml (SI, 7 to
140 µg/L)
Neonates
– 25 to 200 ng/ml (SI, 25 to 200 µg/L)
Fibrinogen, plasma
200 to 400 mg/dl (SI, 2 to 4 g/L)
Fibrin split products
Screening assay: < 10 µg/ml (SI, < 10 mg/L)
Quantitative assay: < 3 µg/ml (SI, < 3 mg/L)

Fluorescent treponemal antibody absorption, serum
Negative
Folic acid, serum
1.8 to 9 ng/ml (SI, 4 to 20 nmol/L)
Follicle-stimulating hormone, serum
Menstruating females
– *Follicular phase:* 5 to 20 mIU/ml (SI, 5 to 20 IU/L)
– *Ovulatory phase:* 15 to 30 mIU/ml (SI, 15 to 30 IU/L)
– *Luteal phase:* 5 to 15 mIU/ml (SI, 5 to 15 IU/L)
Menopausal females
– 5 to 100 mIU/ml (SI, 50 to 100 IU/L)
Males
– 5 to 20 mIU/ml (5 to 20 IU/L)
Free thyroxine, serum
0.9 to 2.3 ng/dl (SI, 10 to 30 nmol/L)
Free triiodothyronine
0.2 to 0.6 ng/dl (SI, 0.003 to 0.009 nmol/L)

G

Galactose 1-phosphate uridyl transferase
Qualitative: negative
Quantitative: 18.5 to 28.5 U/g of hemoglobin
Gamma-glutamyl transferase
Males
– ≥ *16 years:* 6 to 38 U/L (SI, 0.10 to 0.63 µkat/L)
Females
– *16 to 45 years:* 4 to 27 U/L (SI, 0.08 to 0.46 µkat/L)
– > *45 years:* 6 to 38 U/L (SI, 0.10 to 0.63 µkat/L)
Children
– 3 to 30 U/L (SI, 0.05 to 0.51 µkat)
Gastric acid stimulation
Males: 18 to 28 mEq/hour
Females: 11 to 21 mEq/hour
Gastric secretion, basal
Males: 1 to 5 mEq/hour
Females: 0.2 to 3.3 mEq/hour
Gastrin, serum
50 to 150 pg/ml (SI, 50 to 150 ng/L)
Globulin, peritoneal fluid
30% to 45% of total protein
Glucose, amniotic fluid
< 45 mg/dl (SI, < 2.3 mmol/L)
Glucose, cerebrospinal fluid
50 to 80 mg/dl (SI, 2.8 to 4.4 mmol/L)
Glucose, peritoneal fluid
70 to 100 mg/dl (SI, 3.5 to 5 mmol/L)
Glucose, plasma, fasting
70 to 100 mg/dl (SI, 3.9 to 6.1 mmol/L)
Glucose-6-phosphate dehydrogenase
4.3 to 11.8 U/g (SI, 0.28 to 0.76 mU/mol) of hemoglobin

Glucose tolerance, oral
Peak at 160 to 180 mg/dl (SI, 8.8 to 9.9 mmol/L) 30
to 60 minutes after challenge dose
Growth hormone suppression
Undetectable to 3 ng/ml (SI, undetectable to 3 µg/L)
after 30 minutes to 2 hours

H

Ham test
Negative
Haptoglobin, serum
40 to 180 mg/dl (SI, 0.4 to 1.8 g/L)
Heinz bodies
Negative
Hematocrit
Males
– 42% to 52% (SI, 0.42 to 0.52)
Females
– 36% to 48% (SI, 0.36 to 0.48)
Children
– *10 years:* 36% to 40% (SI, 0.36 to 0.40)
Infants
– *3 months:* 30% to 36% (SI, 0.30 to 0.36)
– *1 year:* 29% to 41% (SI, 0.29 to 0.41)
Neonates
– *At birth:* 55% to 68% (SI, 0.55 to 0.68)
– *1 week:* 47% to 65% (SI, 0.47 to 0.65)
– *1 month:* 37% to 49% (SI, 0.37 to 0.49)
Hemoglobin (Hb) electrophoresis
Hb A: 95% (SI, 0.95)
Hb A$_2$: 1.5% to 3% (SI, 0.015 to 0.03)
Hb F: < 2% (SI, < 0.02)
Hemoglobin, unstable
Heat stability: negative
Isopropanol: stable
Hemoglobin, urine
Negative
Hemosiderin, urine
Negative
Hepatitis B surface antigen, serum
Negative
Herpes simplex antibodies, serum
Negative
Heterophil agglutination, serum
Normal titer < 1:56
Hexosaminidase A and B, serum
Total: 5 to 12.9 U/L (hexosaminidase A constitutes
55% to 76% of total)
Histoplasmosis antibody, serum
Normal titer < 1:8
Homovanillic acid, urine
< 10 mg/24 hours (SI, < 55 µmol/d)

Human chorionic gonadotropin, serum
  < 4 IU/L
Human chorionic gonadotropin, urine
  Pregnant women
    – *First trimester:* 500,000 IU/24 hours
    – *Second trimester:* 10,000 to 25,000 IU/24 hours
    – *Third trimester:* 5,000 to 15,000 IU/24 hours
Human growth hormone, serum
  Males: undetectable to 5 ng/ml (SI, undetectable to
    5 µg/L)
  Females: undetectable to 10 ng/ml (SI, undetectable to
    10 µg/L)
  Children: undetectable to 16 ng/ml (SI, undetectable
    to 16 µg/L)
Human immunodeficiency virus antibody, serum
  Negative
Human placental lactogen, serum
  Males and nonpregnant females: < 0.5 µg/ml
  Pregnant females at term: 9 to 11 µg/ml
17-hydroxycorticosteroids, urine
  Males
    – 4.5 to 12 mg/24 hours (SI, 12.4 to 33.1 µmol/d)
  Females
    – 2.5 to 10 mg/24 hours (SI, 6.9 to 27.6 µmol/d)
  Children
    – *8 to 12 years:* < 4.5 mg/24 hours (SI, < 12.4 µmol/d)
    – *<8 years:* < 1.5 mg/24 hours (SI, < 4.14 µmol/d)
5-hydroxyindoleacetic acid, urine
  2 to 7 mg/24 hours (SI, 10.4 to 36.6 µmol/d)
Hydroxyproline, total, urine
  1 to 9 mg/24 hours (SI, 1.0 to 3.4 IU/d)

IJ

Immune complex, serum
  Negative
Immunoglobulins (Ig), serum
  IgG: 800 to 1,800 mg/dl (SI, 8 to 18 g/L)
  IgA: 100 to 400 mg/dl (SI, 1 to 4 g/L)
  IgM: 55 to 150 mg/dl (SI, 0.55 to 1.5 g/L)
Insulin, serum
  0 to 35 µU/ml (SI, 144 to 243 pmol/L)
Insulin tolerance test
  10- to 20-ng/dl (SI, 10- to 20-µg/L) increase over
    baseline levels of human growth hormone and
    adrenocorticotropic hormone
Iron, serum
  Males: 60 to 170 µg/dl (SI, 10.7 to 30.4 µmol/L)
  Females: 50 to 130 µg/dl (SI, 9 to 23.3 µmol/L)
Iron, total binding capacity, serum
  300 to 360 µg/dl (SI, 54 to 64 µmol/L)

K

17-ketogenic steroids, urine
  Males: 4 to 14 mg/24 hours (SI, 13 to 49 µmol/d)
  Females: 2 to 12 mg/24 hours (SI, 7 to 42 µmol/d)
  Infants to 11 years: 0.1 to 4 mg/24 hours (SI, 0.3 to
    14 µmol/d)
  11 to 14 years: 2 to 9 mg/24 hours (SI, 7 to 31 µmol/d)
Ketones, urine
  Negative
17-ketosteroids, urine
  Males: 10 to 25 mg/24 hours (SI, 35 to 87 µmol/d)
  Females: 4 to 6 mg/24 hours (SI, 4 to 21 µmol/d)
  Infants to 10 years: < 3 mg/24 hours (SI, < 10 µmol/d)
  10 to 14 years: 1 to 6 mg/24 hours (SI, 2 to 21 µmol/d)

L

Lactate dehydrogenase (LD)
  Total: 71 to 207 IU/L (SI, 1.2 to 3.52 µkat/L)
  LD_1: 14% to 26% (SI, 0.14 to 0.26)
  LD_2: 29% to 39% (SI, 0.29 to 0.39)
  LD_3: 20% to 26% (SI, 0.20 to 0.26)
  LD_4: 8% to 16% (SI, 0.08 to 0.16)
  LD_5: 6% to 16% (SI, 0.06 to 0.16)
Lactic acid, blood
  0.93 to 1.65 mEq/L (SI, 0.93 to 1.65 mmol/L)
Leucine aminopeptidase
  Males: 80 to 200 U/ml (SI, 80 to 200 kU/L)
  Females: 75 to 185 U/ml (SI, 75 to 185 kU/L)
Leukoagglutinins
  Negative
Lipase, serum
  < 160 U/L (SI, < 2.72 µkat)
Lipids, fecal
  Constitute < 20% of excreted solids; < 7 g excreted in
    24 hours
Lipoproteins, serum
  High-density lipoprotein cholesterol
    – *Males:* 37 to 70 mg/dl (SI, 0.96 to 1.8 mmol/L)
    – *Females:* 40 to 85 mg/dl (SI, 1.03 to 2.2 mmol/L)
  Low-density lipoprotein cholesterol:
    – *In individuals who don't have coronary artery disease:*
      < 130 mg/dl (SI, < 3.36 mmol/L)
Long-acting thyroid stimulator, serum
  Negative
Lupus erythematosus cell preparation
  Negative

Luteinizing hormone, serum
  Menstruating women
  – *Follicular phase:* 5 to 15 mIU/ml (SI, 5 to 15 IU/L)
  – *Ovulatory phase:* 30 to 60 mIU/ml (SI, 30 to 60 IU/L)
  – *Luteal phase:* 5 to 15 mIU/ml (SI, 5 to 15 IU/L)
  Postmenopausal women
  – 50 to 100 mIU/ml (SI, 50 to 100 IU/L)
  Males
  – 5 to 20 mIU/ml (SI, 5 to 20 IU/L)
  Children
  – 4 to 20 mIU/ml (SI, 4 to 20 IU/L)
Lyme disease serology
  Nonreactive
Lysozyme, urine
  0 to 3 mg/24 hours

M

Magnesium, serum
  1.3 to 2.1 mg/dl (SI, 0.65 to 1.05 mmol/L)
Magnesium, urine
  6 to 10 mEq/24 hours (SI, 3.0 to 5.0 mmol/d)
Manganese, serum
  0.4 to 1.4 µg/ml
Melanin, urine
  Negative
Myoglobin, urine
  Negative

N

5′-nucleotidase
  2 to 17 U/L (SI, 0.034 to 0.29 µkat/L)

O

Occult blood, fecal
  < 2.5 ml
Oxalate, urine
  ≤ 40 mg/24 hours (SI, ≤ 456 µmol/d)

PQ

Parathyroid hormone, serum
  Intact: 10 to 50 pg/ml (SI, 1.1 to 5.3 pmol/L)
  N-terminal fraction: 8 to 24 pg/ml (SI, 0.8 to 2.5 pmol/L)
  C-terminal fraction: 0 to 340 pg/ml (SI, 0 to 35.8 pmol/L)
Partial thromboplastin time
  21 to 35 seconds (SI, 21 to 35 s)

Pericardial fluid
  Amount: 10 to 50 ml
  Appearance: clear, straw-colored
  White blood cell count: < 1,000/µl (SI, < 1.0 x 10⁹/L)
  Glucose: approximately whole blood level
Peritoneal fluid
  Amount: < 50 ml
  Appearance: clear, straw-colored
Phenylalanine, serum
  < 2 mg/dl (SI, < 121 µmol/L)
Phosphates, serum
  Adults: 2.7 to 4.5 mEq/L (SI, 0.87 to 1.45 mmol/L)
  Children: 4.5 to 6.7 mEq/L (SI, 1.45 to 1.78 mmol/L)
Phosphates, urine
  < 1,000 mg/24 hours
Phospholipids, plasma
  180 to 320 mg/dl (SI, 1.80 to 3.20 g/L)
Plasma renin activity
  Normal sodium diet: 1.1 to 4.1 ng/ml/hour (SI, 0.30 to 1.14 ng LS)
  Restricted sodium diet: 6.2 to 12.4 ng/ml/hour (SI, 1.72 to 3.44 ng LS)
Phosphate, tubular reabsorption, urine and plasma
  80% reabsorption
Plasminogen, plasma
  Immunologic method: 10 to 20 mg/dl (SI, 0.10 to 0.20 g/L)
Platelet aggregation
  3 to 5 minutes (SI, 3 to 5 m)
Platelet count
  Adults: 140,000 to 400,000/µl (SI, 140 to 400 × 10⁹/L)
  Children: 150,000 to 450,000/µl (SI, 150 to 450 × 10⁹/L)
Potassium, serum
  3.5 to 5 mEq/L (SI, 3.5 to 5 mmol/L)
Potassium, urine
  Adults: 25 to 125 mmol/24 hours (SI, 25 to 125 mmol/d)
  Children: 22 to 57 mmol/24 hours (SI, 22 to 57 mmol/d)
Pregnanediol, urine
  Nonpregnant females
  – 0.5 to 1.5 mg/24 hours (during the follicular phase of the menstrual cycle)
  Pregnant females
  – *First trimester:* 10 to 30 mg/24 hours
  – *Second trimester:* 35 to 70 mg/24 hours
  – *Third trimester:* 70 to 100 mg/24 hours
  Postmenopausal females
  – 0.2 to 1 mg/24 hours
  Males
  – 0 to 1mg/24 hours

Pregnanetriol, urine
Males ≥ 16 years: 0.4 to 2.5 mg/24 hours (SI, 1.2 to 7.5 µmol/d)
Females ≥ 16 years: 0 to 1.8 mg/ hours (SI, 0.3 to 5.3 µmol/d)

Progesterone, plasma
Menstruating females
– *Follicular phase:* < 150 ng/dl (SI, < 5 nmol/L)
– *Luteal phase:* 300 to 1,200 ng/dl (SI, 10 to 40 nmol/L)
Pregnant women
– *First trimester:* 1,500 to 5,000 ng/dl (SI, 50 to 160 nmol/L)
– *Second and third trimesters:* 8,000 to 20,000 ng/dl (SI, 250 to 650 nmol/L)

Prolactin, serum
Undetectable to 23 ng/ml (SI, undetectable to 23 µg/L)

Prostate-specific antigen
40 to 50 years: 2 to 2.8 mg/ml (SI, 2 to 2.8 µg/L)
51 to 60 years: 2.9 to 3.8 mg/ml (SI, 2.9 to 3.8 µg/L)
61 to 70 years: 4 to 5.3 mg/ml (SI, 4 to 5.3 µg/L)
≥ 71 years: 5.6 to 7.2 mg/ml (SI, 5.6 to 7.2 µg/L)

Protein, cerebrospinal fluid
15 to 50 mg/dl (SI, 0.15 to 0.5 g/L)

Protein C, plasma
70% to 140% (SI, 0.70 to 1.40)

Protein, total, peritoneal fluid
0.3 to 4.1 g/dl (SI, 3 to 41 g/L)

Protein, urine
50 to 80 mg/24 hours (SI, 50 to 80 mg/d)

Prothrombin time
10 to 14 seconds (10 to 14 s)

Pulmonary artery pressures
Right atrial: 1 to 6 mm Hg
Left atrial: approximately 10 mm Hg
Systolic: 20 to 30 mm Hg
Systolic right ventricular: 20 to 30 mm Hg
Diastolic: 10 to 15 mm Hg
End-diastolic right ventricular: < 5 mm Hg
Mean: < 20 mm Hg
Pulmonary artery wedge pressure: 6 to 12 mm Hg

Pyruvate kinase
Ultraviolet: 9 to 22 U/g of hemoglobin
Low substrate assay: 1.7 to 6.8 U/g of hemoglobin

Pyruvic acid, blood
0.08 to 0.16 mEq/L (SI, 0.08 to 0.16 mmol/L)

R

Red blood cell count
Males: 4.5 to 5.5 million/µl (SI, 4.5 to 5.5 × 10^{12}/L)
Females: 4 to 5 million/µl (SI, 4 to 5 × 10^{12}/L)

Neonates: 4.4 to 5.8 million/µl (SI, 4.4 to 5.8 × 10^{12}/L)
2 months: 3 to 3.8 million/µl (SI, 3 to 3.8 × 10^{12}/L) (increasing slowly)
Children: 4.6 to 4.8 million/µl (SI, 4.6 to 4.8 × 10^{12}/L)

Red blood cell survival time
25 to 35 days

Red blood cells, urine
0 to 3 per high-power field

Red cell indices
Mean corpuscular volume: 84 to 99 µm^3
Mean corpuscular hemoglobin: 26 to 32 pg/cell
Mean corpuscular hemoglobin concentration: 30 to 36 g/dl

Respiratory syncytial virus antibodies, serum
Negative

Reticulocyte count
Adults: 0.5% to 2.5% (SI, 0.005 to 0.025)
Infants (at birth): 2% to 6% (SI, 0.02 to 0.06), decreasing to adult levels in 1 to 2 weeks

Rheumatoid factor, serum
Negative or titer < 1:20

Ribonucleoprotein antibodies
Negative

Rubella antibodies, serum
Titer of 1:8 or less indicates little or no immunity; titer more than 1:10 indicates adequate protection against rubella

S

Semen analysis
Volume: 0.7 to 6.5 ml
pH: 7.3 to 7.9
Liquefaction: within 20 minutes
Sperm count: 20 to 150 million/ml

Sickle cell test
Negative

Sjögren's antibodies
Negative

Sodium chloride, urine
110 to 250 mEq/L (SI, 100 to 250 mmol/d)

Sodium, serum
135 to 145 mEq/L (SI, 135 to 145 mmol/L)

Sodium, urine
Adults: 40 to 220 mEq/L/24 hours (SI, 40 to 220 mmol/d)
Children: 41 to 115 mEq/L/24 hours (SI, 41 to 115 mmol/d)

Sporotrichosis antibody, serum
Normal titers < 1:40

T

Terminal deoxynucleotidyl transferase, serum
Bone marrow: < 2%
Blood: undetectable
Testosterone, plasma or serum
Males: 300 to 1,200 ng/dl (SI, 10.4 to 41.6 nmol/L)
Females: 20 to 80 ng/dl (SI, 0.7 to 2.8 nmol/L)
Thrombin time, plasma
10 to 15 seconds (10 to 15 s)
Thyroid-stimulating hormone, neonatal
≤2 days: 25 to 30 µIU/ml (SI, 25 to 20 mU/L)
>2 days: < 25 µIU/ml (SI, < 25 mU/L)
Thyroid-stimulating hormone, serum
Undetectable to 15 µIU/ml (SI, undetectable to 15 mU/L)
Thyroid-stimulating immunoglobulin, serum
Negative
Thyroxine-binding globulin, serum
Immunoassay: 16 to 32 µg/dl (SI, 120 to 180 mg/ml)
Thyroxine, total, serum
5 to 13.5 µg/dl (SI, 60 to 165 mmol/L)
T-lymphocyte count
1,500 to 3,000/µl
Transferrin, serum
200 to 400 mg/dl (SI, 2 to 4 g/L)
Triglycerides, serum
Males: 44 to 180 mg/dl (SI, 0.44 to 2.01 mmol/L)
Females: 11 to 190 mg/dl (SI, 0.11 to 2.21 mmol/L)
Triiodothyronine, serum
80 to 200 ng/dl (SI, 1.2 to 3 nmol/L)

U

Uric acid, serum
Males: 3.4 to 7 mg/dl (SI, 202 to 42 µmol/L)
Females: 2.3 to 6 mg/dl (SI, 143 to 357 µmol/L)
Uric acid, urine
250 to 750 mg/24 hours (SI, 1.48 to 4.43 mmol/d)
Urinalysis, routine
Color: straw to dark yellow
Appearance: clear
Specific gravity: 1.005 to 1.035
pH: 4.5 to 8.0
Epithelial cells: 0 to 5 per high-power field
Casts: none, except 1 to 2 hyaline casts per low-power field
Crystals: present
Urine osmolality
24-hour urine: 300 to 900 mOsm/kg
Random urine: 50 to 1,400 mOsm/kg
Urobilinogen, fecal
50 to 300 mg/24 hours (SI, 100 to 400 EU/100 g)

Urobilinogen, urine
0.1 to 0.8 EU/2 hours (SI 0.1 to 0.8 EU/2 h)
or
0.5 to 4.0 EU/24 hours (SI, 0.5 to 4.0 EU/d)
Uroporphyrinogen I synthase
≥ 7 nmol/second/L

V

Vanillylmandelic acid, urine
1.4 to 6.5 mg/24 hours (SI, 7 to 33 µmol/day)
Venereal Disease Research Laboratory test, cerebrospinal fluid
Negative
Venereal Disease Research Laboratory test, serum
Negative
Vitamin A, serum
30 to 80 µg/dl (SI, 1.05 to 2.8 µmol/L)
Vitamin B$_2$, serum
3 to 15 µg/dl
Vitamin B$_{12}$, serum
200 to 900 pg/ml (SI, 148 to 664 pmol/L)
Vitamin C, plasma
0.2 to 2 mg/dl (SI, 11 to 114 µmol/L)
Vitamin C, urine
30 mg/24 hours
Vitamin D$_3$, serum
10 to 60 ng/ml (SI, 25 to 150 nmol/L)

WXY

White blood cell count, blood
4,000 to 10,000/µl (SI, 4 to 10 × 10^9/L)
White blood cell count, peritoneal fluid
< 300/µl (SI, < 300 × 10^9/L)
White blood cell count, urine
0 to 4 per high-power field
White blood cell differential, blood
Adults
– *Neutrophils:* 54% to 75% (SI, 0.54 to 0.75)
– *Lymphocytes:* 25% to 40% (SI, 0.25 to 0.40)
– *Monocytes:* 2% to 8% (SI, 0.02 to 0.08)
– *Eosinophils:* 1% to 4% (SI, 0.01 to 0.04)
– *Basophils:* 0 to 1% (SI, 0 to 0.01)

Z

Zinc, serum
70 to 120 µg/dl (SI, 10.7 to 18.4 µmol/L)

Selected references

2002 Test Catalog. Rochester, Minn.: Mayo Medical Laboratories, 2002.

Ahya, S.N., ed. *The Washington Manual of Medical Therapeutics,* 30th ed. Philadelphia: Lippincott Williams & Wilkins, 2001.

Beers, M.H., and Berkow, R., eds. *The Merck Manual,* 17th edition. Merck and Co., 1999.

Black, E., et al. *Diagnostic Strategies for Common Medical Problems.* Philadelphia: American College of Physicians, 1999.

Clinical Laboratory Tests: Values and Implications, 3rd ed. Springhouse, Pa.: Springhouse Corp., 2001.

Desai, S.P., and Isa-Pratt, S. *Clinician's Guide to Laboratory Medicine,* 2nd ed. Hudson, Ohio: Lexi-Comp, Inc., 2002.

Diagnostics: An A-to-Z Nursing Guide to Laboratory Tests & Diagnostic Procedures. Springhouse, Pa.: Springhouse Corp., 2001.

Fischbach, F. *A Manual of Laboratory and Diagnostic Tests,* 6th edition. Philadelphia: Lippincott Williams & Wilkins, 2000.

Fischbach, F. *Nurses Quick Reference To Common Laboratory and Diagnostic Tests,* 3rd ed. Philadelphia: Lippincott Williams & Wilkins, 2002.

Handbook of Diagnostic Tests, 3rd ed. Philadelphia: Lippincott Williams & Wilkins, 2003.

Kee, J.L. *Handbook of Laboratory and Diagnostic Tests with Nursing Implications,* 4th ed. Upper Saddle River, N.J.: Prentice Hall Health, 2001.

Pagana K.D., and Pagana, T.J. *Mosby's Manual of Diagnostic and Laboratory Tests,* 2nd ed. St. Louis: Mosby–Year Book, Inc., 2002.

Tierney, L., et al. *Current Medical Diagnosis and Treatment 2003.* New York: McGraw-Hill Book Co., 2002.

Wallach, J. B. *Interpretation of Diagnostic Tests,* 7th ed. Philadelphia: Lippincott Williams & Wilkins, 2000.

Index

A

AAT. *See* Alpha$_1$-antitrypsin.

Abdominal aortic aneurysm
  key diagnostic findings in, 482
  ultrasonography in, 382

Abdominal aortic disease, radionuclide renal imaging in, 324

Abdominal injuries, blunt and penetrating, key diagnostic findings in, 492

Abdominal trauma, peritoneal fluid analysis in, 278

Abetalipoproteinemia
  serum triglyceride levels in, 375
  small-bowel biopsy in, 344

ABG analysis. *See* Arterial blood gas analysis.

ABO blood types, 27t

ABO blood typing, 26-27

Abortion, threatened
  plasma progesterone levels in, 298
  urine human chorionic gonadotropin levels in, 201
  urine pregnanediol levels in, 294

Abruptio placentae
  amniocentesis in, 42
  key diagnostic findings in, 483
  ultrasonography in, 387

Absorptive disorders, fecal lipids in, 223, 224

Accelerated idioventricular rhythm, 458
  electrocardiogram characteristics of, 458i

Acceleration-deceleration cervical injuries, key diagnostic findings in, 483

ACE. *See* Angiotensin-converting enzyme.

Acetest tablet. *See* Ketone.

Acetylcholine receptor antibodies, 27-28

Achalasia, upper gastrointestinal and small-bowel series in, 391

Achlorhydria
  gastric acid stimulation test in, 169
  gastrin levels in, 170

Acid-base disorders
  arterial blood gas analysis in, 57
  chloride levels in, 100

Acidoses
  anion gap in, 50
  carbon dioxide levels in, 81
  pulmonary function tests in, 309t
  urinalysis in, 395, 397

Acid perfusion, 28-29

Acquired immunodeficiency syndrome, key diagnostic findings in, 483

Acromegaly
  fasting plasma glucose in, 171
  luteinizing hormone levels in, 238
  serum creatinine levels in, 123
  serum follicle-stimulating hormone levels in, 163
  serum human growth hormone levels in, 180
  serum phosphate levels in, 281-282

Acromegaly *(continued)*
  skull radiography in, 343
  2-hour postprandial plasma glucose in, 175

Actinomycosis, key diagnostic findings in, 483

Activated clotting time, 29-30

Acute poststreptococcal glomerulonephritis
  complement assays in, 111
  cryoglobulin level in, 124t
  key diagnostic findings in, 483-484

Acute respiratory failure in chronic obstructive pulmonary disease, key diagnostic findings in, 484

Acute transverse myelitis, key diagnostic findings in, 529

Acute tubular necrosis
  creatinine clearance in, 122
  key diagnostic findings in, 484
  radionuclide renal imaging in, 324
  urea clearance in, 393
  urinalysis in, 395

Addison's disease
  blood cell count in, 415t
  chloride levels in, 100
  corticotropin levels in, 31
  human leukocyte antigen testing in, 203
  oral glucose tolerance test in, 173
  plasma cortisol levels in, 118
  plasma renin activity in, 328
  rapid corticotropin in, 116
  serum aldosterone levels in, 33

i refers to an illustration; t refers to a table.

Addison's disease *(continued)*
  serum magnesium levels in, 247
  serum potassium levels in, 292
  urine aldosterone levels in, 34
Adenoid hyperplasia, key diagnostic findings in, 484
Adenomas, thyroid imaging in, 316t
Adenomyoma, oral cholecystography in, 102
ADH. *See* Antidiuretic hormone.
Adrenal disorders, glucose urinalysis in, 177
Adrenal hormone production, sites of, 33i
Adrenal hyperfunction, corticotropin levels in, 31
Adrenal hyperplasia
  corticotropin levels in, 31
  urine pregnanediol levels in, 295
Adrenal hypofunction. *See also* Addison's disease.
  corticotropin levels in, 31
  key diagnostic findings in, 484-485
  plasma cortisol levels in, 118
  rapid corticotropin in, 116
Adrenal insufficiency
  fasting plasma glucose in, 171
  insulin tolerance in, 211
  serum sodium levels in, 347
  serum calcium levels in, 79
  test selection guide for, 419i
  2-hour postprandial plasma glucose in, 175
Adrenal tumors
  kidney-ureter-bladder radiography in, 216
  renal computed tomography scan in, 322-323
  testosterone levels in, 362
Adrenocortical hyperplasias, plasma progesterone levels in, 297-298
Adrenocortical hypofunction, blood cell count in, 415t
Adrenocortical tumor, androstenedione in, 48
Adrenocorticotropic hormone, 30-31, 114-115

Adrenogenital syndrome, key diagnostic findings in, 485
Adrenoleukodystrophy, visual evoked potentials in, 148
AFP. *See* Alpha-fetoprotein.
Agammaglobulinemia, serum immunoglobulin levels in, 208t
Agranulocytosis, bone marrow biopsy in, 74t
Alanine aminotransferase, 31-32
Albinism, key diagnostic findings in, 485
Alcohol intoxication, myoglobin levels in, 258
Alcoholism
  D-xylose absorption in, 134
  folic acid level in, 162
  key diagnostic findings in, 485
  serum magnesium levels in, 248
  serum triglyceride levels in, 375
Alcohol withdrawal syndrome, aspartate aminotransferase levels in, 59
Aldosterone
  serum, 32-34
  urine, 34-35
Aldosteronism, 33
  carbon dioxide levels in, 81
  chloride levels in, 100
  plasma renin activity in, 328
  serum aldosterone levels in, 33
  serum magnesium levels in, 248
  serum potassium levels in, 292
  serum sodium levels in, 347
  urine aldosterone levels in, 34
  urine potassium levels in, 293
Alkaline phosphatase, 35-36
Alkaptonuria, urinalysis in, 395, 397
Allergic angiitis, key diagnostic findings in, 561
Allergic rhinitis, key diagnostic findings in, 485

Alpha$_1$-antitrypsin, 36-37
Alpha-fetoprotein, 37-38
  presence of, in amniotic fluid, 44
Alpha$_1$-globulin deficiency, alpha$_1$-antitrypsin in, 37
Alport's syndrome, key diagnostic findings in, 485
ALP. *See* Alkaline phosphatase.
ALT. *See* Alanine aminotransferase.
Alzheimer's disease, key diagnostic findings in, 485
Amblyopia, visual evoked potentials in, 148
Ambulatory electrocardiography, 197-198. *See also* Electrocardiogram.
Amebiasis
  blood cell count in, 415t
  key diagnostic findings in, 486
  sputum, 38
  stool, 39
Amenorrhea
  luteinizing hormone levels in, 238
  plasma progesterone levels in, 298
  prolactin levels in, 298-299
  test selection guide for, 420i
  urine pregnanediol levels in, 295
Ammonia, plasma, 40-41
Amniocentesis, 41-46, 44t
Amniotic fluid analysis. *See* Amniocentesis.
Amputation, traumatic, key diagnostic findings in, 486
Amylase, serum, 46-47
Amyloidosis
  key diagnostic findings in, 486
  kidney-ureter-bladder radiography in, 216
  synovial membrane biopsy in, 358
  urinalysis in, 397
  urine protein levels in, 304
Amyotrophic lateral sclerosis
  electromyography in, 138
  key diagnostic findings in, 486
Anabolic steroid use, antithrombin III in, 56

i refers to an illustration; t refers to a table.

i refers to an illustration; t refers to a table.

Aspergillosis *(continued)*
key diagnostic findings in, 489
Asphyxia, key diagnostic findings in, 489
Asthma
blood cell count in, 415t
chest X-ray in, 97t
key diagnostic findings in, 489
AST. *See* Aspartate aminotransferase.
Asystole, key diagnostic findings in, 489
Ataxia-telangiectasia
alpha-fetoprotein levels in, 38
delayed hypersensitivity skin tests in, 205
key diagnostic findings in, 489
serum immunoglobulin levels in, 208t
Atelectasis
chest X-ray in, 96t, 97t
key diagnostic findings in, 489
Atherosclerosis
chest X-ray in, 96t
total homocysteine levels in, 199
AT III. *See* Antithrombin III.
Atopic dermatitis, key diagnostic findings in, 489-490
Atresia, amniocentesis in, 45
Atrial fibrillation, 451
electrocardiogram characteristics of, 451i
key diagnostic findings in, 490
Atrial flutter, 450
electrocardiogram characteristics of, 450i
key diagnostic findings in, 490
Atrial natriuretic factor, plasma, 60
Atrial natriuretic hormone, 60
Atrial septal defect, key diagnostic findings in, 490
Atrial tachycardia, key diagnostic findings in, 490-491
Atrionatriuretic peptide, 60
Atriopeptin, 60
Australia antigen, 190-191

Autoimmune disorders
antinuclear antibodies in, 54, 54t
autoantibodies in, 236-237t
immune complex assays in, 206-207
Raji cell assay in, 317
Automated coagulation time, 29-30

B

Bacteremia, blood culture in, 68
Bacterial infection, cerebrospinal fluid analysis in, 93t
Bacterial meningitis antigen, 61
Barium enema, 61-63
Barium swallow, 63-65
Bartter's syndrome, plasma renin activity in, 328
Basal cell carcinoma
key diagnostic findings in, 491
skin biopsy in, 342
Basophils, influence of disease on, 415t. *See also* White blood cell differential.
Bayes' formula, application of, to predictive values, 10i
B-cell deficiency, key diagnostic findings in, 491
Bee sting, key diagnostic findings in, 519
Bell's palsy, key diagnostic findings in, 491
Benign prostatic hyperplasia
key diagnostic findings in, 491
prostate-specific antigen levels in, 301
Benzene poisoning
protein levels in, 303i
urine porphyrin levels in, 291
Bernard-Soulier syndrome
platelet aggregation in, 285
platelet count in, 286
Bernstein test, 28-29
Berylliosis, key diagnostic findings in, 492
Bile duct cancer, key diagnostic findings in, 507

Biliary obstruction
alkaline phosphatase levels in, 35-36
aspartate aminotransferase levels in, 59
cholesterol levels in, 103
fecal lipids in, 223, 224
5'-nucleotidase levels in, 263
hepatic iminodiacetic scan in, 193
leucine aminopeptidase levels in, 222
oral cholecystography in, 102
serum amylase levels in, 46
serum bilirubin levels in, 66
serum triglyceride levels in, 375
ultrasonography in, 383
urinalysis in, 397
urine pregnanediol levels in, 295
Biliary tumors, alpha-fetoprotein levels in, 38
Bilirubin
presence of, in amniotic fluid, 43
serum, 65-66
urine, 66-68
Black widow spider bite, key diagnostic findings in, 520
Bladder abnormalities, excretory urography in, 149
Bladder cancer, key diagnostic findings in, 492
Bladder infection, urinalysis in, 397
Blastomycosis
fungal serology in, 164t
key diagnostic findings in, 492
Bleeding disorders, platelet count in, 286
Blepharitis, key diagnostic findings in, 492
Blood, presence of, in amniotic fluid, 42, 45
Blood compatibility
ABO blood typing for, 26-27
antibody screening for, 51
Blood culture, 68-69
Blood dyscrasias
protein levels in, 303i
urinalysis in, 397-398

i refers to an illustration; t refers to a table.

i refers to an illustration; t refers to a table.

i refers to an illustration; t refers to a table.

i refers to an illustration; t refers to a table.

i refers to an illustration; t refers to a table.

i refers to an illustration; t refers to a table.

i refers to an illustration; t refers to a table.

i refers to an illustration; t refers to a table.

i refers to an illustration; t refers to a table.

Gas gangrene, key diagnostic findings in, 507
Gastrectomy
  fasting plasma glucose in, 171
  2-hour postprandial plasma glucose in, 175
Gastric acid stimulation, 168-169
Gastric carcinoma, key diagnostic findings in, 507. *See also* Gastrointestinal cancer.
Gastric resection, vitamin D_3 levels in, 409
Gastrin, 169-170
Gastritis
  esophagogastroduodenoscopy in, 143
  key diagnostic findings in, 508
Gastroenteritis
  barium enema in, 63
  key diagnostic findings in, 508
  small-bowel biopsy in, 345
Gastroesophageal reflux disease
  key diagnostic findings in, 508
  upper gastrointestinal and small-bowel series in, 391
Gastroesophageal reflux scanning, 64
Gastrointestinal bleeding
  causes of, 152i
  common sites of, 152i
  fecal occult blood in, 153
Gastrointestinal cancer
  alpha-fetoprotein levels in, 38
  CA 19-9 in, 380
  CA-125 in, 380
  CA-50 in, 380
  fecal occult blood in, 153
  gallium scan in, 167
  gastric acid stimulation test in, 169
  gastrin levels in, 170
  plasma fibrinogen levels in, 159
  serum human chorionic gonadotropin levels in, 200
  upper gastrointestinal and small-bowel series in, 391-392

Gastrointestinal cancer *(continued)*
  urine human chorionic gonadotropin levels in, 201
Gastrointestinal disorders
  protein levels in, 303i
  stool examination for ova and parasites in, 350-351
Gastrointestinal hemorrhage, plasma ammonia levels in, 41
Gastrointestinal motility study, 65
Gastrointestinal tract
  endoscopic biopsy of, 345
  pathogens of, 351
Gated cardiac blood pool imaging, 82
Gaucher's disease
  angiotensin-converting enzyme levels in, 49
  key diagnostic findings in, 508
Genital herpes
  fluorescent treponemal antibody absorption test in, 161
  key diagnostic findings in, 508
Genital warts, key diagnostic findings in, 508
Genitourinary infections
  nonspecific, key diagnostic findings in, 531
  urinalysis in, 398
German measles, rubella antibodies in, 333. *See also* Rubella.
Germ cell tumors, alpha-fetoprotein levels in, 38
GGT. *See* Gamma-glutamyl transferase.
Giardiasis
  amebiasis, stool, in, 39
  key diagnostic findings in, 508
  small-bowel biopsy in, 344-345
Gigantism
  serum creatinine levels in, 123
  serum human growth hormone levels in, 180
Gilbert's disease, serum bilirubin levels in, 66

Glanzmann's thrombasthenia, platelet aggregation in, 285
Glaucoma, key diagnostic findings in, 508-509
Glomerulonephritis
  creatinine clearance in, 122
  glucose urinalysis in, 177
  immune complex assays in, 207
  key diagnostic findings in, 497
  kidney-ureter-bladder radiography in, 216
  plasma fibrinogen levels in, 159
  renal ultrasonography in, 325
  urea clearance in, 393
  urinalysis in, 395, 397, 398
  urine hemoglobin in, 186
  urine protein levels in, 304
  urine uric acid levels in, 394
Glomerulosclerosis, urinalysis in, 397
Glucose, fasting plasma, 170-171
Glucose, 2-hour postprandial plasma, 174-176
  age as factor in levels of, 176i
  as preferred screening test for diabetes, 175
Glucose in amniotic fluid, 45
Glucose oxidase test, interpreting results of, 177i
Glucose-6-phosphate dehydrogenase, 171-172
Glucose-6-phosphate dehydrogenase deficiency, glucose-6-phosphate dehydrogenase in, 172
Glucose tolerance, oral, 172-174
  interpreting results of, 174t
Glucose urinalysis, 176-178
Glycogen storage diseases, key diagnostic findings in, 509
Glycosylated hemoglobin, 178
Goiter
  key diagnostic findings in, 510
  radioactive iodine uptake in, 315
  thyroid biopsy in, 367
  thyroid imaging in, 316t

i refers to an illustration; t refers to a table.

i refers to an illustration; t refers to a table.

i refers to an illustration; t refers to a table.

i refers to an illustration; t refers to a table.

HSV. *See* Herpes simplex virus antibodies, Herpes simplex infections, *and* Herpes simplex virus.
Human chorionic gonadotropin
production of, during pregnancy, 200i
serum, 199-200
urine, 200-201
Human chorionic gonadotropin deficiency, insulin tolerance in, 211
Human immunodeficiency virus antibodies, 201-202
Human immunodeficiency virus infection
blood cell count in, 416t
human immunodeficiency virus antibodies in, 202
transmission of, 201-202
Human leukocyte antigen, 202-203
Huntington's disease
key diagnostic findings in, 513-514
visual evoked potentials in, 148
Hyaline membrane disease, alpha$_1$-antitrypsin levels in, 37
Hydatidiform mole
key diagnostic findings in, 514
serum human chorionic gonadotropin levels in, 200
urine pregnanediol levels in, 295
Hydrocephalus
intracranial computed tomography scan in, 212
key diagnostic findings in, 514
Hydronephrosis
excretory urography in, 149
key diagnostic findings in, 514
kidney-ureter-bladder radiography in, 216
renal ultrasonography in, 325
urinalysis in, 397
Hydrops fetalis, parvovirus B19 antibodies in, 275

Hyperaldosteronism, key diagnostic findings in, 514
Hyperbilirubinemia
fecal/urine urobilinogen levels in, 67t
key diagnostic findings in, 515
serum/urine bilirubin levels in, 67t
Hypercalcemia, test selection guide for, 430-431i
Hypercholesterolemia
cholesterol levels in, 103
vitamin A and carotene levels in, 406-407
Hypercoagulation disorders, antithrombin III levels in, 56
Hyperemesis gravidarum, key diagnostic findings in, 515
Hyperglycemia, cerebrospinal fluid analysis in, 93t
Hyperinsulinemia, serum insulin levels in, 210
Hyperinsulinism
C-peptide assay in, 119
fasting plasma glucose in, 171
2-hour postprandial plasma glucose in, 175
Hyperlipemia, vitamin A and carotene levels in, 406
Hyperlipoproteinemias
fasting plasma glucose in, 171
key diagnostic findings in, 515
lipoprotein phenotyping in, 226-227t
serum triglyceride levels in, 375
2-hour postprandial plasma glucose in, 175
Hypermagnesemia, anion gap in, 50
Hypernatremia, test selection guide for, 432i
Hyperparathyroidism
key diagnostic findings in, 515
parathyroid hormone levels in, 273t
serum calcium levels in, 79
serum magnesium levels in, 248

Hyperparathyroidism *(continued)*
serum phosphate levels in, 281
urine calcium levels in, 78t
urine phosphate levels in, 78t
Hyperpituitarism, key diagnostic findings in, 516
Hypersensitivity skin tests, delayed, 203-205
administering test antigens for, 204i
Hypersensitivity states, blood cell count in, 415t
Hypersensitivity vasculitis, key diagnostic findings in, 562
Hypersplenism, key diagnostic findings in, 516
Hypertension
key diagnostic findings in, 516
plasma renin activity in, 328
protein levels in, 303i
urinalysis in, 395
Hypertensive retinopathy
fluorescein angiography in, 160
key diagnostic findings in, 561
Hyperthyroidism
angiotensin-converting enzyme levels in, 49
blood cell count in, 415t
cholesterol levels and, 103
folic acid level in, 162
free triiodothyronine and free thyroxine levels in, 371
key diagnostic findings in, 516
protein levels in, 303i
radioactive iodine uptake in, 315
testosterone levels in, 362
test selection guide for, 433i
thyroid biopsy in, 367
thyroid imaging in, 316t
thyroxine levels in, 370
thyroid-stimulating hormone levels in, 368
thyroid-stimulating immunoglobulin levels in, 369

i refers to an illustration; t refers to a table.

i refers to an illustration; t refers to a table.

i refers to an illustration; t refers to a table.

i refers to an illustration; t refers to a table.

i refers to an illustration; t refers to a table.

Macular degeneration, age-related, key diagnostic findings in, 485
Magnesium, 247-248
Magnesium imbalance, key diagnostic findings in, 524-525
Magnetic resonance imaging, 248-249. *See also specific type.*
    open units for, 249
Malabsorption syndrome
    D-xylose absorption in, 134
    fasting plasma glucose in, 171
    folic acid levels in, 162
    oral glucose tolerance test in, 173
    protein levels in, 303i
    serum calcium levels in, 79
    serum magnesium levels in, 248
    serum phosphate levels in, 281
    2-hour postprandial plasma glucose in, 175
    upper gastrointestinal and small-bowel series in, 392
    urine potassium levels in, 293
    vitamin B_{12} levels in, 408
Malaria
    blood cell count in, 416t
    cold agglutinins in, 108
    key diagnostic findings in, 525
    mixed lymphocyte culture assay in, 244
    urinalysis in, 397
Male climacteric, serum follicle-stimulating hormone levels in, 163
Malignant hypertension, urinalysis in, 397-398
Malignant hyperthermia, creatine kinase levels in, 120
Mallory-Weiss syndrome
    esophagogastroduodenoscopy in, 143
    key diagnostic findings in, 525
Malnutrition
    alpha$_1$-antitrypsin levels in, 37
    blood urea nitrogen in, 69

Malnutrition *(continued)*
    cholesterol levels and, 103
    protein levels in, 303i
    serum magnesium levels in, 248
    serum phosphate levels in, 281
    serum triglyceride levels in, 375
    small-bowel biopsy in, 345
    triiodothyronine levels in, 376
Mammography, 249-250
Mantoux test, 378-379
Maple syrup urine disease, urinalysis in, 395
Marasmic kwashiorkor. *See* Protein-calorie malnutrition.
Marfan syndrome, key diagnostic findings in, 525
Mastitis, key diagnostic findings in, 525-526
Mastocytosis, blood cell count in, 415t
Mastoiditis, key diagnostic findings in, 526
Maternal abnormalities, ultrasonography in, 387
Maternal urine estriol, 283-284
Mean corpuscular hemoglobin, 319
Mean corpuscular hemoglobin concentration, 319
Mean corpuscular volume, 319
Measles
    blood cell count in, 415t
    delayed hypersensitivity skin tests in, 205
    white blood cell count in, 412
Meconium, presence of, in amniotic fluid, 43
Mediastinitis, chest X-ray in, 96t
Mediastinoscopy, 250, 252
Medullary cystic disease, key diagnostic findings in, 526
Medullary sponge kidney, key diagnostic findings in, 526
Melanoma
    key diagnostic findings in, 525

Melanoma *(continued)*
    skin biopsy in, 342
    urine human chorionic gonadotropin in, 201
Ménière's disease, key diagnostic findings in, 526
Meningitis
    bacterial meningitis antigen in, 61
    cerebrospinal fluid analysis in, 93t
    electroencephalogram in, 136
    key diagnostic findings in, 526
    white blood cell count in, 411-412
Meningococcal infection, key diagnostic findings in, 526
Menopause
    key diagnostic findings in, 526
    luteinizing hormone levels in, 238
    serum follicle-stimulating hormone levels in, 163
Menstrual abnormalities
    androstenedione levels in, 48
    urine pregnanediol levels in, 295
Menstrual cycle, luteinizing hormone secretion peaks at, 239i
Mental distress, blood cell count in, 415t
Metabolic acidosis
    anion gap in, 49, 50
    arterial blood gas analysis in, 58t
    carbon dioxide in, 81
    chloride levels in, 100
    key diagnostic findings in, 527
Metabolic alkalosis
    arterial blood gas analysis in, 58t
    carbon dioxide in, 81
    chloride levels in, 100
    key diagnostic findings in, 527
    urinalysis in, 395
Metabolic disorders, blood cell count in, 415t

i refers to an illustration; t refers to a table.

Metastatic disease
  antidiuretic hormone levels
    in, 52
  aspartate aminotransferase
    levels in, 59
  blood cell count in, 415t
  CA 15-3 (27,29) in, 380
  chest X-ray in, 97t
  gallium scan in, 167
  intracranial computed
    tomography scan in, 212
  liver-spleen scanning in, 230
  lymph node biopsy in, 241
  myelography in, 256
  protein levels in, 303i
  Raji cell assay in, 317
  serum calcium levels in, 79
  serum human growth hor-
    mone levels in, 180
  ultrasonography in, 385
  urine calcium levels in, 78t
  urine phosphate levels in,
    78t
  urine pregnanediol levels in,
    295
MetHb. *See* Methemoglobin.
Methemoglobin, 253
Methemoglobinemia, methe-
    moglobin levels in, 253
Microcytic anemia, test selec-
    tion guide for, 423i. *See
    also* Anemia.
Milk-alkali syndrome
  urine calcium levels in, 78t
  urine phosphate levels in,
    78t
Miscarriage, chromosome
    analysis in, 106t
Mitogen assay, 241-242
Mitral insufficiency, key diag-
    nostic findings in, 527
Mitral stenosis, key diagnostic
    findings in, 527
Mixed lymphocyte culture
    assay, 242
Mobitz I atrioventricular block.
    See Second-degree atri-
    oventricular block, type
    I.
Mobitz II atrioventricular
    block. *See* Second-degree
    atrioventricular block,
    type II.
Monoclonal test for
    cytomegalovirus, rapid,
    194, 253-254

Monocytes, influence of dis-
    ease on, 416t. *See also*
    White blood cell differ-
    ential.
Mononucleosis, infectious
  alanine aminotransferase
    levels in, 32
  aspartate aminotransferase
    levels in, 59
  bone marrow biopsy in, 74t
  cell count in, 415t
  cold agglutinins in, 108
  cryoglobulin level in, 124t
  delayed hypersensitivity skin
    tests in, 205
  Epstein-Barr virus antibodies
    in, 140-141
  haptoglobin levels in, 181
  heterophil antibody tests in,
    196-197
  key diagnostic findings in,
    518
  Monospot test for, 196
  rheumatoid factor titer in,
    330
  white blood cell count in,
    412
Mono-Vacc test, 378-379
Motility disorders, upper
    gastrointestinal and
    small-bowel series in,
    391
Motion sickness, key diagnos-
    tic findings in, 527
MRI. *See* Magnetic resonance
    imaging.
Mucocutaneous lymph node
    syndrome, key diagnos-
    tic findings in, 562
Multiple endocrine neoplasia,
    key diagnostic findings
    in, 528
Multiple-gated acquisition
    scanning, 82-83
Multiple myeloma
  anion gap in, 50
  cold agglutinins in, 108
  complement assays in, 111
  erythrocyte sedimentation
    rate in, 141
  key diagnostic findings in,
    528
  kidney-ureter-bladder radi-
    ography in, 216
  protein levels in, 303i
  serum calcium levels in, 79

Multiple myeloma *(continued)*
  serum immunoglobulin lev-
    els in, 208t
  urinalysis in, 397
  urine calcium levels in, 78t
  urine human chorionic
    gonadotropin levels in,
    201
  urine phosphate levels in,
    78t
  urine uric acid levels in, 394
Multiple pregnancy, amniocen-
    tesis in, 44
Multiple sclerosis
  evoked potentials in, 146i,
    147i, 148
  key diagnostic findings in,
    528
Mumps
  blood cell count in, 415t
  cerebrospinal fluid analysis
    in, 93t
  delayed hypersensitivity skin
    tests in, 205
  key diagnostic findings in,
    528
Muscular dystrophy
  creatine kinase levels in, 120
  electromyography in, 138
  key diagnostic findings in,
    528
  myoglobin levels in, 258
Myasthenia gravis, 27
  acetylcholine receptor anti-
    bodies in, 28
  autoantibodies in, 236t
  electromyography in, 138
  human leukocyte antigen
    testing in, 203
  key diagnostic findings in,
    528-529
  pulmonary function tests in,
    311t
  Tensilon test in, 360
Mycosis fungoides, key diag-
    nostic findings in, 529
Myelitis
  key diagnostic findings in,
    529
  somatosensory evoked
    potentials in, 148
Myelofibrosis, platelet count
    in, 286
Myelography, 254-256
  removing contrast media
    after, 255

i refers to an illustration; t refers to a table.

i refers to an illustration; t refers to a table.

Normocytic anemia, test selection guide for, 424i
5'-NT. See 5'-nucleotidase.
Nuclear medicine scans, 261-262. See also specific nuclear medicine scan.
5'-nucleotidase, 262-263
Nystagmus, key diagnostic findings in, 531

O

Obesity
    free urine cortisol levels in, 117
    key diagnostic findings in, 531-532
    pulmonary function tests in, 309t
Occlusive impedance phlebography, 286-287
Odds ratios, 11
OGTT. See Glucose tolerance, oral.
Old tuberculin test, 378
Omphalocele
    alpha-fetoprotein levels in, 38
    amniocentesis in, 45
One-stage factor assay
    extrinsic coagulation system for, 264-265
    intrinsic coagulation system for, 265-266
Optic atrophy, key diagnostic findings in, 532
Optic neuritis, visual evoked potentials in, 148
Oral infections, key diagnostic findings in, 552
Oral specimens, collecting, 18
Orbital cellulitis, key diagnostic findings in, 532
Orbital computed tomography scan, 266-267
Orbital fracture
    orbital computed tomography scan in, 267
    orbital radiography in, 268
Orbital lesions
    orbital computed tomography scan in, 267
    orbital radiography in, 268
Orbital radiography, 267-269
Ornithosis, key diagnostic findings in, 532

Osgood-Schlatter disease, key diagnostic findings in, 532
Osmolality, urine, 269
Osmotic fragility, 269-270
Osteoarthritis
    key diagnostic findings in, 532
    synovial fluid analysis in, 356-357t
    vertebral radiography in, 305-306
Osteogenesis imperfecta, key diagnostic findings in, 532
Osteomalacia
    urine calcium levels in, 78t
    urine phosphate levels in, 78t
    vitamin D_3 levels in, 409
Osteomyelitis
    blood cell count in, 415t
    key diagnostic findings in, 532
    skull radiography in, 343
Osteoporosis
    bone densitometry and, 69-70
    key diagnostic findings in, 533
    vertebral radiography in, 305-306
Otitis externa, key diagnostic findings in, 533
Otitis media
    blood cell count in, 415t
    key diagnostic findings in, 533
Otosclerosis, key diagnostic findings in, 533
Ovarian agenesis, serum estrogen levels in, 145
Ovarian biopsy, 95t
Ovarian cancer
    androstenedione levels in, 48
    CA 15-3 (27,29) in, 380
    CA-125 in, 380
    carcinoembryonic antigen levels in, 82
    key diagnostic findings in, 533-534
    ovarian biopsy in, 95t
    serum human chorionic gonadotropin levels in, 200

Ovarian cancer (continued)
    urine human chorionic gonadotropin levels in, 201
    urine pregnanediol levels in, 295
Ovarian cysts
    key diagnostic findings in, 534
    plasma progesterone levels in, 297
Ovarian failure
    luteinizing hormone levels in, 238
    serum estrogen levels in, 145
    serum follicle-stimulating hormone levels in, 163
Ovarian tumors, testosterone levels in, 362
Overhydration, blood urea nitrogen in, 69
Ovulation
    blood cell count in, 415t
    plasma progesterone levels in, 297

P

Paget's disease
    alkaline phosphatase levels in, 35-36
    key diagnostic findings in, 534
    serum calcium levels in, 79
    skull radiography in, 343
    urine calcium levels in, 78t
    urine phosphate levels in, 78t
    vertebral radiography in, 305-306
Pancreatectomy, C-peptide assay in, 119
Pancreatic cancer
    alpha-fetoprotein in, 38
    CA 15-3 (27,29) in, 380
    CA 19-9 in, 380
    CA-125 in, 380
    CA-50 in, 380
    key diagnostic findings in, 534
    lipase levels in, 223
    plasma fibrinogen levels in, 159
    serum amylase levels in, 46
    serum human chorionic gonadotropin levels in, 200

i refers to an illustration; t refers to a table.

i refers to an illustration; t refers to a table.

i refers to an illustration; t refers to a table.

i refers to an illustration; t refers to a table.

i refers to an illustration; t refers to a table.

Renal disease *(continued)*
  protein levels in, 303i
  radionuclide renal imaging in, 324
  renal angiography in, 321
  serum calcium levels in, 79
  serum creatinine levels in, 123
  serum sodium levels in, 347
  triiodothyronine levels in, 376
  transferrin levels in, 374
  urinalysis in, 395, 397
  urine protein levels in, 304-305
  vitamin D_3 levels in, 409
Renal failure
  blood cell count in, 415t
  chloride levels in, 100
  creatine kinase levels in, 120
  key diagnostic findings in, 484, 497-498
  myoglobin levels in, 258
  plasma renin activity in, 328
  renal angiography in, 321
  serum calcium levels in, 79
  serum magnesium levels in, 247
  serum phosphate levels in, 281-282
  serum potassium levels in, 292
  urinalysis in, 397
  urine potassium levels in, 293
  urine protein levels in, 304
Renal hypertension, urinalysis in, 397
Renal imaging, radionuclide, 323-324
Renal infarction
  key diagnostic findings in, 545
  urinalysis in, 397-398
Renal insufficiency
  urinalysis in, 397
  urine calcium levels in, 78t
  urine phosphate levels in, 78t
Renal tuberculosis
  creatinine clearance in, 122
  excretory urography in, 149
  urea clearance in, 393
  urinalysis in, 395, 397
  urine culture in, 399
  urine hemoglobin in, 186

Renal tubular acidosis
  key diagnostic findings in, 545
  serum phosphate levels in, 281
  urine calcium levels in, 78t
  urine phosphate levels in, 78t
  urine potassium levels in, 293
Renal tubular function, urine osmolality in, 269
Renal tumors
  nephrotomography in, 261t
  renal angiography in, 321
  renal computed tomography scan in, 322
  renal ultrasonography in, 325
  urine hemoglobin in, 186
Renal ultrasonography, 324-326
Renal vein thrombosis
  key diagnostic findings in, 545
  renal venography in, 327
  urinalysis in, 397
Renal venography, 326-327
Renin activity, plasma, 327-328
Renovascular hypertension
  excretory urography in, 149
  key diagnostic findings in, 545
  plasma renin activity in, 328
  radionuclide renal imaging in, 324
  renal angiography in, 321
  renal venography in, 327
Respiratory acidosis
  arterial blood gas analysis in, 58t
  carbon dioxide in, 81
  key diagnostic findings in, 545
Respiratory alkalosis
  arterial blood gas analysis in, 58t
  carbon dioxide in, 81
  key diagnostic findings in, 545
  urinalysis in, 395
Respiratory distress syndrome
  adult, key diagnostic findings in, 545-546
  child, key diagnostic findings in, 546

Respiratory function, impaired, arterial blood gas analysis in, 57
Respiratory syncytial virus antibodies, 328-329
Respiratory syncytial virus infection
  key diagnostic findings in, 546
  respiratory syncytial virus antibodies in, 329
Respiratory tract infections, nasopharyngeal culture in, 260
Restrictive cardiomyopathy, key diagnostic findings in, 546
Reticulocyte count, 329-330
Retinal detachment, key diagnostic findings in, 546
Retinitis pigmentosa, key diagnostic findings in, 546
Retinopathies, visual evoked potentials in, 148
Reverse blood typing, 27. *See also* ABO blood typing.
Reye's syndrome
  key diagnostic findings in, 546-547
  plasma ammonia levels in, 41
RF. *See* Rheumatoid factor.
Rhabdomyolysis, myoglobin levels in, 258
Rheumatic fever
  antistreptolysin-O titer in, 55
  blood cell count in, 415t
  complement assays in, 111
  erythrocyte sedimentation rate in, 141
  key diagnostic findings in, 547
  synovial fluid analysis in, 356-357t
Rheumatic heart disease, key diagnostic findings in, 547
Rheumatoid arthritis
  alpha$_1$-antitrypsin levels in, 37
  autoantibodies in, 237t
  blood cell count in, 415, 416t t
  complement assays in, 111
  cryoglobulin levels in, 124t
  D-xylose absorption in, 134

i refers to an illustration; t refers to a table.

i refers to an illustration; t refers to a table.

i refers to an illustration; t refers to a table.

i refers to an illustration; t refers to a table.

Systemic lupus erythematosus
(continued)
antinuclear antibodies in,
54, 54t
autoantibodies in, 236t
blood cell count in, 415t,
416t
complement assays in, 111
cryoglobulin level in, 124t
fluorescent treponemal antibody absorption test in,
161
human leukocyte antigen
testing in, 203
immune complex assays in,
206-207
lupus erythematosus cell
preparation in, 235, 237
myoglobin levels in, 258
pericardial fluid analysis in,
276
protein levels in, 303i
rheumatoid factor titer in,
330
serum immunoglobulin lev-
els in, 209t
synovial fluid analysis in,
356-357t
synovial membrane biopsy
in, 358

T

T_4. See Thyroxine, total.
Taeniasis, key diagnostic find-
ings in, 554
Takayasu's arteritis, key diag-
nostic findings in,
561-562
Tay-Sachs disease, key diagnos-
tic findings in, 554
TdT. See Terminal deoxynu-
cleotidyl transferase.
Tearing deficiency, Schirmer
test in, 335
Telangiectasia, chromosome
analysis in, 106t
Temporal arteritis, key diag-
nostic findings in, 561
Tendinitis, key diagnostic find-
ings in, 554
Tensilon test, 359-360
Tension pneumothorax, chest
X-ray in, 96t
Terminal deoxynucleotidyl
transferase, 360-361

Tes-Tape, 176, 177t. See also
Glucose urinalysis.
Testes, undescended, key diagnostic findings in, 559
Testicular cancer
alpha-fetoprotein levels in,
38
androstenedione in, 48
gallium scan in, 167
key diagnostic findings in,
554
testosterone levels in, 362
urine human chorionic
gonadotropin levels in,
201
Testicular failure, serum
follicle-stimulating hor-
mone levels in, 163
Testicular torsion, key diagnostic findings in, 554
Testosterone, 361-362
Test results, 21-22
factors that affect, 6-7, 8t, 9
drug interference with,
576-580t
Test/treat threshold, 9-11
Tetanus, key diagnostic findings in, 554-555
Tetralogy of Fallot
alpha-fetoprotein levels in,
38
key diagnostic findings in,
555
Thalassemia
hemoglobin electrophoresis
in, 185t
key diagnostic findings in,
555
osmotic fragility in, 270
Thallium imaging, 362-364
Thallium scintigraphy,
362-364
Therapeutic drug monitoring
guidelines, 568-575t
Third-degree atrioventricular
block, 462
electrocardiogram characteristics of, 462i
key diagnostic findings in,
491
Thoracentesis, 288-290, 289t
Thoracic aortic aneurysm, key
diagnostic findings in,
555

Thoracic disorders, transesophageal echocardiog-
raphy in, 373
Threshold levels, 9-11
Throat abscesses, key diagnostic findings in, 555
Throat culture, 364-365
Thrombin time, plasma,
365-366
Thrombocythemia, platelet
count in, 286
Thrombocytopenia
bone marrow biopsy in, 74t
folic acid levels in, 162
key diagnostic findings in,
555
Thrombocytopenic purpura,
bone marrow biopsy in,
74t
Thromboembolic disorders,
antithrombin III levels
in, 56
Thrombophlebitis
as cardiac catheterization
complication, 86t
key diagnostic findings in,
556
Thyroid biopsy, 366-367
Thyroid cancer
calcitonin stimulation testing in, 77
chest X-ray in, 96t
key diagnostic findings in,
556
plasma calcitonin levels in,
77
thyroid biopsy in, 367
thyroid imaging in, 316t
thyroid-stimulating hor-
mone levels in, 368
Thyroid disorders, glucose
urinalysis in, 177
Thyroiditis. See also
Hashimoto's thyroiditis.
complement assays in, 111
key diagnostic findings in,
556
radioactive iodine uptake in,
315
thyroid biopsy in, 367
thyroid-stimulating hor-
mone levels in, 368
Thyroid replacement therapy,
triiodothyronine levels
in, 376

i refers to an illustration; t refers to a table.

i refers to an illustration; t refers to a table.

Tuberculosis *(continued)*
  rheumatoid factor titer in, 330
  serum immunoglobulin levels in, 209t
  synovial membrane biopsy in, 358
  tuberculin skin tests in, 379
Tuberculous arthritis, synovial fluid analysis in, 356-357t
Tubular reabsorption, impaired, urinalysis in, 397
Tularemia
  blood cell count in, 415t
  febrile agglutination test for, 151
  key diagnostic findings in, 559
Tumor marker tests, 379-380
Turner's syndrome, 338t
  alpha-fetoprotein levels in, 38
  amniocentesis in, 45
  luteinizing hormone levels in, 238
  serum estrogen levels in, 145
  serum follicle-stimulating hormone levels in, 163
12-lead electrocardiograms
  electrical axis and, 463-466, 467i, 469
  interpreting, 468, 469-471i, 471
  leads for, 463
    placement of, 463
  purpose of, 463
Typhoid fever
  blood cell count in, 41t
  white blood cell count in, 412
Typhus
  epidemic, key diagnostic findings in, 559
  Weil-Felix test for, 151

U

Ulcerative colitis
  barium enema in, 63
  blood cell count in, 415t
  colonoscopy in, 109
  complement assays in, 111
  fecal occult blood in, 153
  gallium scan in, 167

Ulcerative colitis *(continued)*
  key diagnostic findings in, 559
  Raji cell assay in, 317-318
Ulcers. *See also* Duodenal ulcer *and* Peptic ulcer.
  esophagogastroduodenoscopy in, 143
  perforated, chest X-ray in, 97t
  upper gastrointestinal and small-bowel series in, 391-392
Ultrasonography
  of abdominal aorta, 381-382
  of gallbladder and biliary system, 382-383
  of liver, 383-385
  of pancreas, 385-386
  of pelvis, 386-387
  of spleen, 387-389
  of vagina, 389-390
Universal precautions. *See* Standard precautions.
Upper gastrointestinal and small-bowel series, 390-392
Urea clearance, 392-393
Urea formation, 393
Uremia
  blood cell count in, 415t
  delayed hypersensitivity skin tests in, 205
  platelet aggregation in, 285
Ureteral abnormalities, excretory urography in, 149
Ureteral calculi
  excretory urography in, 149
  urine hemoglobin in, 186
Ureteral obstruction
  radionuclide renal imaging in, 324
  urea clearance in, 393
Ureterocele, voiding cystourethrography in, 410
Urethral stricture, voiding cystourethrography in, 410
Urethritis
  urinalysis in, 398
  urine hemoglobin in, 186
Uric acid
  presence of, in amniotic fluid, 45
  urine, 393-394
Urinalysis, 394-395, 396t, 397-398

Urinary tract infections
  key diagnostic findings in, 524
  urinalysis in, 395, 397
  urine culture in, 399
  urine protein levels in, 304-305
Urinary tract obstruction, blood urea nitrogen in, 69
Urine culture, 398-399
Urine specimens, collecting, 18
Urticaria, key diagnostic findings in, 559
Uterine bleeding, dysfunctional
  endometrial biopsy in, 95t
  key diagnostic findings in, 502
Uterine cancer
  gallium scan in, 167
  key diagnostic findings in, 559
Uterine fibroids, ultrasonography in, 387
Uterine leiomyomas, key diagnostic findings in, 559-560
Uveitis, key diagnostic findings in, 560

V

Vagal response as cardiac catheterization complication, 86t
Vaginal cancer
  colposcopy in, 110
  gallium scan in, 167
  key diagnostic findings in, 560
Vaginal smear, 272, 400-401
Vaginismus, key diagnostic findings in, 560
Vaginitis
  urinalysis in, 398
  vaginal smear in, 401
Validity of test as influencing factor, 7
Valvular heart disease, cardiac catheterization in, 88
Vanillylmandelic acid, 401-402
Varicella, key diagnostic findings in, 560
Varices
  barium swallow in, 65
  fecal occult blood in, 153

i refers to an illustration; t refers to a table.

i refers to an illustration; t refers to a table.

Whooping cough
  key diagnostic findings in,
    564
  throat culture in, 364
Widal's test, 150-151
Wilms' tumor
  gallium scan in, 167
  key diagnostic findings in,
    565
Wilson's disease
  key diagnostic findings in,
    565
  urine uric acid levels in, 394
Wiskott-Aldrich syndrome
  delayed hypersensitivity skin
    tests in, 205
  key diagnostic findings in,
    565
Wound culture, 413-414, 416
Wounds, open trauma, key
    diagnostic findings in,
    565

X
X-linked infantile hypogam-
    maglobulinemia, key
    diagnostic findings in,
    565

Y
Yellow fever, key diagnostic
    findings in, 565
Yellow jacket sting, key diag-
    nostic findings in, 519

Z
Zinc deficiency, key diagnostic
    findings in, 565
Zollinger-Ellison syndrome
  gastric acid stimulation test
    in, 169
  gastrin levels in, 170

i refers to an illustration; t refers to a table.